AF783123

Down Syndrome: Diagnosis, Treatment and Management

Down Syndrome: Diagnosis, Treatment and Management

Editor: Luke Stanton

FOSTER ACADEMICS

www.fosteracademics.com

www.fosteracademics.com

FOSTER ACADEMICS

Cataloging-in-Publication Data

Down syndrome : diagnosis, treatment and management / edited by Luke Stanton.
p. cm.
Includes bibliographical references and index.
ISBN 978-1-63242-540-9
1. Down syndrome. 2. Down syndrome--Diagnosis. 3. Down syndrome--Treatment.
4. Down syndrome--Prevention. I. Stanton, Luke.
RC571 .D69 2018
616.858 842--dc23

Foster Academics,
118-35 Queens Blvd., Suite 400,
Forest Hills, NY 11375, USA

ISBN 978-1-63242-540-9 (Hardback)

Printed and bound in China.

Contents

Preface

Down syndrome is a genetic disorder caused because of the 47th chromosome. The children born with this syndrome usually have distinctive features, lower IQ and impaired physical growth. Down syndrome can be detected during pregnancy by screening tests or by diagnostic tests. This book provides comprehensive insights into the field of down syndrome. It aims to shed light on current diagnostic and management techniques associated with this disorder. The readers would gain knowledge that would broaden their perspective about the topic.

The researches compiled throughout the book are authentic and of high quality, combining several disciplines and from very diverse regions from around the world. Drawing on the contributions of many researchers from diverse countries, the book's objective is to provide the readers with the latest achievements in the area of research. This book will surely be a source of knowledge to all interested and researching the field.

In the end, I would like to express my deep sense of gratitude to all the authors for meeting the set deadlines in completing and submitting their research chapters. I would also like to thank the publisher for the support offered to us throughout the course of the book. Finally, I extend my sincere thanks to my family for being a constant source of inspiration and encouragement.

Editor

1

Memory Decline in Down Syndrome and Its Relationship to iPF2alpha, a Urinary Marker of Oxidative Stress

Panagiotis Zis[1]*, Patrick McHugh[2], Andrew McQuillin[3], Domenico Praticò[4], Mark Dickinson[5], Sima Shende[1], Zuzana Walker[1], Andre Strydom[1]

1 University College London, Division of Psychiatry, London, United Kingdom, **2** Division of Pharmacy and Pharmaceutical Sciences, School of Applied Sciences University of Huddersfield, Queensgate, Huddersfield, United Kingdom, **3** University College London, Molecular Psychiatry Laboratory, London, United Kingdom, **4** Department of Pharmacology and Center for Translational Medicine, Temple University, Philadelphia, Pennsylvania, United States of America, **5** Enfield Integrated Learning Disability Team, Enfield, United Kingdom

Abstract

Background: Lipid peroxidation may be a marker of free-radical-mediated injury associated with Alzheimer's disease (AD). We aimed to investigate whether changes in lipid peroxidation is associated with cognitive decline in individuals with Down syndrome over a 4-year period.

Methods: Thirty-two adults with DS participated in a longitudinal study with urinary isoprostane 8,12-iso-iPF2alpha (iPF2alpha) assays at baseline and four years follow-up. Informants rated their functional ability and memory function and the adults with DS attempted assessments of language skills and memory. Twenty-six individuals completed assessments of memory (Modified Memory Object Task, MOMT), adaptive behavior (ABAS), and receptive vocabulary (British Picture vocabulary, BPVS) at both time-points.

Results: Overall change in iPF2alpha level was negatively correlated with change in the MOMT score (Spearman's Rho = −0.576, p = 0.006), i.e., increased lipid peroxidation was correlated with worse memory functioning over time. An increase of ≥0.02 ng/mg creatinine iPF2α had good sensitivity (85.7%), positive predictive value (75%,), specificity (85.7%) and negative predictive value (92.3%) for memory decline.

Conclusion: Change in iPF2alpha over time may have potential as a biomarker for memory decline in Down syndrome and potentially also help to track progression of MCI to AD in the general population.

Editor: Stephan N. Witt, Louisiana State University Health Sciences Center, United States of America

Funding: Funding for the baseline work was provided by the north central London research consortium (NoCloR). The funders had no role in study design, data collection and analysis, decision to publish, or preparation of the manuscript.

Competing Interests: The authors have declared that no competing interests exist.

* E-mail: takiszis@gmail.com

Introduction

Oxidative stress reflects the biological imbalance between oxidant production and the ability to detoxify the system of reactive oxygen species (ROS) and repair the damage they cause. Although low levels of ROS are physiologically important, high concentrations above the clearance capacity cause mitochondrial dysfunction, cellular damage, and cell death [1], implicating oxidative stress as an important mechanism of age-related pathology [2] such as the cognitive decline associated with Alzheimer's Disease (AD) [3].

Down syndrome (DS) has been associated with disturbed oxidative metabolism, which is assumed to be due to a variety of mechanisms [4], and most adults with DS will eventually show the clinical or neuropathological hallmarks of AD [5]. Although this may be in large part due to the triplication of the APP gene in DS, increasing evidence suggests that oxidative stress and inflammation may also play a role in AD pathogenesis associated with the syndrome [6].

Lipid peroxidation is one of the major outcomes of oxidative stress following free-radical-mediated injury, leading to the generation of various end products [7]. Isoprostane 8,12-iso-iPF2alpha (iPF2alpha) are isomers of the prostagladin F2alpha produced by ROS attack on polyunsaturated fatty acids. They are chemically stable, sensitive and specific biomarkers of lipid peroxidation in vivo [8] and have been shown to be increased in Alzheimer's disease, and may mediate the neuronal response to oxidative stress [9]. Elevated levels of iPF2alpha have been demonstrated in living adults in DS [10].

Given the DS population's much increased risk for dementia, they are an important population in which to study biomarkers of AD. We aimed to investigate (in an existing research cohort of adults with DS) whether a peripheral marker of oxidative stress, specifically a change over time in lipid peroxidation (measured with urinary iPF2alpha) is associated with cognitive decline in people with DS, and whether this is related to anti-oxidative enzyme levels, including Cu/Zn Superoxide dismutase (SOD1).

Materials and Methods

Study Population, iPF2alpha, Enzyme Assays and Psychometric Measurements

We used a within-syndrome design to examine the association between urinary markers of oxidative stress and changes in cognitive functioning over time in adults with DS. We have previously established a cohort of 32 individuals with DS who underwent cognitive testing and donated urine samples for isoprostane 8,12-iso-iPF2alpha (iPF2alpha) analysis and blood samples for Cu/Zn superoxide dismutase (SOD1), overall superoxide dismutase activity (SOD) and glutathione peroxidase (GPx) analysis. Assays for SOD1, SOD, GPx were measured at baseline, using methods described elsewhere [11,12].

Urine iPF2alpha levels (corrected for creatinine concentrations) were measured at both baseline and at follow-up four years later (mean length of follow up 55.46 months, range 46 to 61 months). Collection of and processing of urine samples were similar at both time points. At baseline, urine ipf2alpha levels were measured using methods described elsewhere [11]. At follow-up, urine samples were hydrolysed with a 1/10 volume of 1N HCL and diluted 1:4 with PBS prior to analysis. All reagents for subsequent 8-iso-PGF2alpha analysis were obtained from Cell Biolabs, Inc. 8-iso-PGF2alpha standards ranging from 200 μg/mL to 0.2 μg/mL were used to generate a standard curve. Urine samples or standards were mixed with a 8-iso-PGF2alpha-HRP conjugate for 1 hour at room temperature in a 96-well plate. Wells were washed 5 times with 300 μL wash buffer (1X PBS, 0.05% Tween-20). One hundred microlitres of HRP substrate was added to each well and mixed for 30 mins at room temp. The enzyme reaction was stopped with 100 μl 1 M phosphoric acid the enzyme reaction by adding 100 μL of Stop Solution to each well. The absorbance was determined for each well at 450 nM (POLARstar OPTIMA plate-reader, BMG) and quantified by comparing with the known predetermined standard curve.

To determine creatinine levels, urine samples were diluted 1:20 with Milli-Q water. Creatinine standards ranging from 20 mg/dl to 0.078 mg/dl were used to generate a standard curve. Fifty microliters of standards and samples were added to a 96-well plate with 200 μl creatinine reaction reagent (Cell Biolabs, Inc.) and incubated for 30 mins with shaking at room temp. Initial absorbance values were determined for each well at 490 nM (POLARstar OPTIMA plate-reader). Fifty microliters creatinine quencher (Cell Biolabs, Inc.) was added to each well, mixed thoroughly and incubated for 10 mins at room temp. A final absorbance value was determined at 490 nM and subtracted from the initial absorbance giving a corrected absorbance value. Samples were quantified using by comparing the corrected absorbance against the known predetermined standard curve.

Details of the psychometric assessments and population characteristics have also been described elsewhere [11,12]. In brief, informants (who were in most cases family members) completed a measure of adaptive behavior (Adaptive Behaviour Assessment Scale; ABAS [13]) and a dementia screen (the cognitive scale of the Dementia Scale for people with Learning Disabilities; DLD [14]). Participants who were able to, completed a measure of receptive vocabulary (British picture vocabulary scale; BPVS II [15]), and a modification of an object memory task (MOMT) based on the Fuld object memory test [16,17]. We modified the task by reducing the number of objects to 6, and the number of trials to two.

Ethics Statement and Consent Procedures

The study was approved by the National NHS research ethics committee and we followed the Mental Capacity Act, UK (2005) if participants did not have the capacity to consent for themselves, by gaining agreement from carers. Written informed consent was obtained for all participants.

Data Analyses

Data was analysed with Statistical Package for the Social Sciences (SPSS) version 14 [18]. The SOD/GPx activity ration was calculated from the logarithms of the activities because of the different orders of magnitude [19]. Correlations between urinary iPF2alpha levels and baseline factors were examined using Spearman's correlations. Correlations between the changes in psychometric and functional assessments scores (BPVS, ABAS, MOMT) were examined using Spearman's correlations. Mann Whitney U tests were used to compare scores between groups. The significance level was set at 0.05.

Results

Demographics and Psychometric Tests

Twenty-six out of 32 individuals with DS completed psychometric testing at both time points. Two of the original participants refused to participate again, and four were lost to follow-up. We have previously described the demographic features of this cohort [12]. In summary, the 26 participants had a mean age of 36.65±7.05 years, and half of them where males. None were diagnosed with Alzheimer's disease at baseline or during the follow-up period.

Table 1 summarizes the average scores of all psychometric tests and subtests at follow up and shows the mean change of each score between baseline and follow-up.

Although total MOMT scores remained relatively stable, 7(33.3%) participants showed decline on MOMT scores between T1 and T2.

iPF2alpha Measurements and Enzyme Assays

Data on urinary iPF2α were available for 24 patients at baseline and follow-up. For these 24 patients, at baseline, the range of iPF2alpha was 0.16 to 3.18 ng/mg creatinine (mean 1.39±0.79) and at follow-up 0.52 to 5.27 ng/mg creatinine (mean 1.38±1.23). The change between iPF2α levels at follow up and at baseline ranged from −2.60 to +4.30 ng/mg creatinine (mean 0.003±1.56). Table 2 presents individual values for all patients, at both baseline and follow-up.

The mean change in the iPF2α levels did not correlate with age (Spearman's rho = 0.074, p = 0.731), nor did it differ between males and females (Student's t-test, t value = −0.715, p = 0.482), patients with thyroid disorder and those without (Mann-Whitney U, Z value = −0.400, p = 0.689), mild ID or moderate to severe ID (Mann-Whitney U, Z value = −0.306, p = 0.760), and white UK or those of other ethnicity (Mann-Whitney U, Z value = −1.333, p = 0.182). However, those receiving vitamins and supplements at baseline presented with increased urinary levels of iPF2α (mean change +0.882 ng/mg) compared to those who were not (mean change −0.404 ng/mg); t value = −1.975; p = 0.02.

Relationship between Oxidative Enzymes and Urinary iPF2alpha

Table 3 summarizes the correlations between baseline enzyme assays, urine iPF2alpha at follow-up, and change in iPF2alpha over time. Correlations between baseline enzyme assays and

Table 1. Mean scores and 95% confidence intervals of psychometric tests at baseline, follow up and change between time points.

	Baseline (t1)	Follow-up (t2)	Mean change i.e. t2-t1
ABAS			
Functional academics	30.4 (21.6–39.2)	25.1 (17.9–32.3)	−5.3 (−9.3–−1.4)
Total score	366.8 (312.7–421.0)	317.9 (263.9–371.8)	−49.0 (−71.1–−26.9)
BPVS			
Raw score	61.6 (53.1–70.2)	55.7 (46.3–65.1)	−6.0 (−9.1–−2.8)
Age equivalent, in months	73.1 (62.3–83.9)	66.4 (54.4–78.4)	n/a
MOMT			
Delayed recall	4.7 (4.3–5.2)	4.8 (4.4–5.3)	0.1 (−0.4–0.6)
Total score	12.6 (11.9–13.4)	13.0 (12.3–13.7)	0.4 (−0.4–1.2)

baseline urine iPF2alpha have been presented elsewhere [11]. Enzyme assays at baseline were not correlated significantly with urinary iPF2alpha at follow up, or the change in urinary iPF2alpha levels over the 4-year period. However, there was a trend towards a negative relationship between overall SOD function at baseline and change in iPF2alpha over time. A trend towards a similar relationship was also noted for GPx (i.e. better SOD function and higher GPx levels may be related to less change in iPF2alpha over 4 years).

Relationship between Urinary iPF2alpha and Cognitive Ability Changes

Table 4 lists the correlations between levels of iPF2alpha and performance over 4 years on tests of functional ability, memory or language ability. Correlations between baseline psychometric measures and baseline urine iPF2alpha have been presented elsewhere [11]. There were no statistically significant correlations between levels of ipF2alpha level at follow up or its change over 4 years and ABAS total score, or with ABAS functional academic

Table 2. Individual values of urinary ipf2alpha for both baseline and follow up.

Patient	Gender	Age at baseline, in years	Ipf2a at baseline, in ng/mg creatinine	Ipf2a at follow up, in ng/mg creatinine
#1	Female	40	.22	.89
#2	Female	22	1.19	.87
#3	Female	33	1.75	.87
#4	Male	45	1.04	4.42
#5	Female	27	1.22	.57
#6	Female	30	.86	1.16
#7	Male	26	3.18	.58
#8	Male	31	1.45	1.16
#9	Female	36	1.31	.62
#10	Male	35	2.12	1.79
#11	Female	30	1.05	1.04
#12	Female	25	1.24	3.49
#13	Male	32	.97	5.27
#14	Female	22	1.75	.67
#15	Male	36	1.12	.90
#16	Male	39	2.86	1.41
#17	Female	35	3.16	1.06
#18	Female	40	1.33	.68
#19	Male	35	.72	.97
#20	Male	27	1.51	.52
#21	Female	24	.16	1.44
#22	Female	30	1.55	.62
#23	Male	18	.60	1.27
#24	Male	41	.93	.95

Table 3. Correlations between anti-oxidant enzymes in blood and urinary iPF2alpha.

		iPF2alpha at follow-up (t2)	Change in iPF2alpha (t2–t1)
SOD function	Spearman's Rho	−0.406	−0.444
	p	0.076	0.065
	N	20	18
SOD enzyme units	Spearman's Rho	−0.128	−0.065
	p	0.612	0.811
	N	18	16
GPx	Spearman's Rho	−0.400	−0.420
	p	0.081	0.082
	N	20	18
SOD function/GPx	Spearman's Rho	0.186	0.207
	p	0.431	0.409
	N	20	18

score. However, overall change in iPF2alpha level was negatively correlated with change in the MOMT total score (Spearman's Rho = −0.516, p = 0.017) and MOMT delayed recall score (Spearman's Rho = −0.576, p = 0.006). Increases in lipid peroxidation were correlated with worse memory functioning over time. An increase equal to or more than 0.02 ng/mg creatinine in iPF2alpha identified 6 out of 7 participants who showed declines on memory tasks (sensitivity = 85.7%; positive predictive value = 75%) and included only 2 of 14 participants who did not show memory decline (specificity = 85.7%; negative predictive value = 92.3%).

Discussion

Findings

We have previously shown that serum levels of SOD predicts memory decline over time [12]. In the present study, we have explored the relationship between cognitive change over time in adults with DS and urinary markers of oxidative stress, which suggests that there is a correlation between increased oxidative stress measured with lipid peroxidation and memory decline in adults with DS over time. Our results suggest that an increase in iPF2alpha, but not absolute iPF2alpha titers, is an early marker of progression to AD in DS, and that increased lipid peroxidation can predict decline on memory tests in this population with good sensitivity and specificity.

Table 4. Correlations between changes in psychometric measures (scores at follow up minus score at baseline), and urinary iPF2alpha titers.

		iPF2alpha at follow-up	Change in iPF2alpha
Change in ABAS total score	Spearman's Rho	0.215	0.188
	p	0.292	0.379
	N	26	24
Change in ABAS functional academic score	Spearman's Rho	0.118	−0.241
	p	0.566	0.256
	N	26	24
Change in BPVS raw score	Spearman's Rho	−0.204	−0.178
	p	0.363	0.440
	N	22	21
Change in MOMT total score	Spearman's Rho	−0.195	−0.516
	p	0.397	0.017*
	N	21	21
Change in MOMT delayed recall score	Spearman's Rho	−0.258	−0.576
	p	0.259	0.006**
	N	21	21

*means p<0.05 when **means p<0.01.

Implications

Our results suggest that increases in urinary iPF2alpha over time are associated with the memory decline that is typical of AD in adult participants with DS, an ultra-high risk group for developing dementia.

In keeping with our results, a general population study of AD found that an increase in isoprostane levels in CSF (rather than absolute values) was associated with progression of mild cognitive impairment (MCI) to AD and with cognitive decline over time, and that this marker was more predictive of progression than other AD biomarkers [20]. Taken together, our study (in adults with DS) and the CSF study (with participants without DS) suggest that markers of oxidative stress have considerable potential as a biomarkers of the cognitive decline suggestive of MCI, and of progression of AD symptoms. Although absolute values of isoprostanes may not have much value in screening for AD, increased levels over time have considerable potential to track progression of disease. Given that urine samples are easier to obtain than CSF, our results have important practical implications.

It has been suggested that oxidative stress is an important consequence of the specific biology of DS, and is likely to play a role in some of the co-morbidities associated with DS, including the tendency to develop AD [4]. Oxidative damage may lead to enhanced amyloid beta peptide (Aβ) production [21–24] and in a recent study, Cenini et al. showed that soluble and insoluble Aβ and oligomers increase as a function of age in DS frontal cortex, and that Aβ40 correlated with protein carbonyls (an oxidative stress marker), which suggests that oxidative damage may contribute to the onset and progression of AD pathogenesis in DS [25]. The exact mechanism is still unknown, but Yang et al. showed that ROS enhanced amyloid toxicity in the neurons of APP/PS1 mice [26], an AD mouse model with excessive amyloid production which is also found in DS, while Di Domenico et al demonstrated that oxidation of proteins is an early event in DS and might contribute to neurodegenerative phenomena [27].

Peripheral biomarkers of oxidative stress in Down syndrome include SOD [12,26,28], GPx [6,29], uric acid [29], plasma melatonin, urinary kynurenine [30], gelsolin [31], nitric oxide [32,33] and neopterin [34]. However, oxidative stress or lipid peroxidation may not necessarily be increased in DS. Tolun et al. compared the levels of urinary allantoin and F2-isoprostanes between individuals with DS and controls without finding any significant difference [35]. Moreover, Campos et al assessed a set of urinary oxidative stress biomarkers in children with DS including 8-hydroxy-2′-deoxyguanosine (8-OHdG), isoprostane 15-F2t-IsoP, thiobarbituric acid-reacting substances (TBARS), advanced glycation end products (AGEs), dityrosine (diTyr), hydrogen peroxide (H2O2) and nitrite/nitrate (NOx) and found that only levels of diTyr were increased in DS, although no differences were obtained when hypothyroid DS children were excluded [36]. In another study, Campos et al, aimed to assess the same set of oxidative and nitrosative stress biomarkers in urine samples of adolescents and adults with DS, with and without hypothyroidism and concluded that some biomarkers such as 8-OHdG, 15-F2t-IsoP and TBARS may be prone to age effects, renal function, and thyroid function [37]. In contrast, we did not find any correlation between changes in iPF2alpha over time and age, nor an effect for thyroid disorder.

It has been demonstrated that premature aging in kidneys of DS patients could lead to an impaired renal function [38]. For this reason, not only the oxidative status but also the alteration of the glomerular filtration rate could affect nitrite and nitrate levels in DS patients. Therefore, Ripoll et al conducted a comparative study assessing nitrosative stress biomarkers in plasma samples from adult DS patients [39], concluding that the increased levels of nitrates found in urine samples of adult DS patients [37] are also found in plasma samples, which confirms the use of nitrogen reactive species as stress biomarkers in adult DS patients.

Increases in the anti-oxidant systems in DS (such as SOD) help to protect against increased oxidative stress [40]. Our results are in keeping with these studies – we have previously demonstrated a positive relationship between SOD1 and better memory function, while the present results indicate that when the protective mechanisms fail over time and lipid peroxidation increases, it is associated with decline in memory function.

Lastly, increased lipid peroxidation has been shown to precede amyloid plaque formation in some studies of animal models [24] and lipid peroxidation may trigger neurodegeneration [22]; reduction of oxidative stress could therefore be a potential treatment target in the DS population.

Strengths and Limitations

We undertook a prospective cohort study of adults with DS, in which we managed to follow up 80% of the initial study group over an unusually long period (4 years). We have included participants with the full range of cognitive abilities associated with DS, and our sample is therefore representative of the wide variation in intellectual phenotype. However, our sample size was relatively small, and our results need to be confirmed with a replication study.

We were not able to control for all possible confounders as, for example, cognitive performance may be influenced by educational exposure, though in the UK all adults with DS have equal access to education. Moreover, it is likely that dietary intake of food with antioxidant properties varied across participants and we did not collect sufficient detail on compliance with vitamin supplementation during the follow-up period to include this in our analysis.

The technique of measurement of ipf2alpha at follow up was different at follow-up compared to baseline (where gas chromatography and mass spectrometry i.e. GC/MS was used). When immunoassays are performed under appropriate conditions, values obtained for isoprostanes obtained by immunoassay often correlate well ($r^2 > 0.8$) with values obtained by the standard GC/MS method [41].

Among the followed-up population, there were no patients with translocation, and there was only one patient with mosaicism. Therefore, we were not able to study the relationship between iPF2alpha levels and these categories in more detail. The study was powered to detect correlations of moderate strength and it is therefore possible to have missed more subtle relationships. For example, a significant relationship between SOD and GPx and changes in lipid peroxidation may become apparent in larger studies.

Conclusion

For the first time, it is suggested that change in urinary iPF2alpha over time is associated with memory decline in people with DS, suggesting that sequential measurements of urinary iPF2alpha may have potential as biomarker for cognitive decline and progression to AD in this population. This preliminary finding adds to similar studies in the general population, which showed increased isoprostanes in the CSF of people with MCI who have progressed to full-blown AD. Furthermore, the association between an increase in lipid peroxidation and cognitive decline in relatively young adults with DS suggests that reduction of oxidative stress and consequent lipid peroxidation may be a potential treatment strategy to reduce the high risk for AD in this population.

Acknowledgments

Blood samples were analyzed at BioLab, London. Marsha Lewis and Ahmad Srour contributed to assessment of participants at baseline. We wish to thank the Down Syndrome Association (UK) for their assistance with recruitment, and all the participants and their carers for their time and efforts.

Author Contributions

Conceived and designed the experiments: PZ AS. Performed the experiments: PZ AS. Analyzed the data: PZ AS. Wrote the paper: PZ PM AM DP MD SS ZW AS.

References

1. Patten DA, Germain M, Kelly MA, Slack RS (2010) Reactive oxygen species: stuck in the middle of neurodegeneration. J Alzheimers Dis 20(2): S357–S367.
2. Kregel KC, Zhang HJ (2007) An integrated view of oxidative stress in aging: basic mechanisms, functional effects, and pathological considerations. Am J Physiol Regul Integr Comp Physiol. 292(1): R18–R36.
3. Cardoso SM, Santana I, Swerdlow RH, Oliveira CR (2004) Mitochondria dysfunction of Alzheimer's disease cybrids enhances Aβ toxicity. J Neurochem 89(6): 1417–1426.
4. Lott IT (2012) Antioxidants in Down syndrome. Biochim Biophys Acta. 1822(5): 657–63.
5. Millan Sanchez M, Heyn SN, Das D, Moghadam S, Martin KJ, et al. (2012) Neurobiological elements of cognitive dysfunction in Down syndrome: exploring the role of APP. Biol Psychiatry. 71(5): 403–9.
6. Yang H, Zhuo JM, Chu J, Chinnici C, Praticò D (2010) Amelioration of the Alzheimer's disease phenotype by absence of 12/15-lipoxygenase. Biol Psychiatry. 68(10): 922–9.
7. Ferreiro E, Baldeiras I, Ferreira IL, Costa RO, Rego AC, et al. (2012) Mitochondrial- and endoplasmic reticulum-associated oxidative stress in Alzheimer's disease: from pathogenesis to biomarkers. Int J Cell Biol. 2012: 735206.
8. Praticò D (1999) F(2)-isoprostanes: sensitive and specific non-invasive indices of lipid peroxidation in vivo. Atherosclerosis 147(1): 1–10.
9. Praticò D (2010) The neurobiology of isoprostanes and Alzheimer's disease. Biochim Biophys Acta. 1801(8): 930–3.
10. Praticò D, Iuliano L, Amerio G, Tang LX, Rokach J, et al. (2000) Down's syndrome is associated with increased 8,12-iso-iPF2alpha-VI levels: evidence for enhanced lipid peroxidation in vivo. Ann Neurol. 48(5): 795–8.
11. Strydom A, Dickinson MJ, Shende S, Pratico D, Walker Z (2009) Oxidative stress and cognitive ability in adults with Down syndrome. Prog Neuropsychopharmacol Biol Psychiatry. 1; 33(1): 76–80.
12. Zis P, Dickinson M, Shende S, Walker Z, Strydom A (2012) Oxidative stress and memory decline in adults with Down syndrome: longitudinal study. J Alzheimers Dis. 31(2): 277–83.
13. Harrison PT, Oakland T (2000) Adaptive Behaviour Assessment System (ABAS), Harcourt Assessment, USA.
14. Evenhuis HM (1996) Further evaluation of the Dementia Questionnaire for Persons with Mental Retardation (DMR). J Intel Dis Res 40, 369–373.
15. Dunn LM, Dunn LM (1997) British Picture Vocabulary Scale. 2nd edition, NFER-Nelson, London.
16. Fuld PA, Masur DM, Blau AD, Crystal H, Aronson MK (1990). Object-memory evaluation for prospective detection of dementia in normal functioning elderly: predictive and normative data. J Clin Exp Neuropsychol. 12(4): 520–8.
17. Burt DB, Aylward EH (2000). Test battery for the diagnosis of dementia in individuals with intellectual disability. Journal of Intellectual Disability Research, 44(2), 175–180.
18. SPSS inc. SPSS for Windows Release 11.0.0. SPSS Inc; 2001.
19. Pastor MC, Sierra C, Doladé M, Navarro E, Brandi N, et al. (1998) Antioxidant enzymes and fatty acid status in erythrocytes of Down's syndrome patients. Clin Chem 44, 924–929.
20. Kester MI, Scheffer PG, Koel-Simmelink MJ, Twaalfhoven H, Verwey NA, et al. (2012) Serial CSF sampling in Alzheimer's disease: specific versus non-specific markers, Free Radic Biol Med. 62: 157–69.
21. Nunomura A, Perry G, Pappolla MA, Friedland RP, Hirai K, et al. (2000). Neuronal oxidative stress precedes amyloid β deposition in Down syndrome, J. Neuropathol. Exp. Neurol. 59, 1011–1017.
22. Sultana R, Perluigi M, Butterfield DA (2012) Lipid peroxidation triggers neurodegeneration: A redox proteomics view into the Alzheimer disease brain, Free Radic Biol Med. 62: 157–69.
23. Reddy PH (2006), Amyloid precursor protein-mediated free radicals and oxidative damage: implications for the development and progression of Alzheimer's disease, J. Neurochem. 96(1): 1–13.
24. Praticò D, Uryu K, Leight S, Trojanoswki JQ, Lee VM (2001) Increased lipid peroxidation precedes amyloid plaque formation in an animal model of Alzheimer amyloidosis, J. Neurosci. 21, 4183–4187.
25. Cenini G, Dowling AL, Beckett TL, Barone E, Mancuso C, et al. (2012), Association between frontal cortex oxidative damage and beta-amyloid as a function of age in Down syndrome. Biochim Biophys Acta. 1822(2): 130–8.
26. Yang B, Sun X, Lashuel H, Zhang Y (2012) Reactive oxidative species enhance amyloid toxicity in APP/PS1 mouse neurons. Neurosci Bull. 28(3): 233–9.
27. Di Domenico F, Coccia R, Cocciolo A, Murphy MP, Cenini G, et al. (2013). Impairment of proteostasis network in Down syndrome prior to the development of Alzheimer's Disease neuropathology: Redox proteomics analysis of human brain. Biochim Biophys Acta. 1832(8): 1249–1259.
28. Brugge K, Nichols S, Saitoh T, Trauner D (1999) Correlations of glutathione peroxidase activity with memory impairment in adults with Down syndrome. Biol Psychiatry 46(12): 1682–9.
29. Campos C, Guzmán R, López-Fernández E, Casado A (2010). Urinary uric acid and antioxidant capacity in children and adults with Down syndrome, Clin. Biochem. 43, 228–233.
30. Uberos J, Romero J, Molina-Carballo A, Muñoz-Hoyos A (2010). Melatonin and elimination of kynurenines in children with Down's syndrome, J. Pediatr. Endocrinol. Metab. 23, 277–282.
31. Ji L, Chauhan V, Mehta P, Wegiel J, Mehta S, et al. (2010). Relationship between proteolytically cleaved gelsolin and levels of amyloid-beta protein in the brains of Down syndrome subjects, J. Alzheimer's Dis. 22, 609–617.
32. Akomolafe A, Lunetta KL, Erlich PM, Cupples LA, Baldwin CT, et al. (2006) Genetic association between endothelial nitric oxide synthase and Alzheimer disease, Clin. Genet. 70, 49–56.
33. Coppus AM, Fekkes D, Verhoeven WM, Tuinier S, van Duijn CM (2010) Plasma levels of nitric oxide related amino acids in demented subjects with Down syndrome are related to neopterin concentrations, Amino acids 38, 923–928.
34. Coppus AW, Fekkes D, Verhoeven WM, Tuinier S, Egger JI, et al. (2007), Plasma amino acids and neopterin in healthy persons with Down's syndrome. J. Neural. Transm. 114, 1041–1045.
35. Tolun AA, Scarbrough PM, Zhang H, McKillop JA, Wang F, et al. (2012) Systemic oxidative stress, as measured by urinary allantoin and F(2)-isoprostanes, is not increased in Down syndrome. Ann Epidemiol. 22(12): 892–4.
36. Campos C, Guzmán R, López-Fernández E, Casado A (2011) Evaluation of urinary biomarkers of oxidative/nitrosative stress in children with Down syndrome. Life Sci. 24; 89(17–18): 655–61.
37. Campos C, Guzmán R, López-Fernández E, Casado A (2011) Evaluation of urinary biomarkers of oxidative/nitrosative stress in adolescents and adults with Down syndrome. Biochim Biophys Acta. 1812(7): 760–8.
38. Guzmán R, Campos C, López-Fernández E, Casado A (2011) Biomarkers of age effect on renal function in Down syndrome. Biomarkers. 16(8): 679–85.
39. Ripoll C, Dairou J, Stora S, Delabar JM, Janel N (2013) Plasma nitrate levels are increased in adult Down syndrome patients. Biomarkers. 18(4): 373–4.
40. Garlet TR, Parisotto EB, de Medeiros GDS, Pereira LCR, Moreira EAM, et al. (2013). Systemic oxidative stress in children and teenagers with Down syndrome. Life Sci.; 93(16): 558–63.
41. Callewaert DM, Sloan C (2010). Enzyme immunoassay of isoprostanes. In Free Radicals and Antioxidant Protocols (435–449). Humana Press.

2

Development, Problem Behavior, and Quality of Life in a Population Based Sample of Eight-Year-Old Children with Down Syndrome

Helma B. M. van Gameren-Oosterom*, Minne Fekkes, Simone E. Buitendijk, Ashna D. Mohangoo, Jeanet Bruil, Jacobus P. Van Wouwe

Department Child Health, Netherlands Organization for Applied Scientific Research (TNO), Leiden, The Netherlands

Abstract

Objective: Children with Down syndrome (DS) have delayed psychomotor development. We investigated levels of development, problem behavior, and Health-Related Quality of Life (HRQoL) in a population sample of Dutch eight-year-old children with DS. Developmental outcomes were compared with normative data of eight-year-old children from the general population.

Method: Over a three-year-period all parents with an eight-year-old child with DS were approached by the national parent organization. Developmental skills were assessed by means of the McCarthy Scales of Children's Ability. To measure emotional and behavioral problems we used the Child Behavior Checklist. HRQoL was assessed with the TNO-AZL Children's Quality of Life questionnaire. Analyses of variance were applied to compare groups.

Results: A total of 337 children participated. Mean developmental age was substantially lower than mean calendar age (3.9 years, SD 0.87 and 8.1 years, SD 0.15 respectively). Mean developmental age was significantly lower among boys than girls (3.6 (SD 0.85) and 4.2 years (SD 0.82) respectively; $p<0.001$). Compared with the general population, children with DS had more emotional and behavioral problems ($p<0.001$). However on the anxious/depressed scale, they scored significantly more favorably ($p<0.001$). Significantly lower HRQoL scores for the scales gross motor skills, autonomy, social functioning and cognitive functioning were found (p-values<0.001). Hardly any differences were observed for the scales physical complaints, positive and negative emotions.

Conclusion: Eight-year-old children with DS have an average developmental delay of four years, more often have emotional and behavioral problems, and have a less favorable HRQoL compared with children from the general population.

Editor: James G. Scott, The University of Queensland, Australia

Funding: This study was financially supported by grant #2200.0061 from the Netherlands Organization for Health Research and Development (ZonMw). The funders had no role in study design, data collection and analysis, decision to publish, or preparation of the manuscript.

Competing Interests: The authors have declared that no competing interests exist.

* E-mail: helma.vangameren@tno.nl

Introduction

An important feature of children with Down syndrome (DS) is their delayed development. DS is known as the most prevalent cause of intellectual impairment associated with a chromosomal anomaly (Trisomy 21). In the United States prevalence of DS is estimated to be 12 per 10,000 live births; in 2002 83,400 children with DS aged 0–19 years lived in the United States [1]. In the Netherlands the prevalence of DS seems higher: 14 per 10.000 live births (approximately 270 children per year) [2–4]. Children with DS have a well-recognized phenotype, including external characteristics, specific physical problems (such as congenital heart defects, gastro-intestinal disorders, thyroid dysfunction and visual impairment) and intellectual impairment with delayed cognitive and motor development [5,6].

This delayed development has frequently been studied during the past 50 years. Results indicated that children with DS have a lower IQ and have difficulties with expressive language [7–14]. In particular, they have difficulties with verbal working memory, receptive language, reading, writing and arithmetic [7,8,12,14,15]. Studies on behavior problems indicate on average one quarter to one third of the children with DS to have significant emotional and behavior problems [6,10,16]. Most studies observe that children with DS frequently have speech problems, attention deficit and concentration problems, social withdrawal, stubbornness, as well as oppositional and disobedient behavior [9–11,16,17]. A substantial number of studies found that 8–23% of the children with DS have significant psychopathology [10]. Specifically, 7% are diagnosed with autism, 6% to 9% with attention deficit/hyperactivity disorder (ADHD), and 10% to 15% with conduct or oppositional disorders [6,10,16–20].

The vast majority of the above-mentioned studies are not population based and included fewer than 50 children with DS. Studies that included larger numbers of children with DS date back to the 1970s and 1980s, when the children grew up under different circumstances. Improvement of medical care and general support could have enhanced overall development of children with DS or specific aspects of their development. Our sample is studied between 2000 and 2003, and since no major changes in the approach to the developmental aid, medical care and upbringing of children with DS have taken place since then, in our opinion these results are still valid.

When a child with DS is born, parents want to be informed reliably on the expected development of their child. Most of the current available information focuses on the medical aspects like concomitant congenital anomalies and organic disorders, which children with DS are at high risk for. Hardly any information is available on the actual expected development. In this study we aimed to investigate the developmental skills, problem behavior, and Health-Related Quality of Life (HRQoL) in a large population based sample of Dutch children with DS at the age of eight years old, compared to normative data from same-age-children from the general population. Subsequently, we aimed to provide valuable information for families, health care and educational professionals all involved in the care for children with DS.

Methods

Ethics statement

The study protocol was approved by the Medical Ethics Committee of the Leiden University Medical Centre, and written informed consent was obtained from parents/next of kin of all participants.

Subjects

Dutch families, who were member of the Dutch Down Syndrome Foundation and who parent a child with DS born in 1992, 1993 or 1994, were invited to participate in the study. The Dutch Down Syndrome Foundation manages a database which includes most Dutch children with DS. In the Netherlands, about 80% of all parents with a child with DS in the age up to 12 year join this organization, routinely advised by their pediatrician [21].

The selected parents received a written request from the Dutch Down Syndrome Foundation to participate. Parents, who signed up to participate, received a set of questionnaires and an appointment for a home visit. Between June 2000 and February 2003 a professional, experienced and trained psychological assistant visited the children at home and administered the McCarthy Scales of Children's Ability (MSCA) [22]. Developmental testing was conducted following their eighth birthday. If the test was not completed during one visit, the child was rescheduled for further testing within a few weeks. The set of parent questionnaires contained two formal tests: the Child Behavior Checklist (CBCL) and the TNO-AZL Children's Quality of Life (TACQOL) [23–25]. Questions on background, demographic variables and medical condition of the child were included in the set of questionnaires.

Measures

The Dutch version of the MSCA developed for children aged 2.5 to 8.5 years was used [26]. The MSCA contains 18 subtests, grouped into the scales: verbal, perceptual, quantitative, memory and motor skills. The verbal, perceptual and quantitative scales are combined to form the general cognitive scale. A developmental age is calculated based on the various scale scores. To prevent an excessive influence of one of the subscales on the developmental age, the 18 subtests are each representing one competence in order to test a specific ability of the child and not a broad range of abilities, i.e. the test is developed so that level of verbal ability will minimally influence test-scores on other domains measured.

The CBCL measures emotional and behavior problems. The Dutch version of the CBCL for four to twelve years old children was used [27]. The CBCL is suitable for children with developmental delay [28–30]. It contains 118 problem behavior items rated from 0 (not true) to 2 (very true or often true), covering nine scales: withdrawn, somatic complaints, anxious/depressed, social problems, thought problems, attention problems, delinquent behavior, aggressive behavior and sexual problems. These scales combined form the scales internalizing problems (containing withdrawn, somatic complaints and anxious/depressed) and externalizing problems (containing delinquent and aggressive behavior).

The TACQOL, developed in the Netherlands for children aged six to fifteen years old, was used to measure HRQoL. It assesses functional problems weighted by the degree to which a child shows negative emotions to such problems. The questionnaire contains 56 items divided over seven scales: physical complaints, gross motor skills, autonomy, cognitive functioning, social functioning, positive emotions and negative emotions.

Statistical analysis

All questionnaires and test results were collected and merged into one dataset. The levels of developmental skills, problem behaviour and HRQoL were calculated for each outcome measure, according to the accompanying (supplementary) test manuals. The test results of the DS-sample were – for each outcome measure – compared with normative data from the general population, matched on calendar age. Analyses of variance (ANOVA) were used to evaluate differences between mean values. All statistical tests were 2-tailed and statistical significance was defined at $p<0.05$. The effect sizes were estimated by dividing the differences in mean scores between the subgroups by the pooled SD. Cohen's effect sizes (d) were used for interpretation of relevant differences: $d<0.2$ is considered a negligible difference, $0.2\leq d<0.5$ a small, $0.5\leq d<0.8$ a moderate, $0.8\leq d<1.3$ a large, and $d\geq1.3$ a very large difference [31]. Means for the total DS-sample were weighted for gender. All analyses were performed using Statistical Package for the Social Sciences, version 17.0 for Windows (SPSS Inc, Chicago, Illinois).

Analyses of the MSCA scales were carried out with raw scale scores. The norms for children of 8.25 years of age, as available in the accompanying manual and based on a nationwide sample from the United States, were used for comparison with the DS-sample [22]. In addition, developmental age was calculated and compared for boys and girls, using ANOVA.

For the CBCL, normative data were derived from a Dutch sample of 661 children aged seven to nine years (mean 7.9 years, SD 0.40) [32]. In addition to the comparison of scale scores, the proportions of subjects with a scale score in the clinical area were compared between DS-sample and the normative sample, using Chi-Square test.

The TACQOL was analyzed by comparing the scale scores of the DS-sample with data from a Dutch reference population of 519 children aged eight or nine years [25].

Results

A total of 531 parents with a child with DS born in 1992, 1993 or 1994 were approached via the Dutch Down Syndrome Foundation to participate in the present study, which holds 78% of all living children of this birth cohort in the Netherlands (based on a 84% survival rate) [33]. A total of 380 parents (72%) signed up to participate; 337 parents provided actual data for the present study (response rate: 63%; equaling 50% of this birth cohort). Gender and age were known of all 337 participating children. Background characteristics were known of 325 children. The number of subjects participating in the formal tests was 325 for the TACQOL, 320 for the CBCL and 285 for the MSCA. Overall, 266 parents and their children completed all questionnaires and tests.

Background characteristics are presented in Table 1. Mean age was 8.1 years (SD = 0.15, range 7.8–9.1); 52.0% of the subjects were boys and 94.6% of the children were of Dutch origin. A total of 156 children (48.0%) attended regular education at the age of eight years; more girls than boys (60.3% versus 36.7%; $p<.001$). Above 90% of the children with DS were diagnosed and/or treated for one or more concomitant chronic diseases, mainly visual impairment, chronic airway infection, heart defect or hearing impairment.

Developmental skills

The psychological assistants visited 285 children at home to administer the MSCA. Table 2 shows mean scores of the test scales. Higher values reflect more favorable results.

On all measures the DS-sample scored significantly lower than the normative sample, with very large effect sizes. The largest effect sizes were found for the memory scale ($d = 5.1$) and the quantitative scale ($d = 4.8$). Within the DS-sample, boys had significantly lower scale scores than girls; effect sizes ranged from 0.5 to 0.7, indicating a moderate effect by gender.

In addition, developmental age was calculated for each child. In Figure 1 the developmental age of the subjects is plotted stratified for gender. In 33 children (82% boys), who had very low test scores, developmental age could not be calculated exactly, but was estimated to be at a level of under 2.5 years, according to the MSCA test manual. By calculating mean age these children were ranked as having a developmental age of 2.4 years. For the total sample, mean developmental age for boys was 3.6 years (SD = 0.85) and for girls 4.2 years (SD = 0.82), showing a difference of 0.53 years ($p<0.001$). In all children the highest developmental age scored was 6.8 years.

Emotional and behavior problems

A total of 320 questionnaires of the CBCL were completed. Mean scores are shown in Table 3, whereby higher values reflect more problems. On almost all subscales children in the DS-sample scored significantly more problem behavior than the normative

Table 1. Characteristics of the studied population of children with DS, as reported by their parents, arranged by gender (n = 325).

	Total		Boys		Girls		
General characteristics	n	%	n	%	n	%	p*
Number of subjects	325	*100.0*	169	*52.0*	156	*48.0*	
Education at 8 years old							
Regular primary school	156	*48.0*	62	*36.7*	94	*60.3*	.000
Special school or day-care centre	169	*52.0*	107	*63.3*	62	*39.7*	.000
Ever enrolled in regular primary school	240	*73.8*	112	*66.3*	128	*82.1*	.001
Level of regular primary school at 8 years old							
Preschool	31	*9.5*	17	*10.1*	14	*9.0*	.614
First grade	95	*29.2*	35	*20.7*	60	*38.5*	.000
Second grade	30	*9.2*	10	*5.9*	20	*12.8*	.032
Age in years (range)	7.8 – 9.1		7.9 – 9.1		7.8 – 9.0		
Age in years (mean ± SD)	8.14 ± 0.15		8.15 ± 0.15		8.13 ± 0.15		.193
Concomitant chronic diseases							
Visual impairment	158	*48.6*	76	*45.0*	82	*52.6*	.172
Chronic Airway Infections	149	*45.8*	85	*50.3*	64	*41.0*	.094
Congenital heart defect	137	*42.2*	63	*37.3*	74	*47.4*	.064
Hearing impairment	98	*30.2*	55	*32.5*	43	*27.6*	.330
Gastrointestinal tract abnormality	45	*13.8*	27	*16.0*	18	*11.5*	.248
Thyroid dysfunction	39	*12.0*	22	*13.0*	17	*10.9*	.558
Asthma	34	*10.5*	25	*14.8*	9	*5.8*	.008
Diabetic Mellitus	3	*0.9*	2	*1.2*	1	*0.6*	.611
Other chronic disease	81	*24.9*	46	*27.2*	35	*22.4*	.758
Number of concomitant chronic diseases							
No chronic disease	26	*8.0*	18	*10.7*	8	*5.1*	.067
Only one chronic disease	81	*24.9*	39	*23.1*	42	*26.9*	.423
Two or more chronic diseases	218	*67.1*	112	*66.3*	106	*67.9*	.748

Abbreviation: SD – standard deviation.
*Boys with DS compared to girls with DS.

Table 2. Developmental skills, measured by the MSCA in a population of eight-year-old children with DS (n = 285), compared to the normative sample (NS, n = 238); raw scale scores are reported; higher scores denote more favorable skills.

	Total sample (male and female)			DS sample		
	DS	NS		Male	Female	
	(n = 285)	*(n = 106)*		*(n = 153)*	*(n = 132)*	
	Mean ± SD	Mean ± SD	Effect size[1]	Mean ± SD	Mean ± SD	Effect size[1]
Verbal	37.32±18.11	89.00±10.75	−3.15***	33.29±18.73	41.36±16.57	−0.46***
Perceptual-Performance	29.84±15.89	76.00±7.00	−3.29***	24.88±15.69	34.80±14.53	−0.66***
Quantitative	10.98±6.78	44.00±7.00	−4.84***	9.09±6.71	12.86±6.33	−0.58***
Memory	12.56±7.81	50.00±6.25	−5.06***	10.52±7.30	14.60±7.80	−0.54***
Motor	25.79±21.42	64.00±5.50	−2.07***	22.35±12.49	29.23±11.39	−0.58***
General Cognitive	78.15±38.13	209.00±20.00	−3.84***	67.26±38.37	89.05±34.75	−0.60***

*p<0.05,
**p<0.01,
***p<0.001.
[1]Cohen's *d* effect size: *d*<0.2 negligible; 0.2≤*d*<0.5 small; 0.5≤*d*<0.8 moderate; 0.8≤*d*<1.3 large; *d*≥1.3 very large.
Abbreviations: MSCA – McCarthy Scales of Children's Ability, DS – Down syndrome, NS – Normative sample, SD – standard deviation.

sample. The highest effect size was found for the subscale social problems (*d* = 1.55), followed by the subscale attention problems (*d* = 1.15 for boys and 1.30 for girls), indicating large to very large effects. The effect size of the difference in total problem score between the children with DS and the normative sample indicated a moderate effect (*d* = 0.72 for boys and *d* = 0.63 for girls).

For the scale anxious/depressed an opposite score was observed: the DS-sample showed significantly fewer problems with a moderate effect size (*d* = 0.60 for boys and *d* = 0.53 for girls).

Additionally, scale scores were arranged in the normal or clinical area of the scale (Table 3). For the subscales somatic complaints, social, thought, attention and sexual problems, and the total problem scale the children with DS scored significantly more within the clinical areas. An exception again was the subscale anxious/depressed, where fewer children with DS scored within the clinical area (*p*<0.05).

Health-Related Quality of Life

Mean scores of the TACQOL – evaluating the influence of having DS in daily life – are summarized in Table 4, whereby higher values reflect better HRQoL. Compared with the normative population, children with DS had significantly lower

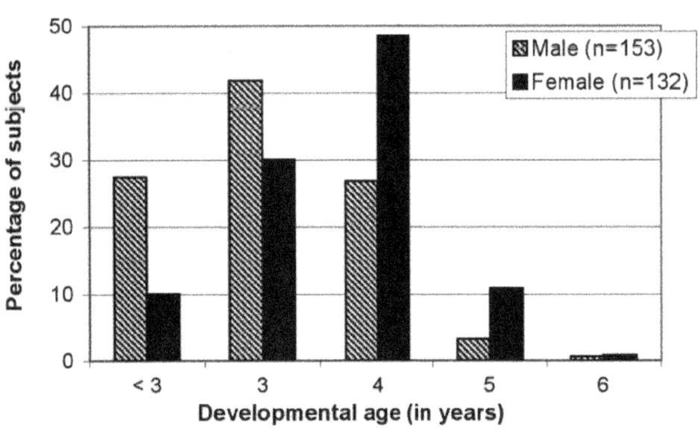

Figure 1. Distribution of MSCA developmental age in eight-year-old children with DS, arranged by gender (n = 285).

scores with very large effects on autonomy (*d* = 1.90) and cognitive functioning (*d* = 1.51); with a large effect on the gross motor skills (*d* = 0.89), and with a small effect on social functioning (*d* = 0.46) scales.

For the scale negative emotions we observed a significant favorable outcome for boys, but the effect size was small (*d* = *0.21*). For the other scales – physical complaints, positive emotions and (for girls) negative emotions – there were no differences observed.

Discussion

The aim of the present study was to investigate the development of a population based sample of Dutch children with DS at the age of eight years. The study included a large nationwide cohort of children with DS born in 1992, 1993 or 1994, approximately 50% of all children with DS of this birth cohort living in the Netherlands [2–4]. We measured a wide spectrum of developmental skills, emotional and behavior problems and HRQoL. Previous studies indicated that children with DS have a delayed development [7–12,14,15]. However, detailed aspects of development and quality of life have not been quantified in a population based sample.

The large sample of our study presented an opportunity to study differences between boys and girls. Few studies addressed gender differences with regard to developmental skills and cognition. Most observed no significant differences, probably due to their small sample size [10].

Furthermore the present study is different from most others in defining the comparison groups. Previous studies compared their DS-sample with participants matched for mental age and gender or used siblings [9–12,17]. We compared the selected DS-sample with randomly selected children from the general population with identical chronological age and same gender.

Our sample is born in 1992, 1993 and 1994, after the era (the 1980's) in which major changes in the care for the children with DS have taken place; i.e. medical care has been optimized; early intervention was introduced, and the majority of the children was no longer raised in institutions but at home.

Results

One of the main findings of our study is that children with DS have a substantial delay in developmental skills in comparison with

Table 3. Emotional and behavioral problems, measured by the CBCL, in a population of eight-year-old children with DS (n = 320): scale scores and proportion of children scoring in the clinical area of the scales, compared to the normative sample (NS, n = 661), arranged by gender; higher scores denote more problems.

	Total DS sample		Male					Female				
	Scale score	Clinical score	Scale score			Clinical score		Scale score			Clinical score	
	(*n* = 320)		DS (*n* = 169)	NS (*n* = 325)		DS	NS	DS (*n* = 151)	NS (*n* = 336)		DS	NS
	Mean ± SD	%	Mean ± SD	Mean ± SD	Effect size[1]	%	%	Mean ± SD	Mean ± SD	Effect size[1]	%	%
Withdrawn	2.54±2.66	5.9	2.61±2.75	1.63±1.85	0.45***	7.1**	1.5	2.46±2.55	1.65±1.84	0.39***	4.6	2.1
Somatic complaints	1.35±1.92	6.9	1.29±1.85	0.77±1.24	0.35***	7.7**	2.2	1.42±2.00	1.04±1.49	0.23*	6.0*	2.1
Anxious/Depressed	0.88±1.42	0.3	0.78±1.33	2.40±3.20	−0.60***	0.6*	4.3	0.99±1.50	2.50±3.26	−0.53***	0.0*	3.6
Social problems	4.38±2.15	21.6	4.57±2.17	1.51±1.83	1.57***	18.9***	1.9	4.17±2.11	1.30±1.76	1.53***	24.5***	2.7
Thought problems	1.18±1.66	8.8	1.30±1.76	0.35±0.92	0.75***	10.7***	1.9	1.03±1.53	0.27±0.67	0.75***	6.6***	0.9
Attention problems	6.50±3.15	12.2	6.76±3.19	3.22±3.02	1.15***	12.4***	2.5	6.22±3.10	2.61±2.62	1.30***	11.9***	2.1
Delinquent behavior	1.47±1.57	3.1	1.55±1.60	1.11±1.43	0.30**	2.4	1.5	1.38±1.53	0.78±1.23	0.45***	4.0	1.5
Aggressive behavior	7.27±5.69	4.4	8.13±6.06	6.66±6.11	0.24*	5.9	4.3	6.30±5.11	5.07±5.05	0.24*	2.6	2.4
Sexual problems	0.37±0.83	3.8	0.42±0.89	0.15±0.52	0.40***	3.6	1.2	0.30±0.76	0.11±0.42	0.35***	4.0**	0.3
Internalizing problems[2]	4.71±4.55	10.6	4.62±4.54	4.69±4.96	-	11.2	11.4	4.82±4.58	5.09±5.32	-	9.9	11.0
Externalizing problems[3]	8.73±6.84	15.3	9.68±7.25	7.77±7.17	0.27**	12.4	11.1	7.68±6.21	5.85±5.95	0.30**	18.5	13.4
Total problems	30.08±18.06	26.9	32.05±18.81	19.78±15.96	0.72***	27.8***	10.8	27.87±16.97	17.98±15.28	0.63***	25.8***	11.9

*$p<0.05$,
**$p<0.01$,
***$p<0.001$.
[1]Cohen's d effect size: $d<0.2$ negligible; $0.2\le d<0.5$ small; $0.5\le d<0.8$ moderate; $0.8\le d<1.3$ large; $d\ge1.3$ very large.
[2]Combined from the subscales withdrawn, somatic complaints and anxious/depressed.
[3]Combined from the subscales delinquent and aggressive behavior.
Abbreviations: CBCL – Child Behavior Checklist, DS – Down syndrome, NS – Normative sample, SD – standard deviation.

Table 4. HRQoL, measured by the TACQOL, in a population of eight-year-old children with DS (n = 325), compared to the normative sample (NS, n = 519), arranged by gender; higher scores denote better HRQoL.

	Total DS sample	**Male**			**Female**		
		DS	**NS**		**DS**	**NS**	
	(n = 325)	*(n = 169)*	*(n = 260)*		*(n = 156)*	*(n = 259)*	
	Mean ± SD	**Mean ± SD**	**Mean ± SD**	**Effect size[1]**	**Mean ± SD**	**Mean ± SD**	**Effect size[1]**
Physical complaints	27.26±3.48	27.14±3.56	27.29±3.92	-	27.39±3.39	26.66±4.05	-
Gross motor skills	27.85±3.92	27.76±4.21	30.78±2.50	−0.90***	27.95±3.61	30.72±2.85	−0.88***
Autonomy	26.28±3.59	26.06±3.72	31.10±1.90	−1.84***	26.51±3.45	31.32±1.60	−1.96***
Cognitive functioning	22.76±3.54	22.75±3.89	28.39±3.98	−1.43***	22.77±3.12	28.62±4.00	−1.58***
Social functioning	28.25±3.54	27.95±3.72	29.36±2.82	−0.44***	28.57±3.33	29.91±2.49	−0.47***
Positive emotions	15.06±1.64	15.01±1.70	14.73±2.01	-	15.11±1.58	14.81±2.05	-
Negative emotions	11.71±1.99	11.70±2.18	11.18±2.78	0.21	11.73±1.78	11.45±2.30	-

*p<0.05,
**p<0.01,
***p<0.001.
[1]Cohen's *d* effect size: $d<0.2$ negligible; $0.2 \le d<0.5$ small; $0.5 \le d<0.8$ moderate; $0.8 \le d<1.3$ large; $d \ge 1.3$ very large.
Abbreviations: HRQoL – Health-related quality of life, TACQOL – TNO-AZL Children's Quality of Life questionnaire, DS – Down syndrome, NS – Normative sample, SD – standard deviation.

the normative sample. The mean developmental age of the children with DS was 3.9 years (SD = 0.87), which is four years behind their average calendar age of 8.1 years (SD = 0.15). A substantial delay in development was recorded in all children. However, the range was wide, with some children indicating a developmental delay of only one or two years, and other children indicating a developmental delay of more then five years. Girls with DS scored on average more favorably on all skills and had a higher developmental age in comparison to boys with DS.

Our results further indicate that children with DS had more emotional and behavior problems in comparison to the normative sample on almost all domains measured, with the exception of the scale anxious/depressed. Some previous studies with a small number of children (less than 50) and a wide range of age, found also more behavior problems in children with DS [11]. Our finding that children with DS score significantly better on the problem scale anxious/depressed in comparison to the normative sample has not been reported in previous studies [9,11,16]. Only among adults with DS, several studies report more depression compared to the general population [6,18,19]. The internalizing problem scale score – which is composed of withdrawn, somatic complaints and anxious/depressed – did not differ significantly from the normative sample, as a result from the opposite score for the anxious/depressed scale.

The children with DS scored a lower HRQoL on the scales gross motor skills, autonomy, social and cognitive functioning in comparison with the normative sample. These domains determine the main topics in everyday life of children with DS, as reported by parents. Remarkably, HRQoL of children with DS showed no significant difference on the physical complaints scale, even though 92% of the children indicated one or more concomitant chronic conditions.

In our sample a high percentage (46%) of chronic airway infections was observed. Prospective studies on the exact incidence of chronic airway infections are lacking. A recent national health survey showed that in children with DS in the age of 6–10 years parents reported 38% to have head or chest cold in the previous two weeks [34]. A study among Dutch children showed that 24% of the children with DS were hospitalized twice or more for pulmonary infection or use inhalation medication for more than six months [35]. In our study parents were asked "Does your child suffer from chronic airway infections (often severe common cold/ bronchitis)" and "Was your child diagnosed with asthma?" to evaluate respiratory complaints. Therefore, the higher number of reported chronic airway infections in our study could be explained by the broader definition used. For other concomitant disorders, like congenital heart defects, hearing impairment and thyroid dysfunction, the incidences in our sample are in accordance with earlier studies [6].

The data of this study were collected between 2000 and 2003. Despite this data collection occurred several years ago, these data will be valid for the current generation of children with DS, because no major changes in the approach of (medical) care for children with DS has taken place since the measurement of this study.

Of the parents with a child with DS who were approached, about 63% participated in the study. Unfortunately, we were not able to carry out a non-response analysis. It is possible that parents whose child had more serious developmental problems than most of the children with DS, more frequently refused to participate. These factors may have resulted in an underestimation of the problem behavior of these children and an overestimation of the developmental level. However, we observed a wide range in developmental level and more than 50 children to have a developmental age below three years, showing also children with more serious developmental problems are included in our study.

Implications

The results of this study provide reference information for pediatricians and other health care professionals when they inform parents of the expected development of a child with DS. They may assist parents in gaining realistic expectations about the future of their children.

Currently children with DS in the Netherlands are encouraged to attend regular education in primary school. Studies showed that attending regular education provides more positive peer relationships and can improve social skills [36,37]. However, low mean developmental age at the calendar age of eight years can be an important obstacle to enroll them in regular primary education. In order to keep them in regular education, additional support is needed to provide adequate learning conditions. If adequate support can not be guaranteed, special education is needed.

The children with DS indicated more social, attention and thought problems than the normative sample. These problems should be recognized as they form obstacles in learning conditions. In particular the high level of social problems suggests that this is an area where significant improvement may be made. From an early age onwards, children with DS should be stimulated to develop social skills, confirming the need for adequate support in primary school.

For the children themselves HRQoL was mainly decreased for their level of autonomy and cognitive functioning. Current medical care for children with DS focuses on the physical conditions of the children, as advised in the guidelines of the American Academy of Pediatrics, and the Pediatric Association of the Netherlands [38,39]. Medical professionals should extend their care with supportive coaching on autonomy and cognitive functioning, to improve quality of life for the children with DS.

Conclusion

Eight-year-old children with DS have an average developmental delay of four years. This finding has important implications for (parents of) children with DS and professionals. These children have more emotional and behavioral problems, and have on some domains a less favorable HRQoL compared with children from the general population.

It is recommended to investigate the factors influencing the social participation and development of children with DS, as well as the relation between developmental level and problem behavior, and its influence on quality of life. Population based longitudinal cohort studies are needed to gain insights in all aspects of functioning and social participation of children with DS.

Acknowledgments

We thank the psychological assistants, who visited all children at home and administered the tests: Petra Buijs and Nicolette van Kessel. We thank the Dutch Down Syndrome Foundation for inviting all participants, and their efforts in enabling the present study.

Author Contributions

Conceived and designed the experiments: MF JB JPW. Performed the experiments: MF JB. Analyzed the data: HBMG MF JB. Contributed reagents/materials/analysis tools: MF JB. Wrote the paper: HBMG MF SEB ADM JPW.

References

1. Shin M, Besser LM, Kucik JE, Lu C, Siffel C, et al. (2009) Prevalence of Down syndrome among children and adolescents in 10 regions of the United States. Pediatrics 124: 1565–1571.
2. Anthony S, Dorrepaal CA, Kateman H, Pal van der-Bruin KM (2005) TNO report on Congenital defects in the Netherlands 1996–2003. Leiden: Netherlands Organisation for Applied Scientific Research, TNO, Quality of Life, TNO-rapport KvL/JPB/2005.152.
3. Mohangoo AD, Buitendijk SE (2009) TNO report on congenital defects in the Netherlands 1997–2007. Leiden: Netherlands Organisation for Applied Scientific Research, TNO, Quality of Life, TNO-rapport KvL/P&Z/2009.112.
4. Weijerman ME, van Furth AM, Vonk NA, Van Wouwe JP, Broers CJ, et al. (2008) Prevalence, neonatal characteristics, and first-year mortality of Down syndrome: a national study. J Pediatr 152: 15–19.
5. Weijerman ME, de Winter JP (2010) Clinical practice. The care of children with Down syndrome. Eur J Pediatr 169: 1445–1452.
6. Roizen NJ, Patterson D (2003) Down's syndrome. Lancet 361: 1281–1289.
7. Carr J (1988) Six weeks to twenty-one years old: a longitudinal study of children with Down's syndrome and their families. Third Jack Tizard memorial lecture. J Child Psychol Psychiatry 29: 407–431.
8. Chapman RS, Hesketh LJ (2000) Behavioral phenotype of individuals with Down syndrome. Ment Retard Dev Disabil Res Rev 6: 84–95.
9. Dykens EM, Kasari C (1997) Maladaptive behavior in children with Prader-Willi syndrome, Down syndrome, and nonspecific mental retardation. Am J Ment Retard 102: 228–237.
10. Dykens EM (2007) Psychiatric and behavioral disorders in persons with Down syndrome. Ment Retard Dev Disabil Res Rev 13: 272–278.
11. Pueschel SM, Bernier JC, Pezzullo JC (1991) Behavioural observations in children with Down's syndrome. J Ment Defic Res 35(Pt 6): 502–511.
12. Silverman W (2007) Down syndrome: cognitive phenotype. Ment Retard Dev Disabil Res Rev 13: 228–236.
13. Stores R, Stores G, Fellows B, Buckley S (1998) Daytime behaviour problems and maternal stress in children with Down's syndrome, their siblings, and non-intellectually disabled and other intellectually disabled peers. J Intellect Disabil Res 42(Pt 3): 228–237.
14. Turner S, Alborz A (2003) Academic attainments of children with Down's syndrome: A longitudinal study. Journal of Educational Psychology 73: 563–583.
15. Jarrold C, Baddeley AD, Phillips C (1999) Down syndrome and the phonological loop: the evidence for, and importance of, a specific verbal short-term memory deficit. Downs Syndr Res Pract 6: 61–75.
16. Coe DA, Matson JL, Russell DW, Slifer KJ, Capone GT, et al. (1999) Behavior problems of children with Down syndrome and life events. J Autism Dev Disord 29: 149–156.
17. Gath A, Gumley D (1986) Behaviour problems in retarded children with special reference to Down's syndrome. Br J Psychiatry 149: 156–161.
18. Myers BA, Pueschel SM (1991) Psychiatric disorders in persons with Down syndrome. J Nerv Ment Dis 179: 609–613.
19. Capone G, Goyal P, Ares W, Lannigan E (2006) Neurobehavioral disorders in children, adolescents, and young adults with Down syndrome. Am J Med Genet C Semin Med Genet 142C: 158–172.
20. Kent L, Evans J, Paul M, Sharp M (1999) Comorbidity of autistic spectrum disorders in children with Down syndrome. Dev Med Child Neurol 41: 153–158.
21. De Graaf G (2006) A historic demographic model for Down syndrome with a number of applications. Down&Up 76: 37–48.
22. McCarthy D (1972) Manual for the McCarthy scales for children's abilities. San AntonioTX: The Psychological Corporation.
23. Vogels T, Verrips GH, Verloove-Vanhorick SP, Fekkes M, Kamphuis RP, et al. (1998) Measuring health-related quality of life in children: the development of the TACQOL parent form. Qual Life Res 7: 457–465.
24. Achenbach TM (1991) Manual for the Child Behaviour Checklist and 1991 Profile. Burlington: University of Vermont.
25. Verrips GH, Vogels T, Koopman HM, Theunissen NCM, Kamphuis RP, et al. (1999) Measuring health-related quality of life in a child population. European Journal of Public Health 9: 188–193.
26. Meulen van der BF, Smrkovsky M (1985) Mos 2,5–8,5, McCarthy ontwikkelingsschalen. Lisse: Swets & Zeitlinger B.V.
27. Verhulst FC, Ende van der J, Koot HM (1996) Manual for the CBCL/4–18 (in Dutch). Rotterdam: Erasmus University/Dept of Child and Adolescent Psychiatry, Sophia Childrens' Hospital.
28. Noterdaeme M, Minow F, Amorosa H (1999) [Applicability of the Child Behavior Checklist in developmentally delayed children]. Z Kinder Jugendpsychiatr Psychother 27: 183–188.
29. de Ruiter KP, Dekker MC, Verhulst FC, Koot HM (2007) Developmental course of psychopathology in youths with and without intellectual disabilities. J Child Psychol Psychiatry 48: 498–507. JCPP1712 [pii];10.1111/j1469-7610(06)01712.x [doi].
30. Dekker MC, Koot HM, van der Ende J, Verhulst FC (2002) Emotional and behavioral problems in children and adolescents with and without intellectual disability. J Child Psychol Psychiatry 43: 1087–1098.
31. Cohen J (1997) Statistical power analysis for the behavioral sciences. New York: Academic Press.
32. Reijneveld SA, Brugman E, Verhulst FC, Verloove-Vanhorick SP (2005) Area deprivation and child psychosocial problems–a national cross-sectional study among school-aged children. Soc Psychiatry Psychiatr Epidemiol 40: 18–23.
33. Tennant PW, Pearce MS, Bythell M, Rankin J (2010) 20-year survival of children born with congenital anomalies: a population-based study. Lancet 375: 649–656. S0140-6736(09)61922-X [pii];10.1016/S0140-6736(09)61922-X [doi].
34. Schieve LA, Boulet SL, Boyle C, Rasmussen SA, Schendel D (2009) Health of children 3 to 17 years of age with Down syndrome in the 1997–2005 national health interview survey. Pediatrics 123: e253–e260. 123/2/e253 [pii];10.1542/peds.2008-1440 [doi].

35. van Trotsenburg AS, Heymans HS, Tijssen JG, de Vijlder JJ, Vulsma T (2006) Comorbidity, hospitalization, and medication use and their influence on mental and motor development of young infants with Down syndrome. Pediatrics 118: 1633–1639. 118/4/1633 [pii];10.1542/peds.2006-1136 [doi].
36. Buckley S, Bird G, Sacks B, Archer T (2006) A comparison of mainstream and special education for teenagers with Down syndrome: implications for parents and teachers. Downs Syndr Res Pract 9: 54–67.
37. Davis AS (2008) Children with Down syndrome: Implications for assessment and intervention in the school. School Psychology Quarterly 23: 271–281.
38. Committee of Genetics (2001) Health supervision for children with Down syndrome. Pediatrics 107: 442–449.
39. Van Wouwe JP, Siderius EJ, Borstlap R, Nijenhuis TA, Hirasing RA (2001) [Optimal medical care for children with Down syndrome and their parents]. Ned Tijdschr Geneeskd 145: 1617–1621.

3

Prenatal Treatment Prevents Learning Deficit in Down Syndrome Model

Maddalena Incerti[1,2]*, Kari Horowitz[1,3], Robin Roberson[1], Daniel Abebe[1], Laura Toso[1], Madeline Caballero[1], Catherine Y. Spong[1]

1 Unit on Perinatal and Developmental Neurobiology, National Institute of Child and Human Development, National Institute of Health, Bethesda, Maryland, United States of America, 2 Department of Obstetrics and Gynaecology, University of Milano-Bicocca, Ospedale S. Gerardo, Fondazione MBBM, Monza, Italy, 3 Department of Obstetrics and Gynecology, University of Connecticut, Groton, Connecticut, United States of America

Abstract

Down syndrome is the most common genetic cause of mental retardation. Active fragments of neurotrophic factors release by astrocyte under the stimulation of vasoactive intestinal peptide, NAPVSIPQ (NAP) and SALLRSIPA (SAL) respectively, have shown therapeutic potential for developmental delay and learning deficits. Previous work demonstrated that NAP+SAL prevent developmental delay and glial deficit in Ts65Dn that is a well-characterized mouse model for Down syndrome. The objective of this study is to evaluate if prenatal treatment with these peptides prevents the learning deficit in the Ts65Dn mice. Pregnant Ts65Dn female and control pregnant females were randomly treated (intraperitoneal injection) on pregnancy days 8 through 12 with saline (placebo) or peptides (NAP 20 µg +SAL 20 µg) daily. Learning was assessed in the offspring (8–10 months) using the Morris Watermaze, which measures the latency to find the hidden platform (decrease in latency denotes learning). The investigators were blinded to the prenatal treatment and genotype. Pups were genotyped as trisomic (Down syndrome) or euploid (control) after completion of all tests. Statistical analysis: two-way ANOVA followed by Neuman-Keuls test for multiple comparisons, $P<0.05$ was used to denote statistical significance. Trisomic mice who prenatally received placebo (Down syndrome -placebo; $n=11$) did not demonstrate learning over the five day period. DS mice that were prenatally exposed to peptides (Down syndrome-peptides; $n=10$) learned significantly better than Down syndrome -placebo ($p<0.01$), and similar to control-placebo ($n=33$) and control-peptide ($n=30$). In conclusion prenatal treatment with the neuroprotective peptides (NAP+SAL) prevented learning deficits in a Down syndrome model. These findings highlight a possibility for the prevention of sequelae in Down syndrome and suggest a potential pregnancy intervention that may improve outcome.

Editor: Judith Homberg, Radboud University, The Netherlands

Funding: This research was supported by the Division of Intramural Research Program, United States National Institutes of Health, NICHD. The funders had no role in study design, data collection and analysis, decision to publish, or preparation of the manuscript.

Competing Interests: The authors have declared that no competing interests exist.

* E-mail: maddalena.incerti@gmail.com

Introduction

Down Syndrome (DS) is the most common genetic cause of mental retardation due to triplication of all or part of chromosome 21 [1] and occurs in 1 in 800 live births. In the newborn period, infants with DS have hypotonia and delay in achievement of developmental motor [2] and sensory milestones [3,4]. At the neuropathological level, neonates with DS have a smaller brain, delayed myelination of neurons and glial alterations [5]. These early developmental anomalies may predispose to abnormalities in adulthood including mental retardation and early onset of Alzheimer disease.

The Ts65Dn mouse is a well-characterized model for DS [6], with triplication of a segment of chromosome 16 which includes over 55% of the genes present on human chromosome 21.

In the newborn period, Ts65Dn mice mimic the human condition, including developmental delay [7]. Microscopically, Ts65Dn neonates have fewer granule cells in the hippocampus, reduced Long Term Potentiation (LTP) and abnormal synaptic plasticity [8–10]. In adulthood, Ts65Dn mice have a deficit in short and long term memory, deficits in learning, and early onset of the neuropathology of Alzheimer disease [7,11–14]. The mechanisms underlying the neuropathology of DS are not well understood.

Vasoactive Intestinal Peptide (VIP) is a neuropeptide crucial for the development of the brain [15,16]. In human studies the level of VIP is increased in neonatal blood of children with DS [17,18]; Ts65Dn mice have elevated brain VIP mRNA [19], and cortical astrocytes from postnatal day 8 brains show a defect in the signal transduction mechanism of the VIP receptor VPAC-1 with astrocyte dysfunction [20]. Furthermore, blockade of VIP during embryogenesis is followed by postnatal hypotonia, growth restriction and developmental delay [21] in both human DS and Ts65Dn mice. It is hypothesized that the up-regulation of VIP in DS may be an attempt to compensate for the loss of neuronal function [19], which may explain the high levels of VIP [17,18].

VIP stimulation of astrocytes results in the release of neurotrophic factors, including Activity Dependent Neuroprotective Protein (ADNP) and Activity Dependent Neurotrophic Factor (ADNF), which have been demonstrated to be neuroprotective [22]. Active fragments of ADNP and ADNF, NAPVSIPQ (NAP) and SALLRSIPA (SAL) respectively, have shown therapeutic potential for developmental delay [23,24] and learning deficits [25,26]. Addition of SAL or NAP to DS cortical neurons resulted in a 2-fold increase in neuronal survival as well as a reduction of degenerative morphological changes [27].

To date, there is no therapy for the prevention of developmental delays in DS (MEDLINE from 1963, keywords: Down syndrome, treatment, development, fetus; all languages). Our hypothesis was that prenatal treatment with NAP+SAL may prevent the learning deficit in the Ts65Dn mouse model for Down syndrome.

Materials and Methods

Pregnant Ts65Dn females were randomly assigned to NAP+ SAL or control groups, and treated by investigators blinded to group and genotype from gestational day 8 to 12. This time period was chosen based on previous studies that showed that this is a critical time for VIP action during in utero development [28]. Offspring were weighed and tested from postnatal day (P) 5 to 21 for motor and sensory milestones with standardized tests [7]. The pup's genotype was determined after completion of all tests. The offspring were tested at 8–10 months of age for learning assessment. The mice were typed for the ability to see as ¼ of these would have carried the rd mutation in a homozygous state and would have been blind. Operators blinded to the offspring's treatment and genotype performed all the tests.

Animals

Ts65Dn female mice (The Jackson Laboratory, Bar Harbor, ME) were kept in a 12-hour light/12-hour dark regimen, with food (6% fat diet) and water available at all times. The mice received humane animal care in compliance with the National Institutes of Health (NIH) guidelines for care and use of experimental animals. The protocol was approved by the National Institute of Child Health and Human Development (NICHD) Animal Care and Use Committee. Females were mated with B6EiC3SnFi male mice; the animals were checked twice daily and the day of appearance of a vaginal plug was considered day 0 (E0) of pregnancy.

Treatment

Ts65Dn (DS) and control pregnant females were treated (intraperitoneal injection) on pregnancy days 8 through 12 (a typical mouse gestation is 18–21 days) with saline (placebo) or peptides (NAP 20 µg +SAL 20 µg) daily. NAP and SAL were obtained from SynPep, Dublin, CA. NAP was diluted in 50 µL of dimethyl sulfoxide and diluted in filtered Dulbecco's phosphate-buffered saline (DPBS); SAL was dissolved and diluted in filtered DPBS.

Learning Assessment

The Morris watermaze is a well-established test that evaluates spatial learning, a measure of cognitive function [29]. The apparatus consists of a circular pool with a water level of approximately 30 cm and maintained at 24–26°C. Nontoxic Tempura paint is added to make the water opaque and blend with the colour of the pool wall. External cues (arrow, star, circle, and rectangle) are placed around the pool as a reference for the mice. A transparent platform is placed in the pool and kept in a fixed location throughout the testing period. The platform surface is hidden, submerged under the water surface. Each day, the mouse was positioned on the platform for 15 seconds before being placed into the pool. The mouse was placed into the water at the same location for each trial and allowed to swim freely to find the hidden platform using the external visual cues. On the first day of testing, animals were allowed to remain on the platform for 60 seconds. Each animal underwent 4 consecutive trials daily, with the average time or latency required to find the platform recorded over 5 consecutive days. The animal was given 90 seconds to find the platform, if the animal could not they were rescued and 90 seconds was recorded. Each trial was tracked using an overhead camera interfaced with a computer which recorded the time and path travelled. The latency to find the hidden platform for each trial was recorded and the average of the trials was calculated for each of the five days.

Genotyping of the Ts65Dn Mice

For genotyping, tail tips (2 mm/sample) from adult mice were collected after the completion of the watermaze. A previously published method was used [23,30]. All examiners were blinded to the treatment groups and genotype.

Statistical Analysis

Two-way ANOVA followed by Neuman-Keuls test for multiple comparisons was used for analysis. A P value less than 0.05 was used to denote statistical significance.

Results

Given the difficulty breeding these animals, the breeding occurred between 2008 and 2010 with four separate watermaze experiments performed as the animals reached the appropriate age for the testing (8–10 months of age). In all, 33 control animals from 9 litters receiving placebo, 30 control animals from 8 litters receiving peptides, 11 DS animals from 4 litters receiving placebo and 10 DS animals from 6 litters receiving prenatal peptides were tested.

Trisomic mice who prenatally received placebo (DS-placebo; $n = 11$) did not demonstrate learning over the five day period. DS mice that were prenatally exposed to peptides (DS-peptides; $n = 10$) learned significantly better than DS-placebo ($p < 0.01$), and similar to control-placebo ($n = 33$) and control-peptide ($n = 30$) (Figure 1).

Discussion

Prenatal treatment with the neuroprotective peptides NAP and SAL prevented the learning deficits in adult mice, with learning similar to control animals. Our findings are novel in that we propose the possibility of an intervention during pregnancy that may prevent or reverse the learning deficits of DS. These results extend the benefit shown with prenatal treatment in the Ts65Dn model where NAP and SAL prevented developmental delay in the DS offspring and with postnatal treatment where NAP and SAL prevented learning deficit in Ts65Dn animals treated during adulthood [23,26]. The results are consistent with studies of learning enhancement with NAP and SAL from our group in a model of fetal alcohol syndrome [25] and in normal animals [31]. Others have also shown that neonatal mice treated with intraperitoneal NAP had increased performance in the Morris watermaze and that VIP is dysregulated in the Ts65Dn partial trisomy model for DS [32,33].

These results may, at least in part, be explained by our findings of alterations in the N-methyl-D-aspartate (NMDA) receptors. Using this DS mouse model we have shown that prenatal administration of NAP and SAL during pregnancy has long-lasting effects, specifically increasing NR2B and GABAAα3 expression in adult Ts65Dn mice to levels similar to wild-type

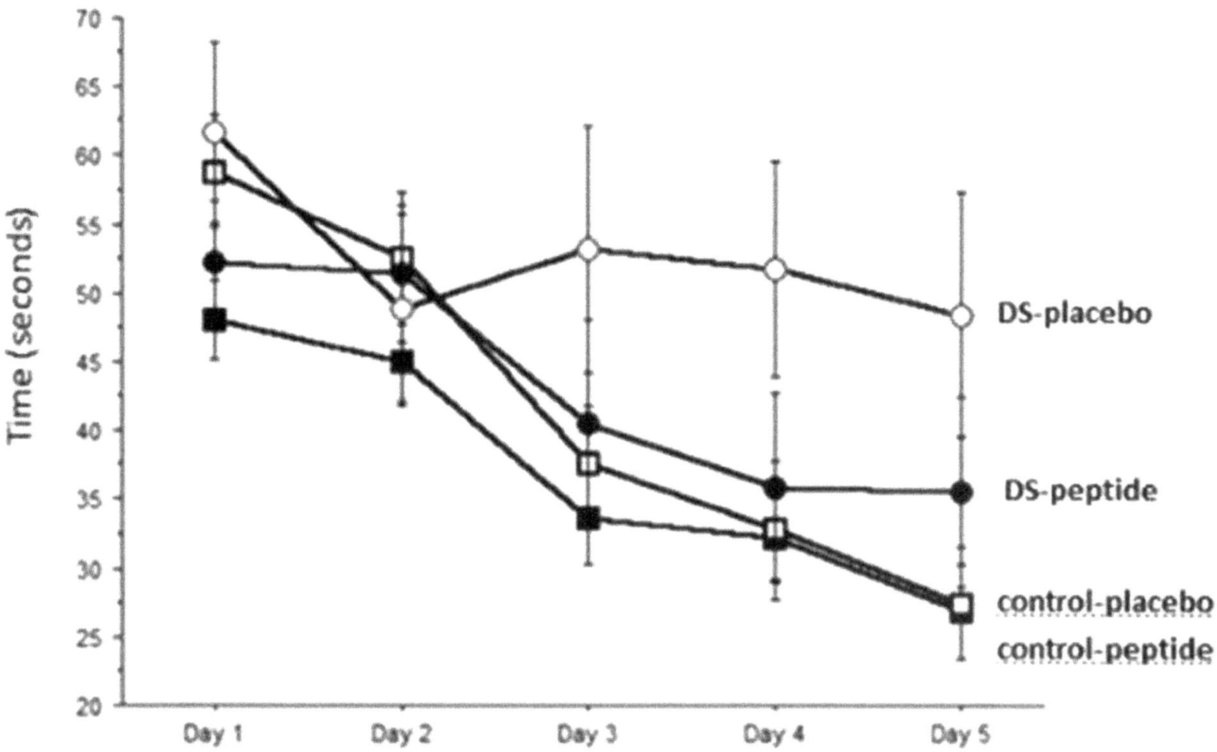

Figure 1. Assessment of spatial learning in the Morris watermaze. Learning was assessed by the latency in seconds to find the hidden platform. Animals with DS who prenatally received saline (placebo, open circles) did not learn over the 5 day period. Control animals (open squares) who prenatally received saline (placebo) did learn with an approximate halving of their latency. Control animals who prenatally received NAP+SAL (closed squares) also learned over the five day period. Animals with DS who prenatally received NAP+SAL (closed circles) learned over the five day period, similar to controls and significantly better than DS-placebo ($p<0.01$).

controls. In the NMDA receptors, the NR2B receptor is the more plastic subunit, thus a decrease in NR2B would make the synapse less plastic. Given the interaction between the GABA and NMDA receptors, a decrease in GABAAα3 would provide less inhibitory tone on the synapse causing overexcitation and ultimately termination of this neural synapse. Restoring the levels of these receptors to the level in controls may in part explain how the peptides NAP and SAL prevent adult learning impairment in the mouse model [34]. Fernandez et al. [35] demonstrated that chronic systemic treatment of Ts65Dn mice with GABAA antagonists causes a persistent post-drug recovery of cognition and LTP. The results support the hypothesis that excessive GABA-mediated inhibition in the Ts65Dn brain actively interferes with declarative memory in Ts65Dn mice [35].

Regarding the protective effects of the peptides on learning and memory, previous studies of hippocampal cultures demonstrated that the peptides alter glutamate release and NMDA receptors [36], both of which are important in learning and memory. Particularly, treatment of hippocampal neurons with SAL controls NR2A and NR2B subunit stability of the NMDA receptor in neurons that have yet to establish efficient synaptic connections [36]. Although the exact mechanism by which SAL influences the synaptogenesis and neurotransmission used by glutamate remains unknown, in vitro studies strongly suggest that the peptide interacts with and regulates the glutaminergic synapses in developing neural systems. Kleschevnikov et al. found that LTP could not be elicited in the dentate gyrus of Ts65Dn mice. They suggested that excessive inhibition of dentate granule cells was shown to restrict synaptic activation of NMDA receptors and to inhibit LTP [37].

One of the neuropathologic characteristics of DS is a glial deficit that likely induces alterations in VIP and its related neuropeptides. In the Ts65Dn mouse, we and others have showen a decrease in ADNP and an upregulation of VIP [20,23]. Prenatal treatment with NAL and SAL resulted in a normalization of ADNP and of the glial marker GFAP in Ts65Dn adult brains [23]. Treatment with the peptides may have overcome the glial deficit by restoring the appropriate neuropeptides. Nonetheless, treatment did not prevent VIP upregulation; it is possible that other mechanisms regulate VIP release [23].

Previous studies have shown that ADNF and ADNP are neuroprotective in the presence of toxins associated with neurodegenerative disorders, and that neonatal treatment with ADNP attenuated head injury–related dysfunctions in adulthood [38]. Numerous studies have shown the protective effects of VIP-related peptides against alcohol developmental effects [24,25,39–42]. Here we confirm the role of NAP and SAL in the prevention of learning impairment in a model of DS.

The strengths of this work include the study design and the validation of the results in three different sets of animals. Moreover, this work confirms that the Ts65Dn is a model that is particularly useful in understanding the biological basis for some of the developmental abnormalities and learning deficits of DS subjects.

The high mortality of the DS animals reduced the number of animals available, and consequently the pathway to test to understand the mechanism of action of the VIP related peptides.

We encourage further studies to delineate pathways underlying the mechanism behind learning enhancement in the Ts65Dn mouse model of Down syndrome.

Conclusion

In conclusion, these findings highlight a possibility for the prevention of sequelae in DS and other conditions with learning deficit. Because DS can be diagnosed prenatally, an intervention during pregnancy that may improve cognitive function is an attractive option.

Author Contributions

Conceived and designed the experiments: MI LT CYS. Performed the experiments: MI KH RR LT DA MC. Analyzed the data: MI KH LT CYS. Contributed reagents/materials/analysis tools: MI LT RR DA CYS. Wrote the paper: MI KH CYS.

References

1. Dolk H, Loane M, Garne E, De Walle H, Queisser-Luft A, et al. (2005) Trends and geographic inequalities in the prevalence of Down syndrome in Europe, 1980–1999. Rev Epidemiol Sante Publique 53: 2S87–2S95.
2. Vicari S (2006) Motor development and neuropsychological patterns in persons with Down syndrome. Behavior Genetics 36: 355–364.
3. Chen YJ, Fang PC (2005) Sensory evoked potentials in infants with Down syndrome. Acta Pediatrica 94: 1615–1618.
4. Toledo C, Alembik Y, Aguirre JA, Stoll C (1999) Growth curves of children with Down syndrome. Ann Genet 42: 81–90.
5. Nadel L (2003) Down's syndrome: a genetic disorder in biobehavioral perspective Genes. Brain and Behavior 2: 156–166.
6. Davisson MT, Schmidt C, Akeson EC (1990) Segmental trisomy of murine chromosome 16: a new model system for studying Down syndrome. Prog Clin Biol Res 360: 263–280.
7. Holtzman DM, Santucci D, Kilbridge J, Chua-Couzens J, Fontana DJ, et al. (1996) Developmental abnormalities and age-related neurodegeneration in a mouse model of Down syndrome. Proc Natl Acad Sci 93: 13333–13338.
8. Belichenko PV, Masliah E, Kleschevnikov AM, Villar AJ, Epstein CJ, et al. (2004) Synaptic structural abnormalities in the Ts65Dn mouse model of Down Syndrome. J Comp Neurol 480: 281–298.
9. Contestabile A, Fila T, Ceccarelli C, Bonasoni P, Bonapace L, et al. (2007) Cell cycle alteration and decreased cell proliferation in the hippocampal dentate gyrus and in the neocortical germinal matrix of fetuses with Down syndrome and in Ts65Dn mice. Hippocampus 17: 665–678.
10. Best TK, Siarey RJ, Galdzicki Z (2007) Ts65Dn, a mouse model of Down syndrome, exhibits increased GABAB-induced potassium current. J Neurophisiol 97: 892–900.
11. Reeves RH, Irving NG, Moran TH, Wohn A, Kitt C, et al. (1995) A mouse model for Down Syndrome exhibits learning and behaviour deficits. Nat Genet 11: 177–84.
12. Demas GE, Nelson RJ, Krueger BK, Yarowsky PJ (1996) Spatial memory deficits in segmental trisomic Ts65Dn mice. Behav Brain Res 82: 85–92.
13. Demas GE, Nelson RJ, Krueger BK, Yarowsky PJ (1998) Impaired spatial working and reference memory in segmental trisomy (Ts65Dn) mice. Behav Brain Res 90: 199–201.
14. Escorihuela RM, Vallina IF, Martinez-Cue' C, Baamonde C, Dierssen M, et al. (1998) Impaired short- and long-term memory in Ts65Dn mice, a model for Down syndrome. Neurosci Lett 247: 171–4.
15. Brenneman DE, Eiden LE (1986) Vasoactive intestinal peptide and electrical activity influence neuronal survival. Proc Natl Acad Sci U S A 83: 1159–62.
16. Hill JM, Mervis RF, Politi J, McCune SK, Gozes I, et al. (1994) Blockade of VIP during neonatal development induces neuronal damage and increases VIP and VIP receptors in brain. Ann N Y Acad Sci 31: 211–225.
17. Nelson KB, Grether JK, Croen LA, Dambrosia JM, Dickens BF, et al. (2001) Neuropeptides and neurotrophins in neonatal blood of children with autism or mental retardation. Ann Neurol 49: 597–606.
18. Nelson PG, Kuddo T, Song EY, Dambrosia JM, Kohler S, et al. (2006) Selected neurotrophins, neuropeptides, and cytokines: developmental trajectory and concentrations in neonatal blood of children with autism or Down syndrome. Int J Dev Neurosci 24: 73–80.
19. Hill JM, Ades AM, McCune SK, Sahir N, Moody EM, et al. (2003) Vasoactive intestinal peptide in the brain of a mouse model for Down syndrome. Exp Neurol 183: 56 65.
20. Sahir N, Brenneman DE, Hill JM (2006) Neonatal mice of the Down syndrome model, Ts65Dn, exhibit upregulated VIP measures and reduced responsiveness of cortical astrocytes to VIP stimulation. J Mol Neurosci 30: 329–40.
21. Wu JY, Henins KA, Gressens P, Gozes I, Fridkin M, et al. (1997) Neurobehavioral development of neonatal mice following blockade of VIP during the early embryonic period. Peptides 18: 1131–1137.
22. Brenneman DE, Spong CY, Hauser JM, Abebe D, Pinhasov A, et al. (2004) Protective peptides that are orally active and mechanistically nonchiral. JPET 309: 1190–1197.
23. Toso L, Cameroni I, Roberson R, Abebe D, Bissell S, et al. (2008) Prevention of developmental delays in a Down syndrome model. Obstet Gynecol 112: 1242–1251.
24. Endres M, Toso L, Roberson R, Park J, Abebe D, et al. (2005) Prevention of alcohol-induced developmental delays and learning abnormalities in a model of fetal alcohol syndrome. Am J Obstet Gynecol 193: 1028–1034.
25. Vink J, Auth J, Abebe D, Brenneman DE, Spong CY (2005) Novel peptides prevent alcohol-induced spatial learning deficits and proinflammatory cytokine release in a mouse model of fetal alcohol syndrome. Am J Obstet Gynecol 193: 825–829.
26. Incerti M, Toso L, Vink J, Roberson R, Nold C, et al. (2011) Prevention of Learning Deficit in a Down Syndrome Model. Obstet Gynecol 117: 354–361.
27. Busciglio J, Pelsman A, Helguera P, Ashur-Fabian O, Pinhasov A, et al. (2007) NAP and ADNF-9 protect normal and Down's syndrome cortical neurons from oxidative damage and apoptosis. Curr Pharm Des 13: 1091–1098.
28. Spong CY, Lee SJ, McCune SK, Gibney G, Abebe DT, et al. (1999) Maternal regulation of embryonic growth: the role of vasoactive intestinal peptide. Endocrinology 140: 917–924.
29. Morris RG, Garrud P, Rawlins JN, O'Keefe J (1982) Place navigation in rats with hippocampal lesions. Nature 297: 681–683.
30. Liu DP, Schmidt C, Billings T, Davisson MT (2003) Quantitative PCR genotyping assay for the Ts65Dn mouse model of Down syndrome. Biotechniques 35: 1170–1179.
31. Toso L, Endres M, Vink J, Abebe DT, Brenneman DE (2006) Learning enhancement with neuropeptides. Am J Obstet Gynecol 194: 1153–8.
32. Gozes I, Giladi E, Pinhasov A, Bardea A, Brenneman DE (2000) Activity-dependent neurotrophic factor: intranasal administration of femtomolar-acting peptides improve performance in a water maze. Pharmacol Exp Ther 293: 1091–1098.
33. Hill JM (2000) Vasoactive intestinal peptide in neurodevelopmental disorders: therapeutic potential. Curr Pharm Des 13: 1079–1089.
34. Vink J, Incerti M, Toso L, Roberson R, Abebe D, et al. (2009) Prenatal NAP_SAL prevents developmental delay in a mouse model of Down syndrome through effects on N-methyl-D-aspartic acid and gamma-aminobutyric acid receptors. Am J Obstet Gynecol 200: 524.e1–524.e4.
35. Fernandez F, Morishita W, Zuniga E, Nguyen J, Blank M, et al. (2007) Pharmacotherapy for cognitive impairment in a mouse model of Down syndrome. Nat Neurosci 10: 411–413.
36. Blondel O, Collin C, McCarran WJ, Zhu S, Zamostiano R, et al. (2000) A glia-derived signal regulating neuronal differentiation. J Neurosci 20: 8012–8020.
37. Kleschevnikov AM, Belichenko PV, Villar AJ, Epstein CJ, Malenka RC, et al (2004) Hippocampal long-term potentiation suppressed by increased inhibition in the Ts65Dn mouse, a genetic model of Down syndrome. J Neurosci 24: 8153–8160.
38. Zaltman R, Beni SM, Giladi E, Pinhasov A, Steingart RA, et al. (2003) Injections of the neuroprotective peptide NAP to newborn mice attenuate head-injury-related dysfunction in adults. Neropharm Toxicol 14: 481–484.
39. Spong CY, Abebe D, Gozes I, Brenneman DE (2001) Prevention of fetal demise and growth restriction in a mouse model of fetal alcohol syndrome. J Pharmacol Exp Ther 297: 774–779.
40. Chen SY, Charness MF, Wilkemeyer MF, Sulik KKP, Zouh F, et al. (2004) A neuroprotective peptide antagonizes fetal alcohol exposure-compromised brain growth. J Mol Neurosci 24: 189–199.
41. Poggi SH, Goodwin KM, Hill JM, Brenneman DE, Tendi E, et al. (2003) The role of activity-dependent neuroprotective protein in a mouse model of fetal alcohol syndrome. Am J Obstet Gynecol 189: 790–793.
42. Spong CY, Auth J, Vink J, Goodwin K, Abebe DT, et al. (2003) Vasoactive intestinal peptide mRNA and immunoreactivity are decreased in fetal alcohol syndrome model. Regul Pept 108: 143–147.

4

Maternal Methylenetetrahydrofolate Reductase C677T Polymorphism and Down Syndrome Risk

Vandana Rai[1]*, Upendra Yadav[1], Pradeep Kumar[1], Sushil Kumar Yadav[1], Om Prakesh Mishra[2]

1 Human Molecular Genetics Laboratory, Department of Biotechnology, VBS Purvanchal University, Jaunpur, India, **2** Department of Pediatrics, Institute of Medical Sciences, Banaras Hindu University, Varanasi, India

Abstract

Background: Methylenetetrahydrofolate reductase (*MTHFR*) is a key enzyme of folate metabolic pathway which catalyzes the irreversible conversion of 5, 10-methylenetetrahydrofolate to 5-methyltetrahydrofolate. 5-methyltetrahydrofolate donates methyl group for the methylation of homocysteine to methionine. Several studies have investigated maternal MTHFR C677T polymorphism as a risk factor for DS, but the results were controversial and inconclusive. To come into a conclusive estimate, authors performed a meta-analysis.

Aim: A meta-analysis of published case control studies was performed to investigate the association between maternal MTHFR C677T polymorphism and Down syndrome.

Methods: PubMed, Google Scholar, Elsevier, Springer Link databases were searched to select the eligible case control studies using appropriate keywords. The pooled odds ratio (OR) with 95%confidence interval were calculated for risk assessment.

Results: Thirty four studies with 3,098 DS case mothers and 4,852 control mothers were included in the present meta-analysis. The pooled OR was estimated under five genetic models and significant association was found between maternal *MTHFR* 677C>T polymorphism and Down syndrome under four genetic models except recessive model (for T vs. C, OR = 1.26, 95% CI = 1.09–1.46, p = 0.001; for TT vs. CC, OR = 1.49, 95% CI = 1.13–1.97, p = 0.008; for CT vs. CC, OR = 1.29, 95% CI = 1.10–1.51, p = 0.001; for TT+CT vs. CC, OR = 1.35, 95% CI = 1.13–1.60, p = 0.0008; for TT vs. CT+CC, OR = 0.76, 95% CI = 0.60–0.94, p = 0.01).

Conclusion: The results of the present meta-analysis support that maternal *MTHFR* C677T polymorphism is a risk factor for DS- affected pregnancy.

Editor: Balraj Mittal, Sanjay Gandhi Medical Institute, India

Funding: The authors have no support or funding to report.

Competing Interests: The authors have declared that no competing interests exist.

* Email: raivandana@rediffmail.com

Introduction

Down syndrome (DS) is the most common chromosomal disorder with the prevalence of 1/700–1000 live birth. It is characterized by the trisomy 21, which results from maternal meiotic nondisjunction in majority (90%) of cases. The established risk factor for DS is advanced (>35 years) maternal age at the time of conception. However, a fairly high number of DS children born to younger mothers suggest that risk factors other than advanced maternal age might be involved in predisposing younger mothers to DS-affected pregnancy [1,2]. The molecular and biochemical mechanism of maternal meiotic non-disjunction is still not known. James et al. [3] reported that methylenetetrahydrofolate reductase (*MTHFR*) C677T polymorphism might be a risk factor for maternal meiotic non-disjunction. Since then several studies have investigated the risk of DS to variants of folate pathway genes like *MTHFR*, Methionine synthase (*MTR*) and Methionine synthase reductase (*MTRR*) in Asian [1,2,4,5] and Caucasian [6–8] populations. Folate deficiency and dysfunctional MTHFR causes abnormal DNA methylation [9,10] and chromosomal segregation [11,12]. Hypomethylation of the centromeric DNA has been suggested as the causative mechanism of meiotic non-disjunction. Abnormal DNA methylation of centromere lead to aberrant kinetochore formation that results into abnormal segregation of chromosomes during meiosis [3,13].

MTHFR is a key enzyme in folate metabolism, which catalyzes the reduction of 5, 10-methylenetetrahydrofolate to the predominant circulating form of folate i.e. 5-methyltetrahydrofolate (5-THF). 5-THF donates methyl group for the conversion of homocysteine to methionine, which is further converted into S-adenosylmethionine (SAM). SAM is the main methyl group donor for all cellular methylation reactions. Folate deficiency and/or dysfunctional MTHFR reduces the conversion of 5, 10-methylene THF to 5-methyl THF, and elevates plasma homocysteine

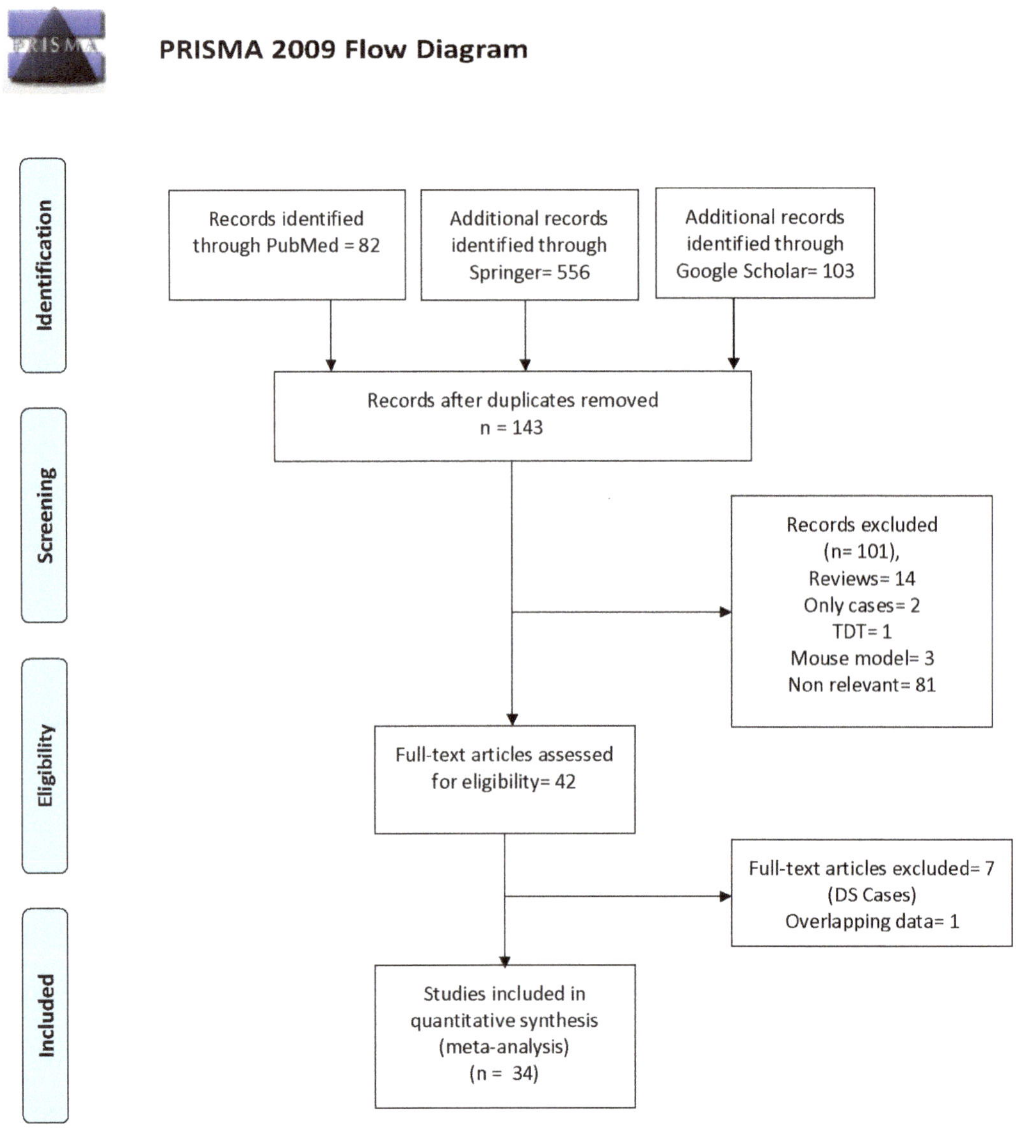

Figure 1. Flow Diagram of Study Searching and Selection Process.

concentration. Both folate and MTHFR are involved in many complex biochemical reactions like DNA synthesis, repair and methylation.

There are more than 40 polymorphisms reported in *MTHFR* gene and among them C677T variant is the most studied and clinically important. The C677T variant (rs 1801133; Ala 222 Val) has been associated with a decreased activity of MTHFR, and increased homocysteine level [14–16]. Mutant homozygous (TT) individuals have a decreased enzymatic activity ~ 70% and the heterozygote by 40%. A dysfunctional MTHFR leads to lower levels of SAM resulting into DNA hypomethylation. DNA hypomethylation increases the risk of many diseases and disorders like- neural tube defects [17], cleft lip and palate [18], Alzheimer disease [19], cardiovascular diseases [14], diabetes [20] and psychiatric disorders [21] etc. Several epidemiological studies have investigated the associations of the maternal *MTHFR* C677T polymorphism with Down syndrome. However, the results were conflicting and inconclusive. In light of the above facts, we conducted a meta-analysis of published case control studies relating the C677T polymorphism of the maternal *MTHFR* gene to the risk of having DS offspring.

Materials and Methods

Selection of studies

Electronic searches were conducted using PubMed, Google Scholar, Elsevier and Springer link and all published manuscripts up to January, 2014 were considered in present meta-analysis. The following index terms were used for search '*MTHFR*' 'Methylenetetrahydrofolate reductase', and 'C677T polymorphism', 'maternal risk' and 'Down syndrome'. In addition, bibliographies of all articles and reviews were hand searched for additional suitable studies.

Table 1. Characteristics of the eligible studies included in the meta-analysis.

Study	Year	Country	Case	Control	Quality Score	Reference
James et al.	1999	Canada	50	57	7	Am J Clin Nutr 70:495-50
Hobbs et al.	2000	America	157	140	7	Am J Hum Genet 67:623–630
Chadeaux-Vekemans et al.	2002	France	85	70	5	Pediatr Res 51:766–767
O'Leary et al.	2002	Ireland	41	192	5	Am J Med Genet A 107:151–155
Stuppia et al.	2002	Italy	64	112	7	Eur J Hum Genet 10:388–390
Boduroglu et al.	2004	Turkey	158	91	5	Am J Med Genet 127A: 5–10
Acacio et al.	2005	Brazil	70	88	8	Prenat Diagn 25:1196–1199
Da Silva et al.	2005	Brazil	154	158	7	Am J Med Genet Part A 135A: 263–267
Coppede et al.	2006	Italey	79	111	7	Am J Med Genet A 140(10): 1083–1091
Liang et al.	2006	China	30	70	7	China J Modern Medicine 20:011
Rai et al.	2006	India	149	165	6	J Hum Genet 51:278–283
Scala et al.	2006	Italy	94	256	8	Genet Med 8:409–416
Wang et al.	2007	China	100	100	8	Zhonghua Yi Xue Yi Chuan Xue Za Zhi 24:533–537
Biselli et al.	2008	Brazil	82	134	8	Genet Mol Res 7:33–42
Kohli et al.	2008	India	103	109	6	Downs Syndr Res Pract 12:133–137
Martinez-Frias et al.	2008	Spain	146	188	4	Am J Med Genet A 146A(11): 1477–1482
Meguid et al.	2008	Egypt	42	48	7	Dis Markers 24:19–26
Santos-Reboucas et al.	2008	Brazil	103	108	7	Dis Markers 25:149–157
Wang et al.	2008	China	64	70	8	J Zhejiang Univ Sci B 9(2): 93–99
Brandalize et al.	2009	Brazil	239	197	6	Am J Med Genet 149A (10): 2080–2087
Coppede et al.	2009	Italy	94	113	8	Neurosci Lett 449:15–19
Cyril et al.	2009	India	36	60	6	Indian J Hum Genet 15:60–64
Kokotas et al.	2009	Denmark	177	984	6	Dis Markers 27:279–285
Pozzi et al.	2009	Italy	74	184	8	Am J Obstet Gynecol 63: e1–e6
Coppede et al.	2010	Italy	29	32	5	BMC Med Genomics 3:42
Liao et al.	2010	China	60	68	7	Yi Chuan 32(5): 461–466
Vranekoviz et al.	2010	Croatia	111	141	7	Dis Markers 28:293–298
Bozovic et al.	2011	Croatia	112	221	7	Pediatr Int 53(4): 546–550
Sadiq et al.	2012	Jordan	53	29	6	Genet Test Mol Biomarker 15:1–7
Tayeb	2012	Saudi Arabia	30	40	5	Egyptian J Med Hum Genet 13(3): 263–268
Zampieri et al.	2012	Brazil	105	185	8	Dis Markers 32(2): 73–81
Kaur and Kaur	2013	India	110	111	6	Indian J Hum Genet 19(4): 412–414
Pandey et al.	2013	India	81	99	6	Int J Pharm Bio Sci; 4(2):(B)249–256
Elsayed et al.	2014	Egypt	26	61	9	The Egyptian J Med Hum Genet 15(1): 39–44

Table 2. Distributions of MTHFR C677T genotypes and allele frequencies in DS case mothers and control mothers reported in different included studies.

		CC		CT		TT		C		T	
Study	**Country**	**Case**	**Control**	**Case**	**Control**	**Case**	**Control**	**Case**	**Control**	**Case**	**Control**
James et al., 1999	Canada	24	15	22	34	4	8	70	64	30	50
Hobbs et al., 2000	America	51	67	84	59	22	14	186	193	128	87
Chadeaux-Vekemans et al., 2002	France	36	29	42	30	7	11	114	88	56	52
O'Leary et al., 2002	Ireland	18	90	21	84	2	18	57	264	25	120
Stuppia et al., 2002	Italy	20	27	32	62	12	23	72	116	56	108
Boduroglu et al., 2004	Turkey	86	58	55	30	17	3	227	146	89	36
Acacio et al., 2005	Brazil	35	54	30	25	5	9	100	133	40	43
Da Silva et al., 2005	Brazil	67	84	72	67	15	7	206	235	102	81
Coppede et al., 2006	Italey	20	39	43	54	16	18	83	132	75	90
Liang et al., 2006	China	7	16	20	34	3	20	34	66	26	74
Rai et al., 2006	India	97	124	40	39	12	2	234	287	64	43
Scala et al., 2006	Italy	31	74	39	125	24	57	101	273	87	239
Wang et al., 2007	China	28	48	52	42	20	10	108	138	92	62
Biselli et al., 2008	Brazil	29	100	35	77	8	17	93	229	71	39
Kohli et al., 2008	India	74	71	29	32	0	6	177	174	29	44
Martinez-Frias et al., 2008	Spain	61	76	61	85	24	27	183	237	109	139
Meguid et al., 2008	Egypt	20	33	17	12	5	3	57	78	27	18
Santos-Reboucas et al., 2008	Brazil	51	49	43	47	9	12	145	145	61	71
Wang et al., 2008	China	14	36	32	29	18	5	60	101	68	39
Brandalize et al., 2009	Brazil	94	86	113	93	32	18	301	265	177	129
Coppede et al., 2009	Italy	25	40	52	55	17	18	102	135	86	91
Cyril et al., 2009	India	33	60	3	0	0	0	69	120	3	0
Kokotas et al., 2009	Denmark	92	445	72	449	13	90	256	1339	98	629
Pozzi et al., 2009	Italy	28	62	30	93	16	29	86	217	62	151
Coppede et al., 2010	Italy	5	11	19	17	5	4	29	39	29	25
Liao et al., 2010	China	12	23	26	33	22	12	50	79	70	57
Vranekoviz et al., 2010	Croatia	49	66	49	64	13	11	147	196	75	86
Bozovic et al., 2011	Croatia	46	101	55	97	11	23	147	299	77	143
Sadiq et al., 2011	Jordan	23	23	27	5	3	1	73	51	33	7
Tayeb, 2012	Saudi Arabia	16	22	10	14	4	4	42	58	18	22
Zampieri et al., 2012	Brazil	40	94	55	73	10	18	135	261	75	109
Kaur & Kaur, 2013	India	86	89	22	22	2	0	194	200	26	22
Pandey et al., 2013	India	67	87	12	9	2	3	146	183	16	15
Elsayed et al., 2014	Egypt	11	30	12	24	3	7	34	84	18	38

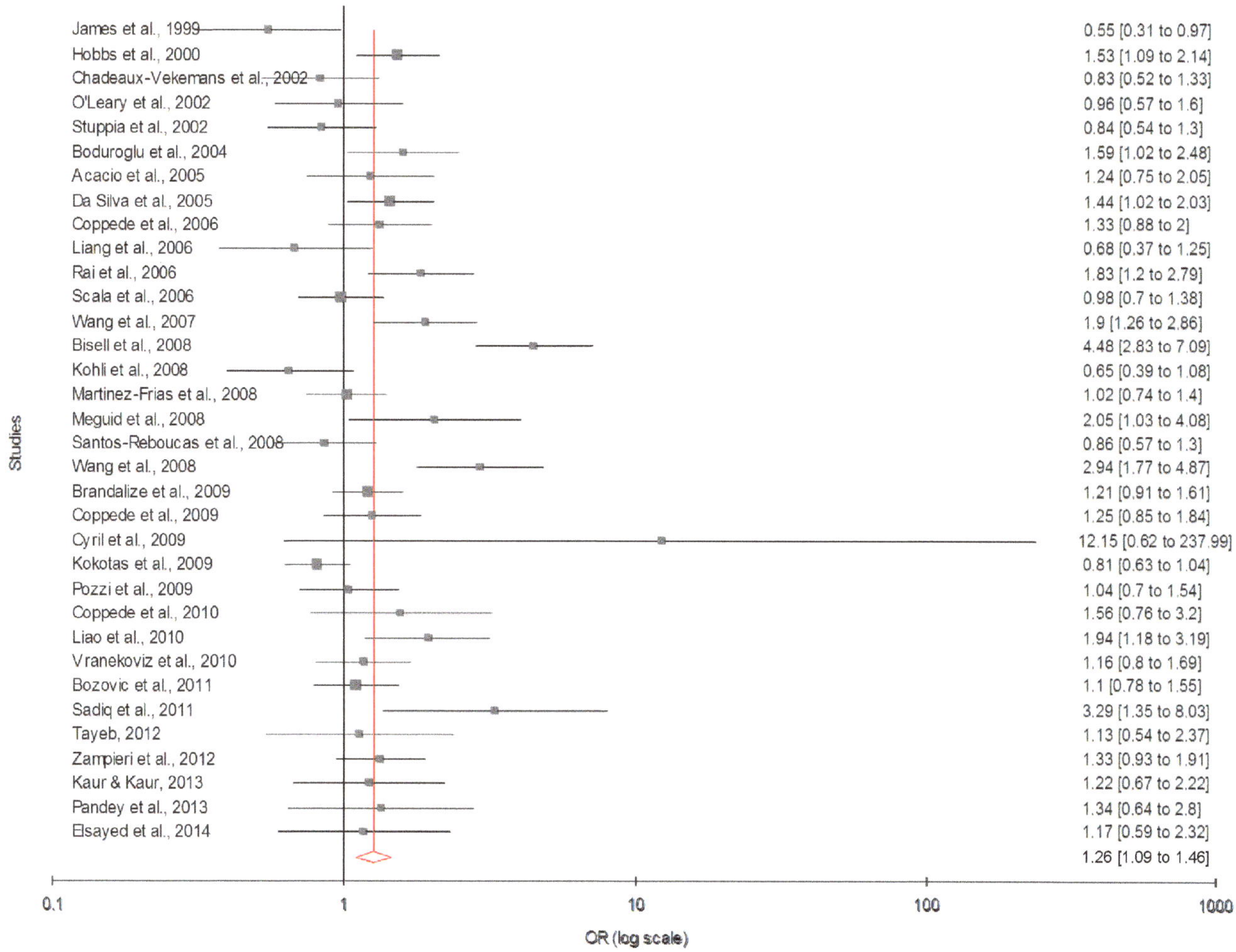

Figure 2. Forest plots (Random effect) showed significant association between MTHFR C677T polymorphism and risk of Down syndrome using allele contrast model (C versus T). Results of individual and summary OR estimates and 95% CI of each study were shown. Horizontal lines represented 95% CI, and dotted vertical lines represent the value of the summary OR.

Inclusion criteria

Included studies had to meet the following criteria: (1) article should be published; (2) article should have sufficient data to calculate the odds ratio with 95% CI; (3) article should be case control association study; and (4) author should describe the genotyping protocols.

Data extraction

The following data were extracted from each study: first author's name, publication year, journal name, country name, genotyping method, and different *MTHFR* genotype numbers.

Meta-analysis

Statistical analysis of maternal *MTHFR* C677T polymorphism and DS risk was estimated by Odds ratio (ORs) with 95% confidence intervals (CIs). The heterogeneity was tested by the Q-statistics with p-values <0.05. Subgroup analysis was done to know the source of heterogeneity. If higher heterogeneity ($I^2>$ 50%) would be observed, the random effect model [22] would be applied. Otherwise, fixed-effect model [23] was applied to obtain the summary OR and 95% CI. All p values were two-sided and a p value of less than 0.05 was considered statistically significant. All analyses were performed using the computer program MIX version 1.7 [24]. The control genotypes were tested for Hardy-Weinberg equilibrium (HWE) using the Goodness of fit Chi-square test. The quality of the included studies was measured according to the scoring system for randomized controlled association studies proposed by Clark and Baudouin [25]. Case control studies scoring <5 were defined as low quality study and those ≥5 were defined as high quality study.

Publication bias

Funnel plots of precision by log (OR) and standard error by log (OR) were plotted to determine publication bias and asymmetrical funnel plots represent publication bias. Begg and Mazumdar rank correlation [26] and Egger's regression intercept [27] tests were adopted to assess the publication bias.

Results

Eligible Studies

With our original search criterion, 85 articles were found. After reviewing each original article, 50 publications were excluded including reviews, case studies, editorials etc. (Figure 1). Following these exclusions, 34 individual case-control studies with a total of

Table 3. Summary estimates for the odds ratio (OR) of MTHFR C677T in various allele/genotype contrasts, the significance level (p value) of heterogeneity test (Q test), the I^2 metric and publication bias p-value (Egger Test) in total studies, Asian, American and European studies.

Genetic Contrast		Fixed effect OR (95% CI), p	Random effect OR (95% CI), p	Heterogeneity p-value (Q test)	I^2 (%)	Publication Bias (p of Egger's test)
All	Allele Contrast (T vs. C)	1.22 (1.13−1.31), <0.0001	1.26 (1.09−1.46), 0.001	<0.0001	69.42	0.14
	Co-dominant (CT vs. CC)	1.23 (1.11−1.36), <0.0001	1.29 (1.10−1.51), 0.001	0.0002	52.49	0.02
	Homozygote (TT vs. CC)	1.44 (1.22−1.69), <0.0001	1.49 (1.13−1.97), 0.008	<0.0001	57.3	0.56
	Dominant (TT+CT vs. CC)	1.28 (1.16−1.41), <0.0001	1.35 (1.13−1.60), 0.0008	<0.0001	63.56	0.05
	Recessive (CT+CC vs. TT)	0.76 (0.65−0.88), 0.0004	0.76 (0.60−0.94), 0.01	0.0044	43.68	0.926
Asian	Allele Contrast (T vs. C)	1.53 (1.29−1.82), <0.0001	1.52 (1.09−2.1), 0.01	0.0003	69.43	0.82
	Co-dominant (CT vs. CC)	1.52 (1.21−1.91), 0.0003	1.57 (1.14−2.14), 0.005	0.09	38.05	0.11
	Homozygote (TT vs. CC)	2.41 (1.62−3.59), <0.0001	2.21 (1.03−4.74), 0.0411	0.0074	60.04	0.204
	Dominant (TT+CT vs. CC)	1.64 (1.32−2.0), <0.0001	1.70 (1.18−2.4), 0.004	0.01	56.67	0.30
	Recessive (CT+CC vs. TT)	0.54 (0.37−0.78), <0.0001	0.58 (0.29−1.16), 0.12	0.0094	58.77	0.334
American	Allele Contrast (T vs. C)	1.23 (1.07−1.39), 0.003	1.19 (0.99−1.44), 0.06	0.06	47.69	0.11
	Co-dominant (CT vs. CC)	1.42 (1.17−1.71), 0.0002	1.42 (0.97−2.06), 0.066	0.0005	73.15	0.908
	Homozygote (TT vs. CC)	1.68 (1.24−2.28), 0.0008	1.58 (0.84−2.95), 0.148	0.0007	72.07	0.667
	Dominant (TT+CT vs. CC)	1.48 (1.24−1.76), <0.0001	1.44 (0.95−2.19), 0.078	<0.0001	80.11	0.782
	Recessive (CT+CC vs. TT)	0.69 (0.51−0.92), 0.0136	0.72 (0.44−1.18), 0.203	0.0159	59.42	0.753
European	Allele Contrast (T vs. C)	1.03 (0.93−1.15), 0.482	1.04 (0.93−1.16), 0.451	0.3576	8.81	0.084
	Co-dominant (CT vs. CC)	0.99 (0.85−1.16), 0.956	1.00 (0.85−1.17), 0.992	0.3774	6.87	0.050
	Homozygote (TT vs. CC)	1.09 (0.87−1.37), 0.422	1.09 (0.85−1.40), 0.455	0.3715	7.45	0.329
	Dominant (TT+CT vs. CC)	1.02 (0.88−1.17), 0.787	1.03 (0.87−1.21), 0.704	0.308	13.58	0.041
	Recessive (CT+CC vs. TT)	0.90 (0.73−1.10), 0.322	0.90 (0.72−1.11), 0.339	0.570	0	0.948

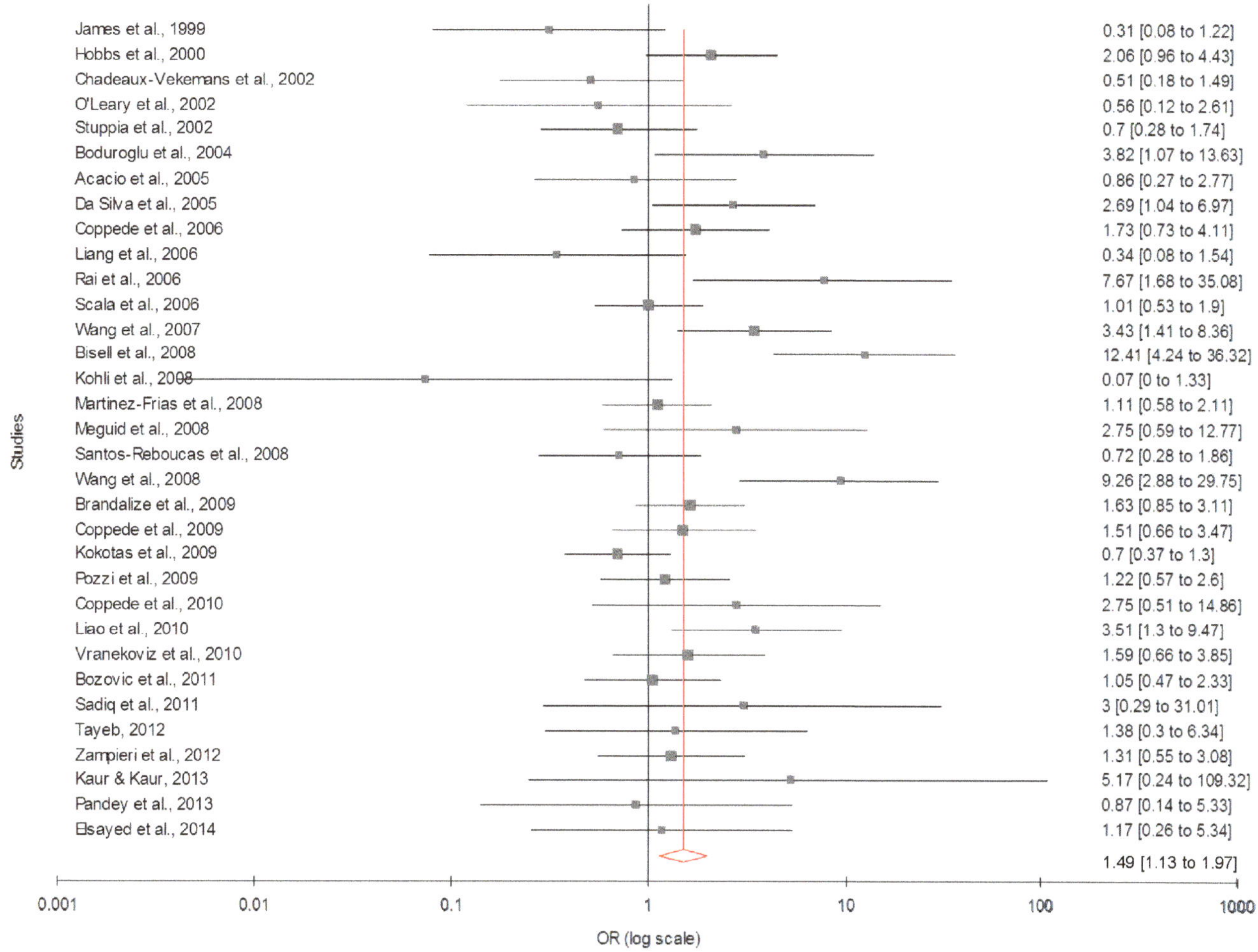

Figure 3. Forest plots (Random effect) showed significant association between MTHFR C677T polymorphism and risk of Down syndrome. Results of individual and summary OR estimates and 95% CI of each study were shown using homozygote model (TT versus CC).

3,098 cases and 4,852 controls were found to be suitable for inclusion into meta-analysis and listed in Table 1 (Figure 1).

These studies were published between 1999 and 2013. All these thirty four studies were performed in different countries- Brazil [28–33], China [4,34–36], Croatia [8,37], Egypt [38,39], France [40], India [1,5,41–43], Ireland [44], Italy [7,13,45–48], Jordan [49], Netherlands [50], Saudi Arabia [2], Spain [51], Turkey [52] and USA [3,6] (Table 1).

Characteristics of included studies

In thirty four studies included in the present meta-analysis, the smallest case sample size was 26 [39] and highest sample size was 239 [32]. ORs for more than one were reported in twenty four articles [1,2,4–6,8,13,28–30,32,33,35–39,42,43,46–49,51,52]. Except two studies [28,43], control populations of all articles were in Hardy-Weinberg equilibrium.

In all thirty four studies, total cases were 3,098 with CC (1,396), CT (1,326) and TT (376), and controls were 4,852 with CC (2,329), CT (2,015), and TT (508) genotypes. In controls genotypes, percentage of CC, CT and TT were 48.00%, 41.53%, and 10.47% respectively. In total cases, genotype percentage of CC, CT, and TT was 45.06%, 42.8% and 12.14% respectively. Frequencies of CC and CT genotypes were highest in both cases and controls (Table 2). In cases and controls, the allele C was the most common. All five genetic models; -allele contrast (T vs C) homozygote (TT vs CC), codominant (CT vs CC), dominant (TT+CT vs CC) and recessive (TT vs CT+CC) models were used to evaluate C677T polymorphism as DS risk.

Meta-analysis

Meta-analysis with allele contrast showed significant association between maternal 677T allele and DS with both fixed effect ($OR_{TvsC} = 1.22$; 95% CI = 1.13–1.31; $p = <0.0001$) and random effect models ($OR_{TvsC} = 1.26$; 95% CI = 1.09–1.45; $p = 0.001$) (Figure 2) (Table 3). In cumulative meta-analysis using random effect model, the association of maternal T allele with DS turned statistically significant with the addition of study of Wang et al. (2008) and remained significant thereafter.

Table 3 summarizes the ORs with corresponding 95% CIs for association between maternal C677T polymorphism and risk of DS in dominant, recessive, homozygote and co-dominant models. With our primary analysis, there was an increased risk of DS among mutant homozygote variants (TT), with both fixed ($OR_{TTvs.CC} = 1.44$; 95% CI = 1.22−1.69, $p = <0.0001$) and ran-

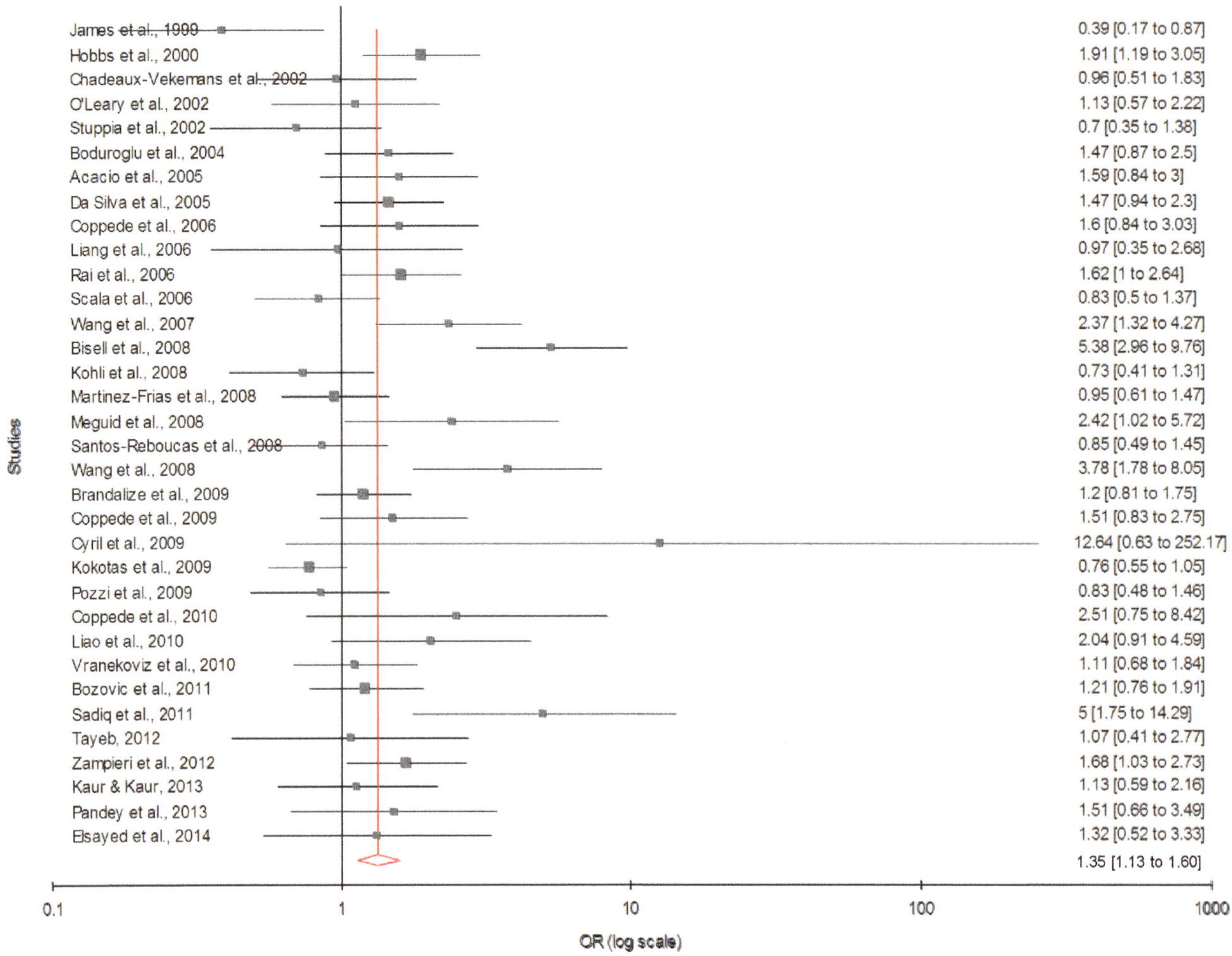

Figure 4. Forest plots (Random effect) showed significant association between MTHFR C677T polymorphism and risk of Down syndrome using dominant model (TT+CT versus CC). Results of individual and summary OR estimates and 95% CI of each study were shown.

dom ($OR_{TTvs.CC} = 1.49$; 95% CI = 1.13 − 1.97, p = 0.008) effect models with moderate statistical heterogeneity between-study (Figure 3). Association of mutant heterozygous genotype (CT vs. CC) was observed significant with fixed ($OR_{CTvs.CC} = 1.23$; 95% CI = 1.11 − 1.36; p = <0.0001) and random ($OR_{CTvs.CC} = 1.29$; 95% CI = 1.10 − 1.51; p = 0.001) effect models. Similarly combined mutant genotypes (TT+CT vs. CC) showed significant association with DS using both fixed ($OR_{TT+CTvs.CC} = 1.28$; 95% CI = 1.16 − 1.41; p = <0.0001) and random ($OR_{TT+CTvs.CC} = 1.35$; 95% CI = 1.13 − 1.60; p = 0.0008) effect models (Figure 4).

Stratified analysis

We also performed sub-group analysis which is based on geographic distribution of population. Out of 34 studies included in present meta-analysis, 11 studies were from Asia, 13 from Europe, 8 from America and 2 from Africa. The subgroup analysis by geographical regions revealed that the significant association between the maternal *MTHFR* C677T polymorphism and DS existed in Asian population (for T vs. C: OR = 1.51; 95% CI = 1.09 − 2.10; p = 0.01; $I^2 = 69.43\%$; $P_{heterogeneity} = 0.0003$; $P_{Pb} = 0.82$) (Figure 5; Table 3). Except allele contrast model of American population (T vs. C: OR = 1.23; 95% CI = 1.07 − 1.39; p = 0.003; $I^2 = 47.69\%$; $P_{heterogeneity} = 0.06$; $P_{Pb} = 0.11$) (Figure 6) no significant association was found in American and European population (for T vs. C: OR = 1.03; 95% CI = 0.93 − 1.15; p = 0.482; $I^2 = 8.81\%$; $P_{heterogeneity} = 0.357$; $P_{Pb} = 0.084$) (Figures 7; Table 3).

Heterogeneity and Sensitive analysis

A true heterogeneity existed between studies for allele ($P_{heterogeneity} = <0.0001$, Q = 107.92, df = 33, $I^2 = 69.42\%$, $t^2 = 0.12$) and mutant genotypes ($P_{heterogeneity} = <0.0001$, Q = 74.90, df = 32, $I^2 = 57.3\%$, $t^2 = 0.10$) comparisons. The 'I^2' value of more than 50% for between studies comparison in both allele and genotype analysis shows high level of true heterogeneity. In Asian ($P_{heterogeneity} = 0.0003$, $I^2 = 67.43\%$) and American ($P_{heterogeneity} = <0.0001$, $I^2 = 83.25\%$) allele contrast meta-analysis significant high heterogeneity was observed, in European sub-group meta-analysis low heterogeneity was observed ($P_{heterogeneity} = 0.357$, $I^2 = 8.81$) in allele contrast model.

In allele contrast meta-analysis, sensitivity analysis performed by exclusion of the studies in which control population was not in Hardy Weinberg equilibrium, studies with small sample size and studies with high p values. Control population of only two studies

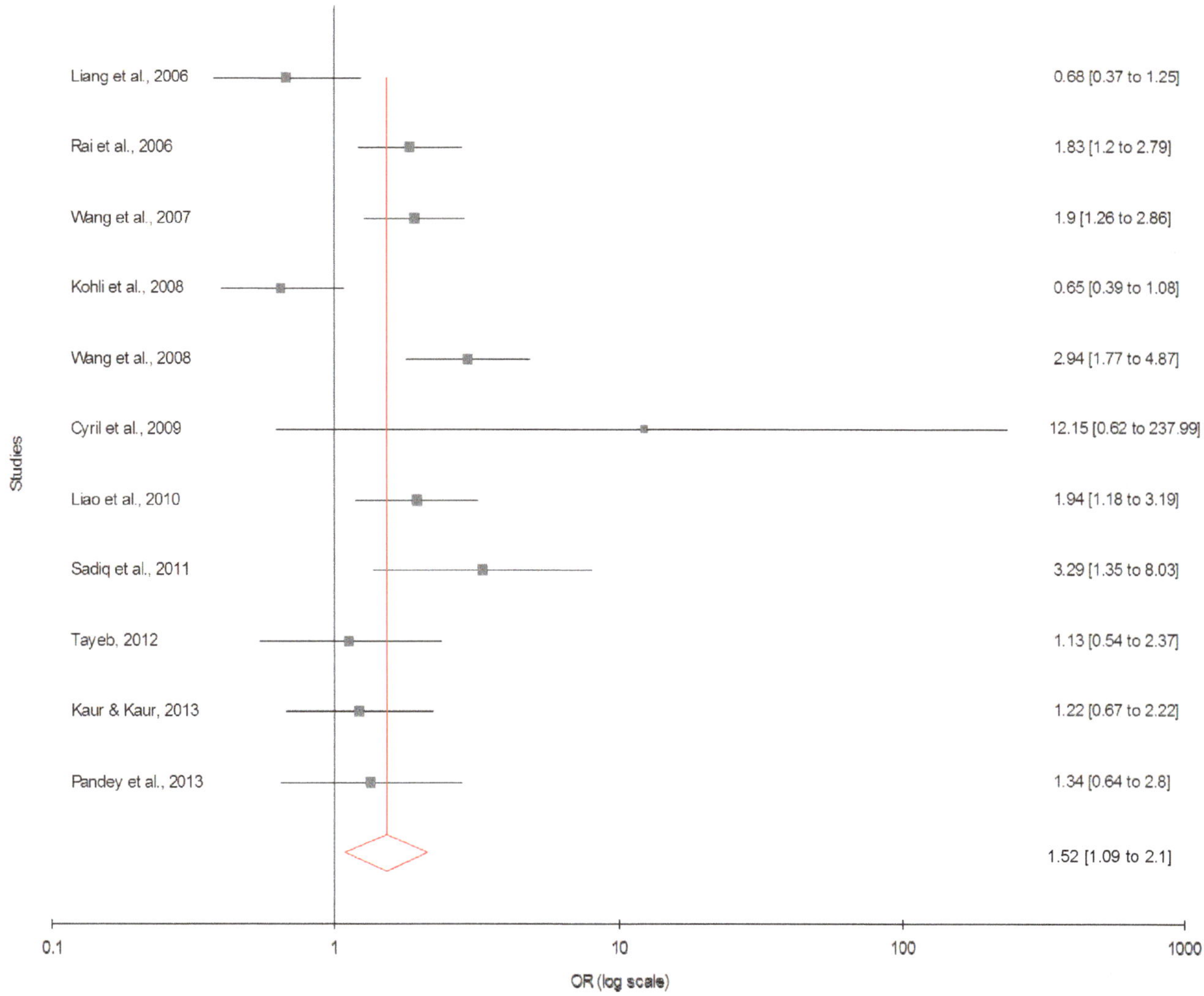

Figure 5. Forest plots (Random effect) showed significant association between MTHFR C677T polymorphism and risk of Down syndrome in Asian studies using allele contrast model (T versus C). Results of individual and summary OR estimates and 95% CI of each study were shown.

[28,43] were not in HW equilibrium and heterogeneity did not decreased after exclusion of these studies ($p = <0.0001$, $I^2 = 70.00\%$). Exclusion of seven studies with small sample size, less than 50 (O'Leary et al. [44], n = 41; Liang et al. [34], n = 30; Mequid et al [38], n = 42; Cyril et al. [42], n = 36; Coppede et al. [48], n = 29; Tayeb [2], n = 30; Elsayed et al. [39], n = 26), also did not decreased heterogeneity ($P_{heterogeneity} = <0.0001$, $I^2 = 72.98\%$). Similarly exclusion of eleven studies with very high p value (O'Leary et al. [44], p = 0.87; Acacio et al. [28], p = 0.40; Scala et al. [7], p = 0.91; Martinez-Frias et al. [51], p = 0.90; Pozzi et al. [13], p = 0.84;Vranekoviz et al. [37], p = 0.43; Bozovic et al. [8], p = 0.58; Tayeb [2], p = 0.74; Elsayed et al. [39], p = 0.65; Kaur and Kaur [5], p = 0.52; Pandey et al. [43], p = 0.44) did not decrease heterogeneity but increased odds ratio (OR = 1.29, 95% CI = 1.18−1.41, $p = <0.0001$).

Publication bias

Publication bias was not observed in allele contrast, homozygote, dominant and recessive models (Begg's p = 0.28, Egger's p = 0.14 for T vs. C; Begg's p = 0.38, Egger's p = 0.56 for TT vs. CC; Begg's p = 0.13, Egger's p = 0.05 for TT+CT vs. CC and Begg's p = 0.19, Egger's p = 0.0.05 for TT vs. CC+CT) but publication bias was observed in co-dominant model (Begg's p = 0.04, Egger's p = 0.02 for CT vs. CC) of overall by using Begg's and Egger's test (Table 3). Funnel plots were showed in Figures 8 and 9.

Discussion

In 1999, James et al [3] reported that genetic polymorphism of folate and homocysteine pathway enzymes predispose a woman to abnormal chromosome segregation, which act as risk factor for DS pregnancy. In subsequent years, several in vivo studies in humans suggested that chronic folate deficiency has been associated with abnormal DNA methylation [11,53,54], and aberrant chromosome segregation [6,55−59]. Population-based studies have shown that folic acid intake during fetal development has a protective effect, resulting in a significant reduction in the

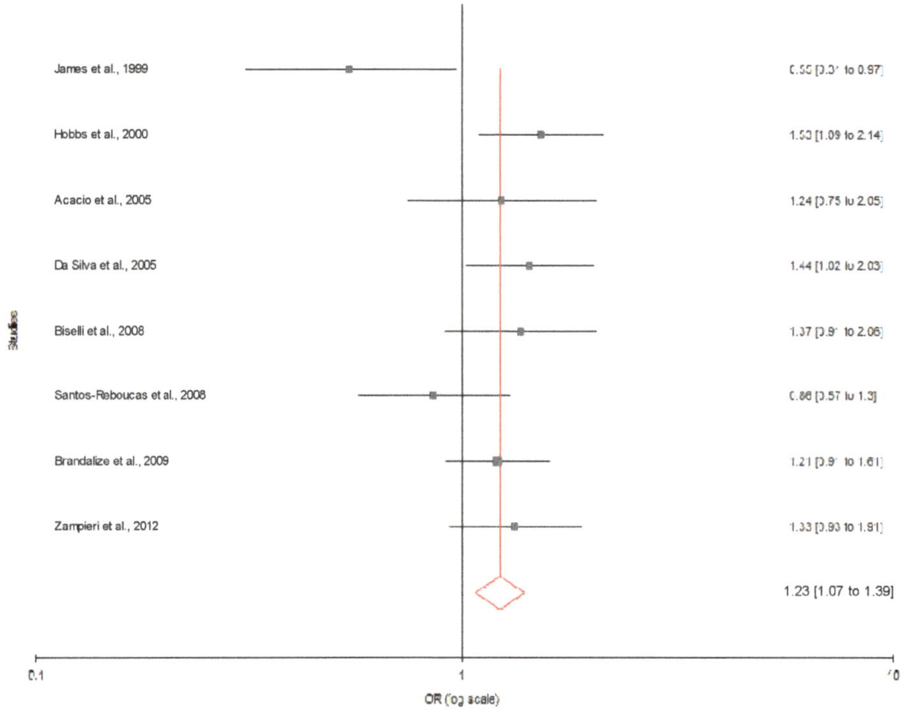

Figure 6. Forest plots (Random effect) showed no association between MTHFR C677T polymorphism and risk of Down syndrome in American studies using allele contrast model (T versus C). Results of individual and summary OR estimates and 95% CI of each study were shown.

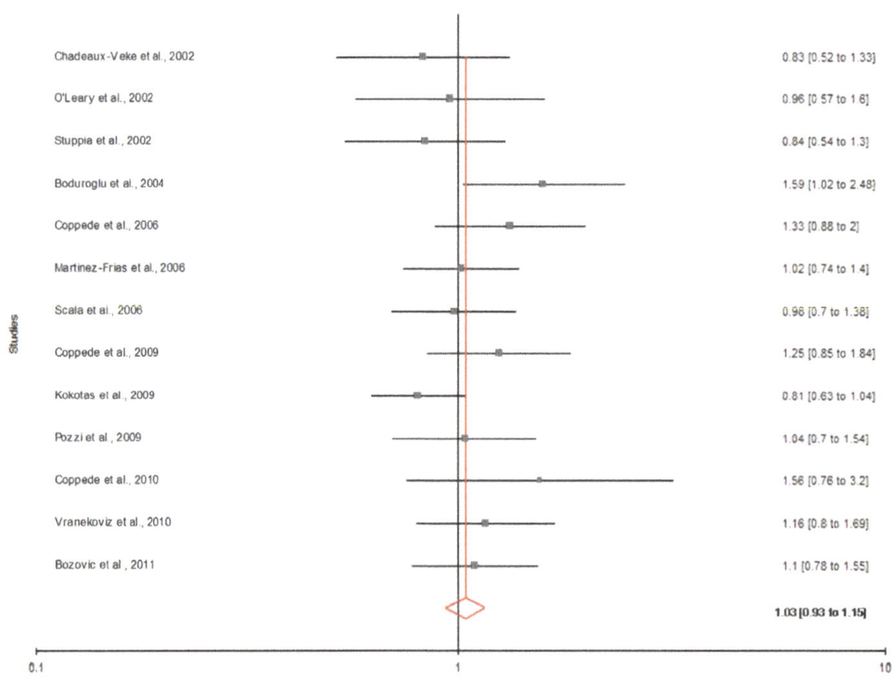

Figure 7. Forest plots (Fixed effect) showed no association between MTHFR C677T polymorphism and risk of Down syndrome in European studies using allele contrast model (T versus C). Results of individual and summary OR estimates and 95% CI of each study were shown. Horizontal lines represented 95% CI, and dotted vertical lines represent the value of the summary OR.

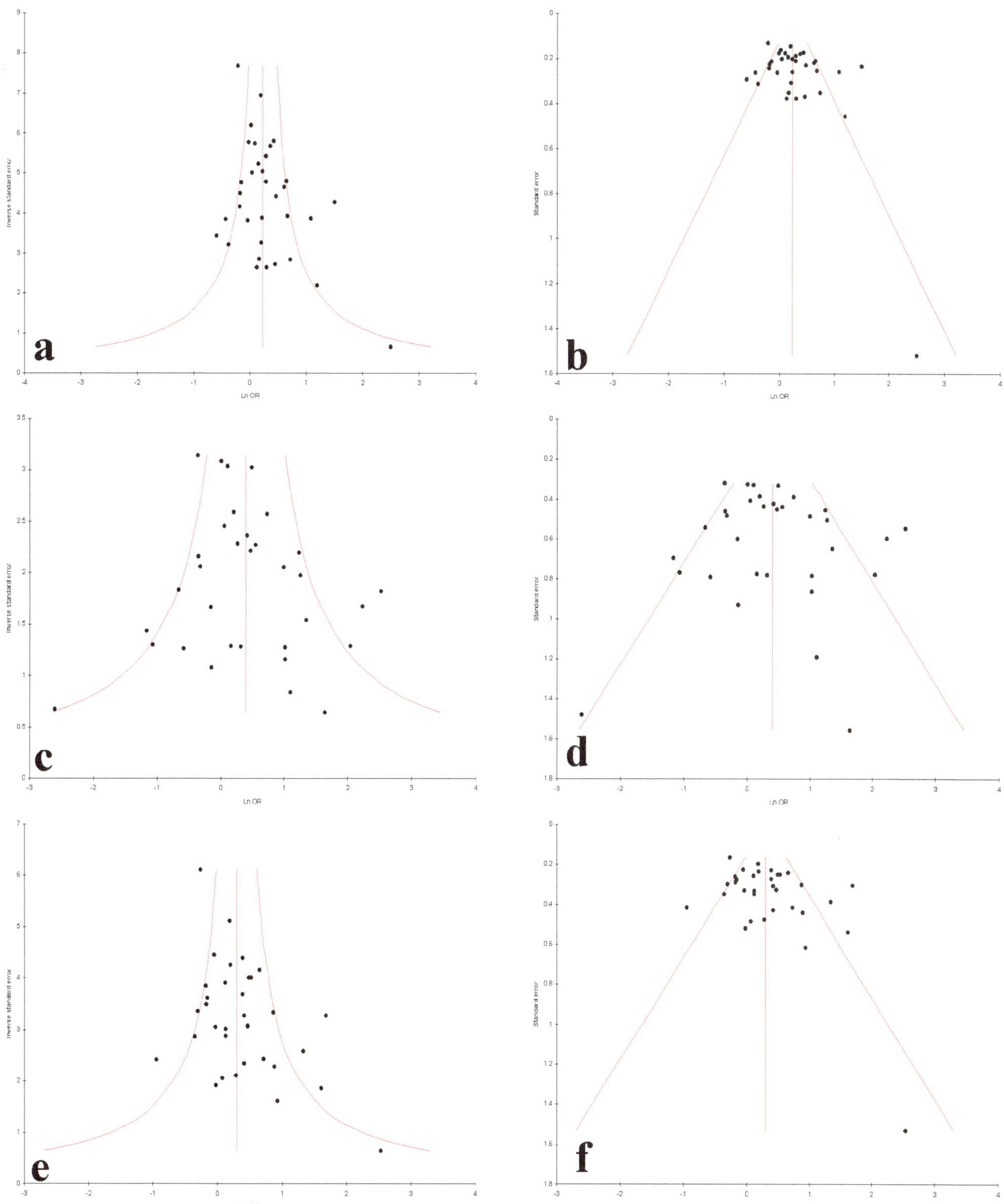

Figure 8. Funnel plots a–f. a. Precision by log odds ratio for additive model; **b.** standard error by log odds ratio for additive model; **c.** precision by log odds ratio for co-dominant model; **d.** standard error by log odds ratio for co-dominant model; **e.** precision by log odds ratio for dominant model; **f.** standard error by log odds ratio for Dominant model.

occurrence of developmental defects, like neural tube defects (NTD), congenital heart defects, limb defects, and orofacial clefts [60].

Meta-analysis is a powerful tool for analyzing cumulative data with small and low power studies. Several meta-analyses were published accessing *MTHFR* as risk factor to various diseases/

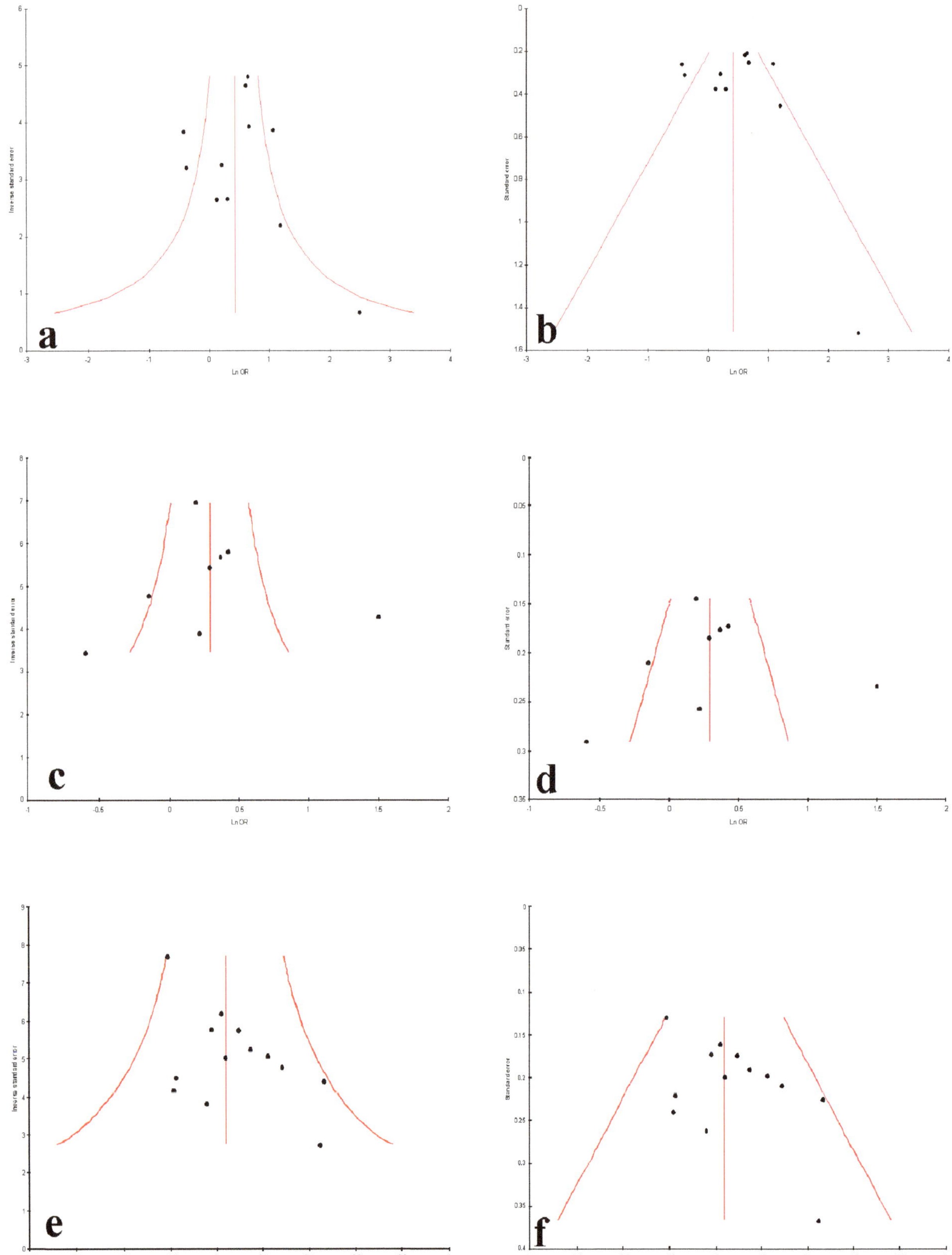

Figure 9. Funnel plots a–f. a. Precision by log odds ratio for additive model; **b.** standard error by log odds ratio for additive model for Asian studies; **c.** precision by log odds ratio for additive model; **d.** standard error by log odds ratio for additive model for American studies; **e.** precision by log odds ratio for additive model; **f.** standard error by log odds ratio for additive model for European studies.

Table 4. A comparative analysis of details of Odds Ratio, 95% CI, genetic models reported in total 5 (including present) meta-analysis published so far analyzing case-control studies of *MTHFR* C677T polymorphism and Down syndrome.

Study	Number of Studies	Cases	Controls	I^2 (%)	Heterogeneity p-value (Q test)	OR (95% CI), p-value	Model	Subgroup analysis
Zintaras, 2007	11	1129	1489	49	0.03	1.20 (1.06–1.35)	Allelic contrast	Not reported
Medica et al., 2009	16	1545	2052	–	–	1.40 (1.16–1.70), 0.0006	Dominant model	Not reported
Yang et al., 2013	26	2458	3144	58.2	<0.01	1.28 (1.11–1.47)	Allelic contrast	Reported
Wu et al., 2013	28	2806	4597	48.0	0.0	1.224 (1.085–1.38), 0.001	Dominant model	Reported
Present Study, 2014	34	3048	4852	69.42	<0.0001	1.26 (1.09–1.46), 0.001	Allelic contrast	Reported

disorders like- neural tube defects [61,62], cleft lip and palate [63], stroke [64], psychiatric disorders [65]. During literature search, we identified four meta-analyses [66–69] published between 2007 and 2013. They examined the effect of maternal *MTHFR* C677T as DS risk, but no consistent conclusion was achieved. Zintzaras [66] performed a meta-analysis based on eleven studies and did not find any significant association between the maternal *MTHFR* polymorphisms and DS risk. Medica et al. [67] aggregated sixteen studies and reported significant relationship between the maternal mutant genotypes (TT+CT vs CC) and risk of DS child. Recently, Wu et al. [68] published a meta-analysis (included twenty eight studies with 2806 cases/4597 controls), and found statistical association with dominant model ($OR = 1.305$, 95% $CI = 1.125$–1.514, $p = 0$, $p = 0.003$). Yang et al. [69] performed a meta-analysis which was based on twenty six studies (2458 cases/3144 controls) and found statistically significant association in allele contrast model ($OR = 1.28$; 95% CI: 1.11–1.47) (Table 4). Several newly published studies were not included in the previous published meta-analyses. So authors conducted a comprehensive meta-analysis with the largest number of studies (34 studies). In the present meta-analysis significant association was found between maternal C677T polymorphism and DS risk in total 34 studies using all five genetic models. Whereas in stratified analysis, except allele contrast model in American population, no significant association was observed in European and American population but significant higher risk was found in Asian population. Such phenomenon probably could be ascribed to the folate metabolism profile and dietary structure of different regions.

There are few limitations of the present meta-analysis like- i) we used crude ORs in the pooled analysis without adjustment; ii) the relatively small sample size in some of the included studies, especially those from Asia; iii) we considered only one gene polymorphism (*MTHFR* C677T) of folate pathway. Present meta-analysis had several advantages/strength to the previous published meta-analyses like- (i) the publication bias was not detected in present meta-analysis, (ii) pooled number of cases and controls from different studies significantly increased the statistical power of the analysis, (iii) largest number of studies (34 studies) with largest sample size (3,098 cases and 4,852 controls) was included in the present meta-analysis, (iv) controls included in the present meta-analysis was mothers of healthy child, (v) distribution of genotypes in control mothers except two studies was in Hardy-Weinberg equilibrium, (vi) significant association was found between maternal *MTHFR* C677T polymorphism and DS risk in allelic contrast, homozygote, co-dominant and dominant genetic models and (vii) in addition we did sub-group analysis according to geographical regions.

In conclusion, results of present meta-analysis suggest that the maternal *MTHFR* 677T allele is a risk factor for development of DS pregnancy. However the results of present meta-analysis were based on single gene polymorphism and significant heterogeneity was also observed; hence results should be interpreted with caution.

Supporting Information

Checklist S1 PRISMA checklist.

Author Contributions

Conceived and designed the experiments: VR PK OPM. Performed the experiments: UY SKY. Analyzed the data: VR UY. Contributed reagents/materials/analysis tools: VR UY. Wrote the paper: VR.

References

1. Rai AK, Singh S, Mehta S, Kumar A, Pandey LK, et al. (2006) MTHFR C677T and A1298C polymorphisms are risk factors for Down's syndrome in Indian mothers. J Hum Genet 51: 278–283.
2. Tayeb MT (2012) The methylenetetrahydrofolate reductase gene variant (C677T) in risk mothers with Down syndrome among Saudi population. Egyptian J Med Hum Genet 13(3): 263–268.
3. James SJ, Pogribna M, Pogribny IP, Melnyk S, Hine RJ, et al. (1999) Abnormal folate metabolism and mutation in the methylenetetrahydrofolate reductase gene may be maternal risk factors for Down syndrome. Am J Clin Nutr 70: 495–50.
4. Wang SS, Qiao F, Feng L, Juan-Juan LV (2008) Polymorphisms in genes involved in folate metabolism as maternal risk factors for Down syndrome in China. J Zhejiang Univ Sci B 9(2): 93–99.
5. Kaur A, Kaur A (2013) Prevalence of methylenetetrahydrofolate reductase 677 C-T polymorphism among mothers of Down syndrome children. Indian J Hum Genet 19(4): 412–414.
6. Hobbs CA, Sherman SI, Yi P, Torfs CP, Hine RJ, et al. (2000) Polymorphism in genes involved in folate metabolism as maternal risk factors for Down syndrome. Am J Hum Genet 67: 623–630.
7. Scala I, Granese B, Sellitto M, Salome S, Sammartino A, et al. (2006) Analysis of seven maternal polymorphisms of genes involved in homocysteine/folate metabolism and risk of Down syndrome offspring. Genet Med 8: 409–416.
8. Božović IB, Vraneković J, Cizmarević NS, Mahulja-Stamenković V, Prpić I, et al. (2011) MTHFR C677T and A1298C polymorphisms as a risk factor for congenital heart defects in Down syndrome. Pediatr Int 53(4): 546–550.
9. James SJ, Melnyk S, Pogribna M, Pogribny IP, Caudill MA (2002) Elevation in S-adenosylhomocysteine and DNA hypomethylation: potential epigenetic mechanism for homocysteine-related pathology. J Nutr 132(8 Suppl): 2361S–2366S.
10. Pogribny IP, James SJ, Jernigan S, Pogribna M (2004) Genomic hypomethylation is specific for preneoplastic liver in folate/methyl deficient rats and does not occur in non-target tissues. Mutat Res. 548(1–2): 53–59.
11. Pogribna M, Melnyk S, Pogribny I, Chango A, Yi P, et al. (2001) Homocysteine metabolism in children with Down syndrome: in vitro modulation. Am J Hum Genet 69: 88–95.
12. Parry EM, Parry JM, Corso C, Doherty A, Haddad F, et al. (2002) Detection and characterization of mechanisms of action of aneugenic chemicals. Mutagenesis. 17(6): 509–521.
13. Pozzi E, Vergani P, Dalpra' L, Combi R, Silvestri D, et al. (2009) Maternal polymorphisms for methyltetrahydrofolate reductase and methionine synthetase reductase and risk of children with Down syndrome. Am J Obstet Gynecol 63: e1–e6.
14. Frosst P, Blom HJ, Milos R, Goyette P, Sheppard CA, et al. (1995) A candidate genetic risk factor for vascular disease: a common mutation in methylenetetrahydrofolate reductase. Nat Genet 10: 111–113.
15. Bagley PJ, Selhub J (1998) A common mutation in the methylenetetrahydrofolate reductase gene is associated with an accumulation of formylated tetrahydrofolates in red blood cells. Proc Natl Acad Sci USA 95(22): 13217–13220.
16. Brattström L, Wilcken DE, Ohrvik J, Brudin L (1998) Common methylenetetrahydrofolate reductase gene mutation leads to hyperhomocysteinemia but not to vascular disease: the result of a meta-analysis. Circulation 98(23): 2520–2526.
17. van der Put NM, Eskes TK, Blom HJ (1997) Is the common 677CT mutation in the methylenetetrahydrofolate reductase gene a risk factor for neural tube defects? A meta-analysis. QJ Med 90: 111–115.
18. Blanton SH, Henry RR, Yuan Q, Mulliken JB, Stal S, et al. (2011) Folate pathway and nonsyndromic cleft lip and palate. Birth Defects Res A Clin Mol Teratol 91: 50–60.
19. Hua Y, Zhao H, Kong Y, Ye M (2011) Association between the MTHFR gene and Alzheimer's disease: a meta-analysis. Int J Neurosci 121(8): 462–71.
20. Benes P, Kankova K, Muzik J, Groch L, Benedik J et al. (2001) Methylenetetrahydrofolate reductase polymorphism, typeII diabetes mellitus, coronary artery disease, and essential hypertension in the Czech population. Mol Genet Metab 73: 188–195.
21. Jönsson EG, Larsson K, Vares M, Hansen T, Wang AG, et al. (2008) Two methylenetetrahydrofolate reductase gene (MTHFR) polymorphisms, schizophrenia and bipolar disorder: an association study. Am J Med Genet B Neuropsychiatr Genet 147B: 976–982.
22. DerSimonian R, Laird N (1986) Meta-analysis in clinical trials. Controlled Clinical Trials. 7: 177–188.
23. Mantel N, Haenszel W (1959) Statistical aspects of the analysis of data from retrospective studies of disease. J Natl Cancer Inst 22: 719–748.
24. Bax L, Yu LM, Ikeda N, Tsuruta H, Moons KG (2006) Development and validation of MIX: comprehensive free software for meta-analysis of causal research data. BMC Med Res Methodol. 2006;6: 50.
25. Clark MF, Baudouin SV (2006) A systematic review of the quality of genetic association studies in human sepsis. Intensive Care Med 32(11): 1706–1712.
26. Begg CB, Mazumdar M (1994) Operating characteristics of a rank correlation test for publication bias. Biometrics 50(4): 1088–1101.
27. Egger M, Davey Smith G, Schneider M, Minder C (1997) Bias in meta-analysis detected by a simple, graphical test. BMJ 315: 629–634.
28. Acácio GL, Barini R, Bertuzzo CS, Couto EC, Annichino-Bizzacchi JM, et al. (2005) Methylenetetrahydrofolate reductase gene polymorphisms and their association with trisomy 21. Prenat Diagn 25: 1196–1199.
29. da Silva LRJ, Vergani N, Galdieri LC, Porto MPR, Longhitano SB, et al. (2005) Relationship between polymorphisms in genes involved in homocysteine metabolism and maternal risk for Down syndrome in Brazil. Am J Med Genet Part A 135A: 263–267.
30. Biselli JM, Goloni-Bertollo EM, Zampieri BL, Haddad R, Eberlin MN, et al. (2008) Genetic polymorphisms involved in folate metabolism and elevated plasma concentrations of homocysteine: maternal risk factors for Down syndrome in Brazil. Genet Mol Res 7: 33–42.
31. Santos-Reboucas CB, Corre^a JC, Bonomo A, Fintelman-Rodrigues N, Moura KC, et al. (2008) The impact of folate pathway polymorphisms combined to nutritional deficiency as a maternal predisposition factor for Down syndrome. Dis Markers 25: 149–157.
32. Brandalize AP, Bandinelli E, dos Santos PA, Roisenberg I, Schüler-Faccini L (2009) Evaluation of C677T and A1298C polymorphisms of the MTHFR gene as maternal risk factors for Down syndrome and Congenital heart defects. Am J Med Genet 149A (10): 2080–2087.
33. Zampieri BL, Biselli JM, Goloni-Bertollo EM, Vannucchi H, Carvalho VM, et al. (2012) Maternal risk for Down syndrome is modulated by genes involved in folate metabolism. Dis Markers 32(2): 73–81.
34. Liang X, Feng Z, Lan-Fang Z, Guo XX, Xiao GF, et al. (2005) Analysis of Down syndrome screening and antenatal diagnosis of 3195 cases in the middle period of pregnancy. China J Modern Medicine 20: 011.
35. Wang W, Xie W, Wang X (2007) The relationship between polymorphism of gene involved in folate metabolism, homocysteine level and risk of Down syndrome. Zhonghua Yi Xue Yi Chuan Xue Za Zhi 24: 533–537.
36. Liao YP, Bao MS, Liu CQ, Liu H, Zhang D (2010) Folate gene polymorphism and the risk of Down syndrome pregnancies in young Chinese women. Yi Chuan 32(5): 461–466.
37. Vranekovic' J, Babic' Bozovic' I, Starcevic' Cizmarevic' N, Buretic'- Tomljanovic' A, Ristic' S, et al. (2010) Functional inference of methylenetetrahydrofolate reductase gene polymorphisms on enzyme stability as a potential risk factor for Down syndrome in Croatia. Dis Markers 28: 293–298.
38. Meguid NA, Dardir AA, Khass M, Hossieny LE, Ezzat A, et al. (2008) MTHFR genetic polymorphism as a risk factor in Egyptian mothers with Down syndrome children. Dis Markers 24: 19–26.
39. Elsayed GM, Elsayed SM, Ezz-Elarab SS (2013) Maternal MTHFR C677T genotype and septal defects in offspring with Down syndrome: A pilot study. The Egyptian J Med Hum Genet 15(1): 39–44.
40. Chadefaux-Vekemans B, Coude M, Muller F, Oury JF, Chabli A, et al. (2002) Methylenetetrahydrofolate reductase polymorphism in the etiology of Down syndrome. Pediatr Res 51: 766–767.
41. Kohli U, Arora S, Kabra M, Ramakrishnan L, Gulati S, et al. (2008) Prevalence of MTHFR 677C>T polymorphism in north Indian mothers having babies with Trisomy 21 Down syndrome. Downs Syndr Res Pract 12: 133–137.
42. Cyril C, Rai P, Chandra N, Gopinath PM, Satyamoorthy K (2009) MTHFR gene variants C677T A1298C and association with Down syndrome: a case–control study from South India. Indian J Hum Genet 15: 60–64.
43. Pandey SK, Mohanty PK, Polipalli SK, Kapoor S (2013) Genetic polymorphisms of MTHFR (677T and 1298C) and homocysteine metabolism as maternal risk factor for Down's syndrome patients in north indian population. Int J Pharm Bio Sci; 4(2):(B)249–256.
44. O'Leary VB, Parle-McDermott A, Molloy AM, Kirke PN, Johnson Z, et al. (2002) MTRR and MTHFR polymorphism: link to Down syndrome? Am J Med Genet A 107: 151–155.
45. Stuppia L, Gatta V, Gaspari AR, Antonucci I, Morizio E, et al. (2002) C677T mutation in the 5,10-MTHFR gene and risk of Down syndrome in Italy. Eur J Hum Genet 10: 388–390.
46. Coppedè F, Marini G, Bargagna S, Stuppia L, Minichilli F, et al. (2006) Folate gene polymorphisms and the risk of Down syndrome pregnancies in young Italian women. Am J Med Genet A 140(10): 1083–1091.
47. Coppede' F, Migheli F, Bargagna S, Siciliano G, Antonucci I, et al. (2009) Association of maternal polymorphisms in folate metabolizing genes with chromosome damage and risk of Down syndrome offspring. Neurosci Lett 449: 15–19.
48. Coppedè F, Grossi E, Migheli F, Migliore L (2010) Polymorphisms in folate-metabolizing genes, chromosome damage, and risk of Down syndrome in Italian women: identification of key factors using artificial neural networks. BMC Med Genomics 3: 42.
49. Sadiq MF, Al-Refai EA, Al-Nasser A, Khassawneh M, Al-Batayneh Q (2011) Methylenetetrahydrofolate reductase polymorphisms C677T and A1298C as maternal risk factors for Down syndrome in Jordan. Genet Test Mol Biomarker 15: 1–7.
50. Kokotas H, Grigoriadou M, Mikkelsen M, Giannoulia-Karantana A, Petersen MB (2009) Investigating the impact of the Down syndrome related common MTHFR 677C[T polymorphism in the Danish population. Dis Markers 27: 279–285.
51. Martínez-Frías ML (2008) The biochemical structure and function of methylenetetrahydrofolate reductase provide the rationale to interpret the

epidemiological results on the risk for infants with Down syndrome. Am J Med Genet A 146A(11): 1477–1482.
52. Boduroğlu K, Alanay Y, Koldan B, Tunçbilek E (2004) Methylenetetrahydrofolate reductase enzyme polymorphisms as maternal risk for Down syndrome among Turkish women. Am J Med Genet 127A: 5–10.
53. Balaghi M, Wagner C (1993) DNA methylation in folate deficiency: use of CpG methylase. Biochemical and Biophysical Research Communications 193: 1184–1190.
54. Fenech M (2001) The role of folic acid and Vitamin B12 in genomic stability of human cells. Mutat Res 475: 57–67.
55. Libbus BL, Borman LS, Ventrone CH, Branda RF (1990) Nutritional folate deficiency in CHO cells: chromosomal abnormalities associated with perturbations in nucleic acid precursors. Cancer Genet Cytogenet 46: 231–242.
56. Leyton BL, Mergudich D, del la Torre D, Sans J (1995) Impaired chromosome segregation in plant anaphase alter moderate hypomethylation of DNA. Cell Prolif 28: 481–496.
57. Pogribny IP, Basnakian AG, Miller BJ, Lopatina NG, Poirier LA, et al. (1995) Breaks in genomic DNA and within the p53 gene are associated with hypomethylation in livers of folate/methyl-deficient rats. Cancer Res 55(9): 1894–1901.
58. Chen RZ, Pettersson U, Beared C, Jackson-Grusby I, Jaenisch R (1998) DNA hypomethylation leads to elevated mutation rates. Nature 395: 89–93.
59. Titenko-Holland N, Jacob RA, Shang N, Balaraman A, Smith MT (1998) Micronuclei in lymphocytes and exfoliated buccal cells of postmenopausal women with dietary changes in folate. Mutat Res 417: 101–114.
60. Botto LD, Yang Q (2000) 5, 10-methylenetetrahydrofolate reductase variants and congenital anomalies: A huge review. Am J Epidemiol 151: 862–877.
61. Zhang T, Lou J, Zhong R, Wu J, Zou L, et al. (2013) Genetic Variants in the Folate Pathway and the Risk of Neural Tube Defects: A Meta-Analysis of the Published Literature. PLos One 8: e59570.
62. Yadav U, Kumar P, Yadav SK, Mishra OP, Rai V (2014) Polymorphisms in folate metabolism genes as maternal risk factor for Neural Tube Defects: an updated meta-analysis. Metab Brain Dis. [Ahead of Print; DOI: 10.1007/s11011-014-9575-7].
63. Zhao M, Ren Y, Shen L, Zhang Y, Zhou B (2014) Association between MTHFR C677T and A1298C Polymorphisms and NSCL/P Risk in Asians: A Meta-Analysis. Plos One 9(3): e88242.
64. Yadav S, Hasan N, Marjot T, Khan MS, Prasad K, et al. (2013) Detailed Analysis of Gene Polymorphisms Associated with Ischemic Stroke in South Asians. PLos One 8: e57305.
65. Peerbooms OL, van Os J, Drukker M, Kenis G, Hoogveld L, et al. (2011) Meta-analysis of MTHFR gene variants in schizophrenia, bipolar disorder and unipolar depressive disorder: evidence for a common genetic vulnerability? Brain Behav Immun 25(8): 1530–1543.
66. Zintzaras E (2007) Maternal gene polymorphisms involved in folate metabolism and risk of Down syndrome offspring: a meta analysis. J Hum Genet 52: 943–953.
67. Medica I, Maver A, Augusto GF, Peterlin B (2009) Polymorphisms in genes involved in folate metabolism as maternal risk factors for Down syndrome- meta-analysis. Cent Eur J Med 4: 395–408.
68. Wu X, Wang X, Chan Y, Jia S, Luo Y, et al. (2013) Folate metabolism gene polymorphisms MTHFR C677T and A1298C and risk for Down syndrome offspring: a meta-analysis. Eur J Obstet Gynecol Reprod Biol 167(2): 154–159.
69. Yang M, Gong T, Lin X, Qi L, Guo Y, et al. (2013) Maternal gene polymorphisms involved in folate metabolism and the risk of having a Down syndrome offspring: a meta-analysis. Mutagenesis 28(6): 661–671.

5

Postural Stability in Young Adults with Down Syndrome in Challenging Conditions

Ewa Bieć[1], Joanna Zima[1]*, Dorota Wójtowicz[1], Bożena Wojciechowska-Maszkowska[2], Krzysztof Kręcisz[2], Michał Kuczyński[1,2]

1 Faculty of Physiotherapy, University School of Physical Education in Wroclaw, Wroclaw, Poland, **2** Department of Biomechanics, The Opole University of Technology, Opole, Poland

Abstract

To evaluate postural control and performance in subjects with Down syndrome (SwDS), we measured postural sway (COP) in quiet stance in four 20-second tests: with eyes open or closed and on hard or foam surface. Ten SwDS and eleven healthy subjects participated, aged 29.8 (4.8) and 28.4 (3.9), respectively. The time-series recorded with the sampling rate of 100 Hz were used to evaluate postural performance (COP amplitude and mean velocity) and strategies (COP frequency, fractal dimension and entropy). There were no intergroup differences in the amplitude except the stance on foam pad with eyes open when SwDS had larger sway. The COP velocity and frequency were larger in SwDS than controls in all trials on foam pad. During stances on the foam pad SwDS increased fractal dimension showing higher complexity of their equilibrium system, while controls decreased sample entropy exhibiting more conscious control of posture in comparison to the stances on hard support surface. This indicated that each group used entirely different adjustments of postural strategies to the somatosensory challenge. It is proposed that the inferior postural control of SwDS results mainly from insufficient experience in dealing with unpredictable postural stimuli and deficit in motor learning.

Editor: Ramesh Balasubramaniam, University of California, Merced, United States of America

Funding: The authors have no support or funding to report.

Competing Interests: The authors have declared that no competing interests exist.

* E-mail: joannazima@gmail.com

Introduction

Individuals with Down syndrome exhibit several major motor disorders when compared to healthy persons. Slow movements, different gait patterns and an inability to respond rapidly to changes in the environment [1–3] are easily noticed even by casual observers. Much less apparent - although of fundamental importance in the overall motor development of these persons - is deteriorated postural stability [3–5]. Postural stability is a rate-limiting factor and a prerequisite for a great number of gross motor skills. Good stability supports more complicated movements, encourages us to explore new situations, and ultimately leads to optimal motor control, based on growing experience and skill in using a variety of motor synergies. In contrast, poor stability increases the risk of falling and puts constraints on physical activity, which results in very limited motor experience in subjects with Down syndrome (SwDS). Hence, improving postural control may be beneficial for these people for at least two reasons. Firstly, better stability usually leads to decreased sway and increased stability area, which may build self-confidence in SwDS, allowing them to interact with the environment more willingly, with less fear of falling. Secondly, with some of the internal constraints on physical activity presumably lifted, a broader repertoire of movements should occur. Apparently, habitual inactivity and inadequate postural control form a vicious circle in SwDS that must be broken to clear the way for their overall functional improvement.

To achieve this goal, we need to know the mechanisms of deteriorated postural control in SwDS. Once they are deciphered, the premises for adequate therapy will come to light; however, the existing literature seems vague on this subject. Poor postural stability was attempted to be explained through several cognitive and motor deficits found in these patients. Cognitive impairment may cause deteriorated information processing, slower decision making [2] and poorer ability to integrate multimodal sensory input. Other deficits include longer simple motor reaction times [6], excessive grip force [7], poorer capacity to adapt to changes in sensory information, delays in the onset of postural activity and loss of anticipatory postural control [1]. The SwDS also show different responses to novel tasks [8] than healthy subjects. Potentially, all of these deficits may affect postural control system; however, no study has provided a plausible explanation for the role of these deficits in deteriorated postural control in SwDS. It may signify the presence of another antecedent of the altered postural performance in SwDS, which is very likely related to specific postural strategies that have evolved in the process of reciprocal interactions during concurrent development of the postural and motor system.

In light of the aforementioned habitual inactivity and limited motor experience of SwDS, the possible reason for their balance deficit may be linked to an inadequately developed postural control system that does not adequately adjust its responses to the changing levels of postural task requirements. However, the traditional amplitude measures of postural performance are not well suited to assess this issue because of their descriptive character and low specificity. On the other hand, the nonlinear measures of sway dynamics, i.e., sway entropy and fractal dimension, have shown promise in detecting important differences between the groups investigated. The strength of the latter measures lies in their ability to detect between-group differences which may be attributed to different levels of automaticity and/or adaptability that are specifically adjusted according to the balance challenge. The richer the changes in challenge to balance we apply, the more complete the picture of the inter-group differences we might expect.

The main purpose of this study was to assess standing stability in SwDS in a series of trials with increasing postural challenge using traditional and nonlinear measures of the center-of-pressure (COP) time-series and to compare it with standing stability in healthy subjects. We hypothesized that the SwDS would exhibit deteriorated postural performance (higher values of the COP variability and mean velocity) and different postural strategies in comparison with the control subjects. Specifically, with regard to postural strategies, we hypothesized that SwDS would show inadequate changes in these strategies that would account for their insufficient preparation to the more demanding postural tasks. Further elucidation of these differences will help improve our understanding of the antecedents of falls, and provide a rational basis for designing rehabilitation programs for individuals with Down syndrome.

Methods

Subjects

The study was approved by the Senate Ethics Committee for Research at the University School of Physical Education in Wroclaw. All subjects and their guardians provided written informed consent to participate in the research.

Subjects from the Occupational Therapy Workshop participated in the research voluntary and were not disadvantaged in any other way by not participating in the study.

The study involved 10 people with Down syndrome who participated in the Occupational Therapy Workshop in Wroclaw and 11 doctoral students from our university. The basic characteristics of subjects, i.e., age, the type of Down syndrome and level of intellectual disability are presented in Table 1.

Table 1. Characteristics of the subjects with Down syndrome (SwDS, N = 10) and control group (CG, N = 11).

		SwDS	CG
Sex	Male	5	7
	Female	5	4
Age		29.8 (4.8)	28.4 (3.9)
Type of Down syndrome	Trisomy of chromosom 21	10	-
	Trisomy with translocation	-	-
	Mosaicism	-	-
Intellectual disability	Light	-	-
	Moderate	5	-
	Significant	5	-
	Deep	-	-

Procedure

Postural stability was assessed in four 20-second trials of quiet standing on a hard or soft (a 50-kg/m^3 foam pad placed on a platform) support surface with eyes open (EO) or closed (EC). The sequence of trials was fixed: EO followed by EC on a hard surface and then repeated on a soft surface with 1-minute breaks between consecutive trials. The subjects were asked to stand barefoot as motionlessly as possible with feet together and hands at their sides. In the EO trials the subjects were instructed to focus their gaze on a dot placed at eye level at a distance of 2 m. A practice run was allowed prior to the test to ensure that the subjects felt comfortable in the laboratory area. Each recording started 10 seconds after the subject was ready for testing to eliminate possible transients in the COP data.

Data analysis

Data were recorded on a force plate (Kistler 9286 AA) at a sampling frequency of 100 Hz. The COP signal was calculated from the recorded ground reaction forces in the medial-lateral (ML) and anterior-posterior (AP) plane separately. Postural balance was evaluated by five parameters based on the COP signal: standard deviation (SD), mean speed (MV) [9], sample entropy (SE) [10], frequency (FR) and fractal dimension (FD). Measures of COP variability and mean speed determine performance, with lower values of these indices indicating better performance. The SE is the negative natural logarithm of an estimate of the conditional probability that a subseries (an epoch) of length m that matches pointwise within a specific tolerance r also matches at the next point [11]. High values of sample entropy are associated with a low probability of repeated template sequences in the data. In other words, the higher the sample entropy, the greater the irregularity of the time series. The increased values of sample entropy, which indicate larger irregularity of the COP, have been attributed to a reduced amount of attention invested in posture [12] and may be interpreted as an increase in the efficiency or 'automaticity' of postural control [13]. Input parameters for estimating the sample entropy were based on the median value of the relative error [11] resulting in the selection of pattern length of $m = 3$ and error tolerance of $r = 0.02$ as optimal parameters for both ML and AP planes (normalized to unit variance) of all subjects and tasks. A visual guide to optimal selection of the latter two parameters for sample entropy estimation may be found in Roerdink et al. [12] (see Appendix). The fractal dimension of the signal was calculated using custom-written software in Matlab (Higuchi's algorithm, see Appendix). Fractal dimension is an easily accessible measure that could be used for the study of COP complexity, and provides more information about posture control than traditional measures [14,15]. The data were tested for normal distribution and homogeneity of variances. After log-transformation of the non-normally distributed data, all dependent variables were subjected to 2 groups (SwDS and CG)×2 surfaces (hard and compliant)×2 conditions (with eyes open and closed)×2 planes (AP and ML) ANOVA (Statistica 9.0) with repeated measures of the last three factors. Selected pairwise comparisons were explored using follow-up analyses (Tukey test). The level of significance was set at $p<0.05$.

Results

The means and their standard deviation of the variables are shown in Table 2.

Table 2. The means and their standard deviation of the variables.

		Group	Platform		Foam pad	
			EO	EC	EO	EC
AP	SD (mm)	SwDS	3.8+1.2	5.2+0.7	11.3+1.2	16.6+2.1
		CG	3.7+1.9	5.2+1.9	9.3+3.5	14.3+6.8
	MV(mm/s)	SwDS	13.3+4.9	18.9+5.9	54.5+27.5	76.6+25.3
		CG	8.3+0.9	12.1+3.0	16.5+2.5	36.9+9.2
	FR (Hz)	SwDS	0.59+0.26	0.64+0.24	0.77+0.28	0.78+0.27
		CG	0.43+0.17	0.41+0.15	0.32+0.14	0.44+0.12
	SE (-)	SwDS	0.75+0.18	0.72+0.16	0.67+0.10	0.65+0.09
		CG	0.97+0.37	0.80+0.27	0.56+0.17	0.64+0.09
	FD (-)	SwDS	1.46+0.10	1.49+0.08	1.53+0.09	1.55+0.08
		CG	1.38+0.08	1.41+0.07	1.39+0.08	1.44+0.05
ML	SD (mm)	SwDS	4.1+1.5	4.7+2.2	10.2+3.12	12.3+2.9
		CG	3.4+1.1	5.9+2.2	5.5+0.8	13.2+2.4
	MV(mm/s)	SwDS	10.6+2.6	14.5+5.7	43.0+12.4	52.3+18.3
		CG	8.3+1.7	14.7+5.1	16.0+2.6	41.0+7.8
	FR (Hz)	SwDS	0.44+0.13	0.52+0.11	0.68+0.16	0.67+0.18
		CG	0.42+0.15	0.43+0.14	0.47+0.10	0.50+0.06
	SE (-)	SwDS	0.69+0.07	0.75+0.05	0.68+0.03	0.70+0.02
		CG	0.65+0.22	0.60+0.14	0.58+0.07	0.57+0.05
	FD (-)	SwDS	1.41+0.07	1.47+0.05	1.52+0.05	1.52+0.06
		CG	1.42+0.06	1.42+0.06	1.45+0.06	1.46+0.02

(SD- COP standard deviation, MV- COP mean velocity, FR- COP frequency, SE- COP sample entropy, FD- fractal dimension).

COP standard deviation (SD)

Surface, eyes and plane significantly affected COP standard deviation (Figure 1), $F(1, 19) = 208.8$, $p<0.05$; $F(1, 19) = 52.4$, $p<0.05$; $F(1, 19) = 13.9$, $p<0.05$, respectively as did the group×eyes $F(1, 19) = 8.8$, $p<0.05$ and the eyes×plane×group $F(1, 19) = 12.6$, $p<0.05$ interactions. The SD was larger on foam, with EC, and in the AP plane. Eyes closure equally affected both groups in the AP plane significantly increasing the COP amplitude. However, in the ML plane, the two groups behaved differently as depicted in Figure 2, in contrast to the controls, the SwDS displayed no differences between the EO and EC conditions. Additionally Figure 2 demonstrates an 85% higher COP SD in SwDS as compared to controls while standing on foam with EO ($F(1, 19) = 14.0$, $p<0.001$), being the only yet meaningful intergroup difference.

COP mean speed (MV)

Group, surface, plane and eyes significantly affected COP mean speed, $F(1, 19) = 24.8$, $p<0.05$, $F(1, 19) = 343.4$, $p<0.05$, $F(1, 19) = 7.9$, $p<0.05$, $F(1, 19) = 133.9$, $p<0.05$, respectively as did surface×group $F(1, 19) = 15.7$, $p<0.05$, eyes×group $F(1, 19) = 19.7$, $p<0.05$, plane×group $F(1, 19) = 19.1$, $p<0.05$, group×surface×eyes $F(1, 19) = 12.6$, $p<0.05$ and group×eyes×plane $F(1, 19) = 18.2$, $p<0.05$ interaction. Mean speed was larger in SwDS than in CG, on foam than on hard surface, with eyes closed than with eyes open, and in AP than in ML plane. The group×surface interaction ($F(1, 19) = 24.6$, $p<0.0001$) showed that changing the support surface from hard to foam increased MV much more in the SwDS than in controls. The group×surface×plane interaction ($F(1, 19) = 8.3$, $p<0.01$) accounted for much larger contribution from AP than ML plane to this increase in MV on foam. Finally, the group×plane interaction ($F(1, 19) = 17{,}3$ $p<0.001$) revealed that SwDS had much higher MV than controls in AP plane only.

Fractal dimension (FD)

Group, surface and eyes significantly affected fractal dimension (Figure 3), $F(1, 19) = 9.4$, $p<0.05$, $F(1, 19) = 23.3$, $p<0.05$, $F(1, 19) = 14.1$, $p<0.05$, respectively as did group×plane $F(1, 19) = 14.23$, $p<0.05$, group×eyes×surface $F(1, 19) = 6.6$, $p<0.05$, and group×eyes×plane $F(1, 19) = 8.0$, $p<0.05$. The FD was higher in SwDS, on foam pad, and with EC. The group×plane interaction accounted for larger FD intergroup difference in the AP than in ML plane. The group×eyes×surface interaction indicated that the shift from a hard surface to foam pad had larger effect on SwDS in EO than EC without affecting the control group.

COP sample entropy (SE)

Plane and surface significantly affected sample entropy, $F(1, 19) = 8.4$, $p<0.05$ and $F(1, 19) = 11.1$, $p<0.05$, respectively as did the group×plane interaction, $F(1, 19) = 11.6$, $p<0.05$. Higher values of sample entropy on the platform and in AP plane indicated more automatic postural control. The group×plane interaction showed that while the SwDS had the same level of automaticity in both planes, there was a difference in controls in favor of the AP plane. The group×surface×eyes interaction, $F(1, 19) = 8.0$, $p<0.05$, showed that the transition from hard to foam surface decreased SE in controls more in EO than in EC condition. In a similar way, the group×surface×plane interaction, $F(1, 19) = 4.8$, $p<0.05$ indicated that the transition from hard to foam surface significantly decreased SE in controls in AP plane only (Figure 4).

COP frequency (FR)

Group, surface and eyes significantly affected COP frequency (Figure 5), $F(1, 19) = 13{,}6$, $p<0.05$, $F(1, 19) = 14.0$, $p<0.05$, $F(1, 19) = 5.3$, $p<0.05$, respectively as did the group×surface $F(1, 19) = 8.1$, $p<0.05$, the group×plane $F(1, 19) = 14.5$, $p<0.05$, and the group×eyes×surface $F(1, 19) = 13.3$ interactions. The COP frequency was higher in SwDS, on foam pad, and with EC. The group×surface interaction reflected the larger intergroup difference in FR on foam as compared to hard support surface which resulted solely from the FR increase in SwDS while the controls remained unaffected by the change of support surface. The group×plane interaction complemented the latter result indicating that AP plane only contributed to this difference with increased FR in SwDS and decreased FR in controls (Figure 4). The group×eyes×surface interaction indicated that the shift from hard surface to foam pad had larger effect on SwDS in EO than EC without affecting the control group.

Discussion

The purpose of this study was to elucidate the mechanisms responsible for altered postural control in SwDS. We hypothesized that the SwDS would exhibit deteriorated postural performance (higher values of the COP variability and mean velocity) and different postural strategies in comparison with the control subjects. Although existing work on postural control in SwDS seemed to justify these hypotheses, they could be only partly verified.

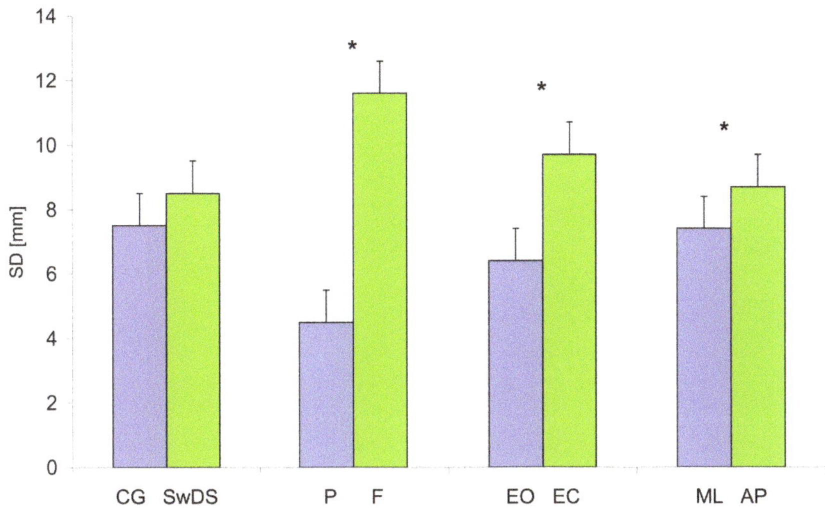

Figure 1. Mean values of the COP standard deviation (SD) collapsed over group, surface, eyes and plane. Vertical bars indicate the standard error. (CG- control group, SwDS- subjects with Down syndrome, P- platform, F- foam, EO- eyes open, CE- eyes closed, ML- medial-lateral plane, AP- anterior-posterior plane. Asterisks indicate significant differences (p<0.05) between conditions.)

Three results seem to be of particular interest. Firstly, postural performance based on the COP variability did not differ between groups in any tasks that might account either for similar postural behavior or effective compensatory strategies used by the SwDS. The only exception was much larger ML COP variability in SwDS during the EO stance on the foam pad. Secondly, the large increase in the COP MV and frequency caused by the foam pad in patients showed that this group might be particularly vulnerable to deteriorated or abundant somatosensory inputs. Thirdly, deteriorated somatosensory input had different effects on the sway measures in both groups. During stances on the foam pad, CON decreased sample entropy, exhibiting more conscious control of posture, while SwDS increased the fractal dimension, evidencing higher complexity of the equilibrium system in comparison to the stances on a hard support surface. This indicated that each group used entirely different adjustments in postural strategies to the somatosensory challenge. Fourth, the sway frequency, mean velocity, and fractal dimension were higher in SwDS than in the control group in the AP plane only. And last, the changes in sway frequency, sample entropy, and fractality, in response to the transition from hard surface to foam, affected only the SwDS in the eyes open condition. This accounts for particular vulnerability of these patients to the incongruent sensory inputs.

The COP variability, represented by standard deviation of postural sway, is a widely accepted measure of postural performance. In this study we did not find differences in COP variability between SwDS and the control group in any trial except the EO stance on the foam pad that revealed greater ML sway in

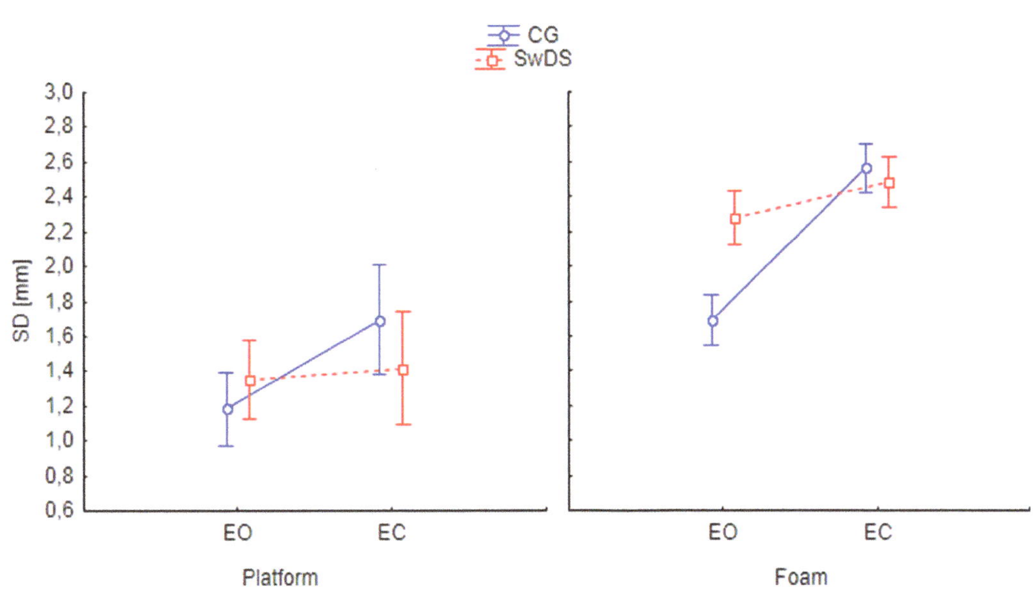

Figure 2. Group, eyes and surface interaction on standard deviation (SD) in medial-lateral plane. (CG- control group, SwDS- subjects with Down syndrome, EO- eyes open, EC- eyes closed.)

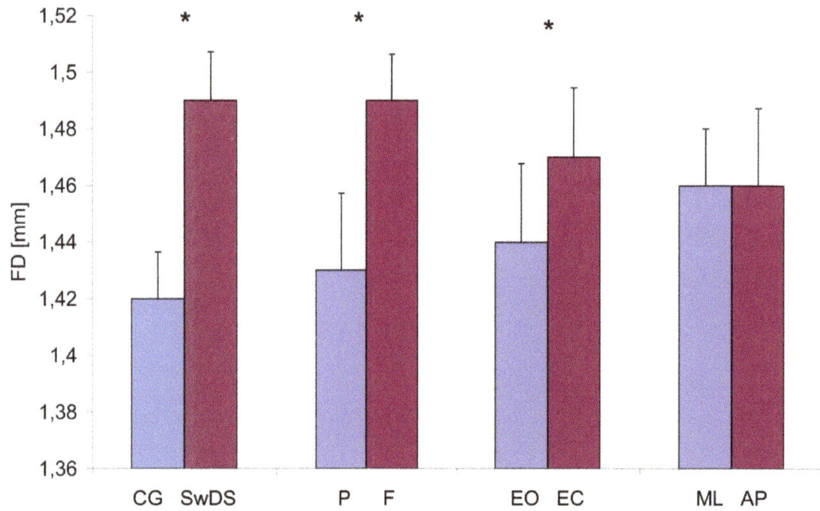

Figure 3. Mean values of the COP fractal dimension (FD) collapsed over group, surface, eyes and plane. Vertical bars indicate the standard error. (CG- control group, SwDS- subjects with Down syndrome, P- platform, F- foam, EO- eyes open, CE- eyes closed, ML- medial-lateral plane, AP- anterior-posterior plane. Asterisks indicate significant differences (p<0.05) between conditions.)

the SwDS. This evidence indicated very similar postural performance in both groups. Our SwDS somehow managed to equal the control group. We must admit that several authors reported poorer performance in subjects with DS [4,16,17], but our results still concur with a recent study by Cabeza-Ruiz et al. [18] who compared COP variability in 27 individuals with DS and 27 healthy adults, and found no differences between both groups in EO or EC stances on a hard support surface. Our study extends these results to stances on a compliant support surface and collectively shows similar patterns of postural performance and similar changes in this performance resulting from altered visual and/or somatosensory inputs. At this point, based on the COP variability only, we would advocate the notion of quantitative rather than qualitative differences in postural control between SwDS and healthy adults [4,17]. This notion argues that postural control mechanisms basically have similar principles in both groups, with a comparable weighting of sensory inputs [4].

The COP amplitude measures provide summary characteristics of the postural control system which have been often used for the general descriptive assessment and classification of postural performance in terms of better or worse. The main disadvantage of these measures is their inability to provide relevant interpretable information about the operation of the physiological control system [16]. Here, based on the COP variability, we found that the postural performance of both groups was about the same. Does this imply that the means undertaken by the CNS to produce the observed performance in both groups were also similar? The evidence gathered by the majority of researchers indicates the contrary, with a much higher COP mean velocity in SwDS than in control groups, reported even in simple standing trials [4,17,18].

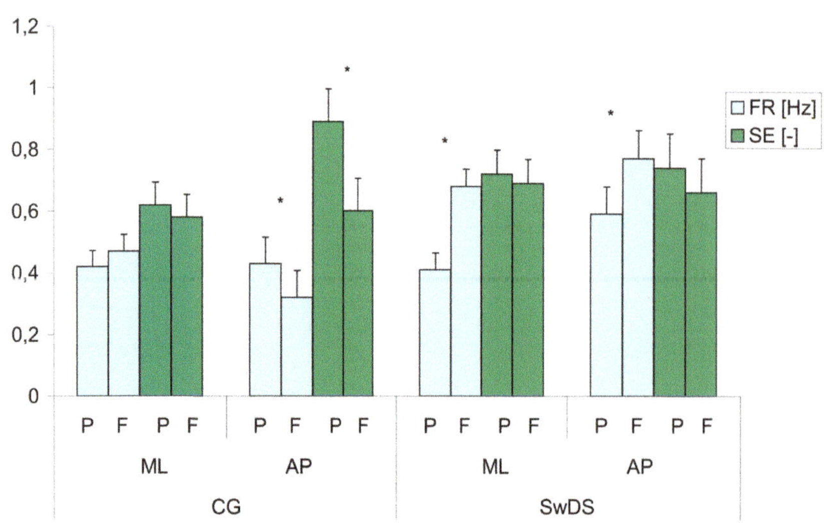

Figure 4. Mean values of the COP frequency (FR) and sample entropy (SE) in subjects with Down syndrome (SwDS) and control group (CG) in the medial-lateral (ML) and anterior-posterior (AP) planes while standing on the platform (P) and foam (F) with eyes open. Vertical bars indicate the standard error. Asterisks indicate significant differences (p<0.05) between stances on platform and foam.

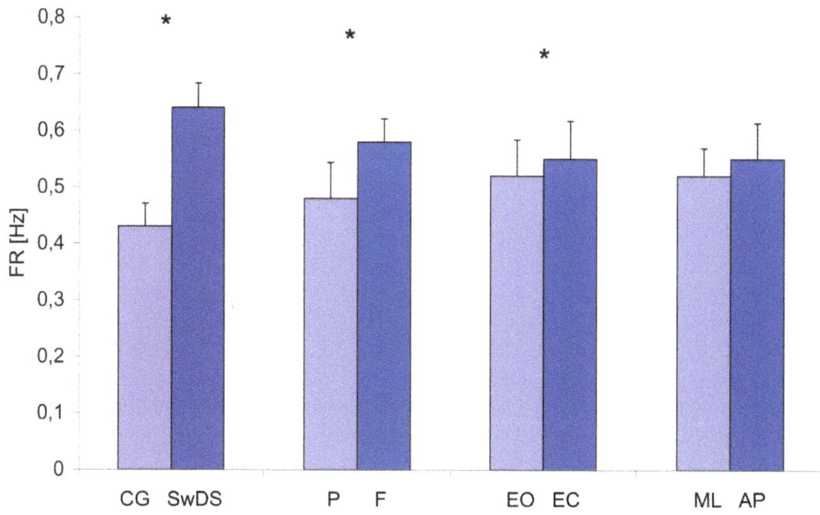

Figure 5. Mean values of the COP frequency (FR) collapsed over group, surface, eyes and plane. Vertical bars indicate the standard error. (CG- control group, SwDS- subjects with Down syndrome, P- platform, F- foam, EO- eyes open, CE- eyes closed, ML- medial-lateral plane, AP- anterior-posterior plane. Asterisks indicate significant differences ($p<0.05$) between conditions.)

Unfortunately, in too many studies the COP mean velocity is regarded as one more measure of postural performance that, if no more dependent variables are available, inevitably cuts out further inferences. Only Vuillerme et al. [4] interpreted higher mean velocity in teenagers with DS as more effort invested in balance control and correctly suggested a link between this effort and the increased sway activity which might be explained by increased cocontraction of antigravity muscles [2,19]. In fact, a coactivation pattern in SwDS that involves the simultaneous increase in activity of agonist and antagonist muscle has been reported by several authors [6,20,21]. In addition, studies on postural control in healthy subjects have shown that this coactivation pattern, induced by specific instructions or experimental setup, has led to higher postural stiffness with accompanying higher frequency of sway [22]. Furthermore, some authors have actually compared sway frequency or stiffness between SwDS and CON. Webber et al. [16] found a positive relationship between sway velocity and postural stiffness, and higher values of these parameters in SwDS. Larger COP frequency with the accompanying larger COP mean velocity was reported by Rigoldi et al. [5] and Cabeza-Ruiz et al. [18].

The former scheme would imply the CNS's ability to perceive and evaluate the threat to stability imposed by alteration in the somatosensory input and to decide which level of postural stiffness and frequency should be selected and used. This gradual adjustment of stiffness and frequency to increasing postural challenge has been observed in healthy individuals [23] and explained as a need to perform faster postural corrections and/or exploratory function. Accordingly, within this scheme, postural control in SwDS would still be qualitatively similar to that of healthy subjects, with inferior stability on the foam pad attributed to very limited practice in this unstable environment. If this is true, it would be good news for SwDS, i.e., an extensive training that involves quick unpredictable changes in somatosensory input might improve stability. Our cautious optimism follows at least three observations in SwDS: (1) the lack of increased frequency on a hard support surface even in trials with EC in this study; (2) the decrease in postural stiffness over consecutive trials [16]; and (3) the improvement in performance and gradual substitution of cocontraction with coactivation patterns of muscle recruitment following intensive practice [6,20]. This belief is further corroborated by Latash et al. [24] who pointed out that "persons with Down syndrome have all the machinery, both muscular and neural, to perform movements with characteristics like those seen in persons without Down syndrome."

On the other hand, the "safety catch" scheme suggests that the CNS selects cocontraction as the best remedy for any disturbance regardless of its direction and (probably) magnitude. This protective strategy is often used by novices in the early stages of acquiring a new motor skill [2] which again implies that postural control in SwDS may not differ much from that of healthy persons. Still, healthy individuals use this simple strategy as a transient protection, which, following the progress in motor learning, is quickly replaced by a more effective reciprocal strategy [2]. Thus, cocontraction seems a common necessary postural strategy which is used by the CNS in more challenging situations. For one thing it manifests a sort of helplessness in establishing the optimal coordination pattern, and for another it provides the room and temporal space to endure and may facilitate adaptation.

In the present experiment, the CG did not need any "safety catch," as can be judged from the lack of increased sway frequency on the foam pad. In contrast, the same trials turned out to be quite challenging for the SwDS, who relied on cocontraction that resulted in increased postural stiffness and frequency of sway. This apparent difference between the two groups may be tentatively explained by a physiological trigger that caused the onset of cocontraction in SwDS only. This was in no way surprising, as persons with poor postural control should detect threats to stability earlier than healthy individuals. In other words, the CNS of the SwDS would shift postural strategy from normal to stiff in response to lower values of sway amplitude or velocity and/or lower perceived distance to stability limits. We believe that these lower thresholds in SwDS are mainly the results of habitual physical inactivity, unwillingness to explore alternative strategies, and the basic goal of remaining safe [24]. When these factors are considered together, the SwDS have very limited experience with proper assessment of atypical stimuli, let alone quick and efficient decision making based on these stimuli. Thus, the "safety catch" strategy which is put into execution before the actual danger to posture arises seems to be an easy, comfortable and safe response to postural threats to SwDS.

To summarize, the traditional parameters of the COP indicate that postural stability (sway amplitude) during well-trained stances on a hard surface is equal in both groups. Yet, to achieve a similar level of performance in a novel environmental condition (standing on a foam pad) the SwDS need to use higher postural stiffness reflected by increased sway frequency and mean velocity. Such means of stabilizing the body are plainly excessive in comparison to control groups and resemble those used by healthy subjects at the early stage of motor development, as well as by subjects who are acquiring new motor skills or adaptations. A common characteristic of this initial stage of motor learning is the involvement of a broad spectrum of available sensory resources in order to select, fine-tune and integrate the optimal set of inputs later used to trigger efficient postural synergies. This implies that the postural control system at this transient developmental or learning stage is particularly plastic, multimodal, adaptive and complex. However, it also suggests that the SwDS may have some delay in motor learning abilities or that these abilities are vulnerable to environmental challenges. The nonlinear stabilographic parameters computed in this study seem to support the above interpretation and shed more light on the possible mechanisms involved in the postural control deficit of the SwDS. Higher levels of complexity and adaptivity have been associated with higher values of the COP fractality [15,25,26]. This fits well with our data which shows an increase in FD in all conditions on the foam pad for SwDS only, indicating that it was the patients but not the control group who treated the more demanding stances as those yet to be learned. In the control group the increased FD was observed only in more challenging conditions, such as in the ML plane with EC, where their postural automaticity was lowest. On the other hand, the decrease in the COP entropy, which was caused in the control group by foam pad stances, occurred only in conditions with the highest level of automaticity (AP plane with EO or EC).

These findings, which manifest an entirely different postural reaction demonstrated by different changes in SE and FD in both groups to the decreased reliability of somatosensory input, provide insight into sensory mechanisms of postural control. Standing on a compliant surface results in a significant challenge to postural balance and is often used to investigate the relative contributions from visual, somatosensory and vestibular systems [27], most frequently to test vestibular patients [28]. However, the additional role of this challenge in the present study was to tax the sensory response of our subjects in terms of automaticity and adaptability. Decreased entropy on a foam pad in healthy individuals concurs with the reports of other authors [29,30] and may account for the selection of an optimal level of automaticity to the difficulty of the postural task. In fact, Strang et al. [30] suggested that the broad, continuous and deliberate sway reflects the most appropriate postural strategy available in this setting. Such a strategy was evident in our control group, who invested more attention in postural control by trying to adjust their postural behavior to the constraints imposed by a compliant surface. This may reflect their willingness to explore the new environment and possibly restructure the respective postural synergies based on perceived feedback. A similar conscious action was missing in the SwDS who, as shown by the increased COP FD, turned to higher complexity and adaptability as a means to deal with the somatosensory challenge. However, the increased complexity in biological signals has been shown to correlate positively with the number of neurons involved [31], suggesting that the SwDS probably used abundant means to cope with the experimentally impaired somatosensory input, which might obstruct their ability to identify relevant features of the task performed. Higher values of the FD have been argued to be associated with the tendency for instability or the use of less stable control strategies [14,15]. Our results extend this proposition by suggesting a tentative yet plausible mechanism which may cause the instability as reflected by the increased FD. Excessive sensory inputs were sending a stream of information that was probably poorly organized and coordinated, and thus could lead to sensory conflict, which instead of being helpful in motor learning, might even endanger a stable stance. Along similar lines, Cimolin et al. [26] have interpreted the higher complexity of the COP in subjects with Prader-Willi syndrome as the inability to synergically modulate the three sensory systems involved in maintaining posture. This notion is further corroborated by the lack of effect of vision on the ML sway variability in SwDS, which accounts for the deficit in sensory integration.

We believe that the relationship between changes in sway performance and strategies in our SwDS, who were exposed to a series of increasingly challenging conditions, indicates mainly central origin or their postural deficit. However, it is known that the peripheral proprioceptive system may be altered in these patients due to hypotonia and ligament laxity [32,33]. This may lead to the reduced proprioceptive acuity and to impaired reflex function. Reduced proprioceptive acuity is an important factor contributing to postural control feedback while the abnormalities of musculoskeletal reflex function may account for particularly large intergroup differences in the stances on foam. It is possible that these impairments may be to some extent compensated by the proper selection of postural strategies. Therefore, the change in postural strategies found in this study may partly underlie a dysfunction of the peripheral proprioceptive system.

Our results regarding the possible differences in postural control between the ML and AP plane seem equivocal. The only intergroup difference in postural performance (indexed by the sway standard deviation) occurred in the ML plane (with eyes open on foam pad), with SwDS performing worse than the controls. On the other hand, SwDS had higher values of sway frequency, mean velocity and fractal dimension than control subjects in the AP plane only, i.e. in the plane where no differences in performance were found. It indicates that the SwDS may have implemented an efficient postural strategy that allowed them to improve their AP stability. However, the adopted changes in the latter sway measures seem to be suboptimal leading to a question whether they should or should not be subjected to therapeutic interventions.

Collectively, it seems plausible that a major difference in postural control between patients with DS and healthy subjects is reflected in novel or relatively unpracticed situations which require either learning or selecting and reweighing the previously stored motor synergies. What can be learned from these findings to make the therapy for SwDS more efficient? It has been suggested as necessary to provide these patients with stimulating and diversified practice conditions in which they may learn how to perform motor tasks optimally. While we generally agree with the significance of such an environment, the present results postulate focusing increased attention on the early stages of acquiring control over novel postural tasks. We believe it is crucial to double-check the patients' understanding of instructions and to provide them with augmented feedback regarding the actual performance or knowledge of results. Furthermore, the process of selection of postural synergies should be actively supported by assessment of how the individual sensory inputs are perceived and how these inputs help in proper decision making. This is related to gaining information about many aspects of movement through inherent feedback compared to the reference of correctness and this process may be inadequately developed in persons with DS. However, our present knowledge on possible relationships between progress in postural learning and nonlinear measures of postural sway is only emerging, and, to avoid unnecessary speculation, further research in this area is warranted.

Supporting Information

Appendix S1 In this appendix we explain choice of the parameters m and r for computation of sample entropy and the parameter k_{max} for computation of Higuchi fractal dimension.

Author Contributions

Conceived and designed the experiments: EB JZ MK DW BWM KK. Performed the experiments: JZ DW MK. Analyzed the data: EB JZ MK KK. Contributed reagents/materials/analysis tools: EB JZ MK DW BWM. Wrote the paper: EB JZ DW BWM KK MK.

References

1. Shumway- Cook A, Woollacott MH (1985) Dynamic of postural control in the child with Down syndrome. Physical Therapy 65(9): 1315–1322.
2. Latash ML, Anson GJ (1996) What are "normal movements" in atypical population? Behavioral and Brain Science 19: 55–106.
3. Galli M, Rigoldi Ch, Mainardi L, Tenore N, Onorati P, et al. (2008) Postural control in patients with Down Syndrome. Disability and Rehabilitation 30(17): 1274–1278.
4. Vuillerme N, Marin L, Debu B (2001) Assessment of static postural control in teenagers with Down syndrome, Adapted Physical Activity Quarterly 18: 417–433.
5. Rigoldi Ch, Galli M, Crivellini M Albertini G (2011) Postural control in children, teenagers and adults with Down Syndrome. Research in Developmental Disabilities 32: 170–175.
6. Latash M.L (1992) Motor control in Down syndrome: The role of adaptation and practice. Journal of Developmental and Physical Disabilities 4: 227–261.
7. Cole KJ, Abbs JH, Turner GS (1988) Deficits in the production of grip forces in Down syndrome. Developmental Medicine & Child Neurology 30(6): 752–758.
8. Ulrich BD, Haehl V, Buzzi UH, Kubo M, Holt KG (2004) Modeling dynamic resource utilization in populations with unique constraints: Preadolescents with and without Down syndrome. Human Movement Science 23(2): 133–156.
9. Prieto TE, Myklebust JB, Hoffmann RG, Lovett EG, Myklebust BM (1996) Measures of postural steadiness: differences between health young and elderly adults. IEEE Trans Biomed Eng 43(9): 956–966.
10. Richman JS, Moorman JR (2000) Physiological time series analysis using approximate entropy and samople entropy. American Journal of Physiology: heart and Circulatory Physiology 278: H2039–H2049.
11. Lake DE, Richman JS, Griffin MP, Moorman JR (2003) Sample entropy analysis of neonatal heart rate variability. American Journal of Physiology: Regulatory, Integrative and Comparative Physiology 283: R798–R797.
12. Roerdink M, Hlavackova P, Vuillerme N (2010) Center-of-pressure regularity as a marker for attentional investment in postural control: A comparison between sitting and standing postures. Human movement science 30: 203–212.
13. Donker SF, Roerdink CM, Greven AJ, Beek PJ (2007) Regularity of center-of-pressure trajectories depends on the amount of attention invested in postural control. Exp Brain Res 181:1–11.
14. Błaszczyk JW, Klonowski W (2001) Postural stability and fractal dynamics. Acta Neurobiologiae Experimentalis 61: 105–112.
15. Doyle TLA, Dugan E,Humphries B, Newton RU (2004) Discriminating between elderly and young using a fractal dimension analysis of center of pressure. International Journal of Medical Science 1(1): 11–20.
16. Webber A, Virji- Babul N, Edwards R, Lesperance M (2004) Stiffness and postural stability in adults with Down syndrome. Experimental Brain Research 155: 450–458.
17. Gomes MM, Barela JA (2007) Postural control on Down syndrome: the use of somatosensory and visual information to attenuate body sway. Motor Control 11: 224–234.
18. Cabeza- Ruiz R, Garcia- Masso X, Centeno- Prada RA, Beas- Jimenez JD, Colado JC, et al. (2011) Time and freauency analysis of the static balance in young adults with Down syndrome. Gait & Posture 3: 23–28.
19. Querner V, Krafczyk S, Dietrich M, Brandt T (2000) Patients with somatoform phobic postural vertigo: The more difficult the balance task, the better the balance performance. Neuroscience Letters 285: 21–24.
20. Almeida GL, Corcos DM, Latash ML (1994) Practice and transfer effects during fast single-joint elbow movements in individuals with Down syndrome. Physical Therapy 74(11): 1000/9–1012/21.
21. Aruin AS, Almeida GL (1997) A co-activation strategy in anticipatory postural adjustments in persons with Down syndrome. Motor Control 1: 178–191.
22. Carpenter MG, Frank JS, Silcher CP, Peyser GW (2001) The influence of postural threat on the control of upright stance. Experimental Brain Research 138: 210–218.
23. Kuczyński M (1999) The second order autoregressive model in the evaluation of postural stability. Gait & Posture 9: 50–56.
24. Latash M,Wood L, Ulrich D (2008) What is currently known about hypotonia, motor skill development, and physical activity in Down syndrome. Down Syndrome Education Online doi:10.3104/reviews.2074.
25. Harbourne RT, Stergiou N (2003) Nonlinear analysis of the development of sitting postural control. Developmental Psychobiology 42(4): 368–377.
26. Cimolin V, Galli M, Grugni G, Vismara L, Precilios H, et al. (2011) Postural strategies in Prader–Willi and Down syndrome patients. Research in Developmental Disabilities 32(2): 669–673.
27. Patel M, Fransson PA, Johansson R, Magnusson M (2010) Foam posturography: standing on foam is not equivalent to standing with decreased rapidly adapting mechanoreceptive sensation. Experimental Brain Research 208(4): 519–527.
28. Furman J M (1995) Role of posturography in the management of vestibular patients. Otolaryngology- Head & Neck Surgery 112: 8–15.
29. Lamoth CJC, van Lummel RC, Beeket PJ (2009) Athletic skill level is rejected in body sway: A test case for accelometry in combination with stochastic dynamics. Gait &Posture 29(4): 546–51.
30. Strang AJ, Haworth J, Hieronymus M, Walsh M, Smart LJ Jr (2011) Structural changes in postural sway lend insight into effects of balance training, vision, and support surface on postural control in a healthy population. European Journal of Applied Physiology 7(11): 1485–1495.
31. Liu JZ, Yang Q, Yao B, Brown RW, Yue GH (2005) Linear correlation between fractal dimension of EEG signal and handgrip force. Biological Cybernetics 93(2):131–140.
32. Galli M, Cimolin V, Vismara L, Grugni G, Camerota F, et al. (2011) The effects of muscle hypotonia and weakness on balance: A study on Prader- Wilii and Ehler-Danlos syndrome patients. Research in Developmental Disabilities 32: 1117–1121.
33. Rigoldi Ch, Galli M, Mainardi L, Albertini G (2012) Evaluation of posture signal using entropy analysis and fractal dimension in adults with Down syndrome. Computer Methods in Biomechanics and Biomedical Engineering 1–6.

6

Which Neurodevelopmental Disorders Get Researched and Why?

Dorothy V. M. Bishop*

Developmental Neuropsychology, University of Oxford, Oxford, United Kingdom

Abstract

Aim: There are substantial differences in the amount of research concerned with different disorders. This paper considers why.

Methods: Bibliographic searches were conducted to identify publications (1985–2009) concerned with 35 neurodevelopmental disorders: Developmental dyslexia, Developmental dyscalculia, Developmental coordination disorder, Speech sound disorder, Specific language impairment, Attention deficit hyperactivity disorder, Autistic spectrum disorder, Tourette syndrome, Intellectual disability, Angelman syndrome, Cerebral palsy, Cornelia de Lange syndrome, Cri du chat syndrome, Down syndrome, Duchenne muscular dystrophy, Fetal alcohol syndrome, Fragile X syndrome, Galactosaemia, Klinefelter syndrome, Lesch-Nyhan syndrome, Lowe syndrome, Marfan syndrome, Neurofibromatosis type 1, Noonan syndrome, Phenylketonuria, Prader-Willi syndrome, Rett syndrome, Rubinstein-Taybi syndrome, Trisomy 18, Tuberous sclerosis, Turner syndrome, Velocardiofacial syndrome, Williams syndrome, XXX and XYY. A publication index reflecting N publications relative to prevalence was derived.

Results: The publication index was higher for rare than common conditions. However, this was partly explained by the tendency for rare disorders to be more severe.

Interpretation: Although research activity is predictable from severity and prevalence, there are exceptions. Low rates of research, and relatively low levels of NIH funding, characterise conditions that are the domain of a single discipline with limited research resources. Growth in research is not explained by severity, and was exceptionally steep for autism and ADHD.

Editor: Rory Edward Morty, University of Giessen Lung Center, Germany

Funding: This work was supported by Wellcome Trust Programme Grant 053335. The funders had no role in study design, data collection and analysis, decision to publish, or preparation of the manuscript.

Competing Interests: The author has declared that no competing interests exist.

* E-mail: dorothy.bishop@psy.ox.ac.uk

Introduction

It is well recognised that there are substantial differences in the amount of research activity concerned with different medical conditions, but the reasons for disparities are not fully understood. Within the field of neurology, Al-Shahi and colleagues found that the amount of research into a condition was not proportionate to the frequency of the disease [1]. Common conditions such as stroke or migraine were under-researched relative to rare diseases such as Wilson's disease or Creutzfeldt-Jakob disease, when assessed using 'publication ratio', a measure of number of publications divided by disease frequency. They suggested that as well as political, economic and scientific interest, research activity might also be influenced by the fashionable nature of some conditions, and recommended that similar analyses should be conducted in other areas. However, their analysis did not take into account the severity of disease, which might be expected to play some part in research priorities. A review of grants awarded by the National Institutes of Health [2] confirmed that research funding was not related to how common a disease was, but it was related to disease burden, as indicated by mortality, years of life lost, and disability-adjusted life years. Thus severity of the impact of a condition seemed to play a larger role in determining research priorities than disease frequency.

The field of neurodevelopmental disorders is a microcosm in which these issues can be further explored. The term neurodevelopmental disorder is used in two ways [3]. The first refers to conditions affecting children's neurological development with a known genetic or acquired etiology, such as Fragile X syndrome or fetal alcohol syndrome. The second use refers to conditions of presumed multifactorial etiology in which certain aspects of neurodevelopment are selectively impaired; this includes such conditions as autistic disorder, developmental dyslexia, and attention-deficit hyperactivity disorder (ADHD). Both types of condition were included in the current analysis. In this article, counts are provided for publications in this field to consider how far the amount of a research on a condition can be explained by (a) frequency of disorder, (b) severity of disorder or (c) the disciplines involved in research. In addition, research activity is evaluated in terms of funding by the National Institutes of Health (NIH) relating to these conditions.

Methods

Conditions included in the analysis

The conditions included in this review are shown in Table 1. These were identified from Rutter's Textbook of Child and

Table 1. Search terms (in title) used to identify neurodevelopmental disorders.

Presumed multifactorial etiology	*Known etiology*
"Developmental dyslex*"	**"Angelman syndrome"**
OR dyslex* NOT (acquired OR deep OR surface)	**"Cerebal pals*"**
OR "specific reading disab*/retard*/impair*/difficulties"	**"Cornelia de Lange syndrome"**
OR "developmental reading disorder*"	OR "Brachmann-de Lange"
"Developmental dyscalcul*"	**"Cri du chat syndrome"**
OR "specific arithmetic*/math* disab*/retard*/disorder*"	OR "deletion 5p"
NOT dyscalcul*	**Down syndrome**[1]
"Developmental coordination disorder"**	"trisomy 21"
OR "developmental co-ordination disorder*"	**"Duchenne muscular dystrophy"**
OR "developmental dysprax*	**"Fetal alcohol syndrome"**
OR "clumsy child*" NOT dysprax*	"foetal alcohol syndrome"
"Speech sound disorder*"	**"Fragile X syndrome" OR FraX**
OR "articulation difficulties" AND child* NOT palate	**Galactosemia OR Galactosaemia**
OR "articulation disorder*" AND child*	**"Klinefelter* syndrome" OR XXY**
OR "apraxia of speech" AND (childhood OR developmental)	**"Lesch-Nyhan syndrome"**
OR ("delayed speech" OR "speech delay") NOT palate	"Lesch Nyhan syndrome"
OR "developmental apraxia of speech"	**"Lowe/Lowe's syndrome"**
OR "developmental articulation/phonological disab*/disorder*"	**"Marfan syndrome"**
OR "developmental phonological impair*/problem*"	**"Neurofibromatosis type 1"**
OR "developmental verbal dyspraxia"	"Neurofibromatosis type I"
OR "phonological disabi*/disorder*/impair*problems" AND child* NOT developmental	**"Noonan syndrome"**
OR "speech difficulties/disorder*/impair*" AND child*	**Phenylketonuria OR PKU**
OR "phonological disabi*/disorder*/impair*problems" AND child* NOT developmental	**"Prader-Willi syndrome"**
OR "speech difficulties/disorder*/impair*" AND child*	**"Rett/Rett's syndrome"**
"Specific language impair*"	**"Rubinstein-Taybi syndrome"**
OR "developmental dysphas*/aphas*"	**"Smith-Magenis syndrome"**
OR "developmental language" AND	**"Trisomy 18"**
disorder*/impair*disab*/difficult*	OR "Edwards syndrome"
OR SLI NOT specific impairment potato* gene elegans battery	**"Tuberous sclerosis"**
flight arithmetic SLI-1 crystal BMT laser somatostatin gastrin	**"Turner* syndrome"** NOT Ullrich
OR "language learning disab*"	**"Velocardiofacial syndrome"**
"Attention deficit hyperactivity disorder*"	OR "Velo-cardio-facial syndrome"
OR "attention deficit" NOT (hyperactiv* OR schiz*)	OR "22q11.2 deletion"
OR ADHD NOT "attention deficit"	**"Williams syndrome"**
Autism OR autistic	OR "Williams-Beuren syndrome"
OR (Asperger OR PDDNOS OR "pervasive developmental	OR "idiopathic infantile
disorder") NOT autis*	hypercalcaemia/calcemia"
"Tourette* syndrome"	**XXX** AND (female* OR karyotype
"Intellectual disability/handicap/retardation"	OR chromosome OR trisomy)
OR "mental handicap/retardation"	**XYY**
OR "learning disab*" NOT specific	

Term in bold is main category; plain text beneath indicates alternative search terms. Asterisk is wildcard symbol.
1 Estimated from rate for 'trisomy 21': see text.

Adolescent Psychiatry, 5th edition [4] and a review of behavioural phenotypes [5]. Those from the latter source were included only if an estimate of prevalence was available. The category of 'intellectual disability' (ID) posed problems, because this can be both a symptom of a known disorder, and a nonsyndromal condition of unknown etiology. Furthermore, in the UK, the term 'learning disability' is used to refer to intellectual disability, whereas elsewhere 'learning disability' is used for specific difficulties in a child of normal IQ. Despite these problems, it was decided to attempt an estimate of publications focusing on ID, but data on this condition need to be treated with particular caution.

Number of people affected

Estimates of prevalence per 100 were computed from Rutter et al. [4] or Udwin and Dennis [5], with the mean being used if a range was given.

Severity of condition

Measures of disease burden used in mainstream medicine focus mainly on mortality and morbidity and are not in general appropriate for neurodevelopmental disorders. It was therefore necessary to derive an ad hoc measure for this study. This was a 4-point scale representing the extent to which an affected individual could be expected to obtain educational qualifications and live independently in adulthood (see Table 2). Nine expert clinicians who saw children with neurodevelopmental disorders were asked to estimate severity for conditions shown in Table 1 on this scale. For some conditions, this scale was difficult to apply because of the wide variation in severity. For instance, a person with autistic disorder is unlikely to fall in category 1, but could fall into category 2, 3 or 4. In such a case, raters were asked to give their best estimate of the average level of severity. The data in Table 3 shows the average across all raters. For rare conditions, few clinicians had sufficient experience of cases to be able to make a judgement, and in those cases, the author provided a rating based on the description of the phenotype in Udwin and Dennis [5].

Estimates of number of publications

Web of Knowledge was the basis for research counts; the search terms used are shown in Table 1; for a paper to be counted, the search term had to appear in the title. This exercise revealed that some disorders lacked consistent terminology and were correspondingly hard to search. Total number of articles for each condition was obtained for 5-year bands from 1985 to 2009. Note that coding of articles was not mutually exclusive, so that if search terms for two conditions were included in the title, the same article would be counted towards toward the total for both conditions. The word 'Down' is not a valid search term in Web of Knowledge, so it was necessary to estimate the number of articles on Down syndrome. From a Google scholar search it was established that 9.9% of articles on Down syndrome include 'trisomy 21' in the title. Thus the number of articles on Down syndrome in Web of Knowledge was estimated by multiplying the number of articles with 'trisomy 21' in the title by 10.1.

Publication index

This was derived in a method similar to that used by Al-Shahi et al [1] by dividing the total number of articles by prevalence. This was scaled so that it could be readily interpreted as a count of the N papers in 25 years per 100 affected cases in a population of 11.56 million, which is an estimate of number of children in the UK [6].

Rate of increase in publications

This measure was derived by computing the slope of the line linking the number of publications in 5-year time bins across the period 1985–2009.

Estimates of amount of genetic/animal research

Preliminary analyses suggested that the amount of research on a condition was partly determined by the disciplines involved; for some conditions, a high proportion of studies involved genetics and/or mouse models. To gain an estimate of how much research on each condition was of this type, searches were re-run to find the proportion of papers on a condition that had the words 'gene', 'genetic', 'mouse', 'mice' or 'chromosome' in the topic field.

Amount of funding by the National Institutes of Health (NIH)

Data on NIH funding were obtained using the Research Portfolio Online Reporting Tools (RePORT) (http://projectreporter.nih.gov/reporter.cfm). For each disorder, the database was interrogated to identify funded projects for the period 2000–2010, and the total funding in thousands of dollars was computed, together with the NIH institute that provided the funds. It is important to note that the RePORT software identifies projects on the basis of keywords, and may include projects that do not have a central focus on the disorder in question. This means that, on the one hand, the amount of funding focused on a specific disorder is likely to be over-estimated, and on the other hand, that the same project is likely to be included in counts for more than one disorder. For this analysis, it proved impossible to obtain realistic estimates of funding for studies of intellectual disability, as the search terms from Table 1 identified numerous projects concerned with a wide range of disorders. This category was therefore omitted from this analysis. For the remaining conditions, a measure of rate of increase in funding between 2000–2010 was computed from the slope of the function for funding by year.

Results

Table 3 shows the estimates of prevalence, severity of condition, number of publications, rate of increase in publications, proportion of genetic/animal papers for each condition, and publication index, with disorders ranked by prevalence. Most variables were skewed, and so nonparametric Spearman correlations were used when assessing association between variables.

The first point to note is that the publications count has only a weakly significant relationship to prevalence of a condition ($r_s = .34$, $N = 35$, $p = .046$). To explore predictors of publications, the publication index was used, i.e. a measure that reflects the number of publications relative to estimated number of affected individuals. It is evident on inspection that there is a general trend for a higher publication index for the rarer conditions; the Spearman correlation between publication index and prevalence is $r_s = -.91$, $N = 35$, $p < .001$. However, when we consider the common conditions, we see that most of them have a relatively low severity index; indeed, there is a significant negative correlation between severity and prevalence, $r_s = -.61$, $N = 35$, $p < .001$. Furthermore, the severe, rare conditions are more likely than common, milder conditions to be monogenic disorders, consistent

Table 2. Coding of severity of impact of condition.

1	Little impact on ability to obtain educational qualifications and live independently
2	Likely to have poorer than average educational qualifications but can live independently
3	Likely to require special schooling; may be employable in adulthood, but likely to need support in daily living
4	Likely to require full-time care and support during childhood and adulthood

Table 3. Prevalence per 100, severity rating, number of publications (1985–2009), rate of increase in publications, % publications with genetic/animal model content, estimated N affected children in the UK, and publication index for each condition, ordered by prevalence.

Condition	Prevalence per 100[1]	Mean severity	N pubs in 25 yr	Rate of increase[2]	% genet.	N cases in UK	Pub. index[3]
Lesch-Nyhan syndrome	0.0005	4.00	428	−14	69	57	750.88
Lowe syndrome	0.0005	4.00	171	1	67	57	300.00
Rubinstein-Taybi syndrome	0.0008	3.50	291	2	48	92	316.30
Cornelia de Lange syndrome	0.0014	4.00	420	20	54	165	254.55
Cri du chat syndrome	0.0020	4.00	162	1	79	231	70.13
Galactosaemia	0.0020	2.50	678	8	46	231	293.51
Angelman syndrome	0.0040	3.79	690	36	80	462	149.35
Williams syndrome	0.0044	3.31	1,349	87	54	513	262.96
Marfan syndrome	0.0067	1.50	1,805	71	53	770	234.42
Prader-Willi syndrome	0.0067	3.17	1,851	82	58	770	240.39
Rett syndrome	0.0080	3.94	1,918	35	59	924	207.58
Phenylketonuria	0.0100	2.00	2,941	9	51	1,156	254.41
Duchenne muscular dystrophy	0.0143	2.50	3,212	−28	64	1,651	194.55
Tuberous sclerosis	0.0167	2.69	3,083	76	42	1,926	160.07
Trisomy 18	0.0250	3.70	661	−1	75	2,890	22.87
Velocardiofacial syndrome	0.0250	2.72	839	83	82	2,890	29.03
Neurofibromatosis type 1	0.0308	2.00	1,840	151	62	3,556	51.74
Turner syndrome	0.0400	1.94	2,485	21	60	4,624	53.74
XYY	0.0545	2.00	251	−6	86	6,300	3.98
XXX	0.0550	1.50	62	−3	87	6,358	0.98
Noonan syndrome	0.0571	2.50	635	44	67	6,605	9.61
Fragile X syndrome	0.0615	3.57	4,008	60	81	7,113	56.35
Klinefelter syndrome	0.0860	1.83	1,312	29	64	9,941	13.20
Fetal alcohol syndrome	0.1000	2.58	1,105	14	16	11,560	9.56
Cerebral palsy	0.1500	2.50	6,988	334	1	17,340	40.30
Down syndrome	0.1667	3.44	15,522	295	70	19,266	80.57
Tourette syndrome	0.5000	1.25	2,071	24	27	57,800	3.58
Autistic spectrum disorder	0.6500	2.90	16,071	1,468	18	75,140	21.39
Developmental dyscalculia	3.0000	1.56	229	15	14	346,800	0.07
Attention deficit hyperactivity disorder	5.0000	1.95	12,631	1,434	13	578,000	2.19
Intellectual disability[4]	5.5000	2.75	17,721	497	19	635,800	2.79
Developmental dyslexia	6.0000	1.90	3,789	128	10	693,600	0.64
Developmental coordination disorder	6.5000	1.50	398	38	0	751,400	0.05
Specific language impairment	7.4000	2.15	1140	84	8	855,440	0.13
Speech sound disorder	10.0000	1.69	387	24	11	1,156,000	0.03

[1]Prevalence has been divided by two if reported for one sex only.
[2]Average N additional publications per 5 yr period.
[3]N publications in 25 yr per 100 affected cases in UK, based on population of 11.56 million children.
[4]Includes 'learning disability' if not specified as 'specific' (see text).

with the fact that they are likely to have a high proportion of publications including terms indicative of genetic studies; the correlation between % genetic papers and prevalence was $r_s = -.52$, $N = 35$, $p = .001$. The correlation between % genetic papers and severity was also significant: $r_s = .41$, $N = 35$, $p = .015$.

Further analysis was conducted to consider how far the publication index for each condition related to severity and genetic content. A regression analysis was conducted to find the best-fitting function relating severity to publication index, and a log-log relationship gave the best fit, with $R = .648$, $p < .001$. Figure 1 shows the scatterplot relating mean log severity to log publication index, together with the line showing predicted log publication index.

Adding the proportion of genetic papers as an independent variable led to a significant increase of fit to give $R = .728$; change in fit: $F(1,32) = 7.51$ $p = .01$. Adding prevalence to the model after including severity and genetic index, accounted for a further 24.3% of the variance, change in fit: $F(1,31) = 33.24$, $p < .001$, bring the multiple R up to .879.

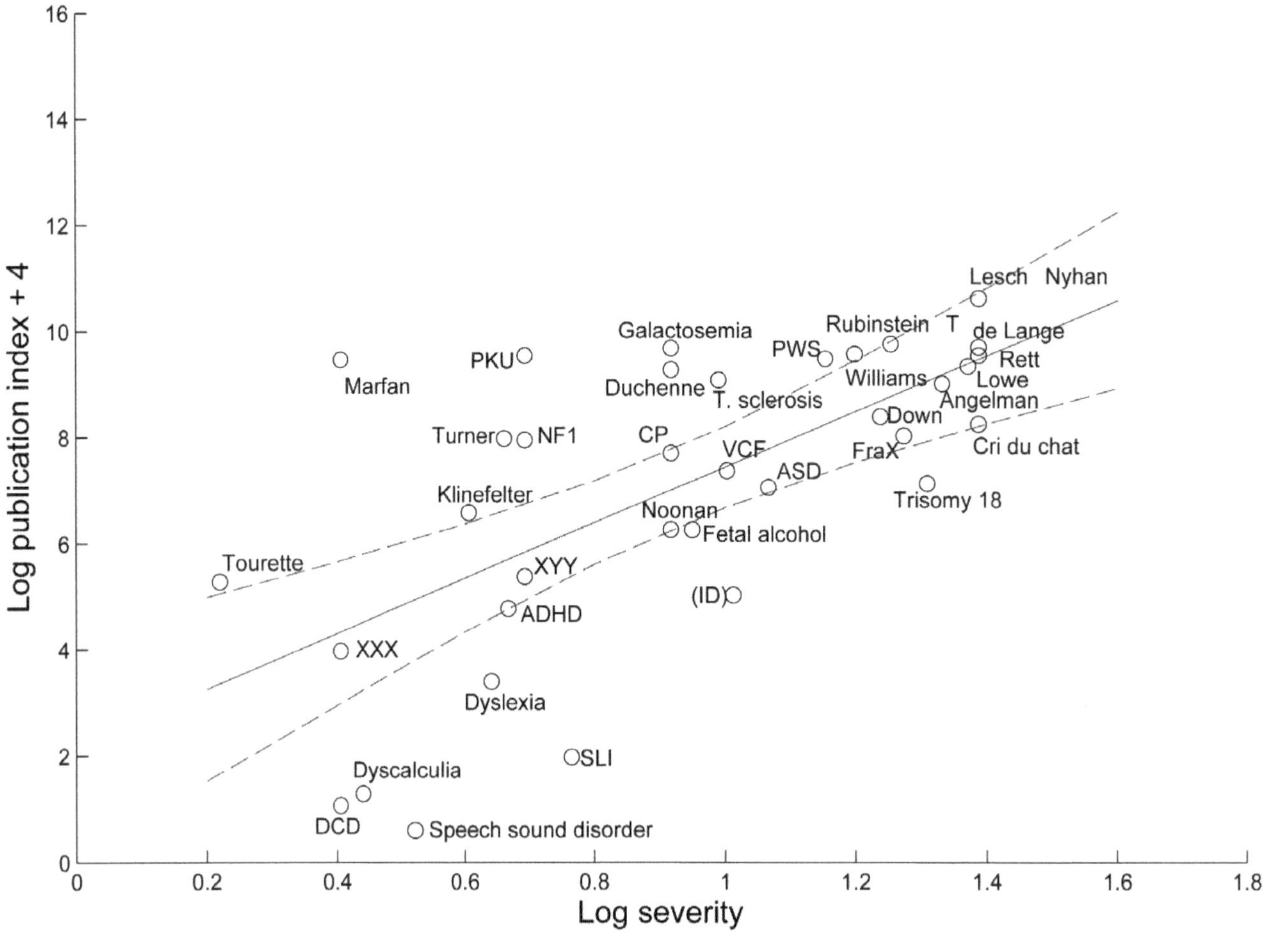

Figure 1. Regression of log publication index on log severity, with 95% confidence interval shown with dotted lines. A constant of 4 is added to log publication index to avoid negative numbers. Abbreviations: ADHD: attention deficit hyperactivity disorder; ASD: autism spectrum disorder; CP: cerebral palsy; DCD: developmental co-ordination disorder; de Lange: Cornelia de Lange syndrome; FraX: fragile X; ID: intellectual disability (shown in brackets to indicate that the publication index is overestimated); NF1: neurofibromatosis type 1; PKU: phenylketonuria; SLI: specific language impairment; T. sclerosis: tuberous sclerosis; VCF: velocardiofacial syndrome.

The rate of increase in publications across the five 5-year age bands is logically independent from the publication index. This measure revealed two clear outliers, autistic spectrum disorder, and ADHD (see Table 3). Autism started from a high baseline, with 1215 publications during 1985–1989, increasing 5-fold by 2005–2009. The increase for ADHD was even more dramatic, from 356 publications in 1985–1989 to 6158 in 2005–2009. In general, rate of increase in publications was positively correlated with N publications in 1985–1989, $r_s = .35$, N = 35, p = .042, but a high initial level of publications did not guarantee rapid growth. For instance, Down syndrome started in 1985–1989 with 2121 publications, more than either ADHD or autism, but this had risen only to 3474 by 2005–2009. It is noteworthy also that Lesch-Nyhan syndrome, which had a remarkably high publication index, showed a slight decrease in number of publications over a 25 year period.

Table 4 shows data on NIH funding per condition by year, and the slope of the function. There are striking parallels with the data on publications. The Spearman correlation between the total N publications from Table 3 and the total funding from Table 4 is .883 (N = 34, p<.0001) and the correlation between the slope indicating increase in publications from 1985 to 2009, and the slope of increase in NIH funding from 2000 to 2010 is .522 (N = 34, p = .002). In a final analysis, the proportion of funding from different NIH institutes was computed for the most common neurodevelopmental disorders. These data are shown in Figure 2.

Discussion

Before discussing the results, it is important to note that the range of conditions investigated is not comprehensive, and the approach adopted here could be extended to include a wider range of disorders. For instance, psychiatric conditions such as antisocial behavior disorder and schizophrenia were not included here, though a case can be made for treating them as neurodevelopmental disorders [3]. Reliance on a textbook of behavior phenotypes as a source book also meant that many neurological disorders without clear genetic etiology, such as congenital hypothyroidism or spina bifida, were also excluded.

It is also important to note that estimates of all of the main variables in this analysis are imprecise. A frustrating feature of this study was that is was hard to be confident that search terms identified all relevant papers without including papers on other conditions. Subsets of identified papers were scrutinised to ensure that they reflected the intended content, but relevant articles would be missed if they did not include the search terms in the title. For

Table 4. Data from NIH RePort showing thousands of US dollars spent on projects relating to each disorder.

	2000–2001	2002–2003	2004–2005	2006–2007	2008–2009	Anuual rate of increase 2000–2010
Developmental dyslexia	18,770	18,199	19,971	22,975	27,283	633
Developmental dyscalculia	0	0	400	369	1,574	151
Developmental coordination disorder	0	623	602	1,379	1,166	55
Speech sound disorder	858	876	501	964	1,116	8
Specific language impairment	16,279	16,219	15,389	18,133	28,611	780
Attention deficit hyperactivity disorder	274,500	346,039	314,232	365,207	532,800	13,042
Autistic spectrum disorder	95,114	171,707	360,765	355,458	851,270	50,978
Tourette syndrome	35,604	42,119	37,031	41,626	59,587	1,150
Angelman syndrome	13,039	12,103	11,156	12,392	21,246	594
Cerebral palsy	18,197	31,412	49,467	66,507	94,578	4,409
Cornelia de Lange syndrome	194	655	677	3,541	5,789	352
Cri du chat syndrome	0	0	0	0	0	25
Down syndrome	52,067	56,561	47,662	63,890	107,390	3,924
Duchenne muscular dystrophy	7,953	14,770	33,192	47,138	62,363	3,582
Fetal alcohol syndrome	40,955	51,783	69,504	83,447	105,668	3,905
Fragile X syndrome	28,316	44,054	54,187	67,584	125,661	5,532
Galactosaemia	2,802	5,737	4,398	4,416	6,060	371
Klinefelter syndrome	686	1,049	329	4,936	9,333	513
Lesch-Nyhan syndrome	1,030	1,803	2,049	1,960	6,601	240
Lowe syndrome	2,335	2,488	3,582	2,101	1,581	−66
Marfan syndrome	3,426	4,825	5,701	9,847	20,455	872
Neurofibromatosis type 1	5,966	9,182	11,625	20,348	30,267	1,230
Noonan syndrome	0	1,138	9,099	10,615	8,650	546
Phenylketonuria	8,782	9,015	6,047	9,426	5,941	−151
Prader-Willi syndrome	14,284	15,512	17,924	17,042	24,802	620
Rett syndrome	5,194	10,235	14,980	24,650	48,575	2,995
Rubinstein-Taybi syndrome	1,023	2,766	2,304	2,648	6,032	225
Trisomy 18	0	0	578	282	0	0
Tuberous sclerosis	10,139	16,243	22,844	39,132	68,944	3,181
Turner syndrome	3,766	6,068	9,175	17,475	7,292	255
Velocardiofacial syndrome	5,042	7,229	6,850	5,632	3,895	−107
Williams syndrome	12,652	17,697	19,506	15,627	18,180	115
XXX	0	0	0	285	4,927	161
XYY	0	384	0	3,239	5,050	329

some conditions, the concern was not of missing relevant papers but of using search terms that would yield false positives. Thus, the acronym SLI (used here for specific language impairment) is associated with 16 meanings in Wikipedia, as well as referring to genes in potatoes and worms. Attempts were made to restrict searches to exclude such usages, but it is nevertheless likely that the estimate for N publications is inflated by occasional errors. Another condition that was difficult to search was XXX trisomy, because XXX is used widely with a range of meanings. Conversely, the estimate for velocardiofacial syndrome will be slightly deflated because it was decided to exclude searches for papers with only the acronym VCF in the title, given that this acronym refers to a host of things other than velocardiofacial syndrome, and only a small minority of publications including it in the title were relevant. As noted above, identifying papers on intellectual disability was particularly problematic, and estimates of research on this topic are inflated because of the difficulty excluding articles on specific learning disabilities. It is noteworthy that nevertheless the amount of research on intellectual disability was below the level predicted from severity and prevalence (see Figure 1).

The second key variable in the analysis is prevalence. Estimates were taken from reputable published sources, but are bound to be imprecise for very rare disorders. Furthermore, for some disorders, especially those with multifactorial etiology, prevalence can vary substantially depending on the severity cutoff used. For instance, the prevalence of fetal alcohol syndrome disorder is estimated at 1 per 1000, but this condition is far less commonly identified in the UK than in North America, where a milder phenotype of 'fetal alcohol spectrum disorder' is recognised and estimated to be nine times as common [7].

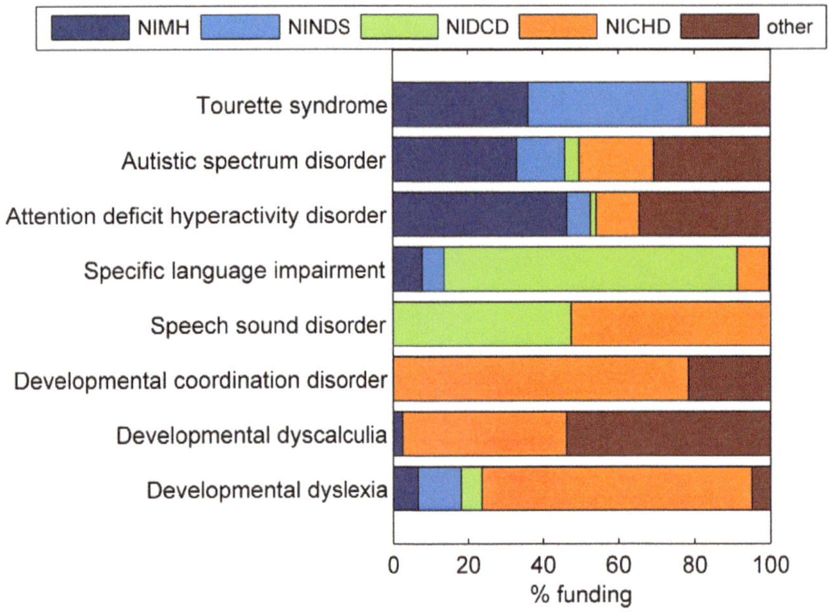

Figure 2. Proportion of grant income from different NIH institutes for the most common neurodevelopmental disorders. Abbreviations: NIMH: National Institute of Mental Health; NINDS: National Institute of Neurological Disorders and Stroke; NIDCD: National Institute on Deafness and Other Communication DIsorders; NICHD: Eunice Kennedy Shriver National Institute of Child Health and Human Development.

A third key variable is severity, which was estimated according to the criteria from Table 2, averaging ratings across a range of experts. All raters agreed that this was difficult to do for those conditions with variable phenotype, such as tuberous sclerosis or autistic spectrum disorder. For a condition such as intellectual disability, severity will also depend on prevalence, with milder forms being more common than more severe. Because it was in general not possible to determine the severity of cases included in specific studies, average estimates were taken, but results for specific conditions need to take into account unreliability that is inevitable when using these fuzzy estimates. Furthermore, the severity scale was devised to assess how far the condition affected educational attainment and adult independence, but did not take into account physical symptoms that characterise some of the rarer conditions. Thus, the majority of females with Turner syndrome do not have significant intellectual impairment and live independent adult lives, and hence this condition is rated as mild. However, the syndrome involves cardiac problems and infertility, which are not trivial symptoms.

Despite these limitations, the analysis gave a striking replication of the findings on neurological conditions [1], namely that, when prevalence is taken into account, the number of publications on rare conditions is greatly in excess of that for common conditions. At the extremes of the distribution considered here, between 1985 and 2009 there were 428 publications on Lesch-Nyhan syndrome, which affects an estimated 57 children in the UK, compared with 340 publications on speech sound disorder, which affects over 1 million. However, these two extremes suggest a reason why this is so: more research is done on more severe conditions. Speech sound disorder can be marked and persistent, but it is usually a relatively mild condition that is often transient and may have little impact on a child's social or educational prospects, whereas Lesch-Nyhan syndrome has severe neurological and cognitive consequences, including self-mutilation as a striking symptom, and is associated with death from renal failure or hypotonia in childhood or young adulthood. Overall, it was possible to show that a high proportion of variance in number of publications could be accounted for in terms of severity.

Furthermore, the amount of research on a given condition will in part depend on the disciplines involved in investigating it. Given the large number of identified publications, it was not possible to classify the discipline of each one, but a rough index was obtained to estimate the proportion of publications that involved genetic investigations. Not surprisingly, these were more common for single-gene disorders, most of which were rare. The amount of genetic research on a disorder was also a significant independent predictor of publication index.

There were some intriguing exceptions where severity failed to predict research activity, which can be seen as outliers in Figure 1. Within the conditions with presumed multifactorial etiology, ADHD and autism spectrum disorder fell within the range of predicted research, with Tourette syndrome slightly above predicted levels. However, the publication indices for dyslexia, dyscalculia, developmental coordination disorder and speech sound disorder fell well below prediction. Dyslexia and SLI are comparable to ADHD in prevalence and severity, yet the number of publications for dyslexia was 4 times lower than for ADHD and that for SLI was 16 times lower than ADHD. It is also interesting to note that there were three times as many studies on developmental dyslexia as on SLI, and nearly ten times as many as on speech sound disorder, although these conditions are similar in terms of rated severity and prevalence. It is perhaps relevant that these latter two conditions posed particular problems when searching for publications, because of the variable terminology used to refer to cases, suggesting that diagnostic uncertainty might be a factor leading to low research rates. This is a field where there is considerable debate about how to diagnose and categorise cases, whether there are disorders that are distinct from normal variation, and where the same terminology that is used to refer to a disorder is also used to refer to symptoms in other disorders.

Even though both disorders feature in the diagnostic classifications of ICD-10 [8] and DSM-IV [9], few researchers adopted definitions or nomenclature from the diagnostic manuals.

Another intriguing contrast is between Turner syndrome and Klinefelter syndrome, both caused by sex chromosome aneuploidies, and both affecting fertility. Table 3 indicates that there were nearly two times as many publications on Turner syndrome as on Klinefelter syndrome, even though Klinefelter syndrome is more than three times as common. Here the discrepancy is likely to relate to the ease of identification of affected individuals. The prevalence rates for Klinefelter syndrome are derived from prenatal and/or newborn surveys, but because the phenotype is not striking, many affected individuals are not identified in childhood. In contrast, the physical phenotype is far more obvious in Turner syndrome. This kind of explanation could also account for the dearth of studies on XYY and XXX trisomies; the majority of affected individuals are not identified because the phenotype is mild [10].

Even after taking into account severity and rates of genetic research, prevalence still was a significant predictor, with higher rates of publication for the rarer disorders. In considering reasons for the higher publication ratios in rare vs. common diseases, Al-Shahi et al.[1] noted that if the publication ratio for stroke were equal to that of variant Creutzfeldt-Jakob disease, clinicians and researchers interested in stroke would have had to read about 10 000 papers per week! One can turn this logic on its head and argue that if rare disorders had a publication index comparable to that for common disorders, there would be too few papers to give a critical mass of evidence in the area. For instance, if we extrapolate from the publication index for SLI (0.13 papers per 100 affected children over the 25 year period), for rare conditions where the national number of affected cases runs into hundreds rather than thousands, there would be no effective research literature. For the even rarer 'orphan' conditions with only a handful of affected individuals, lack of research is recognised as a serious problem [11]. The current analysis indicates that research activity on these disorders would have to occur at a rate well in excess of that predicted by extrapolation from more common disorders, in order to have a critical mass of publications and build research capacity.

The data reported here also suggest a positive effect of critical mass, insofar as the rate of growth in research on a disorder was related to the number of publications recorded in the first time interval, 1985–1989. This is compatible with the idea that a field develops by skilled researchers training their students and postdocs, who are likely to then study the same condition. If each mentor trains several others, then growth will be exponential rather than linear. Nevertheless, there were two conditions – ADHD and autism spectrum disorder – where the growth in research was unexpectedly high. For autism, there are two factors that could be implicated: first, broadening of the diagnostic criteria has led to a dramatic increase in diagnosis [12], and second, research funding has been directed to this area, for instance, by the Combating Autism Act passed in 2006 by the United States Congress, which authorized nearly 1 billion dollars over five years to combat autism and related disorders. For the more classic forms of autism, both prevalence and severity are comparable to Down syndrome, yet funding for autism is six times greater, and the slope showing increase of NIH funding over time is dramatically higher than for any other condition. It seems likely that government initiatives play a large role in explaining the extraordinary rise of publications in autism, though there are in addition several private foundations that provide substantial funding for autism research.

The other condition showing a very high increase in publications over time is ADHD, again with an associated high level of NIH funding. ADHD is comparable in prevalence and severity to SLI and dyslexia, and the proportion of genetic research on ADHD is relatively low, yet it attracts 19 to 21 times as much funding as these two conditions. Figure 2 suggests an explanation in terms of the professional disciplines with primary responsibility for these conditions. ADHD, like autism, is funded through several NIH institutes, but primarily by NIMH, suggesting most researchers in this field are psychiatrists. Dyslexia is funded mainly through NICHD and is the domain of psychologists, whereas SLI is funded mainly through NIDCD and is investigated principally by speech-language pathologists. This analysis suggests that inequities between professional disciplines in access to research training and funding may do a disservice to children who are affected by common yet under-researched neurodevelopmental disorders.

In summary, it is misleading to focus only on prevalence when comparing research activity for different conditions, as this suggests a massive excess of research on rare disorders. If severity is taken into account, the excess reduces considerably, although it is still present. This may, however, have to do with critical mass of research: there have to be proportionately more publications per affected individual for rare than common disorders, to ensure there is a body of work to build on. Nevertheless, even among conditions of similar frequency and severity there are some intriguing discrepancies in levels of research activity. It is suggested that these may have to do with extent of involvement of genetic researchers, specific initiatives in research funding, and lack of research funding in some disciplines working with neurodevelopmental disorders.

Acknowledgments

Thanks to Prisca Middlemiss and Courtenay Frazier Norbury for advice and comments on this paper, and to Andrew Whitehouse for reviewing the manuscript. Also, many thanks to those who assisted with ratings of severity: Gillian Baird, Charles Hulme, Paul Hutchins, Anne O'Hare, Daniel Pine, Emily Simonoff, David Skuse, Margaret Snowling, and Anita Thapar.

Author Contributions

Analyzed the data: DB. Wrote the paper: DB.

References

1. Al-Shahi R, Will RG, Warlow CP (2001) Amount of research interest in rare and common neurological conditions: bibliometric study. Br Med J 323: 1461–2.
2. Gross CP, Anderson GF, Powe NR (1999) The relation between funding by the National Institutes of Health and the burden of disease. New Engl J Med 340: 1881–7.
3. Bishop D, Rutter M (2008) Neurodevelopmental disorders: conceptual approaches. In: M Rutter, D Bishop, D Pine, S Scott, J Stevenson, E Taylor, A Thapar editors. Rutter's Child and Adolescent Psychiatry Oxford: Blackwell.. pp 32–41.
4. Rutter M, Bishop D, Pine D, Scott S, Stevenson J, et al. (2008) Rutter's Child and Adolescent Psychiatry. Oxford: Blackwell.
5. Udwin O, Dennis J (1995) Psychological and behavioural phenotypes in genetically determined syndromes: a review of research findings. In: O'Brien G, Yule W, eds. Behavioural phenotypes. London: Mac Keith Press. pp 90–208.
6. Office for National Statistics (2008) Mid-2008 Estimates of Household Population for England and Wales (experimental). http://www.statistics.gov.uk/statbase/.
7. Harris J (2008) Brain disorders and their effect on psychopathology. In: Rutter M, Bishop D, Pine D, Scott S, Stevenson J, Taylor E, Thapar A, eds. Rutter's Child and Adolescent Psychiatry. Oxford: Blackwell. pp 459–73.
8. World Health Organization (1993) The ICD-10 classification for mental and behavioural disorders: Diagnostic criteria for research. Geneva: WHO.

9. American Psychiatric Association (1994) Diagnostic and statistical manual of mental disorders, 4th edition. Washington, D.C: American Psychiatric Association.
10. Leggett V, Jacobs P, Nation K, Scerif G, Bishop DVM (2010) Neurocognitive outcomes of individuals with a sex chromosome trisomy: XXX, XYY, or XXY: a systematic review. Dev Med Child Neurol 52: 119–29.
11. Ayme S, Schmidtke J (2007) Networking for rare diseases: a necessity for Europe. Bundesgesundheitsblatt-Gesundheitsforschung-Gesundheitsschutz 50: 1477–83.
12. Rutter M (2005) Incidence of autism spectrum disorders: Changes over time and their meaning. Acta Paed 94: 2–15.

7

Assessment of Objectively Measured Physical Activity Levels in Individuals with Intellectual Disabilities with and without Down's Syndrome

Alexander C. Phillips*, Anthony J. Holland

Department of Psychiatry, University of Cambridge, Cambridge, United Kingdom

Abstract

Objective: To investigate, using accelerometers, the levels of physical activity being undertaken by individuals with intellectual disabilities with and without Down's syndrome.

Methods: One hundred and fifty two individuals with intellectual disabilities aged 12–70 years from East and South-East England. Physical activity levels in counts per minute (counts/min), steps per day (steps/day), and minutes of sedentary, light, moderate, vigorous, and moderate to vigorous physical activity (MVPA) measured with a uni-axial accelerometer (Actigraph GT1M) for seven days.

Results: No individuals with intellectual disabilities met current physical activity recommendations. Males were more active than females. There was a trend for physical activity to decline and sedentary behaviour to increase with age, and for those with more severe levels of intellectual disability to be more sedentary and less physically active, however any relationship was not significant when adjusted for confounding variables. Participants with Down's syndrome engaged in significantly less physical activity than those with intellectual disabilities without Down's syndrome and levels of activity declined significantly with age.

Conclusions: Individuals with intellectual disabilities, especially those with Down's syndrome may be at risk of developing diseases associated with physical inactivity. There is a need for well-designed, accessible, preventive health promotion strategies and interventions designed to raise the levels of physical activity for individuals with intellectual disabilities. We propose that there are physiological reasons why individuals with Down's syndrome have particularly low levels of physical activity that also decline markedly with age.

Editor: Tatjana Adamovic, Karolinska Institutet, Sweden

Funding: This study and Dr. Phillips was funded by a grant from the Down's Syndrome Association. Prof. Holland is supported by the Health Foundation and the NIHR Collaboration in Leadership for Applied Health Research and Care (CLAHRC) for Peterborough and Cambridgeshire. The funders had no role in study design, data collection and analysis, decision to publish, or preparation of the manuscript.

Competing Interests: The authors have declared that no competing interests exist.

* E-mail: acp49@medschl.cam.ac.uk

Introduction

When compared with the general population individuals with intellectual disabilities (also referred to as learning disabilities) experience significantly higher rates of morbidity [1], mortality [2], and health inequalities than the general population [3,4]. The term 'intellectual disabilities' refers to a very heterogeneous group of individuals with varied needs and the reasons for these health inequalities are likely to be multiple but low levels of physical fitness [5] and high rates of obesity are contributing factors [6]. For the majority of the population the health benefits of regular physical activity are well established [7–9], however, individuals with intellectual disabilities have not been included in the major epidemiological physical activity studies [10,11] and recent government policy [12,13] and initiatives [14] have not adequately promoted physical activity for this group. Given their possible dependency on others and in the context of the social circumstances where individuals with intellectual disabilities live, physical activity may be a low priority.

To date, there is only a small literature on the physical activity levels of children [15] and of adults [16] with intellectual disabilities, with the data collected being limited due to the fact that mostly self or proxy reports, or pedometers were used. The former methods have well-known methodological weaknesses [17] and, although the latter are better, they do not give information about whether wearers are meeting physical activity recommendations. Accelerometers are more sophisticated motion sensors compared to pedometers [18]. There have been a small number of studies using this methodology in individuals with intellectual disabilities on small sample sizes (<50), and mostly including relatively young participants with mild to moderate intellectual disabilities with few mobility difficulties, or purposively selected participants based on a particular diagnoses (e.g., Down's syndrome, those with obesity) [19–26]. Given these limitations the aims of this study were to investigate, using accelerometers, the levels of physical activity undertaken by a large sample of individuals with intellectual disabilities, to estimate the percentage of participants meeting physical activity recommendations, and to study any association with age, gender, and level of intellectual disabilities. Due to indications from previous research that individuals with Down's syndrome have particularly low levels of physical fitness [5] and high levels obesity [6] we have also compared those with Down's syndrome and those with intellectual disability without Down's syndrome.

Methods

Ethical approval and consent procedures

Ethical approval for the study was granted by the Cambridgeshire 3 Research Ethics Committee in April 2008. The research procedures of the Mental Capacity Act 2005 were adhered to assess participant's capacity to consent to take part in the study. For children (12–15 years), the written consent of their parents was obtained. For adults (>16 years), written consent was obtained from those participants judged to have the capacity to consent. Those participants who were judged to lack the capacity to consent, written agreement for the individual to participate was obtained from either a personal or nominated consultee. Only five adults were not able to provide consent themselves. In each case their mother or father supported their participation in the study. Data were collected between July 2008 and May 2010.

Recruitment

Participants were recruited from the East and South East of England through local care providers, charities, schools, colleges, and clubs. These organisations were asked to identify possible participants based on the selection criteria that participants were known to intellectual disability services, were aged 12 years and above, and could walk unaided (i.e., without a wheel chair or walking aid). Possible participants and their main carer (relative or paid) were sent or given a study information pack and asked to contact the first author (ACP) if they were interested in participating. Unfortunately it was not possible to keep accurate records of how many participants were approached to take part in the study. If participation was agreed then a date was set for the researcher to visit the participant's home residence at a time that was convenient for them. During the home visit several measurements were taken.

Level of intellectual disability

Level of intellectual disability was assessed using the Leicestershire Intellectual Disability tool which is a measure that combines seven questions on writing, dressing, speech, preparing food, feeding, empathy, and community use [27]. Level of intellectual disability is determined by the total score of the tool using the ICD-10 criteria for mild, moderate, severe, and profound intellectual disability. The Leicestershire Intellectual Disability tool has a diagnostic accuracy of 91% as compared to the Vineland Adaptive Behavior Scale [28]. The measure was administered by the researcher to an individual who knew the participant well (e.g., parent or carer).

Measurements of height, weight, body mass index and percentage body fat

Weight and height were measured according to set procedures [29]. Weight was measured to the nearest 0.1 kg with the participant dressed in lightweight weight clothing and with no shoes using a calibrated electronic scale (Seca 813, Seca Ltd, Birmingham, UK). Height was measured by the stretch stature method to the nearest 0.5 cm using a portable stadiometer (Seca Leicester Height Measure, Invicta Plastics, Leicester, UK). Body mass index (BMI) was transferred into age and gender appropriate cut-offs for underweight [30], normal weight, overweight, or obese [31,32].

Assessment of physical activity

Physical activity was assessed using the Actigraph GT1M accelerometer (Actigraph LLC, Pensacola, FL, USA) for seven consecutive days. The accelerometer was distributed to the participant during the home visit and returned by post to the study office. The accelerometer was fitted to an elastic waistband and attached to the participant's right hip. Instructions were given to the participant and carer both verbally and in writing on how to wear the accelerometer during all waking hours except while bathing, showering, swimming, and playing contact sports. Additionally, participants and carers were asked to record the time the accelerometer was put on and taken off each day and the reason for doing so using a time sheet (e.g., to go bed, swimming, or for contact sports, or for any periods of cycling). The time sheet data was not used in the analysis, since subjective interpretation of time sheet data is required. However, observations from the time sheets and observed counts indicate that the degree of underestimation of overall physical activity was minimal.

Data analysis

Data from the accelerometer were downloaded onto a computer upon return and processed using a custom written program (MAHUffe, available at www.mrc-epid.cam.ac.uk). Data from the first seven days of complete recordings were used. If participants missed a day of recording due to unforeseen circumstances they were instructed to wear the accelerometer for an extra day. For inclusion in the analysis each participant needed a minimum wear time of 10 hours per day. Non-wear time was defined as sequences of 10 or more consecutive minutes of zero counts. In case of monitor failure or lack of data, participants were asked to re-wear the monitor for a further week.

Accelerometers were programmed to measure activity in 5 second epochs. Outcome variables were total physical activity (counts/min), steps per day (steps/day), and time spent (mins/day) in sedentary, light, moderate, vigorous, and moderate to vigorous physical activity (MVPA) intensities. Published activity intensity cutpoints for children (12–15 years) and adults (>16 years), which had been used in previous studies, were used to estimate the time spent in different activity intensities [10,11]. Time spent in MVPA was defined as >2802 counts/min for children and >2020 for adults.

Time spent in MVPA and bouts of 10 or more minutes of MVPA were used to estimate the percentage of children and adults with intellectual disabilities meeting physical activity recommendations established by the UK Chief Medical Officers [8]. Briefly children and young people (5–18 years) should accumulate 60 or more minutes of MVPA seven days a week, and adults (>19 years) should accumulate 150 or more minutes of MVPA a week in bouts of at least 10 minutes.

All data analysis was performed using SPSS 15.0 for Windows (Statistical Package for the Social Sciences Inc, Chicago, IL), and significance set at $p<.05$. Each variable was checked for missing data and outliers. Outliers, defined as more than three times the inter-quartile range from the upper quartile boundary, were excluded. Descriptive statistics were calculated for all variables and assessed for normality and homogeneity of variance.

Initial analyses were performed by independent *t*-tests and analysis of variance (ANOVA) to identify differences that could confound comparisons (age, gender, level of intellectual disability, residential setting, and presence of Down's syndrome) between groups. Analysis of covariance (ANCOVA) adjusting for confounding variables as necessary was performed to detect group differences. Partial correlations adjusted for confounding variables were performed to examine the relationship between age and physical activity variables.

Results

Demographics and descriptive data

An initial sample of 171 participants known to services for individuals with intellectual disabilities was recruited. Nineteen participants were eliminated from the final analysis because of not completing all testing, mostly due to a failure to wear the accelerometer for the required time period. The final sample was 152 participants aged between 12 and 70 years with mild to severe levels of intellectual disabilities including 61 with idiopathic intellectual disabilities, 79 with Down's syndrome, nine with autism spectrum conditions, 1 with Russell-Silver syndrome, 1 with Treacher Collins syndrome, and 1 with Beckwith-Wiedemann syndrome. Many participants had one or more health problems that were, when necessary, controlled with medication. Table 1 presents the main descriptive characteristics for males and females who were included in the analyses. Independent samples t-tests revealed statistically significant differences in height [$t(150) = 8.9$, $p < .001$] and BMI [$t(150) = -3.7$, $p < .001$] between male and female participants.

Main physical activity data

Table 2 presents the main physical activity data for male and female participants by age group. The total sample averaged 6334 steps per day over the seven days ranging from a low of 743 to a high of 18,191 steps per day. Regardless of age or gender, on average, most of the waking day was spent being sedentary (608.1 mins/day) followed by light (120.7 mins/day) and then moderate physical activity (33.7 mins/day), with very little time engaged in vigorous physical activity (2.1 mins/day). Most MVPA for both adult males ($M = 1.0$, $SD = 2.3$) and females ($M = 0.4$, $SD = 1.6$) was accrued through short bouts (<10 minutes) and, therefore, does not count towards meeting government physical activity recommendations. No adolescent or adult participants met current UK physical activity recommendations [8].

Physical activity differences by age and gender

Physical activity across age bands are shown in Table 2 with a trend towards an increase in sedentary behaviour and a decrease in physical activity in later life, however, any relationship with age was not significant. Differences in physical activity by gender are shown in Table 3. ANCOVA adjusted for age, presence of Down's

Table 1. Descriptive data for male and female participants.

Category	Subcategory	Males ($n = 74$)	Females ($n = 78$)
Age (years)		33.6 (14.7)	
Age range	12–15 years (%)	4.1	5.1
	16–34 years (%)	50.0	48.7
	35–44 years (%)	23.0	17.9
	45–54 years (%)	12.2	11.5
	55–64 years (%)	10.9	16.7
Presence of Down's syndrome (%)		44.6	59.0
Height (cm)		164.7 (11.1)	149.9 (9.4)*
Weight (kg)		71.9 (16.9)	68.2 (16.0)
BMI (kg/m^2)		26.5 (6.3)	30.3 (6.2)*
BMI category	Underweight (%)	2.7	1.3
	Normal range (%)	34.2	25.3
	Overweight (%)	37.0	29.1
	Obese (%)	26.0	44.3
Level of intellectual disability	Mild (%)	33.8	38.0
	Moderate (%)	39.4	33.8
	Severe (%)	26.8	28.2
Residential setting	With parents (%)	43.2	37.2
	Care home (%)	39.2	50.0
	Supported living (%)	17.6	12.8
Employment/daytime placement	Student (%)	27.0	26.9
	Day centre (%)	14.9	26.9
	Social enterprises (%)	16.2	12.8
	Day centre and social enterprises (%)	21.6	19.2
	Part/full-time work (%)	10.8	7.7
	None (%)	9.6	6.4

Data are mean and (standard deviation) unless stated otherwise.
*statistically significant difference between males and females ($p < .05$).

Table 2. Physical activity data by gender and age group.

MEN					
Variable	**12–15 years (*n* = 3)**	**16–34 years (*n* = 37)**	**35–44 years (*n* = 17)**	**45–54 years (*n* = 9)**	**55+ years (*n* = 8)**
Total physical activity (counts/min)	836.2 (619.0)	694.7 (184.2)	739.0 (418.3)	602.0 (182.7)	585.0 (264.8)
Sedentary (mins/day)	558.3 (61.1)	604.0 (65.2)	586.7 (143.8)	603.6 (96.7)	648.2 (95.1)
Light (mins/day)	151.9 (19.1)	112.9 (30.5)	121.4 (41.5)	131.3 (36.2)	119.9 (52.6)
Moderate (mins/day)	19.8 (4.5)	39.6 (17.3)	42.8 (33.0)	29.5 (18.6)	38.3 (33.9)
Vigorous (mins/day)	8.5 (10.5)	2.6 (2.8)	2.3 (3.2)	1.8 (2.7)	0.7 (0.5)
$MVPA_{all}$ (mins/day)	28.2 (14.9)	42.2 (19.1)	45.2 (34.1)	31.3 (20.1)	39.0 (34.2)
$MVPA_{+10}$	-	0.9 (1.9)	1.6 (3.2)	0.0 (0.0)	1.8 (3.4)
Steps (steps/day)	7181 (179)	6558 (2493)	7376 (4199)	6682 (2831)	7723 (5168)
WOMEN					
Variable	**12–15 years (*n* = 4)**	**16–34 years (*n* = 38)**	**35–44 years (*n* = 14)**	**45–54 years (*n* = 9)**	**55+ years (*n* = 13)**
Total physical activity (counts/min)	680.0 (91.9)	577.0 (138.7)	556.3 (87.7)	577.7 (485.0)	485.0 (170.7)
Sedentary (mins/day)	609.3 (80.6)	644.2 (40.6)	560.4 (84.7)	576.0 (49.5)	605.1 (86.0)
Light (mins/day)	144.2 (49.2)	113.6 (27.8)	139.9 (38.2)	143.2 (54.0)	104.9 (33.2)
Moderate (mins/day)	23.0 (7.5)	30.0 (12.3)	30.8 (9.9)	33.5 (15.3)	20.7 (14.8)
Vigorous (mins/day)	3.9 (1.1)	2.1 (3.3)	1.0 (0.4)	2.0 (2.1)	0.8 (0.4)
$MVPA_{all}$ (mins/day)	26.9 (6.5)	32.1 (13.5)	31.8 (9.9)	35.4 (16.5)	21.5 (14.7)
$MVPA_{+10}$	-	0.4 (1.3)	0.8 (2.9)	0.0 (0.0)	0.0 (0.0)
Steps (steps/day)	6918 (749)	5648 (1831)	6274 (2021)	6751 (2090)	4649 (2126)

Data are displayed as mean and (standard deviation).

syndrome, level of intellectual disability, and residential setting revealed males engaged in significantly more total physical activity [$F(1, 146) = 8.3$, $p = .005$], MVPA [$F(1, 146) = 7.9$, $p = .006$], and steps per day [$F(1, 146) = 6.2$, $p = .014$] than females.

Physical activity differences by level of intellectual disability

Physical activity data by level of intellectual disability are shown in Table 4. There was a general trend towards those with more severe levels of intellectual disability being more sedentary and less physically active, however, ANCOVA adjusted for confounding variables only found a significant trend towards a decreasing number of steps per day as the level of intellectual disability becomes more severe [$F(2, 145) = 6.2$, $p = .003$].

Table 3. Physical activity data for male and female participants.

Variable	**Males (*n* = 74)**	**Females (*n* = 78)**
Total physical activty (counts/min)	665.0 (224.2)	564.1 (146.3)*
Sedentary (mins/day)	605.3 (95.3)	616.0 (70.6)
MVPA (mins/day)	40.4 (24.1)	30.2 (13.7)*
Steps (steps/day)	6978 (3269)	5741 (1918)*
Wear time (mins/day)	767.4 (83.5)	768.5 (66.0)

Data are mean and (standard deviation).
Analysis adjusted for age, presence of Down's syndrome, level of intellectual disability, and residential setting.
*statistically significant difference between male and female participants ($p < .05$).

Physical activity and Down's syndrome

Physical activity data for participants with and without Down's syndrome are shown in Table 5. ANCOVA adjusted for confounding variables found participants with intellectual disabilities without Down's syndrome engaged in significantly more total physical activity [$F(1, 146) = 10.3$, $p < .001$], MVPA [$F(1, 146) = 11.5$, $p < .001$], steps per day [$F(1, 146) = 12.4$, $p < .001$], and were significantly less sedentary [$F(1, 146) = 5.0$, $p = .027$] than participants with Down's syndrome.

Age was more strongly associated with a decrease in total physical activity ($F(1, 146) = 8.9$, $p < .001$) and MVPA ($F(1, 146) = 7.5$, $p = .001$) in those with Down's syndrome than those with intellectual disabilities without Down's syndrome adjusting for gender, level of intellectual disability, and residential setting. This suggested that age was having a more dramatic effect in those with Down's syndrome. This difference is illustrated by the fact that in contrast to those with intellectual disabilities without Down's syndrome, partial correlations adjusted for gender, level of intellectual disability, and residential setting found a statistically significant decrease with age in total physical activity [$r(74) = -.30$, $p = .010$] and MVPA [$r(74) = -.27$, $p = .019$] only for those with Down's syndrome.

Discussion

This study provides the largest published data set on objectively measured physical activity in individuals with intellectual disabilities. The procedures used in this study are consistent with standard accelerometry practices used by researchers in the UK [11] and in other countries [10], and thereby provide valuable information about the physical activity levels of individuals with intellectual disabilities in England.

Table 4. Level of intellectual disability physical activity data.

Variable	Mild (n=54)	Moderate (n=56)	Severe (n=42)
Total physical activty (counts/min)	663.0 (161.9)	615.0 (225.6)	550.6 (175.2)
Sedentary (mins/day)	607.7 (87.6)	604.9 (84.7)	630.0 (60.0)
MVPA (mins/day)	40.1 (19.0)	33.6 (17.5)	28.7 (17.0)
Steps (steps/day)	7323 (2461)	5925 (2379)	5400 (2527)*
Wear time (mins/day)	779.7 (71.8)	765.0 (75.1)	775.0 (65.0)

Data are displayed as mean and (standard deviation).
Analysis adjusted for gender, age, presence of Down's syndrome, and residential setting.
*statistically significant difference between level of intellectual disability ($p<.05$).

Principles findings of the study

Worryingly, no children or adults in the current study met current [8] or former [7] physical activity recommendations. This is lower than the 3.5% of children and 5% of adults in the general population meeting such recommendations with the exception that children and adults were engaged in slightly more MVPA per day than data presented on the general population in the 2008 Health Survey for England [11]. However, children and adults with intellectual disabilities in the current study engaged in more sedentary behaviour than children and adults in the 2008 Health Survey for England. MVPA was very sporadic with few participants managing sustained bouts which is consistent with previous research on individuals with intellectual disabilities [22]. Vigorous physical activity appeared to be non-existent in participants in this study, which is also consistent with previous research on individuals with intellectual disabilities [20,33,34].

In agreement with research from the general population [10,11,35], but in contrast with previous research involving individuals with intellectual disabilities [36,37], males were significantly more physically active than females. This difference in findings with previous intellectual disability research may be explained by methodological differences (e.g., questionnaire, interview, direct observation). Again, in agreement with previous studies from the general population [10,11] and from studies involving individuals with intellectual disabilities [36,37], physical activity decreased with age, however, for the group as a whole this was not significant after adjustment for confounding variables. This study found physical activity decreased with the level of intellectual disability, which is not surprising as it would be expected that individuals with higher ability have, in general, fewer restrictions, less need for staff supervision, and more independence to be physically active [38]. However, after adjusting for potential confounders, a significant decrease was only found in steps per day.

The striking findings of the lower physical activity levels and a marked reduction with age in individuals with Down's syndrome are extremely important. These results shed light on possible reasons why this group has consistently been found to have poorer physical fitness [5] and higher levels of obesity [6] compared to those with intellectual disabilities without Down's syndrome. This would suggest that unique age-related physiological factors maybe at play, which reduce the ability of individuals with Down's syndrome to engage in physical activity. Down's syndrome is associated with conditions that contribute to low levels of physical activity and fitness compared to those with intellectual disabilities without Down's syndrome, e.g., chronotropic incompetence, impaired autonomic function, low muscular strength, and muscle hypotonia [5,39]. We propose that a possible candidate for the above and underlying age-related pathophysiology may be that of mitochondrial dysfunction resulting in energy deficiency and oxidative stress [40,41]. Previous research has found mitochondrial dysfunction in Down's syndrome brain tissue, blood cells, fibroblasts, heart [41], and preliminary work carried out by this research group have found in vivo skeletal muscle mitochondrial dysfunction in adults with Down's syndrome.

Table 5. Physical activity data for participants with and without Down's syndrome.

Variable	ID without DS (n=73)	DS (n=79)
Total physical activty (counts/min)	687.0 (260.8)	570.1 (191.0)*
Sedentary (mins/day)	590.8 (81.0)	627.9 (82.7)*
MVPA (mins/day)	41.6 (23.0)	29.8 (15.6)*
Steps (steps/day)	7301 (3053)	5541 (2214)*
Wear time (mins/day)	751.6 (73.4)	763.0 (73.3)

Data are mean and (standard deviation).
Analysis adjusted for gender, age, level of intellectual disability, and residential setting.
*statistically significant difference between participants with and without DS ($p<.05$).

Comparison with other studies

There have only been two studies to have used the Actigraph to assess physical activity in individuals with intellectual disabilities. Frey [22] assessed 22 adults with intellectual disabilities from the USA using the Actigraph 7164 and found 28% met US physical activity recommendations [42]. Participants engaged in less MVPA (20 mins/day) but more total physical activity (602 counts/min) than this study. Caution is needed when making comparison between the two studies as the studies differ in the Actigraph model used [43], longer epoch length (one minute) [44], sample size, and the inclusion only of participants with mild intellectual disabilities in the previous study. Recently, Melville [26] presented data from a multi-component weight-loss intervention for 45 adults with intellectual disabilities and obesity from Scotland. Baseline physical activity measurement using the Actigraph GT1M found participants engaged in a similar amount of sedentary behaviour(608 mins/day) to this study but far less light physical activity (70 mins/day) and MVPA (13 mins/day). This difference in physical activity levels may be due to the fact that participants in the Melville study were selected on the basis of a BMI of greater than 30 kg/m^2.

Limitations of the study

This study has several limitations which may affect the application of these findings. Physical activity may have been underestimated as the use of a single, waist mounted, uni-axial accelerometer will not measure physical activity during upper-body and non-weight bearing activities (e.g., stereotypy, load carrying, swimming, cycling). However, few participants reported significant amounts of these activities. It is also possible that there may be differences in metabolic equivalent derived cutpoints between individuals with and without intellectual disabilities. To the authors knowledge there has been no published work exploring this issue. However, the use of Actigraph raw scores (counts/min), which are deemed by many researchers to be a more appropriate way of analysing physical activity in a field setting [45], did not change any of the results with respect to age, gender, level of intellectual disability, and Down's syndrome.

Even though all attempts were made to obtain a representative sample, there is the possibility that the participants who volunteered for this study are more active than their average peers with intellectual disabilities, and although the sample size was large for studies on individuals with intellectual disabilities, the sample size for adolescents was small due to difficulties in recruiting this group. Future studies should replicate this study using a larger sample size of adolescents with intellectual disabilities. The cross-sectional nature of results must be considered when interpreting the results of this study. Future studies with a longitudinal design, assessing changes in physical activity over time will be valuable in exploring causal relationships.

The effect of medications on physical activity was not evaluated. Further research is needed to understand the impact of medications on physical activity levels in this population as individuals with intellectual disabilities are prescribed higher amounts of medication compared to the general population [46]. Physical activity is known to show seasonal variation [47] and such variation was not investigated for this study. Examination of seasonal variation in physical activity among individuals with intellectual disabilities may help identify individual and environmental factors that may be targets of tailored strategies to enhance participation.

Conclusions and clinical implications

In recent decades, individuals with intellectual disabilities have experienced many advances in education, work, living arrangements, and human rights [12,13]. Despite these developments, they experience significant health inequalities [3,4] with increased rates of morbidity [1] and mortality [2]. Worryingly, in the current study there were no children or adults that achieved the recommended amount of physical activity for health. Individuals who do not engage in the recommended levels of physical activity present higher rates of mortality and higher incidence rates of many chronic diseases [7–9]. The findings of this study suggest that individuals with intellectual disabilities, especially those with Down's syndrome, may be at risk of developing diseases associated with physical inactivity.

The major epidemiological studies [10,11] and health promotion strategies [14] that have been completed over the last ten years demonstrating the enormous benefit to health derived from physical activity have not included individuals with intellectual disabilities in their designs. This is a group who may be dependent on others for support and whose activities and lifestyle are significantly under the influence of others [48]. There is a need for well-designed, accessible, preventive health promotion strategies and interventions designed to raise the levels of physical activity for individuals with intellectual disabilities which take into account the unique barriers to physical activity this group faces [49,50].

Acknowledgments

We thank all the participants who took part in the study, and to the support workers and parents for supporting the participants during the study. We are grateful to the above and to the care home managers, schools, the Down's Syndrome Association, and voluntary organisations for their help with recruiting participants. Finally we thank Dan Gordon for his comments during the design phase of the study, Dr Peter Watson for his help in reviewing the statistical analysis included in this paper, and to Carys Banks for critically reviewing the manuscript.

Author Contributions

Conceived and designed the experiments: ACP AJH. Performed the experiments: ACP. Analyzed the data: ACP AJH. Wrote the paper: ACP AJH.

References

1. Beange H, McElduff A, Baker W (1995) Medical disorders of adults with mental retardation: A population study. Am J Ment Retard 99: 595–604.
2. Hollins S, Attard MT, von Fraunhofer N, McGuigan S, Sedgwick P (1998) Mortality in people with learning disability: Risks, causes, and death certification findings in London. Dev Med Child Neurol 40: 50–56.
3. Cooper SA, Melville C, Morrison J (2004) People with intellectual disabilities. BMJ 329: 414–415.
4. Michael J (2008) Healthcare for all: Report of the independent inquiry into access to healthcare for people with learning disabilities. London: DoH.
5. Fernhall B, Pitetti KH (2001) Limitations to physical work capacity in individuals with mental retardation. Clin Exer Physiol 3: 176–185.
6. Melville CA, Hamilton S, Hankey CR, Miller S, Boyle S (2007) The prevalence and determinants of obesity in adults with intellectual disabilities. Obes Rev 8: 223–230.
7. Department of Health (2004) At least five a week: Evidence on the impact of physical activity and its relationship to health. London: DoH.
8. Department of Health (2011) Stay active, stay active: A report on physical activity from the four home countries' Chief Medical Officers. London: DoH.
9. Bauman AE (2004) Updating the evidence that physical activity is good for health: An epidemiological review 2000–2003. J Sci Med Sport 7: 6–19.
10. Troiano RP, Berrigan D, Dodd KW, Masse LC, Tilert T, et al. (2008) Physical activity in the United States measured by accelerometer. Med Sci Sports Exerc 40: 181–188.
11. NHS Information Centre for Health and Social Care (2009) Health survey for England 2008: Physical activity and fitness. London: NHS Information Centre for Health and Social Care.
12. Department of Health (2001) Valuing people: A new strategy for learning disability for the 21st century. London: DoH.
13. Department of Health (2009) Valuing people now: A new three-year strategy for learning disabilities. London: DoH.
14. Department of Health (2009) Change4Life: Eat well, move more, live longer. London: DoH.
15. Frey GC, Stanish HI, Temple VA (2008) Physical activity of youth with intellectual disability: Review and research agenda. Adapt Phys Activ Q 25: 95–117.
16. Temple VA, Frey GC, Stanish HI (2006) Physical activity of adults with mental retardation: Review and research needs. Am J Health Promot 21: 2–12.
17. Shephard RJ (2003) Limits to the measurement of habitual physical activity by questionnaires. Br J Sports Med 37: 197–206.
18. Eston RG, Rowlands AV, Ingledew DK (1998) Validity of heart rate, pedometry, and accelerometry for predicting the energy cost of children's activities. J Appl Physiol 84: 362–371.
19. Temple VA, Anderson C, Walkley JW (2000) Physical activity levels of individuals living in a group home. J Intellect Dev Disabil 25: 327–341.
20. Temple VA, Walkley JW (2003) Physical activity levels of adults with intellectual disability. J Intellect Dev Disabil 28: 342–352.
21. Kozub FM (2003) Explaining physical activity in individuals with mental retardation: An exploratory study. Education and Training in Developmental Disabilities 38: 302–313.
22. Frey GC (2004) Comparison of physical activity levels between adults with and without mental retardation. J Phys Act Health 1: 235–245.
23. Whitt-Glover MC, O'Neill KL, Stettler N (2006) Physical activity patterns in children with and without Down syndrome. Pediatr Rehabil 9: 158–164.
24. Foley JT, Bryan RR, McCubbin JA (2008) Daily physical activity levels of elementary school-aged children with and without mental retardation. J Dev Phys Disabil 20: 365–378.

25. Shields N, Dodd KJ, Abblitt C (2009) Do children with Down syndrome perform sufficient physical activity to maintain good health? A pilot study. Adapt Phys Activ Q 26: 307–320.
26. Melville CA, Boyle S, Miller S, Macmillan S, Penpraze V, et al. (2011) An open study of the effectiveness of a multi-component weight-loss intervention for adults with intellectual disabilities and obesity. Br J Nutr 105: 1553–1562.
27. Tyrer F, McGrother CW, Thorp CF, Taub NA, Bhaumik S, et al. (2008) The Leicestershire Intellectual Disability Tool: A simple measure to identify moderate to profound intellectual disability. Journal of Applied Research in Intellectual Disabilities 21: 268–276.
28. Sparrow S, Cichetti DV, Balla DA (2005) Vineland adaptive behavior scale. 2nd ed. Circle PinesMN: American Guidance Service.
29. International Society for the Advancement of Kinanthropometry (2006) International standards for the anthropometric assessment. Potchefstroom, South Africa: International Society for the Advancement of Kinanthropometry.
30. Cole TJ, Flegal KM, Nicholls D, Jackson AA (2007) Body mass index cut offs to define thinness in children and adolescents: International survey. BMJ 335: 194–197.
31. Cole TJ, Bellizzi MC, Flegal KM, Dietz WH (2000) Establishing a standard definition for child overweight and obesity worldwide: International survey. BMJ 320: 1240–1243.
32. World Health Organization (1995) Physical status: The use and interpretation of anthropometry. Report of a WHO Expert Consultation. WHO Technical Report Series Number 854. Geneva: World Health Organization.
33. Draheim CC, Williams DP, McCubbin JA (2002) Prevalence of physical inactivity and recommended physical activity in community-based adults with mental retardation. Ment Retard 40: 436–444.
34. Stanish HI, Draheim CC (2005) Assessment of walking activity using a pedometer and survey in adults with mental retardation. Adapt Phys Activ Q 22: 136–145.
35. Trost SG, Owen N, Bauman AE, Sallis JF, Brown W (2002) Correlates of adults' participation in physical activity: Review and update. Med Sci Sports Exerc 34: 1996–2001.
36. Stanish HI, Temple VA, Frey GC (2006) Health-promoting physical activity of adults with mental retardation. Ment Retard Dev Disabil Res Rev 12: 13–21.
37. Finlayson J, Jackson A, Cooper SA, Morrison J, Melville C, et al. (2009) Understanding predictors of low physical activity in adults with intellectual disabilities. Journal of Applied Research in Intellectual Disabilities 22: 236–247.
38. Peterson JJ, Janz KF, Lowe JB (2008) Physical activity among adults with intellectual disabilities living in community settings. Prev Med 47: 101–106.
39. Mendonca GV, Pereira FD, Fernhall B (2010) Reduced exercise capacity in persons with Down syndrome: Cause, effect, and management. Ther Clin Risk Manag 6: 601–610.
40. Arbuzova S, Hutchin T, Cuckle H (2002) Mitochondrial dysfunction and Down's syndrome. Bioessays 24: 681–684.
41. Pallardo FV, Lloret A, Lebel M, d'Ischia M, Cogger VC, et al. (2010) Mitochondrial dysfunction in some oxidative stress-related genetic diseases: Ataxia-Telangiectasia, Down Syndrome, Fanconi Anaemia and Werner Syndrome. Biogerontology 11: 401–419.
42. US Department of Health and Human Services (1996) Physical activity and health: a report from the Surgeon General. Washington, DC: US Government Printing Office.
43. Thompson D, Batterham AM, Markovitch D, Dixon NC, Lund AJ, et al. (2009) Confusion and conflict in assessing the physical activity status of middle-aged men. PloS One 4: e4337.
44. Rothney MP, Apker GA, Song Y, Chen KY (2008) Comparing the performance of three generations of Actigraph accelerometer. J Appl Physiol 105: 1091–1097.
45. Freedson PS, Pober D, Janz KF (2005) Calibration of accelerometer output for children. Med Sci Sports Exerc 37: S523–530.
46. Straetmans JM, van Schrojenstein Lantman-de Valk HM, Schellevis FG, Dinant GJ (2007) Health problems of people with intellectual disabilities: The impact for general practice. Br J Gen Pract 57: 64–66.
47. Shephard RJ, Aoyagi Y (2009) Seasonal variations in physical activity and implications for human health. Eur J Appl Physiol 107: 251–271.
48. Dunn MC, Clare IC, Holland AJ (2010) Living 'a life like ours': Accounts of substitute decision-making in residential care home for adults with intellectual disabilities. J Intellect Disabil Res 54: 144–160.
49. Messent PR, Cooke CB, Long J (1999) Primary and secondary barriers to physically active healthy lifestyles for adults with learning disabilities. Disabil Rehabil 21: 409–419.
50. Messent PR, Cooke CB, Long J (2000) Secondary barriers to physical activity for adults with mild and moderate learning disabilities. J Learn Disabil 4: 247–263.

8

Model-Based Analysis of Costs and Outcomes of Non-Invasive Prenatal Testing for Down's Syndrome Using Cell Free Fetal DNA in the UK National Health Service

Stephen Morris[1]*, Saffron Karlsen[1], Nancy Chung[2], Melissa Hill[3,4], Lyn S. Chitty[3,4]

1 Department of Applied Health Research, University College London, London, United Kingdom, **2** NHS Fetal Anomaly Screening Programme, University of Exeter, Exeter, United Kingdom, **3** Clinical and Molecular Genetics Unit, UCL Institute of Child Health and Great Ormond Street Hospital for Children NHS Foundation Trust, London, United Kingdom, **4** Fetal Medicine Unit, University College London Hospitals NHS Foundation Trust, London, United Kingdom

Abstract

Background: Non-invasive prenatal testing (NIPT) for Down's syndrome (DS) using cell free fetal DNA in maternal blood has the potential to dramatically alter the way prenatal screening and diagnosis is delivered. Before NIPT can be implemented into routine practice, information is required on its costs and benefits. We investigated the costs and outcomes of NIPT for DS as contingent testing and as first-line testing compared with the current DS screening programme in the UK National Health Service.

Methods: We used a pre-existing model to evaluate the costs and outcomes associated with NIPT compared with the current DS screening programme. The analysis was based on a hypothetical screening population of 10,000 pregnant women. Model inputs were taken from published sources. The main outcome measures were number of DS cases detected, number of procedure-related miscarriages and total cost.

Results: At a screening risk cut-off of 1:150 NIPT as contingent testing detects slightly fewer DS cases, has fewer procedure-related miscarriages, and costs the same as current DS screening (around UK£280,000) at a cost of £500 per NIPT. As first-line testing NIPT detects more DS cases, has fewer procedure-related miscarriages, and is more expensive than current screening at a cost of £50 per NIPT. When NIPT uptake increases, NIPT detects more DS cases with a small increase in procedure-related miscarriages and costs.

Conclusions: NIPT is currently available in the private sector in the UK at a price of £400-£900. If the NHS cost was at the lower end of this range then at a screening risk cut-off of 1:150 NIPT as contingent testing would be cost neutral or cost saving compared with current DS screening. As first-line testing NIPT is likely to produce more favourable outcomes but at greater cost. Further research is needed to evaluate NIPT under real world conditions.

Editor: Reiner A. Veitia, Institut Jacques Monod, France

Funding: This study was funded by the National Institute for Health Research (NIHR) under its Programme Grants for Applied Research scheme (the "RAPID" project; RP-PG-0707-10107), the Central and East London NIHR Comprehensive Local Research Network, the Great Ormond Street Hospital Children's Charity and the NIHR Biomedical Research Centre at Great Ormond Street Hospital. The views expressed are those of the authors and not necessarily those of the NHS, the NIHR or the Department of Health. The funders had no role in study design, data collection and analysis, decision to publish, or preparation of the manuscript.

Competing Interests: The authors have declared that no competing interests exist.

* E-mail: steve.morris@ucl.ac.uk

Introduction

In the UK the National Screening Committee (NSC) sets the standards for antenatal screening and recommends that all pregnant women are offered Down's syndrome (DS) screening. Ideally this is the combined screening test performed between 11 and 14 weeks gestation. In current National Health Service (NHS) practice this has a detection rate of around 85% and a screen postive rate around 2.5% [1]. Women with a risk of 1:150 or greater of the baby having DS are offered an invasive diagnostic test (chorionic villus sampling (CVS) or amniocentesis), providing definitive diagnosis as to whether or not the baby has DS. If full karyotyping or microarray analysis is performed other chromosomal abnormalities may be detected.

Current invasive diagnostic tests have a risk of miscarriage of 0.5–1% [2]. The discovery of cell free fetal DNA (cffDNA) in maternal blood [3] has led to safer non-invasive approaches to prenatal testing where aneuploidies are detected via a maternal blood test from 10 weeks gestation [4]. Several large-scale validity studies have been conducted to evaluate non-invasive prenatal testing (NIPT) for DS based on next generation sequencing [5–12]. Detection rates for DS are typically greater than 99% with a false positive rate of 0.1–1%. NIPT can also detect other aneuploidies including trisomy 18 (99% accurate) and trisomy 13 (up to 90% accurate) [9–12]. The small false positive rate for DS means NIPT should be confirmed by invasive testing [13–15]. NIPT for DS as well as trisomy 18 and 13 is now offered through commercial providers in several countries including the USA,

Germany, Hong Kong and China. It is also available in the private sector in the UK, with prices varying from £400–£900 [16] and samples being sent for testing overseas.

In publicly funded health care systems like the UK NHS, NIPT for DS has the potential to dramatically alter the way prenatal screening and diagnosis is delivered. Before NIPT can be implemented into routine practice, further information is required to identify where it fits in the screening pathway, based on the likely costs and benefits. Several studies have investigated costs and benefits of NIPT for DS using cell free fetal DNA in maternal blood [6,17–21] but there is no evidence that is directly relevant to the UK NHS. Palomaki et al [6] calculated the costs and outcomes of NIPT as contingent testing for DS in the USA. In 100,000 women at high risk for DS, they calculated that invasive testing alone would detect 3,000 DS cases and cost US$100 million with 500 procedure-related losses. NIPT followed by invasive testing in those with positive results would detect 2,958 DS cases at cost of US$3.9 million and 20 procedure-related losses. The authors assumed 100% uptake of NIPT and invasive testing and did not include the cost of NIPT.

Wald and Bestwick [17] investigated the costs and outcomes of a protocol combining DS screening and NIPT, where women at highest risk for DS following screening receive NIPT. Results are presented for different assumptions about the cost of NIPT and the proportion of women eligible for NIPT. The analysis did not include costs and outcomes associated with invasive diagnostic testing.

Garfield and Armstrong [18] assessed the costs and outcomes of NIPT as contingent testing for trisomies 13, 18 and 21 in the USA. In a hypothetical cohort of 100,000 pregnancies they calculated that NIPT as contingent testing reduces the number of procedure-related fetal losses from 60 to 20, increases the number of DS cases detected from 148 to 170, and reduces prenatal testing costs by 1%. They calculated that NIPT as contingent testing is likely to be cost saving at a price of up to US$1,200 per test.

Song et al [19] assessed the cost-effectiveness of NIPT for DS in the USA, comparing first trimester combined screening, integrated screening and NIPT (without conventional screening in women aged 35 years or more, and following a positive screening result in women younger than 35 years). At a cost of US$795, NIPT dominated the other strategies, detecting more DS cases, with fewer procedure-related miscarriages and lower costs. The cost savings were mainly due to reductions in the costs of managing DS during the first five years of life. The authors did not include the medical costs associated with unaffected children during their first five years of life.

Ohno and Caughey [20] analysed the cost-effectiveness of NIPT as contingent testing versus NIPT as a diagnostic test that did not require confirmatory invasive diagnostic testing in the USA. Making assumptions about the quality adjusted life expectancy beyond pregnancy from testing, they concluded that NIPT as contingent testing was cost-effective. The analysis did not compare NIPT versus current practice, so it was not possible to determine if NIPT ought to be adopted.

Cuckle et al [21] investigated factors affecting the cost of avoiding a DS birth using either universal NIPT or NIPT as contingent testing versus conventional screening in the USA. They found that unit costs of NIPT and uptake of NIPT were important factors affecting cost-effectiveness. The high cost of NIPT (US$500-2000 compared with US$150 for the Combined test) meant that universal NIPT was unlikely to be cost-effective.

Our aim was to assess the costs and outcomes of NIPT for DS as contingent testing and as first-line testing compared with the current DS screening programme in the UK NHS. We find that NIPT as contingent testing can produce favourable outcomes at the same cost compared with current DS screening. As first-line testing NIPT is likely to produce more favourable outcomes but at greater cost.

Materials and Methods

Ethics Statement

Data used to populate the model were obtained from publicly available sources listed in Table 1. All the data were group averages taken from multiple previously published sources, based on patient data that were de-identified prior to being used in our study. Hence, ethical approval was not required.

Including NIPT in the DS Screening Pathway

We evaluate two approaches to introducing NIPT into the current DS screening pathway. For current DS screening in the UK, the components most relevant for this study are that all pregnant women are offered DS screening and those who are high risk are offered an invasive test (Figure 1, Figure S1 in Supporting Information). The first alternative we consider is with NIPT as contingent testing. In this case, all pregnant women are offered DS screening as before and those with a risk from DS screening above a pre-specified level are offered NIPT rather than an invasive test (Figure 2, Figure S2 in Supporting Information). Invasive testing is then offered to those with abnormal NIPT results. The second alternative is with NIPT as first-line testing, replacing the current DS screening programme (Figure 3). In this case women are not offered DS screening, but are offered NIPT instead and invasive testing is offered to those with abnormal NIPT results. We focused on DS, and did not consider NIPT for trisomies 18 and 13 as DS is the focus of the National Screening Programme.

Overview of Modelling Approach

The Decision Planning Tool (DPT) is a complex publicly available decision analytic model developed, using Microsoft Excel 1997–2003, by the Peninsula Technology Assessment Group (PenTAG) [22]. It was commissioned by the NHS Fetal Anomaly Screening Programme (FASP), with partial funding from the Knowledge Transfer Partnership (KTP), as a health economic model to support decision-makers and commissioners when assessing the costs and effects of DS screening. The model was developed to include a decision tree structure for six DS screening strategies used within the NHS (double, triple, quadruple, combined, serum integrated and integrated tests) following nationally agreed standards and pathways provided by the NHS FASP. With permission, we amended the DPT to include NIPT as contingent testing and first-line testing. The DPT uses a range of published and publically available national data on the UK costs and estimated prevalence of DS in the UK population as well as the costs of different aspects of DS screening and diagnostic provision. It was specifically designed to assess the costs and benefits of different DS screening tests. For this study, we assumed that all women screened during the first trimester receive the combined test (comprising nuchal translucent measurement combined with analysis of Pregnancy-associated plasma protein-A (PAPP-A) and Free beta-human chorionic gonadotrophin (β-hCG)), and all screened during the second trimester received the quadruple test (Alphafetoprotein (AFP), Free β-hCG or Total hCG, unconjugated oestrial (uE3), and Inhibin-A), since these are recommended tests in the UK [23]. The conclusions do not change when other screening tests are used instead. All stages of the DS screening pathways described in the Figures are accounted for in the adapted DPT model. The perspective was the National

Table 1. Key model inputs.

Parameter	Value	Source/reference
Outcomes		
Maternal age (%)	0.0024–0.0165 by year of maternal age from ≤13 years to ≥50 years	[24]
Prevalence of Down's syndrome (%)	0.1–2.6 by gestational week and maternal age	[25]
Screening late arrivals (%)	15	[1]
Screening uptake (%)	69	[26]
Screening test performance (DR [%]; FPR [%])		
Combined test with screening risk cut-off of 1 in		
150	85.0; 2.5	[27]
500	94.0; 7.0	
1000	96.0; 12.0	
2000	98.0; 19.0	
Quadruple free β-hCG test	80.5; 4.0	[28]
Weekly spontaneous fetal loss (%)		
DS affected pregnancies	0.5–7.1 by gestational week	[29]
Unaffected pregnancies	0.04–0.07 by maternal age	[30]
NT measurement failures (%)	14–19 by gestational week	[31]
Invasive diagnostic test uptake (%)		
Unaffected pregnancies	80	[32]
DS pregnancies	90	[32]
Invasive diagnostic test performance (DR [%]; sample failure rate [%]; procedural miscarriage rate [%])		
CVS/QF-PCR	100; 1.3; 0.5	[33], [30], [33]
Amniocentesis/full karyotyping	100; 0.8; 0.5	[33], [30], [33]
TOP uptake (%)	92.1	[34]
Live birth outcomes (%)		
Vaginal live birth	75.2	[35]
Caesarean live birth	24.8	[35]
Costs		
Costs of screening		
Combined test	27	[22]
Quadruple free β-hCG test	35	[22]
Cost invasive diagnostic test (£)		
CVS/QF-PCR	479	[36]
Amniocentesis/full karyotyping	479	[36]
Cost fetal loss (£)		
Spontaneous	511	[36]
Due to CVS or amniocentesis	511	[36]
Cost TOP (£)		
First trimester	697	[36]
Second trimester	882	[36]
Cost live birth outcomes (£)		
Vaginal live birth	1,341	[36]
Caesarean live birth	2,436	[36]
NIPT		
Uptake of NIPT (%)		
As contingent testing		
Base case		
Unaffected pregnancies	80	Assumption**
DS pregnancies	90	Assumption**

Table 1. Cont.

Parameter	Value	Source/reference
Alternative scenario	100*	Assumption
Alternative scenario	100*, uptake of screening increase from 69% to 79%	Assumption
As first-line screening		
Base case	69	Assumption***
Alternative scenario	79	Assumption
NIPT performance (DR [%]; FPR [%]; sample failure rate [%]; procedural miscarriage rate [%])	99; 1; 5; 0	Assumption based on Table 2
Cost of NIPT	50, 250, 500, 750	Assumption
Cost of taking blood sample	3	[36]

*For both unaffected and DS affected pregnancies.
**As for invasive diagnostic tests.
***As for DS screening. DS = Down's syndrome; NT = nuchal translucency; CVS = chorionic villus sampling; QF-PCR = Quantitative Fluorescence Polymerase Chain Reaction; TOP = termination of pregnancy; DR = detection rate; FPR = false positive rate

DS screening programme in the NHS in the UK. The time horizon over which costs and outcomes are measured is the duration of pregnancy; discounting is therefore unnecessary. As in the DPT, costs are calculated in 2011/12 UK£, inflated from reported values where appropriate.

Model Inputs

All model inputs, except those for NIPT, for DS screening test performance at different risk cut-offs, and procedural miscarriage rates for invasive diagnostic tests, are as used in the original DPT model and taken from published sources [1], [22], [24–36] (Table 1). The screening population is representative of the screening population of England. Maternal age distributions are from the Office for National Statistics' annual maternity statistics [24]. The underlying prevalence of DS varied by maternal age and gestational ages [25].

Eighty-five per cent of women were offered DS screening during the first trimester using the combined test; 15% were booked after 14 weeks' gestation and were offered screening in the second trimester with the quadruple test [1]. The uptake rate for both tests was 69% [26].

The detection rate (DR) and false positive rate (FPR) for the combined test were based on different screening risk cut-offs from 1:150 to 1:2000 [27]. We used the 1:150 risk cut-off to evaluate the

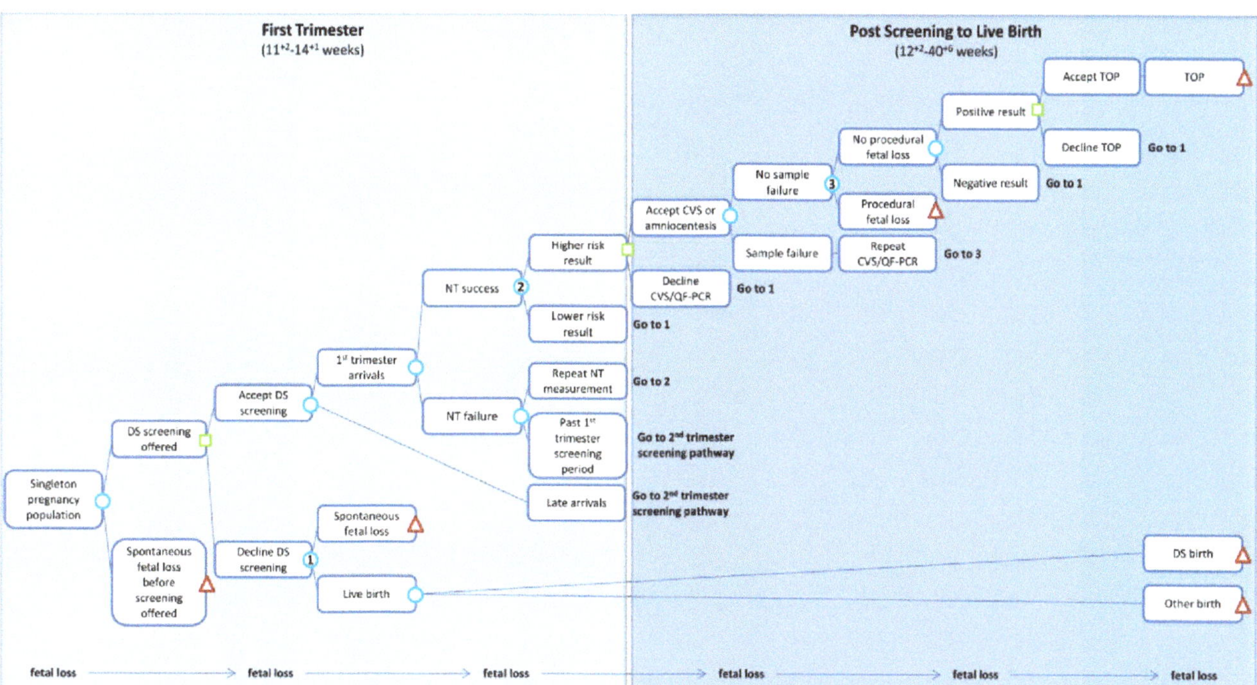

Figure 1 First trimester screening pathway: current DS screening. DS = Down's syndrome; NT = nuchal translucency; CVS = chorionic villus sampling; QF-PCR = Quantitative Fluorescence Polymerase Chain Reaction; TOP = termination of pregnancy. See Figure S1 in Supporting Information for the second trimester screening pathway.

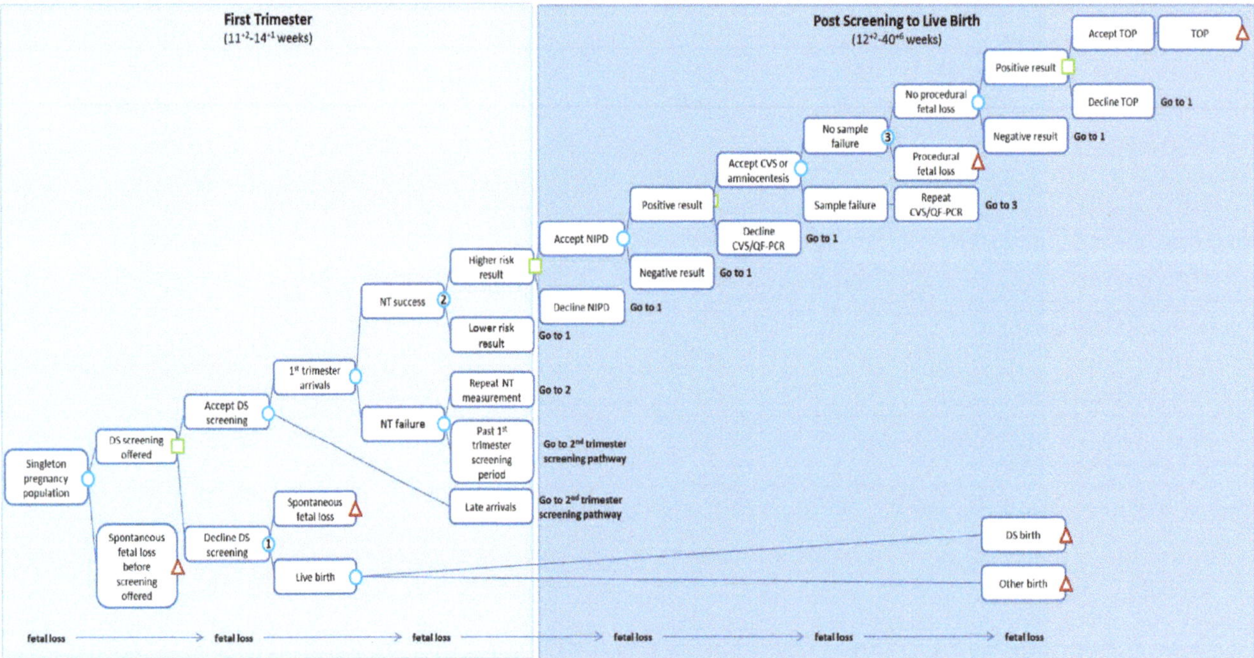

Figure 2 First trimester screening pathway: NIPT as contingent testing. DS = Down's syndrome; NT = nuchal translucency; NIPT = non-invasive prenatal testing; CVS = chorionic villus sampling; QF-PCR = Quantitative Fluorescence Polymerase Chain Reaction; TOP = termination of pregnancy. See Figure S2 in Supporting Information for the second trimester screening pathway.

costs and outcomes associated with current DS screening, and we evaluated NIPT as contingent testing using different screening risk cut-offs from 1:150 to 1:2000. The DR and FPR for the quadruple test were 80.5% and 4%, respectively [28].

CVS (amniocentesis) uptake is the proportion of women who accept a first trimester (second trimester) invasive prenatal diagnostic investigation after receiving a high risk screening result. Evidence suggests that for both tests the uptake is 80% for

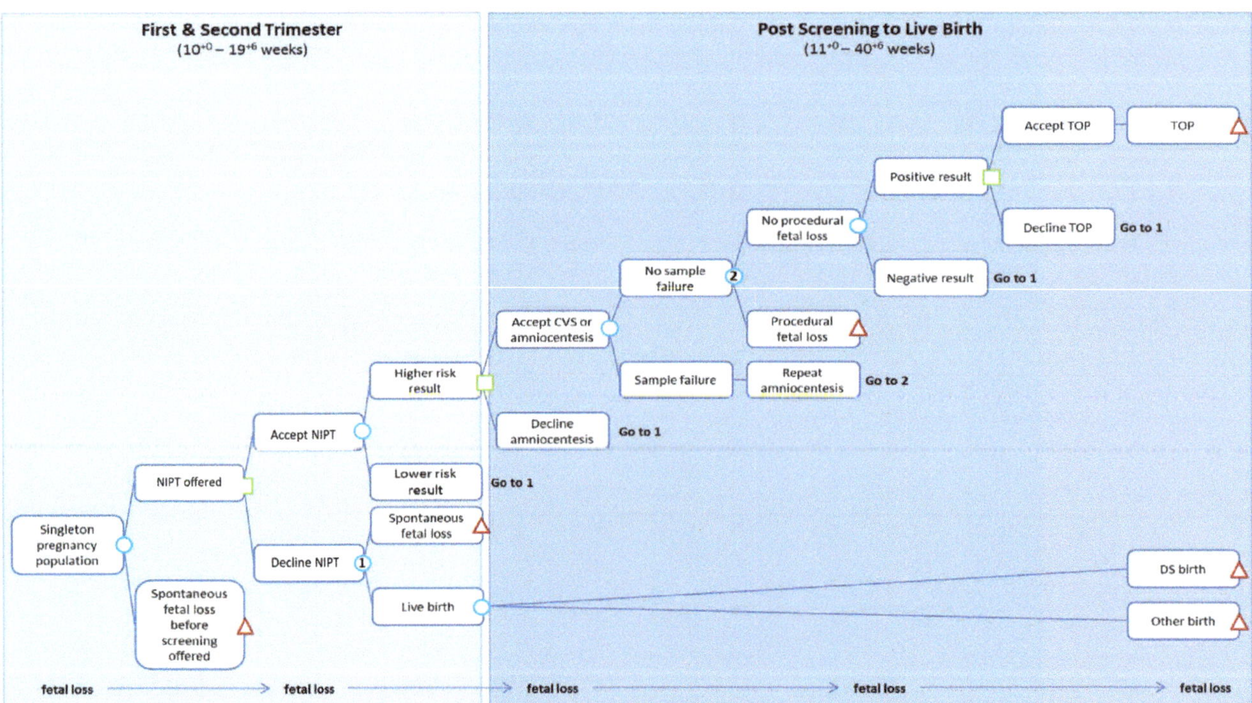

Figure 3 NIPT as first-line testing. DS = Down's syndrome; NT = nuchal translucency; NIPT = non-invasive prenatal testing; CVS = chorionic villus sampling; QF-PCR = Quantitative Fluorescence Polymerase Chain Reaction; TOP = termination of pregnancy.

unaffected pregnancies and 90% for DS affected pregnancies [32]. We use these values in the model of current screening and also, in the absence of data, for uptake of invasive diagnostic testing after NIPT. Values for invasive test detection rates and sample failure rates were taken from published figures [30,33]. The original DPT assumes procedural miscarriage rates of 1% for amniocentesis and 2% for CVS. Based on a recent review [2], which found rates of 0.5–1% for both types of test, we assumed a procedural miscarriage rate for CVS and amniocentesis of 0.5%.

The probability of weekly spontaneous fetal loss for unaffected pregnancies was assumed to be 0.0012 during gestational weeks 10 to 25 and 0.00034 during weeks 26 to 40 [30]. For DS affected pregnancies, it was 0.07067 in weeks 10 to 15 and 0.0051 in weeks 16 to 40 [29]. Termination of pregnancy (TOP) uptake is the proportion of women who accept to terminate their pregnancy after receiving a positive diagnosis for DS and is estimated to be 92.1% [34]. Information on the proportion of women who have a vaginal or caesarean delivery is derived from annual maternity services data [35].

The unit costs of the combined test and the quadruple test were £27 and £35, respectively, including staffing, administration, equipment, overheads, delivery of low risk results via 2nd class mail and high risk results via telephone. The weighted unit cost per CVS/QF-PCR and amniocentesis/full karyotype is estimated to be £479 for each test [36]. The unit cost for spontaneous fetal loss and fetal loss due to an invasive diagnostic procedure are both estimated as £511. The unit cost of TOP was assumed to be £697 in the first trimester and £882 in the second trimester. Unit costs for live birth outcomes were £1,341 for vaginal live birth and £2,436 for caesarean live birth.

A number of studies have reported values for the sensitivity and specificity of NIPT [5–12], with values ranging from 98.6%–100% and 99.7–100%, respectively, and combined values of 99.33% and 99.94%, respectively (Table 2). There were few false negatives, and these occurred in the larger whole genome sequencing studies. We assumed a DR and FPR for NIPT of 99% and 1%, respectively. The sample failure rate for the NIPT was assumed to be 5%. We assumed that when sample failure occurred the cost of another NIPT was incurred; sample failure with NIPT was assumed not to occur more than once in each pregnancy. The procedural fetal loss rate associated with NIPT was 0%. There is limited evidence from the UK to suggest that uptake rate of NIPT in a general DS screening population is higher than current testing [37], a view supported by some small studies of women undergoing NIPT for aneuploidy in the USA [38], but this is currently unproven under real world conditions. For NIPT as contingent screening, we therefore assumed in the base case that uptake of NIPT would be the same as for invasive testing in the current DS screening programme (80% for unaffected pregnancies and 90% for DS affected pregnancies). We also investigated what happened when the NIPT uptake rate increased to 100% and when it increased to 100% with a ten percentage point increase in the uptake of DS screening (69% to 79%). For NIPT as firs- line testing we assumed in the base case that uptake of NIPT would be the same as for DS screening (69%). We also investigated what happened when NIPT uptake increased to 79%. Since NIPT is currently not available via the NHS the actual cost of NIPT is unknown. We therefore used a range of values and present results for costs of NIPT of £50, £250, £500 and £750 per test. In the private sector in the UK, prices for NIPT vary from £400–£900. Figures using a value of £500 are presented, since this represents a threshold value in our results; we do not present results using cost greater than £750 since NIPT is not cost effective above this level; values of £50 and £250 are used to illustrate the cost implications if NIPT costs were to fall substantially beyond current levels in the private sector. We assumed that samples for NIPT were collected at the same time that blood samples for DS screening were collected, and therefore no additional sampling costs were incurred. We also examined an alternative scenario in which women at high risk following DS screening are asked for an additional blood sample for NIPT.

Outcome Measures

Results are reported for a hypothetical screening population of 10,000 pregnant women who are representative of the screening population of England. The main outcomes are the number of DS cases detected, the number of procedure-related miscarriages and the combined cost of screening, NIPT and invasive diagnostic tests. The cost of screening includes the cost of the screening test (combined test in the first trimester, quadruple test in the second trimester), the cost of repeat nuchal translucency measurements and the cost of delivering the screening test results. We also report the number of women undergoing screening, the number undergoing NIPT, the number with a positive NIPT result, the number having an invasive diagnostic test, the cost of screening, the cost of NIPT, and the cost of invasive diagnostic tests. We report each measure by screening risk cut-off and cost per NIPT test, and separately for different scenarios of NIPT uptake. We also report the costs of each strategy including the costs of pregnancy outcomes.

Results

In the current DS screening programme using a screening risk cut-off of 1:150, 6,882 pregnant women would undergo DS screening, 161 would have an invasive diagnostic test, there would be around one procedure-related miscarriage and 13 DS cases detected (Table 3). The total cost would be £279,000 (Table 4). Under base case assumptions concerning NIPT uptake, with NIPT as contingent testing and at a screening risk cut-off of 1:150, 6,882 women would undergo DS screening, 154 would undergo NIPT, 13 would have a positive NIPT result, 11 would have a diagnostic test, there would be fewer than one procedure-related miscarriage and 11 DS cases would be detected. The total cost would be £213,000-£322,000 depending on the cost of NIPT. At a screening risk cut-off of 1:150 NIPT as contingent testing results in fewer procedure-related miscarriages (due to fewer invasive diagnostic tests), slightly fewer DS cases being detected (due to the number of women who are high risk according to NIPT but choose not to have an invasive diagnostic test); and, it costs around the same as current DS screening if the cost per NIPT is £500.

If the screening risk cut-off for NIPT was lowered to 1:500, 1:1000 or 1:2000 there is an increase in the number undergoing NIPT, the number with a positive NIPT result, the number having a diagnostic test, the number of procedure-related miscarriages and the number of DS cases detected. Costs increase such that with a screening risk cut-off of 1:2000 contingent testing with NIPT costs slightly less than current screening if the cost per NIPT is only £50.

With NIPT as first-line screening, 6,882 would undergo NIPT, 28 would have a positive NIPT result, 22 would have an invasive diagnostic test, there would be less than one procedure-related miscarriage and 16 DS cases would be detected. The total cost would be £449,000–£5,266,000 depending on the cost of NIPT. Hence NIPT as first-line screening results in fewer procedure-related miscarriages (due to the lower numbers of invasive diagnostic tests), more DS cases being detected (due to the greater accuracy of NIPT as compared with DS screening as first-line

Table 2. Sensitivity and specificity of NIPT for Down's syndrome: results from eight studies.

	Sequencing approach	Test results				Sensitivity		Specificity	
		TP	FN	TN	FP	%	95% CI (%)	%	95% CI (%)
Enrich et al 2011 [5]	Whole genome	39	0	410	1	100	89–100	99.7	98.5–99.9
Palomaki et al 2011 [6]	Whole genome	212	3	1471	3	98.6	98.6–99.5	99.8	99.4–99.9
Bianchi et al 2012 [7]	Whole genome	89	0	404	0	100	95.9–100	100	99.1–100
Ashoor et al 2012 [8]	Targeted	50	0	297	0	100	92.1–100	100	98.7–100
Sparks et al 2012* [9]	Targeted	36	0	123	0	100	90.4–100	100	97.0–100
Norton et al 2012 [10]	Targeted	81	0	2888	1	100	95.5–99.65	99.97	99.8–99.99
Futch et al 2013 [11]	Whole genome	154	2	5515	1	98.72	95.45–99.65	99.98	99.9–100
Liang et al 2013 [12]	Whole genome	40	0	372	0	100	91.24–100	100	98.98–100
Merged data		736	5	11601	6	99.33	98.43–99.71	99.94	99.88–99.97

*Calculated using the Fetal-fraction Optimized Risk of Trisomy Evaluation (FORTE) algorithm. TP = number of true positive results; FN = number of false negative results; TN = number of true negative results; FP = number of false positive result.

Table 3. Outcomes of testing strategies in a screening population of 10,000 pregnant women.

Testing strategy	Screening risk cut-off (1 in)	Number undergoing screening	Number undergoing NIPT	Number with a positive NIPT result	Number having an invasive diagnostic test	Number of procedure-related miscarriages	Number of DS cases detected
DS screening using the combined test	150s	6,881.66	0		160.59	0.80	13.24
NIPT as contingent testing	150	6,881.66	153.75	13.30	11.48	0.06	11.26
	500	6,881.66	361.43	14.75	12.71	0.06	12.31
	1,000	6,881.66	591.02	15.26	13.13	0.07	12.55
	2,000	6,881.66	912.32	15.85	13.63	0.07	12.78
NIPT as first-line screening		0	6,881.66	28.02	22.03	0.11	16.49

69% uptake of DS screening using the combined test. 80% uptake of NIPT as contingent screening for unaffected pregnancies and 90% for affected pregnancies. 69% uptake of NIPT as first-line screening.
DS = Down's Syndrome; NIPT = non-invasive prenatal testing.

Table 4. Costs of testing strategies in a screening population of 10,000 pregnant women.

Testing strategy	Screening risk cut-off (1 in)	Cost per NIPT test	(A) Cost of screening (£000s)	(B) Cost of NIPT (£000s)	(C) Cost of invasive diagnostic tests (£000s)*	(A)+ (B)+ (C) (£000s)
DS screening using the combined test	150		200	0	79	279
NIPT as contingent testing	150	£50	200	8	6	213
	150	£250	200	39	6	244
	150	£500	200	78	6	283
	150	£750	200	116	6	322
	500	£50	200	18	6	225
	500	£250	200	91	6	298
	500	£500	200	183	6	389
	500	£750	200	274	6	480
	1,000	£50	200	30	6	237
	1,000	£250	200	149	6	356
	1,000	£500	200	298	6	505
	1,000	£750	200	448	6	655
	2,000	£50	200	46	7	253
	2,000	£250	200	230	7	438
	2,000	£500	200	461	7	668
	2,000	£750	200	691	7	898
NIPT as first-line screening		£50	0	438	11	449
		£250	0	1,642	11	1,825
		£500	0	3,535	11	3,546
		£750	0	5,255	11	5,266

69% uptake of DS screening using the combined test. 80% uptake of NIPT as contingent screening for unaffected pregnancies and 90% for affected. pregnancies. 69% uptake of NIPT as first-line screening.
*Including procedural miscarriages. DS = Down's syndrome; NIPT = non-invasive prenatal testing

testing), and costs more even than current DS screening if the cost per NIPT is only £50.

When the costs associated with pregnancy outcomes were included to the base case, these were sufficiently large and similar between the different strategies to mask differences in screening and diagnosis costs between DS screening and NIPT as contingent testing (Table S1 in Supporting Information).

Results are presented using the same methodology but with different assumptions about uptake in Supporting Information. In the case of NIPT as contingent testing, compared with the assumptions made in the base analysis in Tables 3 and 4, when NIPT uptake increases, NIPT detects more DS cases with slightly more procedure-related miscarriages and with a small increase in costs (Tables S2–S3 in Supporting Information). If NIPT uptake increases and the provision of NIPT as contingent testing leads to an increase in uptake of DS screening, NIPT produces fewer invasive diagnostic tests, fewer procedure-related miscarriages, and detects more DS cases compared with current DS screening, for the same or a modest increase in costs depending on the screening risk cut-off (Tables S4–S5 in Supporting Information).

The national average unit cost for a phlebotomist to take a blood sample is £3 [34]. If samples for NIPT were collected for high-risk women following DS screening in a separate visit then the cost associated with NIPT increased by a negligible amount. For example, for NIPT as contingent testing with a screening risk cut-off of 1:150 154 women undergo NIPT and the cost of the extra blood sample is less than £500, making no appreciable difference to the costs in Table 4.

Discussion

Main Findings

We analysed the costs and outcomes of NIPT for DS as contingent testing and first-line testing compared with the current DS screening programme. We found that at a screening risk cut-off of 1:150 NIPT as contingent testing detects slightly fewer DS cases, has fewer procedure-related miscarriages, and costs the same as current DS screening (around UK£280,000) at a cost of £500 per NIPT. NIPT is currently available in the private sector in the UK with prices varying from £400–£900 [16]. If the cost of NIPT in the NHS was at the lower end of this range then at a screening risk cut-off of 1:150 NIPT as contingent testing would be cost neutral or cost saving compared with current DS screening. When the screening risk cut-off is lowered the cost per NIPT would need to fall considerably for NIPT to be cost neutral compared with current DS screening. As first-line testing NIPT detects more DS cases, has fewer procedure-related miscarriages, and is more expensive than current screening at a cost of £50 per NIPT. When NIPT uptake increases, NIPT detects more DS cases with slightly more procedure-related miscarriages and with a modest increase in costs.

Strengths and Limitations

A strength of our study is that we utilised a pre-existing validated cost model of DS screening in the NHS, developed to aid Trusts, commissioners and health professionals plan, improve and monitor DS screening.

A limitation is the lack of data about the cost and uptake of NIPT under real world conditions. Our study is designed to inform the implementation of NIPT and since it is not implemented it is unclear what the cost and uptake of NIPT will be. We present results for a range of values. The £400–£900 price range in the private sector includes the cost of samples being sent and tested overseas; costs are likely to fall if testing is undertaken in the UK, and costs of sequencing are decreasing over time. Further research could evaluate the costs and benefits of UK-based testing and the implications of this for the cost-effectiveness of NIPT.

There is limited evidence to suggest that uptake of NIPT in the general pregnant population may be higher than current DS screening [37] but actual values are unknown. We present results assuming NIPT uptake will be the same as for current DS screening and that it will be 100%, and find that our conclusions are not very sensitive to the uptake rates used. We also assumed that uptake of invasive diagnostic testing after a positive NIPT result is the same as after being found high risk from DS screening. Uptake of invasive diagnostic testing after NIPT may actually be higher because NIPT has a higher positive predictive value than DS screening (Song et al [19] assumed that 99% of patients undergo invasive testing after a positive NIPT). This would mean that the difference in DS cases detected between current DS screening and NIPT as contingent testing will fall.

Another limitation is that NIPT can be used to test for trisomy 18, trisomy 13 and some sex chromosome aneuploidies; we have only looked at NIPT for DS. One shortcoming of NIPT is that it does not detect other chromosomal rearrangements, though this is possible with invasive methods. We have not accounted for this on our model, which focuses on DS. Prenatal diagnosis programmes may need to consider the use of invasive tests in pregnancies where the NIPT test is normal, but increased nuchal translucency or other structural abnormalities suggest other chromosomal rearrangements [39,40]. This requires further evaluation when NIPT is used in clinical practice.

Conclusions

Our study has two main implications. First, at a screening risk cut-off of 1:150 and a cost per NIPT of £500 NIPT as contingent testing appears to offer gains over current DS screening in terms of fewer procedure-related miscarriages and at no additional cost. A cost of £500 per NIPT falls within the range that NIPT is currently offered in the private sector in the UK, and so ought to be achievable in the NHS. Second, while it produces better outcomes in terms of DS cases detected and procedure-related fetal losses, NIPT as first-line screening is more expensive than current DS screening, even at a very low cost per test. Hence, NIPT as first-line testing is unlikely to be attractive to NHS commissioners unless the cost of NIPT was to fall dramatically.

The main uncertainties in our analysis are the uptake of NIPT under real world conditions and the cost of NIPT. We have also assumed that the uptake of invasive diagnostic testing after NIPT is the same as after DS screening. The costs and outcomes of NIPT for DS as contingent testing and first-line testing compared with the current DS screening programme ought to be reassessed once the actual uptake rate of NIPT and the cost of NIPT when delivered at scale in the NHS are known.

Supporting Information

Figure S1 Second trimester screening pathway: current DS screening.

Figure S2 Second trimester screening pathway: NIPT as contingent testing.

Table S1 Costs of testing strategies in a screening population of 10,000 pregnant women including costs of pregnancy outcomes. 69% uptake of DS screening using the combined test. 80% uptake of NIPT as contingent screening for unaffected pregnancies and 90% for affected pregnancies. 69% uptake of NIPT as first line screening.

Table S2 Outcomes of testing strategies in a screening population of 10,000 pregnant women with alternative assumptions for NIPT uptake. 69% uptake of DS screening using the combined test. 100% uptake of NIPT as contingent screening. 79% uptake of NIPT as first line screening.

Table S3 Costs of testing strategies in a screening population of 10,000 pregnant women with alternative assumptions for NIPT uptake. 69% uptake of DS screening using the combined test. 100% uptake of NIPT as contingent screening. 79% uptake of NIPT as first line screening.

Table S4 Outcomes of testing strategies in a screening population of 10,000 pregnant women with alternative assumptions for NIPT uptake. 69% uptake of DS screening using the combined test. 100% uptake of NIPT as contingent screening, plus DS screening uptake increases to 79%. 79% uptake of NIPT as first line screening.

Table S5 Costs of testing strategies in a screening population of 10,000 pregnant women with alternative assumptions for NIPT uptake. 69% uptake of DS screening using the combined test. 100% uptake of NIPT as contingent screening, plus DS screening uptake increases to 79%. 79% uptake of NIPT as first line screening.

Table S6 CHEERS statement.

Acknowledgments

The original DPT model is available from the NHS Fetal Anomaly Screening Programme website: http://fetalanomaly.screening.nhs.uk/. We would like to thank Jan Preece for her editorial assistance.

Author Contributions

Conceived and designed the experiments: SM LSC. Performed the experiments: NC SK SM. Analyzed the data: NC SK SM. Contributed reagents/materials/analysis tools: NC MH LSC. Wrote the paper: SM SK NC MH LSC.

References

1. NHS FASP. Screening for Down's syndrome: UK NSC policy recommendaations (2011) 2011–2014 Model of Best Practice. Exeter, United Kingdom: NHS Fetal Anomaly Screening Programme, UK National Screening Committee.
2. Tabor A, Alfirevic Z (2010) Update on procedure-related risks for prenatal diagnosis techniques. Fetal Diagn Ther 27: 1–7.
3. Lo YMD, Corbetta N, Chamberlain PF, Rai V, Sargent IL, et al. (1997) Presence of fetal DNA in maternal plsma and serum. Lancet 350: 485–487.
4. Boon EM, Faas BH (2013) Benefits and limitations of whole genome versus targeted approaches for non-invasive prenatal testing for fetal aneuploidies. Prenat Diagn 33: 563–568.
5. Ehrich M, Deciu C, Zweifellhofer T, Tynan JA, Cagasan L, et al. (2011) Non-invasive detection of fetal trisomy 21 by sequencing of DNA in maternal blood: a study in a clinical setting. Am J Obstet Gynecol 204; 205.e1–11.
6. Palomaki GE, Kloza EM, Lambert-Messerlian GM, Haddow JE, Neveux LM, et al. (2011) DNA sequencing of maternal plasma to detect Down syndrome: an international clinical validation study. Genet Med 13: 913–920.
7. Bianchi DW, Platt LD, Goldberg JD, Abuhamad AZ, Sehnert AJ on behalf of the MatErnal Blood IS Source to Accurately diagnose fetal aneuploidy (MELISSA) Study Group (2012) Genome-Wide Fetal Aneuploidy Detection by Maternal Plasma DNA Sequencing. Obstet Gynecol 119: 890–901.
8. Ashoor G, Syngelaki A, Wagner M, Birdir C, Nicolaides KH (2012) Chromosome-selective sequencing of maternal plasma cell-free DNA for first-trimester detection of trisomy 21 and trisomy 18. Am J Obstet Gynecol 206: 322.e1–5.
9. Sparks AB, Struble CA, Wang ET, Song K, Oliphant A (2012) Non-invasive prenatal detection and selective analysis of cell-free DNA obtained from maternal blood: evaluation for trisomy 21 and trisomy 18. Am J Obstet Gynecol 206: 319.e1–9.
10. Norton ME, Brar H, Weiss J, Karimi A, Laurent LC, et al. (2012) Non-Invasive Chromosomal Evaluation (NICE) Study: results of a multicentre prospective cohort study for detection of fetal trisomy 21 and trisomy 18. Am J Obstet Gynecol 207: 137.e1–8.
11. Futch T, Spinosa J, Bhatt S, de Feo E, Rava RP, et al. (2013) Initial clinical laboratory experience in non-invasive prenatal testing for fetal aneuploidy from maternal plasma DNA samples. Prenat Diagn 33: 569–574.
12. Liang D, Lv W, Wang H, Xu L, et al. (2013) Non-invasive prenatal testing of fetal whole chromosome aneuploidy by massively parallel sequencing. Prenat Diagn 33: 409–415.
13. ACOG Statement - The American College of Obstetricians and Gynecologists Committee on Genetics; The Society for Maternal-Fetal Medicine Publications Committee (2012) Committee Opinion. Obstet Gynecol 120: 1532–1534.
14. Benn PA, Borrell A, Cuckle H, Dugoff L, Gross S, et al. (2012) Prenatal detection of Down syndrome using massively parallel sequencing (MPS): a rapid response statement from a committee on behalf of the Board of the International Society for Prenatal Diagnosis, 24 October 2011. Prenat Diagn 32: 1–2.
15. Langlois S, Brock JA, Genetics Committee, Wilson RD, Audibert F, et al. (2013) Current status in non-invasive prenatal detection of down syndrome, trisomy 18, and trisomy 13 using cell-free DNA in maternal plasma. J Obstet Gynaecol Can 35: 177–181.
16. Antenatal Results and Choices (2013) Non-invasive prenatal testing for Down's syndrome (NIPT). Available: http://www.arc-uk.org/tests-explained/down-s-syndrome-screening/non-invasive-prenatal-testing-for-down-s-syndrome. Accessed 2013 Sep 30.
17. Wald NJ, Bestwick JP (2013) Incorporating DNA sequencing into current prenatal screening practice for Down's Syndrome. PLoS ONE 8: e58732.
18. Garfield SS, Armstrong SO (2012) Clinical and cost consequences of incorporating a novel non-invasive prenatal test into the diagnostic pathway for fetal trisomies. J Managed Care Med 15; 34–41.
19. Song K, Musci J, Caughey AB (2013) Clinical utility and cost of non-invasive prenatal testing with cfDNA analysis in hi-risk women based on a US population. J Matern Fetal Neonatal Med 26: 1180–1185.
20. Ohno M, Caughey AB (2013) The role of non-invasive prenatal testing as a diagnostic versus a screening tool – a cost-effectiveness analysis. Prenat Diagn 33: 630–635.
21. Cuckle H, Benn P, Pergament E (2013) Maternal cfDNA screening for Down syndrome – a cost sensitivity analysis. Prenat Diagn 33: 636–642.
22. NHS Fetal Anomaly Screening Programme (2012) Decision planning tool. Available: http://fetalanomaly.screening.nhs.uk/costforscreeningstategies#fileid11456. Accessed 2013 Sep 30.
23. NHS Choices (2013). Tests for Down's syndrome. Available: http://www.nhs.uk/conditions/pregnancy-and-baby/pages/screening-amniocentesis-downs-syndrome.aspx#close. Accessed 2014 Feb 6.
24. ONS (2010) Live births in England and Wales by characteristics of mother 2010. Available: http://www.ons.gov.uk/ons/publications/re-reference-tables.html?edition = tcm%3A77-230704. Accessed 2013 Sep 30.
25. Morris JK, Mutton DE, Alberman E (2002) Revised estimates of the maternal age specific live birth prevalence of Down's Syndrome. J Med Screening 9: 2–6.
26. Rowe R, Puddicombe D, Hockley C, Redshaw M (2008) Offer and uptake of prenatal screening for Down syndrome in women from different social and ethnic backgrounds. Prenat Diagn 28: 1245–1250.
27. Chitty LS, Hill M, White H, Wright D, Morris S (2012) Non-invasive prenatal testing for aneuploidy – ready for prime time? Am J Obstet Gynecol 206: 269–275.
28. Wright D (2009) DQASS: detection rates and false positive rates for first and second trimester Down's syndrome screening tests. Plymouth: Down's Syndrome Screening Quality Assurance Support Service (DQASS).
29. Bray I, Wright D (1998) Estimating the spontaneous loss of Down's syndrome fetuses between the times of chorionic villus sampling, amniocentesis and live birth. Prenat Diagn 18: 1045–1054.
30. Gilbert RE, Augood C, Gupta R, Ades AE, Logan S, et al. (2000) Cost-effectiveness and safety effectiveness of first and second trimester screening strategies for Down syndrome. London: Systematic Reviews Training Unit, Centre for Epidemiology and Biostatistics, University of London.
31. Wald NJ, Rodeck CH, Hackshaw AK, Walters J, Chitty LS, et al. (2003) First and second trimester antenatal screening for Down's syndrome: the results of the Serum, Urine and Ultrasound Screening Study (SURUSS). J Med Screen 10: 56–104.
32. Wald NJ, Kennard A, Hackshaw A, McGuire A (1998) Antenatal screening for Down's syndrome. London: NHS R&D Health Technology Assessment (HTA) Programme. Health Technol Assess 2: 1–124.
33. Gray JAM, Ward P (2004) National Downs Syndrome Screening Programme for England: A Handbook for Staff (Version 2.0). London: UK National Screening Committee Programme Directorate.
34. Morris JK (2011) The National Down Syndrome Cytogenetic Register for England and Wales: 2010 Annual Report. London, United Kingdom: Queen Mary University of London, Barts and The London School of Medicine and Dentistry.
35. HESonline. Maternity data 2010–11. Available: http://www.hesonline.nhs.uk/Ease/servlet/ContentServer?siteID = 1937&categoryID = 1815. Accessed 2013 Sep 30.
36. Department of Health (2011) NHS Reference costs 2008–2009: Appendix NSRC01 - NHS Trust Reference Cost Schedules. London, United Kingdom: Crown; 2011 Jan 13. Report No: 15423, 16211.
37. Lewis C, Hill M, Silcock S, Chitty L (2013) Non-invasive prenatal testing for Down's Syndrome – pregnant women's views and likely uptake. Public Health Genomics 16: 223–232.
38. Chetty S, Garabedian MJ, Norton ME (2013) Uptake of non-invasive prenatal testing (NIPT) in women following positive aneuploidy screening. Prenat Diagn 33: 542–546.
39. Chitty LS, Kagan KO, Molina FS, Waters JJ, Nicolaides KH (2006) Fetal nuchal translucency scan and early prenatal diagnosis of chromosomal abnormalities by rapid aneuploidy screening: observational study. BMJ 332: 452–455.
40. Kagan KO, Chitty LS, Cicero S, Eleftheriades M, Nicolaides KH (2007) Ultrasound findings before amniocentesis in selecting the method of analysing the sample. Prenat Diagn 27: 34–39.

Auditory Function in the Tc1 Mouse Model of Down Syndrome Suggests a Limited Region of Human Chromosome 21 Involved in Otitis Media

Stephanie Kuhn[1], Neil Ingham[2], Selina Pearson[2], Susan M. Gribble[2], Stephen Clayton[2], Karen P. Steel[2]*, Walter Marcotti[1]*

1 Department of Biomedical Science, University of Sheffield, Sheffield, United Kingdom, **2** Wellcome Trust Sanger Institute, Wellcome Trust Genome Campus, Hinxton, Cambridge, United Kingdom

Abstract

Down syndrome is one of the most common congenital disorders leading to a wide range of health problems in humans, including frequent otitis media. The Tc1 mouse carries a significant part of human chromosome 21 (Hsa21) in addition to the full set of mouse chromosomes and shares many phenotypes observed in humans affected by Down syndrome with trisomy of chromosome 21. However, it is unknown whether Tc1 mice exhibit a hearing phenotype and might thus represent a good model for understanding the hearing loss that is common in Down syndrome. In this study we carried out a structural and functional assessment of hearing in Tc1 mice. Auditory brainstem response (ABR) measurements in Tc1 mice showed normal thresholds compared to littermate controls and ABR waveform latencies and amplitudes were equivalent to controls. The gross anatomy of the middle and inner ears was also similar between Tc1 and control mice. The physiological properties of cochlear sensory receptors (inner and outer hair cells: IHCs and OHCs) were investigated using single-cell patch clamp recordings from the acutely dissected cochleae. Adult Tc1 IHCs exhibited normal resting membrane potentials and expressed all K^+ currents characteristic of control hair cells. However, the size of the large conductance (BK) Ca^{2+} activated K^+ current ($I_{K,f}$), which enables rapid voltage responses essential for accurate sound encoding, was increased in Tc1 IHCs. All physiological properties investigated in OHCs were indistinguishable between the two genotypes. The normal functional hearing and the gross structural anatomy of the middle and inner ears in the Tc1 mouse contrast to that observed in the Ts65Dn model of Down syndrome which shows otitis media. Genes that are trisomic in Ts65Dn but disomic in Tc1 may predispose to otitis media when an additional copy is active.

Editor: Alice Y. W. Chang, Kaohsiung Chang Gung Memorial Hospital, Taiwan

Funding: This work was supported by grants from the Wellcome Trust (088719) and The Royal Society to WM, and a grant from the Wellcome Trust (077189) to KPS. The funders had no role in study design, data collection and analysis, decision to publish, or preparation of the manuscript.

Competing Interests: The authors have declared that no competing interests exist.

* E-mail: w.marcotti@sheffield.ac.uk (WM); kps@sanger.ac.uk (KPS)

These authors contributed equally to this work.

Introduction

Down Syndrome, a chromosomal disorder caused by the presence of an additional copy (complete or part: trisomy) of chromosome 21, Hsa21, is characterised by some impairment of cognitive ability and physical growth and a particular set of facial characteristics amongst other things [1,2]. About 1 in every 700 newborns is affected with Down Syndrome [1]. One feature often seen and of particular interest to this study, is the relatively high incidence of otitis media (in up to 78% of patients) and conductive hearing impairment in people with Down Syndrome. However, with correct diagnosis and treatment up to 98% of patients have normal hearing [3]. Several mouse models of Down syndrome have been developed [2]. Recently, one of these mouse models for Down Syndrome has been reported exhibiting otitis media (Ts65Dn mice). These mice demonstrated high but variable ABR thresholds, many had middle ear effusion and often showed a thickened middle ear mucosa compared to wildtype controls [4].

In the present study we have examined another mouse model of Down syndrome (Tc1), which carries most of human chromosome 21 (Hsa21) and shows many phenotypic similarities to Down syndrome [5–7], to look for signs of hearing impairment, otitis media and possible defects of the cochlear sensory hair cells. Here we show that despite the increased expression of the K^+ current ($I_{K,f}$) characteristic of mature IHCs, the middle and inner ear structure and functional hearing were indistinguishable between control and Tc1 mice. As only parts of human chromosome 21 have been found to be included in the Tc1 mouse, the predisposition to otitis media in Down syndrome may be associated with genes that are not functionally trisomic in the Hsa21 chromosomal material in Tc1 mice.

Results

Sensitivity of hearing in Tc1 mice

ABRs were recorded and used to determine the threshold of hearing for click and tone pip stimuli in wildtype control

(11.8±0.4 weeks, $n=11$, 7 males, 4 females) and Tc1 mice (11.8±0.4 weeks, $n=10$, 4 males, 6 females). Examples of click-evoked ABR waveforms are shown in Figure 1. There were no obvious or systematic differences in waveforms recorded from the two groups. In all mice, the mean ABR threshold audiograms showed a characteristically normal profile, having a region of highest sensitivity (lowest threshold) in the 12–18 kHz region (Fig. 2). Frequencies above and below this region had typically higher thresholds. In both Tc1 and control groups, thresholds at high frequencies showed considerable variation amongst individuals (Fig. 2A, 2C) which may be associated with the mixed genetic background that includes C57BL/6J and 129S8 and the fact that many mouse strains show progressive hearing loss [8]. Analysis of variance (Two-Way) indicated there were no significant differences between the thresholds of control and Tc1 mice ($F=0.781$, $p=0.634$). Click ABR thresholds were estimated by taking recordings from both the left and right sides of the head. There were no significant asymmetries in click ABR thresholds in either the control or Tc1 mice (Fig. 2) and no significant effect of the addition of human chromosomal material (Two Way ANOVA; $F=0.131$, $p=0.719$).

Input-Output Functions

From click-evoked ABR waveforms, four positive and negative peaks could be discriminated. In Figure 3A, we plotted mean latency of positive peaks 1 and 3 (P1 and P3) as a function of dB SL (sensation level; i.e. dB above threshold) for wildtype and Tc1 mice. The mean positive-negative amplitude of waves 1 and 3 (P1/N1 and P3/N3) were plotted as a function of dB SL in wildtype and Tc1 mice (Fig. 3B–C, respectively). On the whole, there was no systematic effect of addition of extra chromosomal material on these waveform latency and amplitude parameters; the input-output function curves obtained from the mice were largely overlapping.

Middle and inner ear appearance in Tc1 mice

Following ABR recordings, the middle ear was carefully dissected and examined for signs of any inflammation or malformation. Minor anomalies were detected in some individuals such as a small amount of fluid in the middle ear, slight whitening of the bone surrounding the middle ear cavity, or some cerumen accumulating in the external ear canal, but these features were all detected in both Tc1 and control mice and were not correlated with raised thresholds observed at high frequencies. Ossicles showed a normal appearance in Tc1 mice (Fig. 4A, 4B). Sections of the middle ears revealed no evidence of effusion in the middle ear cavities and no signs of thickening of the mucosa lining the middle ear of Tc1 or control mice (Fig. 4C–F). Examples of cleared inner ears from mice of both groups are shown in Figure 5. No gross structural abnormalities were detected in the inner ears of control or Tc1 mice.

The expression of adult-type ion channels in Tc1 mutant hair cells is normal

Sound detection depends on the sensory hair cells present in the cochlea. The role of hair cells is to transduce mechanical acoustic energy into an electrical signal [9]. While IHCs, the primary sensory receptors of the mammalian cochlea, are responsible for relaying sound information to the central nervous system via auditory nerve fibres [10], OHCs act in parallel to enhance the sensitivity and frequency selectivity of the cochlea by active mechanical amplification [11–13].

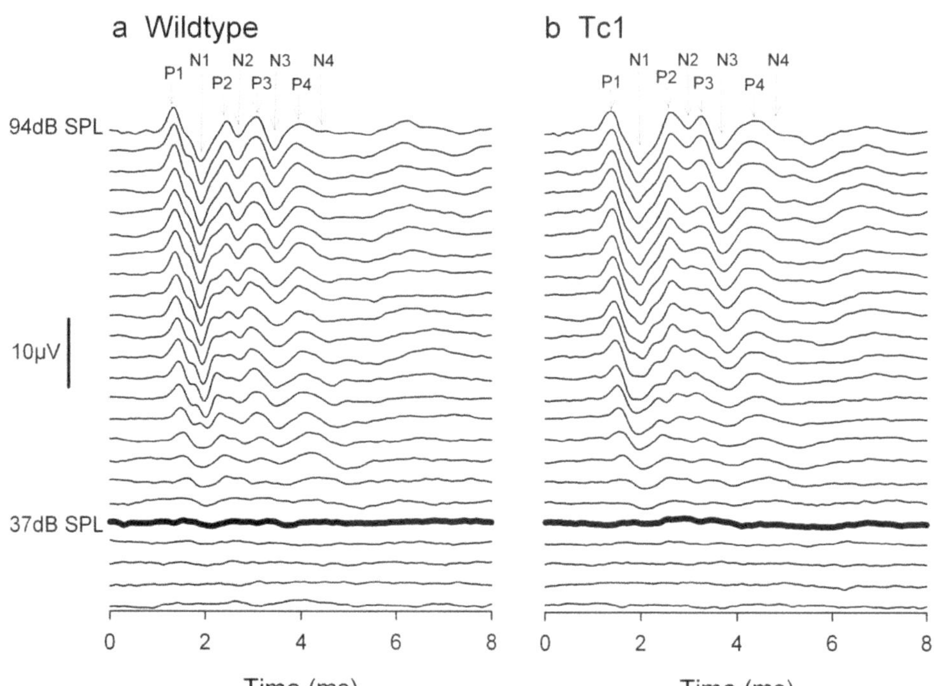

Figure 1. Click-evoked ABR waveforms in control and Tc1 mice. Averaged ABR waveforms recorded in response to clicks in a wildtype (a) and Tc1 (b) mouse. Waveforms are displayed for stimuli in 3 dB incremental steps from 25 dB SPL at the bottom to 94 dB SPL at the top of each panel. Positive peaks 1–4 (P1–P4) and negative peaks (N1–N4) are indicated by arrows at the top of each panel. The heavy black line indicates the visually-determined threshold; 37 dB SPL in both cases. The scale-bar indicates 10 µV amplitude.

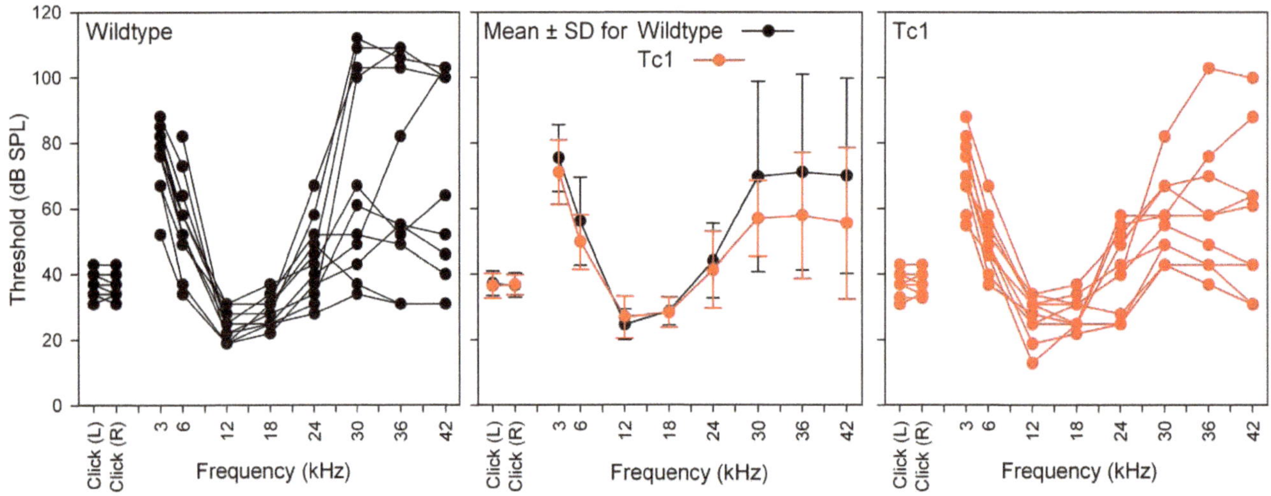

Figure 2. ABR Thresholds in control and Tc1 mice. ABR thresholds for individual control (black circles) and Tc1 (red circles) mice are shown on the left and right panels respectively. The middle panel indicates the mean (± standard deviation, SD) thresholds for control (black) & Tc1 (red) mice, respectively. Tone-evoked ABRs were recorded over the left side of the head only whereas click-evoked ABRs were recorded bilaterally.

We investigated the biophysical properties of adult inner (IHCs) and outer (OHCs) hair cells from Tc1 mice using patch clamp recordings, to test whether additional copy (complete or part) of chromosome 21 (trisomy 21) had any effect on the normal function or development of these cells. Both control and Tc1 IHCs from adult mice exhibited a large K^+ current (Fig. 6A–C). However, the total steady-state outward K^+ current, measured at −25 mV, was found to be significantly larger in Tc1 than that in littermate control IHCs ($p<0.005$: Fig. 6D). When we tested which of the K^+ current characteristics of adult IHCs ($I_{K,f}$ and $I_{K,s}$ [14] and $I_{K,n}$ [15]) was affected by the additional human DNA, we found that only $I_{K,f}$, a large conductance Ca^{2+}-activated K^+ current, was up-regulated in Tc1 IHCs (Fig. 6D, 6E). Despite the larger amplitude the activation of $I_{K,f}$, defined as time to reach half-maximal activation [15], was found to be not significantly different between Tc1 (0.30±0.03 ms, n = 5) and littermate control (0.28±0.04 ms, n = 7) IHCs, suggesting that the additional human DNA is only affecting the expression level and not the intrinsic properties of the channel. We then investigated whether a larger $I_{K,f}$ in mutant IHCs had an effect on the cell's voltage responses. In both control and mutant IHCs, hyperpolarizing and depolarizing current injections from the resting membrane potential, elicited fast, graded voltage responses (Fig. 6F) as previously observed [14,16]. In Tc1 IHCs, current steps appeared to cause significantly smaller voltage responses, which was more evident from the relation between injected current and peak voltage responses ($p<0.0001$, Fig. 6G). Although the increased $I_{K,f}$ affected the receptor potential, the general biophysical properties of Tc1 IHCs (such as resting membrane potentials and linear leak conductance) did not differ from those of control cells (see Table 1). Similar to IHCs, the K^+ current characteristic of adult OHCs, $I_{K,n}$ [17], was also equally expressed in both control and Tc1 OHCs (Fig. 7).

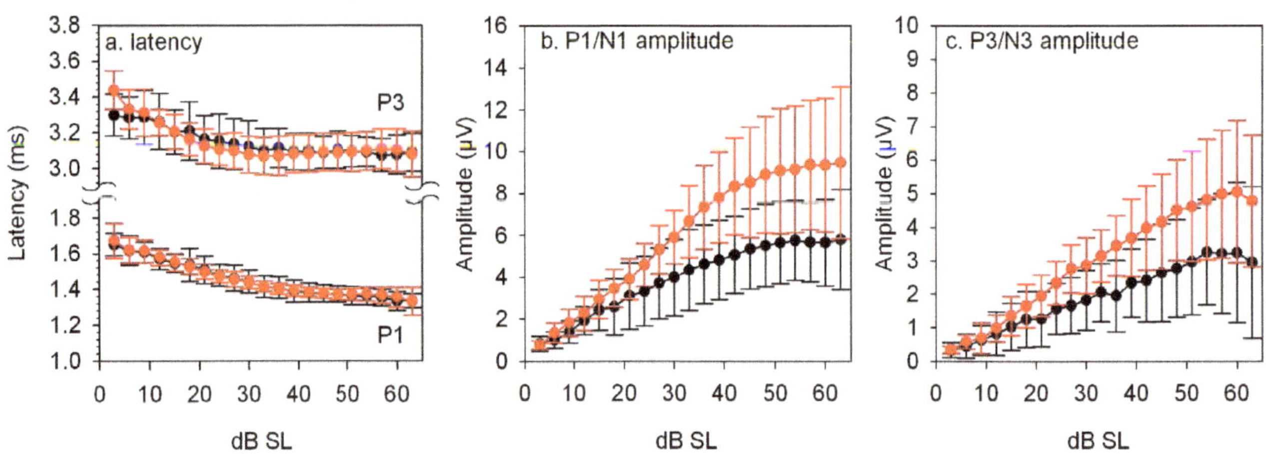

Figure 3. Input-Output Functions of Wave Latency. A, The mean latency (± SD) of 2 positive peaks in the ABR waveform (P1 and P3) are plotted as a function of dB SL (sensation level) for wildtype (black lines) and Tc1 (red lines) mice. B, **C.** The mean amplitude (± SD) of 2 positive-negative (P1-N1 and P3-N3) peaks in the ABR waveform are plotted as a function of dB SL for wildtype (black lines) and Tc1 (red lines) mice.

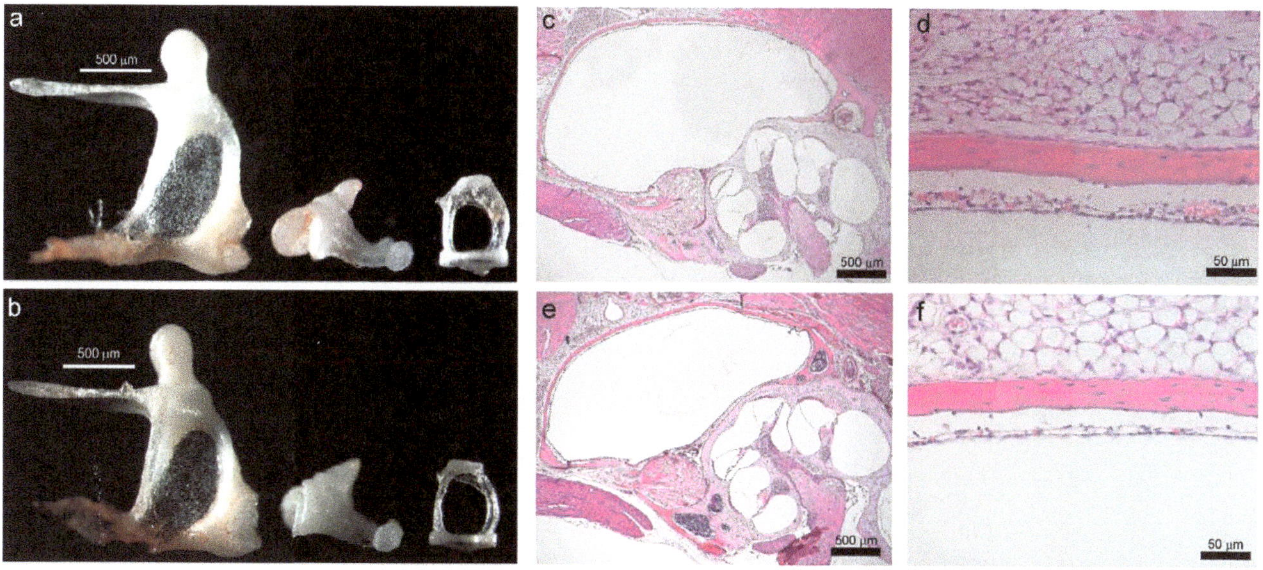

Figure 4. Middle Ears of Control and Tc1 mice. A and B, illustrate the malleus (left), incus (middle) and stapes (right), from a wildtype mouse and a Tc1 mouse, respectively, showing no differences. **C–F** illustrate sections through the mucosal lining of the middle ear (H&E stained) for a wildtype (**C**, **E**) and Tc1 (**D**, **F**) mouse, showing no sign of any middle ear inflammation.

Discussion

Prior to the onset of hearing (postnatal day 12 in most rodents [18]) immature hair cells have to follow a developmental program that consists of the acquisition and/or elimination of different ion channels and synaptic proteins [15,19–21]. One of these channels, which carries the large conductance K^+ current $I_{K,f}$, is characteristic of mature IHCs and enables them to operate fast voltage responses essential for accurate sound encoding. We found that $I_{K,f}$ was slightly up-regulated in IHCs from Tc1 (Fig. 6) mice carrying part of human chromosome 21 (Hsa21), involved in Down syndrome in humans [5]. The gene encoding BK channels, *KCNMA1*, is not located on Hsa21 [22,23], suggesting that the up-regulation of $I_{K,f}$ is a secondary effect caused by activation or modulation of other intracellular signals in Tc1 IHCs. There was no apparent effect of $I_{K,f}$ upregulation on hearing sensitivity, as determined by ABR threshold measurements (Fig. 2).

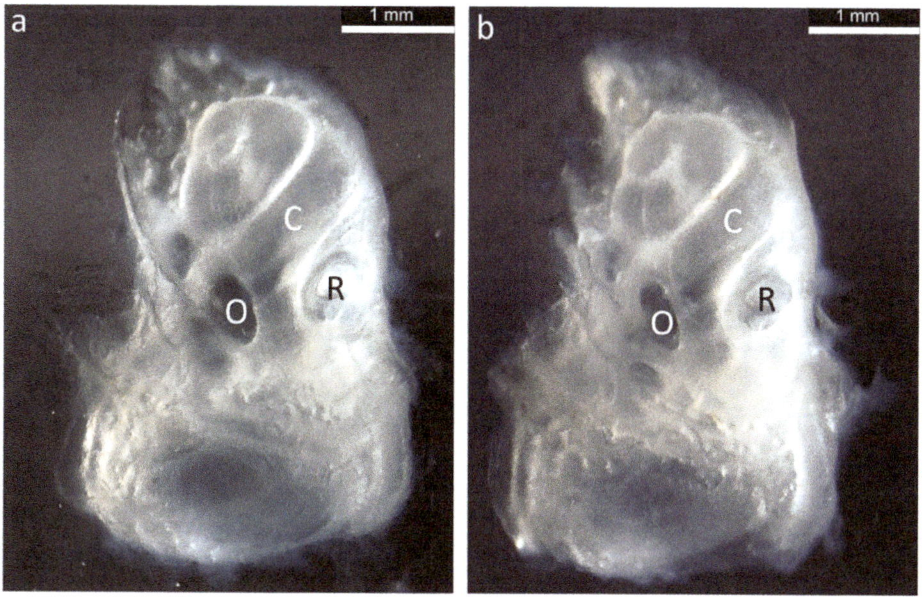

Figure 5. Cleared Inner Ears from Control and Tc1 mice. Gross morphology of the inner ears of a control and Tc1 mouse are shown in **A** and **B**, respectively. The cochlear duct (C) is visible as a spiral structure towards the top of each image. The oval (O) and round (R) windows can be seen in the middle of each panel. The semicircular canals of each inner ear are found in the wider region at the bottom of each image. No abnormalities can be detected in Tc1 inner ears.

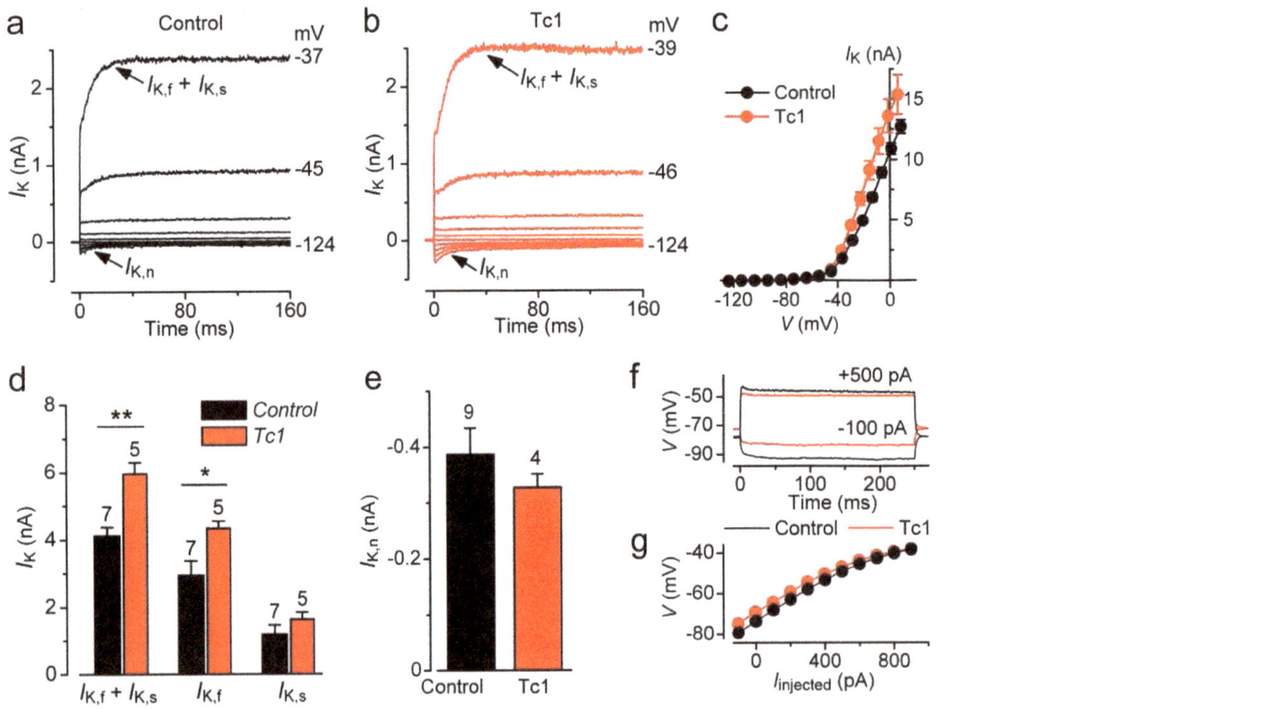

Figure 6. Current and voltage recordings in IHCs from adult Tc1 mice. A and **B**, Membrane currents recorded from adult (P25) control and Tc1 apical coil IHCs. Currents were elicited by depolarizing voltage steps in 10 mV nominal increments from −124 mV to the various test potentials shown by some of the traces (holding potential −84 mV). **C**, Average steady-state current-voltage (*I–V*) curves obtained from control (P25–P26, *n* = 7) and Tc1 (P25–P26, *n* = 5) adult IHCs. **D**, Average total K^+ current ($I_{K,f}$+$I_{K,s}$) and isolated $I_{K,f}$ and $I_{K,s}$ measured at the membrane potential of −25 mV. E, Size of $I_{K,n}$ in control and Tc1 mutant IHCs. **F**, Voltage responses under current clamp from control and Tc1 adult IHCs (P25). Current steps were applied between −100 pA and +900 pA, starting from the resting potential, and for clarity only a few responses are shown. **G**, non-linear behaviour of the peak voltage responses of IHCs, obtained from the protocol described in panel **F**. In this and the following Figure, values are shown as mean ± SEM. Recordings are at body temperature.

Recently, it has been shown that five miRNA genes are overexpressed in the heart and brain of people with Down syndrome [24], three of which (miR-99a, let-7c, miR-125b-2) are expressed in the inner ear [25]. MiRNAs are small non-coding RNAs able to regulate a broad range of genes involved in development, differentiation and human diseases [26,27], including hearing [28–30]. However, the physiological functions for the majority of the known miRNAs are still not understood in most systems. Therefore, one possibility is that overexpression of a human chromosome 21-derived miRNA may exert some degree of gene regulation in cochlear IHCs, affecting BK channel expression. *Mirlet7c-1* (let-7c) is one of the genes on human chromosome 21 that is intact in the Tc1 mouse so may be overexpressed. Upregulation of miR-let-7c is expected to down-regulate miR-17 via downregulation of c-myc [31]; miR-17 in turn is predicted to target Nr4a2 (Targetscan prediction; http://www.targetscan.org/) so downregulation of miR-17 should upregulate Nr4a2; finally, upregulation of Nr4a2 should lead to upregulation of Kcnma1 [32] which could explain the larger K^+ current $I_{K,f}$ in Tc1 IHCs.

Table 1. Electrical properties of IHCs (P25–P26) and OHCs (P13–P14) from control and Tc1 mice.

	Control	Tc1
IHCs (P25–P26)		
C_m, pF	9.9±0.3 (9)	10.5±0.4 (5)
V_m, mV	−73.7±1.2 (9)	−69.8±1.2 (5)
g_{Leak}, nS	1.0±0.2 (9)	1.6±0.4 (5)
V_{Rev}, mV	−59.7±2.62 (7)	−59.7±4.06 (3)
OHC (P13–P14)		
C_m, pF	8.67±0.31 (9)	7.33±0.48 (3)
g_{Leak}, nS	3.07±0.25 (9)	2.60±0.10 (3)

Values are means ± SEM; number of cells is in parentheses. C_m = membrane capacitance; V_m = resting membrane potential; g_{Leak} = resting leak conductance; V_{Rev} = reversal potential of the total current.

Hearing sensitivity of Tc1 mice was comparable to wildtype controls (Figs. 1–3). There were no consistent changes in ABR waveform, amplitude or latency as a function of sound pressure level; a further indication of normal hearing in the Tc1 mice. Some minor anomalies were noted in the middle ears and ossicles of some mice (Fig. 4), but these did not correlate with any functional changes. Gross anatomy of the inner ears, as revealed by clearing of the tissues (Fig. 5), was also normal in both control and Tc1 mice. Thus, we concluded that addition of the majority of human chromosome 21 into the mouse genome does not lead to the otitis media phenotype seen in the Ts65Dn mouse model of Down Syndrome [4] and in Down Syndrome patients [33].

The Ts65Dn mouse model contains just under 60% of the mouse orthologues of the human genes on Hsa21 and produces behavioural and cognitive phenotypes similar to Down Syndrome as well as otitis media [4,34,35]. However, several genes known to

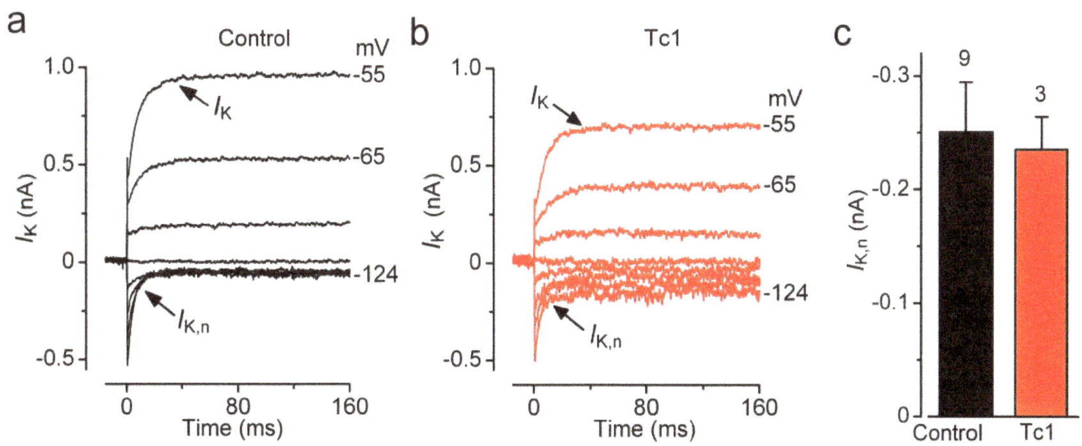

Figure 7. Current recording in OHCs from adult Tc1 mice. A and B, Typical current responses from apical-coil adult control (P14) and Tc1 (P13) OHCs. Currents were elicited by depolarizing voltage steps (10 mV nominal increments) from −124 mV (holding potential of −84 mV). **C**, Steady-state I-V curves for control (P13–P14, $n = 9$) and Tc1 (P13–14, $n = 3$) OHCs. **D**, Average size of the total K^+ current at the steady-state (I_K+$I_{K,n}$) and the isolated $I_{K,n}$.

regulate neuronal function are not triplicated in the Ts65Dn model (eg *S100b* and *Trpm2*) [36,37]. Addition of Hsa21 into mice may also not produce a complete phenotype, for example due to potential differences in expression of human genes in a mouse cell. In the Tc1 line, the extra human DNA is now known to be more disrupted than was originally thought and may lead to inactivation of additional human genes on Hsa21 and consequently lack of trisomy (unpublished data). We carried out a detailed comparison of the genes demonstrating effective trisomy in the Ts65Dn and Tc1 mouse models to investigate which genes might be involved in the susceptibility to otitis media, as Ts65Dn mice show otitis media but Tc1 mice do not. Details of triplicated genes in Ts65Dn mice [38] were compared with the list of intact Hsa21 genes in Tc1 mice (unpublished data). Hsa21 orthologues that are trisomic in Ts65Dn but only disomic in Tc1 might predispose to otitis media when overexpressed, and these are listed in Table 2. Some of these genes appear to be involved in immune function because mouse knockouts show immune defects, including *Ifnar1*, *Ifnar2*, *Il10rb*, *Ifngr2*, *Kcne1*, *Rcan1* and *Runx1*, and these may underlie abnormal (overactive) immune responses to environmental triggers and hence susceptibility to otitis media when overexpressed instead.

A third mouse model for Down syndrome has recently been reported [39] in which Hsa21-syntenic regions on mouse chromosome 10, 16 & 17 (Mmu10, Mmu16 and Mmu17) are duplicated. Here all the mouse orthologs of Hsa21 genes are triplicated with a resulting neurological defect related to Down syndrome; impaired cognitive behaviour, reduced hippocampal LTP and hydrocephalus. Of all the mouse models available, this is perhaps the most similar to the human condition. However, no studies of auditory function have been reported for this mouse model and this could form the basis of a future hearing study.

Materials and Methods

Ethics Statement

All animal studies were licensed by the U.K. Home Office under the Animals (Scientific Procedures) Act 1986 and were approved by the University of Sheffield Ethical Review Committee (Home Office license PPL40/3278) and Wellcome Trust Sanger Institute (Home Office license PPL 80/2163).

Mice

Tc1 mice carrying a copy of human chromosome 21 (HSA 21) were maintained on a mixed C57BL/6J×129S8 background [5].

Auditory Brainstem Response (ABR) recordings

Ten Tc1 and 11 littermate controls were anaesthetised using urethane (ip) and placed on a heating blanket inside a sound attenuating booth. Sub-cutaneous needle electrodes were inserted in the skin on the vertex (active) and overlying the ventral region of the left (reference) and right (ground) bullae to record responses of the left ear. Stimuli were presented as free-field sounds from a speaker (Tucker Davis Technologies, FF1) whose leading edge was 10 cm in front of the mouse's interaural axis at an elevation of 30°. The sound delivery system was calibrated using an ACO Pacific 7017 microphone. For threshold determination, custom software and Tucker Davis Technologies hardware were used to deliver click (0.01 ms duration) and tone pip (3, 6, 18, 24, 30, 36 and 42 kHz of 5 ms duration, 1 ms rise/fall time) stimuli at a range of intensity levels from 10–100+ dB SPL in 3 dB steps. Averaged responses to 256 stimuli, presented at 42.2/s, were analysed and thresholds established as the lowest sound intensity giving a visually-detectable ABR response. For clicks, responses were also recorded from the right ear.

Middle ear analysis

Following ABR, mice were killed by cervical dislocation and the right external and middle ears were examined in detail using a dissecting microscope for any signs of malformation or inflammation, including: appearance of excess cerumen in the external ear canal; thickening, whitening, sponginess or excess vascularisation of the bulla wall; clarity and vascularisation of the tympanic membrane; presence of fluid or white inflammatory material in the middle ear cavity; and solid masses or bony outgrowths of the middle ear wall or ossicles. In addition, following ABR the left side of the head of four Tc1 and four wildtype littermate controls were embedded in paraffin wax, serial sectioned at 8 µm, stained with haematoxylin and eosin and examined.

Inner ear analysis

The right inner ear was dissected out, fixed in Bodian's fixative (75% ethanol, 5% formalin, 5% glacial acetic acid) for 2 hours,

Table 2. Genes trisomic in Ts65Dn but disomic in Tc1.

Name	Start (HG19)	End (HG19)	Human gene	Status of human gene in Tc1	Mouse gene	Mouse mutant reported?	Phenotype of mouse mutant (from MGI)	Candidate for otitis media?
NM_201413	27252860	27543138	APP	rearranged, non functional	*App*	Yes	Mice homozygous for disruptions in this gene exhibit reduced body weight, brain weight, size of forebrain commissures, locomotor activity, forelimb grip strength, spatial learning scores. Many mice also exhibit agenesis of the corpus callosum and extensive reactive gliosis.	
NM_018944	33640529	33651376	C21orf45/ MIS18A	deleted	*2610039C10Rik*	No		
NM_206898	33664123	33687094	MRAP	deleted	*Mrap*	No		
NM_014825	33683329	33765312	URB1	deleted	*Urb1*	No		
NR_002996	33749495	33749631	SNORA80	deleted	Not found	Not found		
NR_026845	33765441	33766266	C21orf119	deleted	Not found	Not found		
NM_058187	33784751	33887697	C21orf63	deleted	*4931408A02Rik*	No		
NM_144659	33947150	33957845	TCP10L	deleted	*Tcp10a*	No		
NM_021254	33973983	33984918	C21orf59	deleted	*1110004E09Rik*	No		
NM_003895	34001068	34100351	SYNJ1	deleted	*Synj1*	Yes	Homozygotes for a targeted null mutation exhibit neurological defects associated with impaired phosphoinositide metabolism and accumulation of clathrin-coated vesicles at nerve endings. Mutants show impaired suckling and most die within 24 hours of birth.	
NM_016631	34106209	34144169	GCFC1	deleted	*Gcfc1*	No		
NR_024622	34144410	34170016	C21orf49	deleted	Not found	Not found		
NM_001162496	34162983	34186053	C21orf62	deleted	*4932438H23Rik*	No		
NM_005806	34398238	34401500	OLIG2	deleted	*Olig2*	Yes	Homozygous mutation of this gene results in neonatal lethality, impaired development of motoneurons and oligodendrocytes, aphagia, hypotonia, abnormal posture and breathing.	
NM_138983	34442449	34444728	OLIG1	deleted	*Olig1*	Yes	Homozygous mutation of this gene results in impaired maturation of oligodendrocytes.	
NR_024102	34537775	34542541	C21orf54	deleted	Not found	Not found		
NM_207585	34602230	34636820	IFNAR2	deleted	*Ifnar2*	Yes	Mice with mutations of this gene have defects in immune responses involving, variously, NK cells, CD4+ and CD8+ T cells and B cells in response to induced and transplanted tumors, viruses, and double stranded DNA. These defects include diminished secretion of type I and type II interferons.	Yes
NM_000628	34638671	34669520	IL10RB	deleted	*Il10rb*	Yes	Most mice homozygous for a ko allele develop moderate to severe colitis without small intestinal involvement and splenomegaly with a hyperproliferative splenic red pulp.	Yes
NM_000629	34697213	34732128	IFNAR1	deleted	*Ifnar1*	Yes	Homozygotes for targeted null mutations exhibit increased susceptibility to viral infection, elevated levels of myeloid lineage cells in the peripheral blood and bone marrow, and reduced immune response to immunostimulatory DNA.	Yes
NM_005534	34775201	34809828	IFNGR2	deleted	*Ifngr2*	Yes	Mice homozygous for disruptions in this gene develop normally. Immune, hematopoietic defects. Diabetes?	Yes
NM_006134	34821447	34852281	TMEM50B	deleted	*Tmem50b*	No		
NM_001040192	34860237	34864023	DNAJC28	deleted	*Dnajc28*	No		
NM_001136006	34876237	34915198	GART	deleted	*Gart*	No		
NM_138927	34915349	34949812	SON	deleted	*Son*	No		
NM_017613	34950210	34961014	DONSON	deleted	*Donson*	No		
NM_145858	34961647	35014160	CRYZL1	deleted	*Cryzl1*	No		

Table 2. Cont.

Name	Start (HG19)	End (HG19)	Human gene	Status of human gene in Tc1	Mouse gene	Mouse mutant reported?	Phenotype of mouse mutant (from MGI)	Candidate for otitis media?
NM_003024	35014783	35261609	ITSN1	deleted	*Itsn1*	Yes	Homozygous for a gene trapped allele exhibit embryonic lethal. Mice homozygous for a null allele exhibit some postnatal lethality and impaired vesicle recycling in surviving mice.	
NM_001697	35275756	35288158	ATP5O	deleted	*Atp5o*	No		
NM_032476	35445822	35515334	MRPS6	deleted	*Mrps6*	No		
NM_006933	35445869	35478561	SLC5A3	deleted	*Slc5a3*	Yes	Homozygous mutation of this gene results in lethality shortly after birth due to respiratory failure and abnormal development of peripheral nerves.	
NR_027266	35552977	35562220	C21orf82/ NCRNA00310	deleted	Not found	Not found		
NM_172201	35736322	35743440	KCNE2	deleted	*Kcne2*	Yes	Digestive/alimentary and homeostasis defects. Gastric hyperplasia and abnormal parietal cell morphology.	
NM_058182	35747748	35761452	FAM165B	deleted	*Fam165b*	No		
NM_000219	35818987	35883613	KCNE1	deleted	*Kcne1*	Yes	Homozygotes for targeted and spontaneous null mutations exhibit head-shaking, circling, ataxia, and severe deafness associated with inner ear defects. Older mutants show increased numbers of T cells. Study of cardiac myocytes in one line showed physiologic defects.	Yes
NM_203418	35888783	35899261	RCAN1	deleted	*Rcan1*	Yes	Unstressed homozygous mutant mice show no overt phenotype other than a slight reduction in heart size and an impaired T helper 1 response. Stress-induced cardiac hypertrophy, however, is attenuated in mutant mice.	Yes
NM_053277	36041687	36090519	CLIC6	deleted	*Clic6*	No		
NR_024351	36096104	36109479	NCRNA00160	deleted	Not found	Not found		
NM_001754	36160097	36421595	RUNX1	partially deleted	*Runx1*	Yes	Mutations affect hematopoiesis, and in some cases result in defective angiogenesis and intraventricular hemorrhage. Null homozygotes die embryonically; heterozygotes have reduced erythroid and myeloid progenitor numbers. Skeletal defects.	Yes

washed in distilled water for 30 mins before being placed in 70% ethanol for 24 hours. Inner ears were left in several changes of 3% KOH over 5 days to dissolve remaining soft tissues, and the bony structures of the ear were cleared by immersion in GEB (2:2:1 ratio of glycerol, 70% ethanol and benzyl alcohol) and thereafter, stored in a 1:1 solution of glycerol and 70% ethanol for further clearing and examination using a dissecting microscope.

Tissue preparation for single-hair cell electrophysiology

Apical-coil inner hair cells (IHCs: $n = 14$) and outer hair cells (OHCs: $n = 12$) from Tc1 mice [5] and their littermate controls were studied in acutely dissected organs of Corti from postnatal day 13–14 (P13–P14) for OHCs and P25–P26 for IHCs, where the day of birth is P0. Cochleae were prepared as previously described [21] in normal extracellular solution (mM): 135 NaCl, 5.8 KCl, 1.3 $CaCl_2$, 0.9 $MgCl_2$, 0.7 NaH_2PO_4, 5.6 d-glucose, 10 Hepes–NaOH, 2 Sodium pyruvate (pH 7.5, osmolality ~308 mmol kg^{-1}). Amino acids and vitamins (Eagle's MEM) were added from concentrates (Invitrogen, UK). Apical coils were transferred into a microscope chamber containing extracellular solution, and immobilized with a nylon mesh fixed to a stainless steel ring. The chamber (volume 2 ml) was perfused at a flow rate of about 10 $ml \cdot h^{-1}$ from a peristaltic pump and mounted on the stage of an upright microscope (Olympus, Japan). The organs of Corti were observed with Nomarski differential interference contrast optics (×60 water immersion objectives). Current and voltage recordings were made by exposing the basolateral surface of the cells using a suction pipette (tip diameter about 4 μm), which was filled with extracellular solution. Tissue samples from all mice were kept for genotyping. All animals were genotyped as previously described [5].

Single-hair cell electrophysiology

IHCs and OHCs were whole cell patch clamped near body temperature (34–37°C) using an Optopatch amplifier (Cairn Research Ltd, Faversham, UK). Patch pipettes were pulled from soda glass capillaries (Harvard Apparatus Ltd., Edenbridge, UK; electrode resistances: 2–3 MΩ) and in order to reduce the electrode resistance coated with surf wax (Mr Zoggs SexWax, Ca, USA). The pipette filling solution contained (in mM): 131 KCl, 3 $MgCl_2$, 1 EGTA-KOH, 5 Na_2ATP, 5 Hepes-KOH, 10 Na_2-phosphocreatine (pH 7.3, 294 mmol kg^{-1}). Data were acquired using pClamp software and Digidata 1320A (Molecular Devices, USA), filtered at 2.5 kHz (8-pole Bessel), sampled at 5 kHz and stored on computer for off-line analysis (Origin: OriginLab, USA). Current recordings were corrected off-line for linear leakage. Membrane potentials were corrected for residual series resistance (R_s) after compensation (1.6 ± 1.1 MΩ, $n = 26$) and for a liquid junction potential (LJP) of −4 mV. The holding currents were plotted as zero current.

The large conductance Ca^{2+} activated K^+ current $I_{K,f}$ was isolated by measuring its amplitude at the membrane potential of −25 mV and at 2 ms from the start of the voltage step [16]. The negatively activating $I_{K,n}$ was measured in isolation as the deactivating tail currents (difference between instantaneous and steady-state inward currents) for voltage steps from the holding potential to −124 mV [15].

Statistical comparisons of means were made by the two-tailed *t*-test. Two-way ANOVA, followed by the Bonferroni test, was used to compare voltage responses from control and Tc1 hair cells. Mean values are quoted ± SEM where $p < 0.05$ indicates statistical significance. In some of the figures statistical significance is indicated by asterisks.

Acknowledgments

We thank Professors E.M.C. Fisher and V.L.J. Tybulewicz for providing the Tc1 mice and comments on the manuscript, Professor K. Gardiner for providing access to new data about trisomy in Ts65Dn mice prior to publication, Dr N. Carter for access to new data about trisomy in the Tc1 mouse, and Dr M. Lewis for advice about microRNA networks. W.M. is a Royal Society University Research Fellow.

Author Contributions

Conceived and designed the experiments: WM KPS. Performed the experiments: SK NI SP. Analyzed the data: SK NI SP. Contributed reagents/materials/analysis tools: SMG SC. Wrote the paper: WM KPS NI SK.

References

1. Mégarbané A, Ravel A, Mircher C, Sturtz F, Grattau Y, et al. (2009) The 50th anniversary of the discovery of trisomy 21: the past, present, and future of research and treatment of Down syndrome. Genet Med 11: 611–616.
2. Wiseman FK, Alford KA, Tybulewicz VL, Fisher EM (2009) Down syndrome—recent progress and future prospects. Hum Mol Genet 18: R75–83.
3. Shott SR, Joseph A, Heithaus D (2001) Hearing loss in children with Down syndrome. Int J Pediatr Otorhinolaryngol 61: 199–205.
4. Han F, Yu H, Zhang J, Tian C, Schmidt C, et al. (2009) Otitis media in a mouse model for Down syndrome. Int J Exp Pathol 90: 480–488.
5. O'Doherty A, Ruf S, Mulligan C, Hildreth V, Errington ML, et al. (2005) An aneuploid mouse strain carrying human chromosome 21 with Down syndrome phenotypes. Science 309: 2033–2037.
6. Dunlevy L, Bennett M, Slender A, Lana-Elola E, Tybulewicz VL, et al. (2010) Down's syndrome-like cardiac developmental defects in embryos of the transchromosomic Tc1 mouse. Cardiovasc Res 88: 287–295.
7. Alford KA, Slender A, Vanes L, Li Z, Fisher EM, et al. (2010) Perturbed hematopoiesis in the Tc1 mouse model of Down syndrome. Blood 115: 2928–2937.
8. Zheng QY, Johnson KR, Erway LC (1999) Assessment of hearing in 80 inbred strains of mice by ABR threshold analyses. Hear Res 130: 94–107.
9. Fettiplace R, Hackney CM (2006) The sensory and motor roles of auditory hair cells. Nat Rev Neurosci 7: 19–29.
10. Ryugo DK (1992) The auditory nerve: peripheral innervation, cell body morphology, and central projections. In: Webster DB, Popper AN, Fay RR, eds. The Mammalian Auditory Pathway: Neuroanatomy. New York: Springer. pp 23–65.
11. Dallos P, Cheatham MA (1992) Cochlear hair cell function reflected in intracellular recordings in vivo. Soc Gen Physiol Ser 47: 371–393.
12. Ashmore JF (1987) A fast motile response in guinea-pig outer hair cells: the cellular basis of the cochlear amplifier. J Physiol 388: 323–347.
13. Kennedy HJ, Crawford AC, Fettiplace R (2005) Force generation by mammalian hair bundles supports a role in cochlear amplification. Nature 433: 880–883.
14. Kros CJ, Ruppersberg JP, Rüsch A (1998) Expression of a potassium current in inner hair cells during development of hearing in mice. Nature 394: 281–284.
15. Marcotti W, Johnson SL, Holley MC, Kros CJ (2003a) Developmental changes in the expression of potassium currents of embryonic, neonatal and mature mouse inner hair cells. J Physiol 548: 383–400.
16. Marcotti W, Johnson SL, Kros CJ (2004) Effects of intracellular stores and extracellular Ca^{2+} on Ca^{2+}-activated K^+ currents in mature mouse inner hair cells. J Physiol 560: 691–708.
17. Marcotti W, Kros CJ (1999) Developmental expression of the potassium current $I_{K,N}$ contributes to maturation of the mouse outer hair cells. J Physiol 520: 653–660.
18. Mikaelian D, Ruben RJ (1965) Development of the hearing in the normal CBA-J mouse. Acta Otolaryngol 59: 451–461.
19. Marcotti W, Johnson SL, Rüsch A, Kros CJ (2003b) Sodium and calcium currents shape action potentials in immature mouse inner hair cells. J Physiol 552: 743–761.
20. Johnson SL, Franz C, Knipper M, Marcotti W (2009) Functional maturation of the exocytotic machinery at gerbil hair cell ribbon synapses. J Physiol 587: 1715–1726.
21. Johnson SL, Franz C, Kuhn S, Furness DN, Rüttiger L, et al. (2010) Synaptotagmin IV determines the linear Ca^{2+} dependence of vesicle fusion at auditory ribbon synapses. Nat Neurosci 13: 45–52.
22. Pallanck L, Ganetzky B (1994) Cloning and characterization of human and mouse homologs of the Drosophila calcium-activated potassium channel gene, slowpoke. Hum Mol Genet 3: 1239–1243.
23. Tseng-Crank J, Foster CD, Krause JD, Mertz R, Godinot N, et al. (1994) Cloning, expression, and distribution of functionally distinct Ca(2+)-activated K+ channel isoforms from human brain. Neuron 13: 1315–1330.
24. Kuhn DE, Nuovo GJ, Martin MM, Malana GE, Pleister AP, et al. (2008) Human chromosome 21-derived miRNAs are overexpressed in down syndrome brains and hearts. Biochem Biophys Res Commun 370: 473–477.
25. Weston MD, Pierce ML, Rocha-Sanchez S, Beisel KW, Soukup GA (2006) MicroRNA gene expression in the mouse inner ear. Brain Res 1111: 95–104.
26. He L, Hannon GJ (2004) MicroRNAs with a big role in gene regulation. Nat Rev Genet 5: 522–531.
27. Stefani G, Slack F (2008) Small non-coding RNAs in animal development. Nat Rev Mol Cell Biol 9: 219–230.
28. Mencía A, Modamio-Høybjør S, Redshaw N, Morín M, Mayo-Merino F, et al. (2009) Mutations in the seed region of human miRNA-96 are responsible for nonsyndromic progressive hearing loss. Nat Genet 41: 609–613.
29. Lewis MA, Quint E, Glazier AM, Fuchs H, De Angelis MH, et al. (2009) An ENU-induced mutation of miR-96 associated with progressive hearing loss in mice. Nat Genet 41: 614–618.
30. Kuhn S, Johnson SL, Furness DN, Chen J, Ingham N, et al. (2011) miR-96 regulates the progression of differentiation in mammalian cochlear inner and outer hair cells. Proc Natl Acad Sci U S A 108: 2355–2360.
31. Shah YM, Morimura K, Yang Q, Tanabe T, Takagi M, et al. (2007) Peroxisome proliferator-activated receptor alpha regulates a microRNA-mediated signaling cascade responsible for hepatocellular proliferation. Mol Cell Biol 27: 4238–4247.
32. Quina LA, Wang S, Ng L, Turner EE (2009) Brn3a and Nurr1 mediate a gene regulatory pathway for habenula development. J Neurosci 29: 14309–14322.
33. Bilgin H, Kasemsuwan L, Schachern PA, Paparella MM, Le CT (1996) Temporal bone study of Down's syndrome. Arch Otolaryngol Head Neck Surg 122: 271–275.
34. Gardiner K, Fortna A, Bechtel L, Davisson MT (2003) Mouse models of Down syndrome: how useful can they be? Comparison of the gene content of human chromosome 21 with orthologous mouse genomic regions. Gene 318: 137–147.
35. Reeves RH, Irving NG, Moran T, Wohn A, Sissodia SS, et al. (1995) A mouse model for Down syndrome exhibits learning and behavior deficits. Nat Genet 11: 177–184.
36. Donato S (2001) S100: a multigenic family of calcium-modulated proteins of the EF-hand type with intracellular and extracellular functional roles. Int J Biochem & Cell Biol 33: 637–669.
37. Olah ME, Jackson MF, Li H, Perez Y, Sun HS, et al. (2009) Ca^{2+}-dependent induction of TRPM2 currents in hippocampal neurons. J Physiol 587: 965–79.
38. Sturgeon X, Gardiner KJ (2011) Transcript catalogs of human chromosome 21 and orthologous chimpanzee and mouse regions. Mamm Genome 22: 261–271.
39. Yu T, Li Z, Jia Z, Clapcote SJ, Liu C, et al. (2010) A mouse model of Down syndrome trisomic for all human chromosome 21 syntenic regions. Hum Mol Genet 19: 2780–2791.

10

Dyrk1A Is Dynamically Expressed on Subsets of Motor Neurons and in the Neuromuscular Junction: Possible Role in Down Syndrome

Gloria Arque[1¤], Anna Casanovas[2], Mara Dierssen[1*]

1 Genes and Disease Program, Center for Genomic Regulation (CRG), Pompeu Fabra University, Barcelona Biomedical Research Park (PRBB) and CIBER de Enfermedades Raras (CIBERER), Barcelona, Spain, 2 Department of Experimental Medicine and IRBLLEIDA, University of Lleida, School of Medicine, Lleida, Catalonia, Spain

Abstract

Individuals with Down syndrome (DS) present important motor deficits that derive from altered motor development of infants and young children. *DYRK1A*, a candidate gene for DS abnormalities has been implicated in motor function due to its expression in motor nuclei in the adult brain, and its overexpression in DS mouse models leads to hyperactivity and altered motor learning. However, its precise role in the adult motor system, or its possible involvement in postnatal locomotor development has not yet been clarified. During the postnatal period we observed time-specific expression of Dyrk1A in discrete subsets of brainstem nuclei and spinal cord motor neurons. Interestingly, we describe for the first time the presence of Dyrk1A in the presynaptic terminal of the neuromuscular junctions and its axonal transport from the facial nucleus, suggesting a function for *Dyrk1A* in these structures. Relevant to DS, *Dyrk1A* overexpression in transgenic mice (TgDyrk1A) produces motor developmental alterations possibly contributing to DS motor phenotypes and modifies the numbers of motor cholinergic neurons, suggesting that the kinase may have a role in the development of the brainstem and spinal cord motor system.

Editor: Yann Herault, IGBMC/ICS, France

Funding: The laboratory of MD is supported by Departament d'Universitats, Recerca i Societat de la Informació (DURSI) (Grups consolidats 09 2009SGR1313). This work was supported by FCT-08-0782, SAF2007-60827, SAF2010-16427, SAF2007-31093-E, Fondo de Investigación Sanitaria (FIS) (PI 082038), Marató TV3, Jerome Lejeune, Reina Sofia and Areces Foundations and EU (LSHG-CT-2006-037627; CureFXS ERare-EU/FIS PS09102673). The CIBER of Enfermedades Raras is an initiative of the ISCIII. The funders had no role in study design, data collection and analysis, decision to publish, or preparation of the manuscript.

Competing Interests: The authors have declared that no competing interests exist.

* E-mail: mara.dierssen@crg.eu

¤ Current address: IST Austria (Institute of Science and Technology Austria), Klosterneuburg, Austria

Introduction

Down syndrome (DS) is the most frequent aneuploidy leading to mental retardation [1]. Motor dysfunction is highly prevalent among individuals with DS, who exhibit clumsy sequences of movements [2], and poor control in programming motor sequences, their timing and force [3]. Delays in achieving motor development milestones are also a constant feature in DS children [4,5]. Babies and young children with DS are late to reach motor milestones such as grasping, rolling, sitting, standing and walking. Some of those DS-associated motor deficits have been reproduced in some mouse models [6,7] and could be contributed by malfunctioning of the cerebellum [6,8,9].

Some candidate genes have been related to DS phenotypes, but few of those could be related to motor dysfunction. *DYRK1A* (dual-specificity tyrosine- (Y)-phosphorylation-regulated kinase 1A) is located on HSA21 [10]. It encodes for a serine threonin kinase, that belongs to an evolutionarily conserved family of proteins involved in functions generally related with growth and development [11].

The role of *DYRK1A* in pathways controlling motor function is supported by its expression pattern and the motor phenotype observed in heterozygous and transgenic *Dyrk1A* mice (TgDyrk1A). Dyrk1A is expressed ubiquitously in the developing nervous system but in adult brain its expression is confined to neurons of the olfactory bulb, the cerebellar cortex, the spinal cord and motor nuclei of the brainstem [12,13,14]. However, little is known of the concrete role of Dyrk1A in motor function or its expression in the postnatal period. This is relevant to DS-related motor dysfunction, since DS motor phenotypes derive to some extent from delays in postnatal motor development. TgDyrk1A overexpressing Dyrk1A show significant levels of motor dysfunction in tasks involving coordination, motor learning and organization of motor behavior [15,16,17] that resemble to some extent the motor phenotypes present in DS patients. Also, both TgDyrk1A and a partial trisomy mouse model (Ts65Dn) of DS present a delay in neuromotor development [15], although this has not been reproduced in a BAC transgenic mouse strain overexpressing human *DYRK1A* [18]. In addition, reduced *Dyrk1A* expression in heterozygous *Dyrk1A* mice leads to a clear hypoactivity [19,20]. Even though altered motor function in DS has been mainly ascribed to dysfunction in the cerebellum, other brain structures, such as the motor nuclei in the brainstem or the spinal cord or the striatum are also crucial in the generation and control of motor behavior. Interestingly, intrastriatal injections of viral vectors expressing shRNA against *Dyrk1A* into TgDyrk1A mice rescued their motor defects [17] suggesting that Dyrk1A expression in various brain regions may contribute to the DS motor alterations.

Here we report time-specific expression of Dyrk1A in discrete subsets of brainstem nuclei and spinal cord motor neurons during the period of craniocaudal motor maturation. Dyrk1A is transported to the presynaptic neuromuscular junction as revealed by experimental axotomy, suggesting a role for the kinase in neuromuscular junction formation and/or function. Relevant to DS, *Dyrk1A* overexpression in transgenic mice (TgDyrk1A) produces motor developmental alterations possibly contributing to DS motor phenotypes. Also Dyrk1A overexpression modifies the numbers of motor cholinergic neurons, suggesting that the kinase may have a role in the development of the brainstem and spinal cord motor system.

Materials and Methods

Animals and General Procedures

In order to study the contribution of *DYRK1A* to Down syndrome phenotypes, we used a single gene transgenic mouse model overexpressing *Dyrk1A* (TgDyrk1A) [15]. The non-transgenic littermates of TgDyrk1A mice served as controls. TgDyrk1A is a single-gene transgenic mouse overexpressing specifically the full-length cDNA of *Dyrk1A* under the control of sheep metallothionein-Ia (*sMT-Ia*) promoter in a C57BL6/SJL genetic background. The genotyping was performed by PCR analysis using the primer pair: DYRK-forward primer, 5′-GTC CAA ACT CAT CAA TGT ATC-3′ and DYRK-reverse primer, 5′-CTT GAG CAC AGC ACT GTT G-3′. Each cycle (32 cycles) consisted of 94°C for 30 s, 52°C for 30 s and 72°C for 45 s. The levels of this transcript were higher in the transgenic mice, in the range of ~1.5–2.2 fold increased. Same-sex littermates were group housed under a 12 h light/dark schedule (lights on at 7:00 a.m.) in controlled environmental conditions of humidity (60%) and temperature (22±1°C) with free access to food and water.

Ethics Statement

All animal procedures were approved by the local ethical committee (Comité Ético de Experimentación Animal del PRBB (CEEA-PRBB); procedure numbers MDS-08-1060P1 and JMC-07-1001P1-MDS), and met the guidelines of the local (law 32/2007) and European regulations (EU directive n° 86/609, EU decree 2001-486) and the Standards for Use of Laboratory Animals n° A5388-01 (NIH). The CRG is authorized to work with genetically modified organisms (A/ES/05/I-13 and A/ES/05/14). All efforts were done to minimize animal suffering.

Behavioral Studies

All the pregnant dams were allowed to deliver spontaneously. The day of delivery was designated as postnatal day 0 (PD0) of age of the neonates. On delivery, the litter size of each dam was recorded and each pup was checked for gross abnormalities. Litters were nursed with their natural dams until weaning at PD21. The pups (wild type: n = 36; TgDyrk1A: n = 39) mice were individually marked with ink at PD7. Behavioral studies to assess neurological and psychomotor development were performed according to Dierssen et al. [21]. Briefly, neuromotor development was assessed on PD7, PD10, PD14 and PD21 by pivoting locomotion test, walking activity, negative geotaxis, climbing ability and wire suspension test. Each experimental day, before the behavioral testing pups were weighed and body/tail length measured, too. Pivoting is an immature locomotion pattern defined by rotations around the hind limbs. Pivoting locomotion test was performed on a flat surface with lines drawn to delineate four 90° segments. The number of pivoting (measured as 90° turns) in 60 seconds was recorded. The ability to walk in a straight line is an indicative of a mature neuromotor development. In the walking test, the latency to walk was measured as the time the mouse waits until it starts moving in a straight line for a distance equal or higher than its own length in less than 60 seconds. To measure negative geotaxis, the mouse is placed on a metallic grid of 45° slope with its head pointing down. It will turn around and crawl up the slope. The score was defined as following: (0) no response, (1) the animal turns around but it doesn't climb, and (2) the animal turns 180° and climb up. The climbing ability was measured when the pup is held against a vertical metallic grid (wire: 0.6 mm in diameter, mesh: 6 mm wide). One behavior is scored as (0) if there is not response and (1) if the animal shows the ability to climb. In the wire suspension test, pups were placed on a wire (4 mm diameter) in an upside-down position. The ability of the animal to remain suspended was measured as the latency to fall. The maximum time allowed was 60 seconds. All the behavioral testing was conducted by the same experimenter in an isolated room and at the same time of the day. Behavioral experimenters were blinded to the genetic status of the animals.

Tissue Preparation and Immunohistochemical Procedures

Mice (PD7, PD10, PD14, PD21 and adults; minimum n = 5 per group) were deeply anesthetized with CO_2 and transcardially perfused with physiological saline solution followed by 4% paraformaldehyde (Sigma, St Louis, MO, USA) in 0.1 M phosphate buffer (PB; pH 7.4). Brain, spinal cord and muscle (caudal portion of digastricus and stylohyoideus muscle) were removed and immersed overnight in fresh fixative at 4°C. Processing of the tissue was different depending on the experiment. Part was transferred to 30% sucrose in 0.1 M PB for 24 hours and frozen, while the rest was embedded in paraffin after dehydration with increasing concentrations of ethanol until arriving to xylene. Frozen spinal cord and brain were sliced in coronal sections (16 μm) whereas muscles were cut into longitudinal sections with the aid of a cryostat.

Tissue sections were processed using streptavidin-biotin-peroxidase complex immunohistochemical method or by immunofluorescence. In both cases, sections were incubated with 10% fetal bovine serum (FBS) and then incubated with the primary antibody overnight at 4°C. Primary antibodies against Dyrk1A (diluted 1:500, [12] and 1:200 AbNova Corporation, Tebu, France), serotonin (diluted 1:35000, DiaSorin, Stillwater, MN, USA), tyrosine hydroxilase (TH, diluted 1:8000, Sigma, St Louis, MO, USA), choline acetyltransferase (ChAT, diluted 1:400, Chemicon, Temeluca, CA, USA), Calbindin D-28K (diluted 1:200, Sigma, St Louis, MO, USA), Calretinin (diluted 1:500, Sigma, St Louis, MO, USA), Parvalbumin (diluted 1:500, Sigma, St Louis, MO, USA), vesicular glutamate transporter 1 (vGlut1, diluted 1:2500, Chemicon, Temeluca, CA, USA), vesicular glutamate transporter 2 (vGlut2, diluted 1:1000, Synaptic Systems, Göttingen, Germany), glutamate decarboxylase (GAD_{65-67}, diluted 1:500, Chemicon, Temeluca, CA, USA) and calcitonin gene related peptide (CGRP, diluted 1:1000, Sigma, St Louis, MO, USA) were used. The sections were then incubated with the appropriate biotinylated secondary antibody or with secondary antibodies labeled either with Alexa Fluor 488 or Alexa Fluor 546 (Molecular Probes, Eugene, OR, USA) for multifluorescent labeling. In the first case, the sections were then incubated with the biotinylated link and the streptavidin-HRP as indicated in the manufacturer's instructions (DAKO, LSAB system, Ely, UK). Peroxidase activity was visualized with 0.05% diaminobenzidine and 0.01% hydrogen peroxide. Sections were dehydrated with increasing concentrations of ethanol until arriving to xylene, and cover slipped with DPX (distyrene, tricresyl phosphate, and xylene; BDH Laboratory Supplies, UK). For immunofluorescence, labeled sections were mounted using Vectashield Mounting medium with DAPI (Vector Laboratories, Burlingame, CA, USA) and stored at 4°C.

Skeletal muscle sections (caudal portion of digastricus and stylohyoideus muscle) that are innervated by facial nerve (VII) were directly incubated with Alexa Fluor 488-conjugated α-bungarotoxin (α-Btx, 1 μg/ml; Molecular Probes, Eugene, OR, USA) to detect the acetylcholine receptors (AchRs) at the neuromuscular synaptic sites and synaptophysin (diluted 1:100; DakoCytomation Glostrup, Denmark) as a pre-synaptic marker.

The sections were examined using a Leica DMR (Leica Microsystems AG, Wetzlar, Germany) microscope with a Leica DC500 digital camera coupled to the microscope. Immunofluorescence sections were captured on a Leica TCS SPE with appropriate lasers. Intensity analysis was performed on images acquired under identical microscope conditions and software settings. For the final published figures, images were assembled, labeled and balanced for optimal brightness and contrast by using either Adobe Photoshop or ImageJ software (National Institutes of Health, Bethesda, MD, USA).

Morphology and Stereological Techniques

To construct the morphological maps we used coronal slices (16 μm). Counterstained with the Nissl technique using 0.1% cresyl violet and other markers (Dyrk1A, ChAT) to characterize specific neuronal populations at PD7, PD10 and PD21. Images of the regions of interest were taken, sections were reconstructed and neuronal maps were drawn. Counts of facial motoneurons were performed on serial Nissl stained paraffin sections (9 μm). Adult mice motoneurons of the facial nucleus are localized in a well-defined region of the brainstem that allows counting their cell bodies. Briefly, a minimum of wild type and TgDyrk1A adult (6 months old) mice (n = 6 per genotype), were transcardially perfused as described above. Sections were stained using the Nissl technique with 0.1% cresyl violet, dehydrated with increasing concentrations of ethanol to xylene, and coverslipped with DPX. Large motoneurons, with clearly defined nucleolus, were counted from every fourth section with the aid of a camera lucida. The area of each motoneuron was also measured.

Axotomy of the Facial Nerve

Adult (6 months old) mice were anesthetized with 3% isoflurane. Using aseptic techniques, the right facial nerve of each animal was exposed and transected at its exit from the stylomastoid foramen [22]. Successful transections were identified by an absence of whisker movement at the left side of the face. The contra lateral side was used as a control. At 2, 7 and 14 days after axotomy, the animals (n = 4 for each time point and genotype) were deeply anesthetized and perfused transcardially as it was described above. The lower brainstem segment was quickly removed and post-fixed in the same fixative. Serial 40 μm thick sections of the brainstem were processed for Dyrk1A immunohistochemistry and for Dyrk1A/CGRP fluorescent labeling, in order to quantify Dyrk1A intensity in the motoneurons of the facial nucleus.

Data Analysis

Simple comparisons between TgDyrk1A and wild type mice in behavioral tasks and morphological/stereological studies were performed using the two-tailed Student's t test or repeated measures ANOVA. Quantitative data are expressed as mean ± standard error (S.E.M.). In all tests, a difference was considered significant at p values <0.05. The statistical analysis was performed using the SPSS 17.0 software.

Results

Neurobehavioral Development

In order to study the contribution of *DYRK1A* to Down syndrome phenotypes, we used a transgenic mouse model for *Dyrk1A* (TgDyrk1A) [15]. TgDyrk1A is a single-gene transgenic mouse overexpressing specifically the full-length cDNA of *Dyrk1A* under the control of sheep metallothionein-Ia (*sMT-Ia*) promoter. The levels of this transcript were higher in the transgenic mice, in the range of ~1.5 to 2.2 fold increased.

No significant differences were detected in weight and body length increase during the preweaning period in wild type (n = 36) versus TgDyrk1A (n = 39) mice (data not shown). TgDyrk1A mice showed no significant differences in the achievements of physical milestones, such as fur appearance, incisor eruption, eyelid opening or permeabilisation of the auditory canal. Also, no differences were detected in sensoriomotor functions, such as forelimb/hind limb placing and grasping, tactile orientation or Preyer's reflex. These data indicate that *Dyrk1A* overexpression did not affect the overall growth or the acquisition of sensoriomotor functions in mice.

Neuromotor Development

Previous data from our lab showed neuromotor developmental delay in TgDyrk1A mice [15]. Thus to get further insight in the effect of *Dyrk1A* overexpression on early postnatal motor development, TgDyrk1A mice were evaluated at four time points important for motor development: PD7, PD10, PD14 and PD21. TgDyrk1A (n = 32) mice showed a similar pivoting activity compared to wild types (n = 32) (Figure 1A). However, we observed a significant delay in the appearance of walking behavior ($F_{(7,56)} = 10.290$, $P = 0.000$, repeated measures ANOVA) (Figure 1B) supporting previous reports. This delay was more apparent at older ages, when the adult walking patterns are fully established. TgDyrk1A also showed a delay in the acquisition of negative geotaxis. At PD7, 21.4% of wild type presented a complete negative geotaxis, compared to only 16.6% of TgDyrk1A mice. However, this impairment was rapidly recovered, so that at PD10, TgDyrk1A mice performed the task even better than the wild type mice ($F_{(5,42)} = 11.016$, $P = 0.000$, repeated measures ANOVA, Figure 1C). TgDyrk1A mice were also slower in acquiring climbing ability (Figure 1D). At PD7, 28% of wild type while no TgDyrk1A was able to climb the screen ($F_{(5,72)} = 32.266$, $P = 0.000$, repeated measures ANOVA), albeit again at PD14 both genotypes correctly performed the task. In the wire suspension test (Figure 1E), TgDyrk1A remained less time hanging in the wire and they fell down earlier than wild type mice ($F_{(7,56)} = 6.875$, $P = 0.000$, repeated measures ANOVA). Finally, no significant alterations in the locomotion pattern between wild type and TgDyrk1A mice were observed in the paw print test at PD21 (data not shown).

Expression Pattern of Dyrk1A during Early Postnatal Development

We next studied the pattern of expression of Dyrk1A in wild type and TgDyrk1A mice during postnatal development (minimum of 6 mice per genotype, age and experiment). Dyrk1A expression is well characterized during embryonic stages [14,23] and in the adult mice [12], but there were no data on the postnatal period. While during development Dyrk1A is ubiquitously expressed, in the adult it is specifically expressed in motoneurons

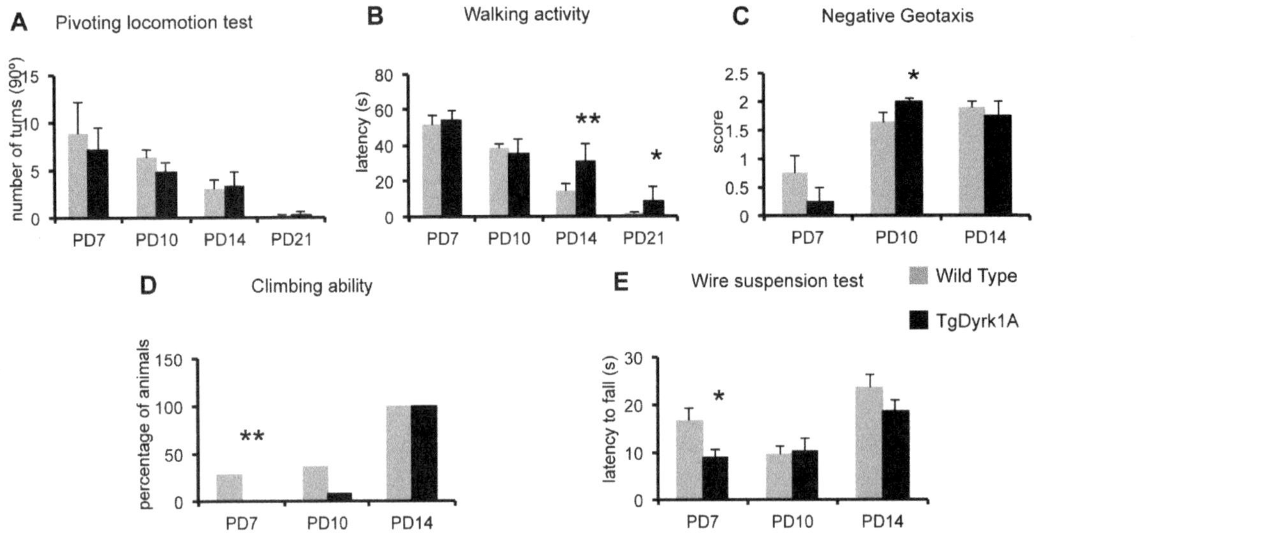

Figure 1. Neuromotor development of TgDyrk1A mice. A) Pivoting activity: TgDyrk1A mice showed a similar number of turns (times the mouse rotated 90 degrees on its hindlimbs) over a 60 sec period in the pivoting test. B) Walking activity: TgDyrk1A mice showed longer latency to initiate walking at PD14 and PD21. C) Negative geotaxis: TgDyrk1A mice exhibited a delay in acquiring negative geotaxis as shown by the impaired performance at PD7 that was recovered at later stages (PD14). D) The percentage of TgDyrk1A mice able to perform the vertical climbing was reduced at PD7 and PD10. E) In the wire suspension test, the latency to fall of TgDyrk1A mice was reduced at P7 developmental stages. Data are presented as mean+SEM, * $P<0.05$, ** $P<0.005$.

of the motor nuclei of the brainstem (i.e. Facial nucleus). Since the motor alterations in DS are established through delays in postnatal motor development, we analyzed the expression of Dyrk1A in the brainstem and spinal cord (SC) at different postnatal days (PD7, PD10, PD14). No differences in the expression pattern of Dyrk1A were detected between genotypes, showing no ectopic expression, but increased Dyrk1A signal intensity in TgDyrk1A mice indicating overexpression of the kinase.

Dyrk1A expression at postnatal day 7. At PD7, immunohistochemistry against choline acetylcholine transferase (ChAT) showed cholinergic neurons mostly in the facial (FN) and trigeminal motor nuclei (Figure 2A,B), although scattered ChAT positive neurons also appeared in other brainstem areas. At this stage, Dyrk1A was not expressed in motoneurons (MTNs) of the FN (Figure 2A, upper panel), but we detected a positive Dyrk1A population in specific nuclei of the reticular formation located around the FN (Figure 2A, lower panel, D): dorsal nucleus paragigantocellular (DPGi), gigantocellular reticular nucleus (Gi), intermediate reticular nucleus (IRT), parvicellular reticular nucleus-alpha part (PCRtA), paragigantocellular lateral nucleus (LPGi) and in the raphe nuclei (nucleus magnum RMC and pale nucleus –RPA). Also, Dyrk1A expression was found in the medial longitudinal fascicle (MLF) and nucleus peripyramidal (ppy) (Figure 2C). In the reticular formation, Dyrk1A was not co-localized with calcium binding proteins, serotonin or tyrosine hydroxylase, but we detected co-immunostaining with GABA, GAD_{65-67}, vGlut1 and vGlut2 (Figure 2D), suggesting that Dyrk1A is expressed in glutamatergic and GABAergic neurons in both genotypes.

Dyrk1A expression at postnatal days 10 and 14. At PD10, Dyrk1A started to be detected in motoneurons (MTNs) of the spinal cord (SC; cervical, dorsal, lumbar; Figure 3A) and FN (Figure 3B), where it remained until adulthood in both genotypes. Double immunofluorescence studies showed co-localization of Dyrk1A positive MTNs with ChAT, confirming their cholinergic phenotype (Figure 3C, left panel), and their localization in the ventral horn of the SC (Figure 3C, right panel).

From PD10 to PD14, Dyrk1A expression disappeared from neurons of the reticular formation and was detected in the MTNs of the FN (Figure 3B) and other motor nuclei of the brainstem, such as the trigeminal nucleus that were positive for Dyrk1A and ChAT (Figure 3D). However, only 70% of the ChAT positive neurons of the FN at PD14 expressed Dyrk1A in both genotypes, although TgDyrk1A showed increased intensity of immunoreactivity against Dyrk1A.

Motoneurons of the SC and the FN showed a strong cytoplasmic granular Dyrk1A immunostaining in the soma and proximal neurites at PD10 and PD14, completely excluding the nucleus, similar to that previously described during adulthood [12]. Although no important genotype-related differences were observed in Dyrk1A expression pattern during postnatal development, adult TgDyrk1A mice showed a 15.5% of significant increase of total number of MTNs ($t=-4.145$, $P=0.003$, Student's t test, Figure 4A,B) in the FN. In addition, MTNs of TgDyrk1A mice had smaller diameters ($t=4.461$, $P=0.000$, Student's t test, Figure 4A,C).

Dyrk1A Expression at the Neuromuscular Junctions

Previous work had described the location of Dyrk1A in neurite terminals, and suggested its involvement in neurotransmission at the synaptic site [24,25]. Thus, we studied Dyrk1A expression at the neuromuscular junctions in adult mice (6 months). Fluorescent α-bungarotoxin (αBtx) conjugate was used to identify postsynaptic ACh receptors, to localize neuromuscular junctions and innervated motor endplates (Figure 5A). Intensity values for Dyrk1A and αBtx fluorescence were plotted for individual endplates on TgDyrk1A mice (Figure 5B). Dyrk1A was not detected with a pre-absorbed anti-Dyrk1A antibody, as a negative control (Figure 5C). To confirm the observation of presynaptic location of Dyrk1A in neuromuscular junctions, a double immunostaining of Dyrk1A and synaptophysin was performed. A clear colocaliza-

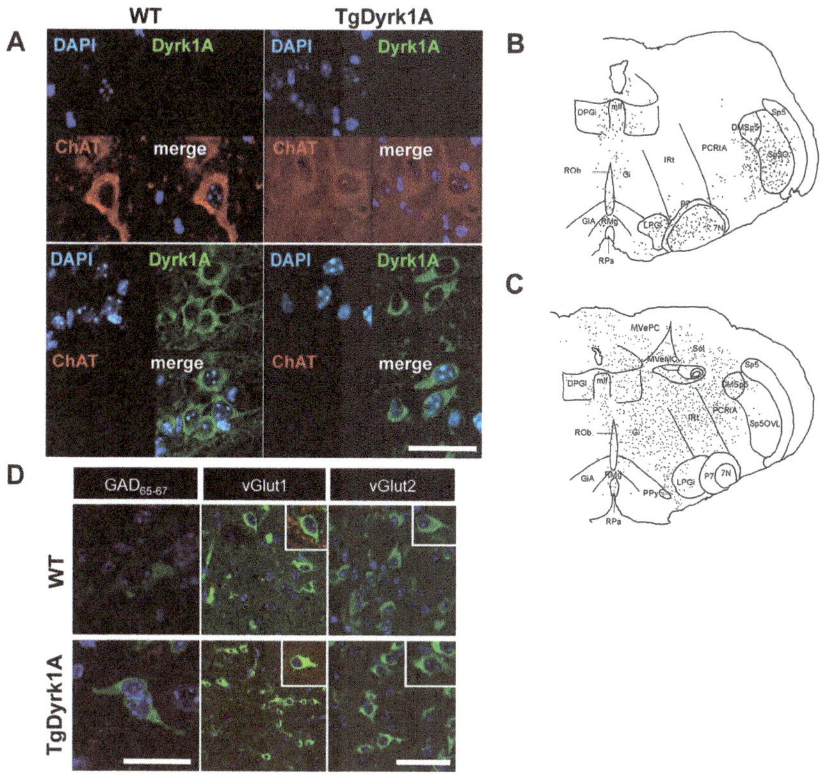

Figure 2. Dyrk1A expression in the brainstem at postnatal day 7. A, D) Collapsed low magnification images of confocal z-stacks of coronal sections (16 μm) of the brainstem from PD7 wild type (left panel) and TgDyrk1A (right panel) mice. A) Double immunofluorescence labeling for Dyrk1A (green) and ChAT (red) and counterstaining with DAPI (blue) showing no positive Dyrk1A cells in MTN of the facial nucleus. Note the typical morphology of ChAT positive MTNs (upper panel). Dyrk1A positive neurons in specific nuclei of the reticular formation located around the facial nucleus (lower panel). B, C) Histological maps showing: B) ChAT positive-Dyrk1A negative neurons mostly localized in the facial (VII) and trigeminal motor (V) nuclei and C) Dyrk1A positive neurons in several nuclei of the reticular formation: dorsal nucleus paragigantocellularis (DPGi), gigantocellularis reticular nucleus (Gi), intermediate reticular nucleus (IRT), parvicellular reticular nucleus-alpha part (PCRtA), paragigantocellularis lateral nucleus (LPGi) and in the raphe nuclei (nucleus magnum –RMG- and pale nucleus –RPA). D) Double immunostaining of Dyrk1A (green) and glutamate decarboxylase (GAD_{65-67}), vesicular glutamate transporter 1 (vGlut1) and vesicular glutamate transporter 2 (vGlut2). Upper panel show wild type and lower panel TgDyrk1A mice. Inserts represent higher magnification images of selected positive neurons. Scale bar (valid for all panels): 10 μm.

tion was observed, indicating Dyrk1A immunostaining associated with presynaptic terminals but not with the post-synaptic marker (αBtx, Figure 5D).

In order to analyze the possible axonal transport of Dyrk1A protein, we performed unilateral facial nerve axotomies in adult mice. The animals were then sacrificed at different time points after surgery (days 2, 7, 14) to determine Dyrk1A accumulation in the FN (Figure 6A). A group of non-axotomized wild type and TgDyrk1A animals were used to determine the basal levels of Dyrk1A expression in the FN. In the non-axotomized group, the expression level of Dyrk1A was higher in TgDyrk1A mice as compared with wild types ($t = -2.937$, $P = 0.043$, Student's t test). For the axotomized groups, the ratio between axotomized and contralateral sides was calculated in each time point after axotomy and ratios were normalized to the basal Dyrk1A expression levels of each genotype.

The ratio of Dyrk1A expression between axotomized and contralateral sides increased 7 days after axotomy and was decreased by day 14 postaxotomy in both genotypes (Figure 6A,B). These results suggested that Dyrk1A is transported along the axons to the neuromuscular junctions since after axotomy Dyrk1A was accumulated in the soma of the FN MTNs. To verify this Dyrk1A accumulation, we analyzed the expression of calcitonin gene related peptide (CGRP), a neuropeptide located in granular vesicles of the Golgi apparatus and smooth endoplasmic reticulum of MTNs [26], at 14 days after surgery. CGRP accumulates in the soma of MTNs 15 hours after axotomy of the FN, reaching a peak at 6 days after surgery, and gradually decreasing to normal levels [27]. In our experiments, Dyrk1A co-localized with CGRP and both genotypes showed a concomitant increase in CGRP expression (Figure 6C).

Discussion

Down syndrome (DS) individuals present important motor deficits that have been classically ascribed to structural and functional deficits in the cerebellum [28]. Genetic dissection studies in mouse models showed the implication of *Dyrk1A,* a candidate gene for DS abnormalities, in the adult DS motor phenotypes [12,16,17,20,29,30,31,32]. However, even though DS motor deficits are the consequence of altered motor development of infants and young children, there are very few studies addressing its pathogenetic mechanisms in this extremely important life period. Here we have explored the postnatal expression pattern of *Dyrk1A* in the brainstem and spinal cord and impact of its overexpression during postnatal motor development in transgenic mice (TgDyrk1A). Our results confirmed and extended

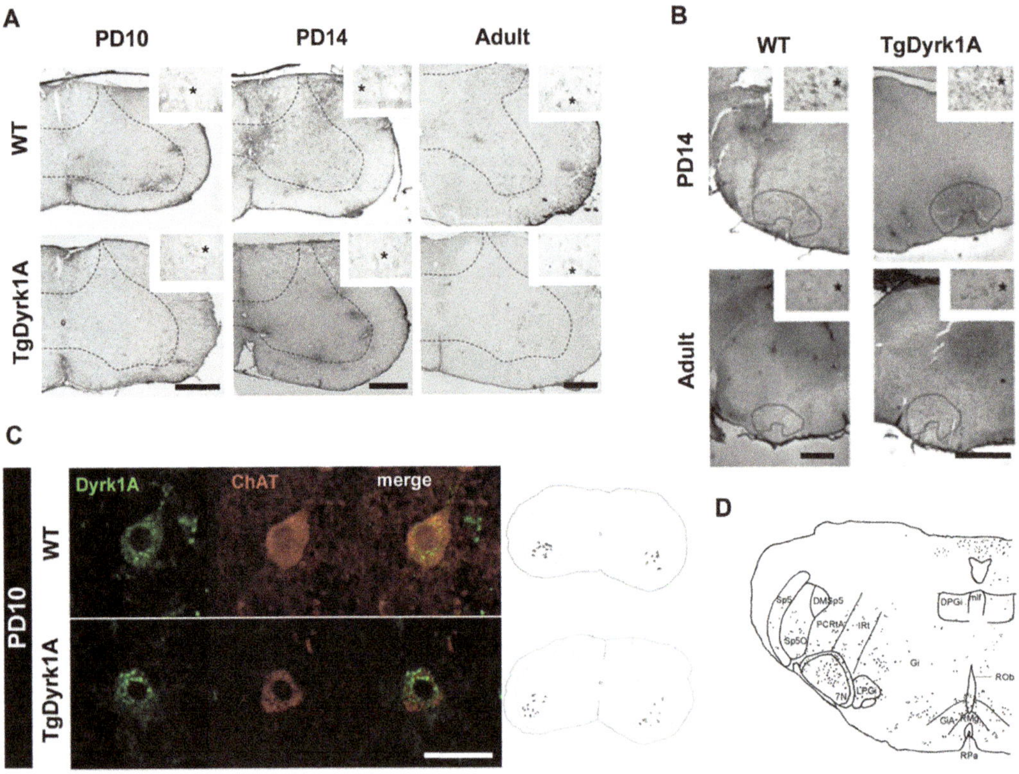

Figure 3. Dyrk1A expression in the spinal cord and facial nucleus at postnatal day 10, postnatal day 14 and adulthood. A) At PD10, Dyrk1A expression started to be detected in MTNs of the spinal cord (left panel), where it remained until adulthood (PD14: middle panel; adult: right panel), in both wild type (upper panel) and TgDyrk1A mice (lower panel). Insert shows MTNs (*) at higher magnification. B) At PD14 (upper panel), Dyrk1A expression disappeared from neurons of the reticular formation and started in the MTNs of the facial nucleus, where it remained until adulthood (lower panel) in wild type (left panel) and TgDyrk1A (right panel). Insert shows Dyrk1A positive MTNs (*) at higher magnification. C) Double immunofluorescence studies at PD10 showed the co-localization of Dyrk1A (green) positive MTNs with ChAT (red) staining in wild type (upper panel) and TgDyrk1A (lower panel) mice that confirmed their cholinergic phenotype. Note the strong Dyrk1A cytoplasmic granular immunostaining in the MTN soma and proximal neurites. Right panel depicts the morphological maps locating Dyrk1A positive neurons in the ventral horn of the spinal cord. D) Mapping of Dyrk1A positive cells showing its location in the MTNs of the FN and other motor nuclei of the brainstem. Abbreviations: DPGi, dorsal nucleus paragigantocellularis; Gi, gigantocellularis reticular nucleus; IRT intermediate reticular nucleus; PCRtA, parvicellular reticular nucleus-alpha part; LPGi, paragigantocellularis lateral nucleus; and raphe nuclei (RMG, nucleus magnum, and RPA, pale nucleus), facial motor (VII) and trigeminal motor (V) nuclei. Scale bar for A and C: 10 μm, Scale bar B: 15 μm.

previous studies [15] indicating a delayed cranio-caudal maturation of the motor system. Dyrk1A showed a time-dependent postnatal expression in specific brainstem nuclei of the reticular formation, and later expression in motoneurons (MTNs) of the facial motor nucleus (FN) and the spinal cord. Importantly, we describe for the first time the presence of Dyrk1A in the presynaptic terminal of the neuromuscular junctions and its axonal transport from the facial nucleus, suggesting a function for Dyrk1A in these structures.

In our experiments, we have confirmed and extended previous observations indicating that Dyrk1A overexpression in TgDyrk1A mice gives rise to neuromotor developmental delay [15]. TgDyrk1A mice showed a delayed development of adult-like walking ability (PD10 and PD14) that was compensated by PD21. The maturation of negative geotaxis required to detecting and to correct body position, was also slightly, though not significantly delayed in TgDyrk1A, suggesting that *Dyrk1A* overexpression could affect propioception and vestibular development. This assumption was reinforced by the significantly slower acquisition of the climbing ability.

In the neonate, immature motor patterns mainly depend on spinal and brainstem control and it is subsequent motor maturation what stems from a growing integration of supraspinal, intraspinal, and sensory control. Previous studies showed ubiquitous spatio-temporal expression of Dyrk1A in the mid/late embryonic (E12–18), the early postnatal (PD0–5) [13,14] that was restricted to the olfactory bulb, some forebrain regions and MTNs of the brainstem (facial nucleus) and spinal cord in the adult mouse brain [12]. In our experiments, a positive Dyrk1A population was detected in specific nuclei of the reticular formation, such as the dorsal nucleus paragigantocellular, gigantocellular reticular nucleus, intermediate reticular nucleus, parvicellular reticular nucleus-alpha part, paragigantocellular lateral nucleus and raphe nuclei, that disappeared from the reticular formation at PD10. *Dyrk1A* transcripts were previously reported in the basal plate of the rhombencephalon during embryonic period, in several pontine nuclei and in the rhombencephalic reticular formation, as well as in the cochlear and vestibular nuclei of the alar plate [13,14]. Our study suggests that its expression persists during early postnatal stages, both in glutamatergic and GABAergic neurons as shown by its co-localization with GABA, GAD_{65-67}, vGlut1 and vGlut2.

At PD10, a period that is crucial for the development of motor patterns such as walking ability, Dyrk1A expression started in

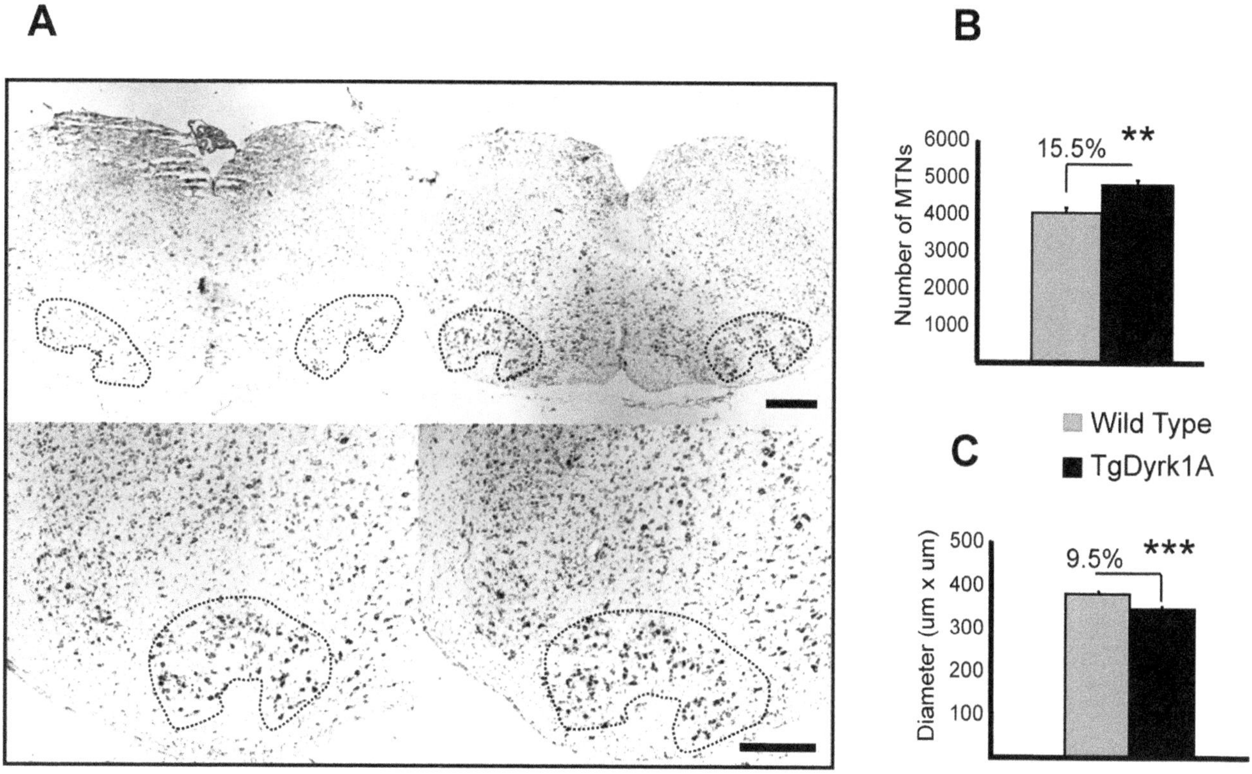

Figure 4. Quantification of the number of motoneurons in the facial nucleus of adult TgDyrk1A. Counting of facial motoneurons was performed on serial Nissl stained paraffin sections (9 μm). A) The number of MTNs in the facial nucleus was quantified in adult wild type (left panel) and TgDyrk1A (right panel) mice. Lower panels show high magnification of the corresponding slice. B) TgDyrk1A mice showed a significant increase of total number of MTNs of the facial nucleus. C) TgDyrk1A MTNs presented a reduction of their diameter. Data in the histograms are represented as means +/− SEM. ** $P<0.005$, *** $P<0.001$. Scale bar (for upper panels): 15 μm, (for lower panels): 1 mm.

MTNs of the facial nucleus and spinal cord (cervical, dorsal, lumbar), where it persisted until adulthood and was co-localized with ChAT. Dyrk1A showed a strong cytoplasmic granular immunostaining in the soma and proximal neurites at PD10 and PD14, completely excluding the nucleus, similar to the subcellular pattern previously described [12].

Interestingly, the number of FN MTNs was significantly increased in TgDyrk1A mice although they were smaller than in wild type mice. *Dyrk1A* has been suggested to control cell proliferation and exit from the cell cycle at precise locations along the neural tube [23]. In a YAC transgenic mouse line (152F7) overexpressing *DYRK1A*, increased brain weight and neuronal size were detected, along with increase in phosphorylation of the transcription factor FKHR and with high levels of cyclin B1 [33]. Our results suggest that Dyrk1A may also affect proliferation of other neuronal populations. However, MTNs' size was decreased in TgDyrk1A that could be interpreted as receiving less terminals contacts [34].

Motor dysfunction in DS is accompanied by hyporeflexia and reduced muscular strength and tone [4,35,36]. Thus, we also studied if Dyrk1A was expressed in at the neuromuscular junctions. We found Dyrk1A in neuromuscular synapses, but it did not co-localized with α-bungarotoxin (αBtx) a post-synaptic marker of acetylcholine receptors (AChRs), indicating that Dyrk1A is located in presynaptic terminals. These results suggested that Dyrk1A could be transported along the axons to the neuromuscular junctions. To proof this hypothesis, we performed facial nerve axotomies, and analyzed expression of Dyrk1A in the FN MTNs. Should Dyrk1A undergo axonal transport, its increased accumulation in the soma would be an indicator of the disruption of transport. In our experiments, the ratio of expression of Dyrk1A between axotomized and contralateral sides was increased 7 days after axotomy in both genotypes, and thereafter reduced at post-axotomy day 14. The expression levels of CGRP, a neuropeptide that accumulates in the soma of motoneurons after axotomy of the facial nerve [27], were also increased after surgery in both wild type and transgenic mice. Interestingly, we observed a co-localization of Dyrk1A with CGRP in granular cytoplasmic vesicles of the MTNs, where it coexists with ChAT, and in the Golgi apparatus and smooth endoplasmic reticulum [26].

In conclusion, we here demonstrate time-specific postnatal Dyrk1A expression in the brainstem, spinal cord and in the neuromuscular junctions where it arrives through anterograde axonal transport. *Dyrk1A* overexpression in TgDyrk1A mice leads delays in motor maturation and increased numbers of small-size MTNs. Interestingly, Dyrk1A was found in the brainstem motor nuclei, which integrity is required for the timely development of motor function. Taken together our work indicates that the role of *Dyrk1A* in motor function may be more complex than previously envisaged and suggest that normalization of its dosage could be a good therapeutic strategy in DS.

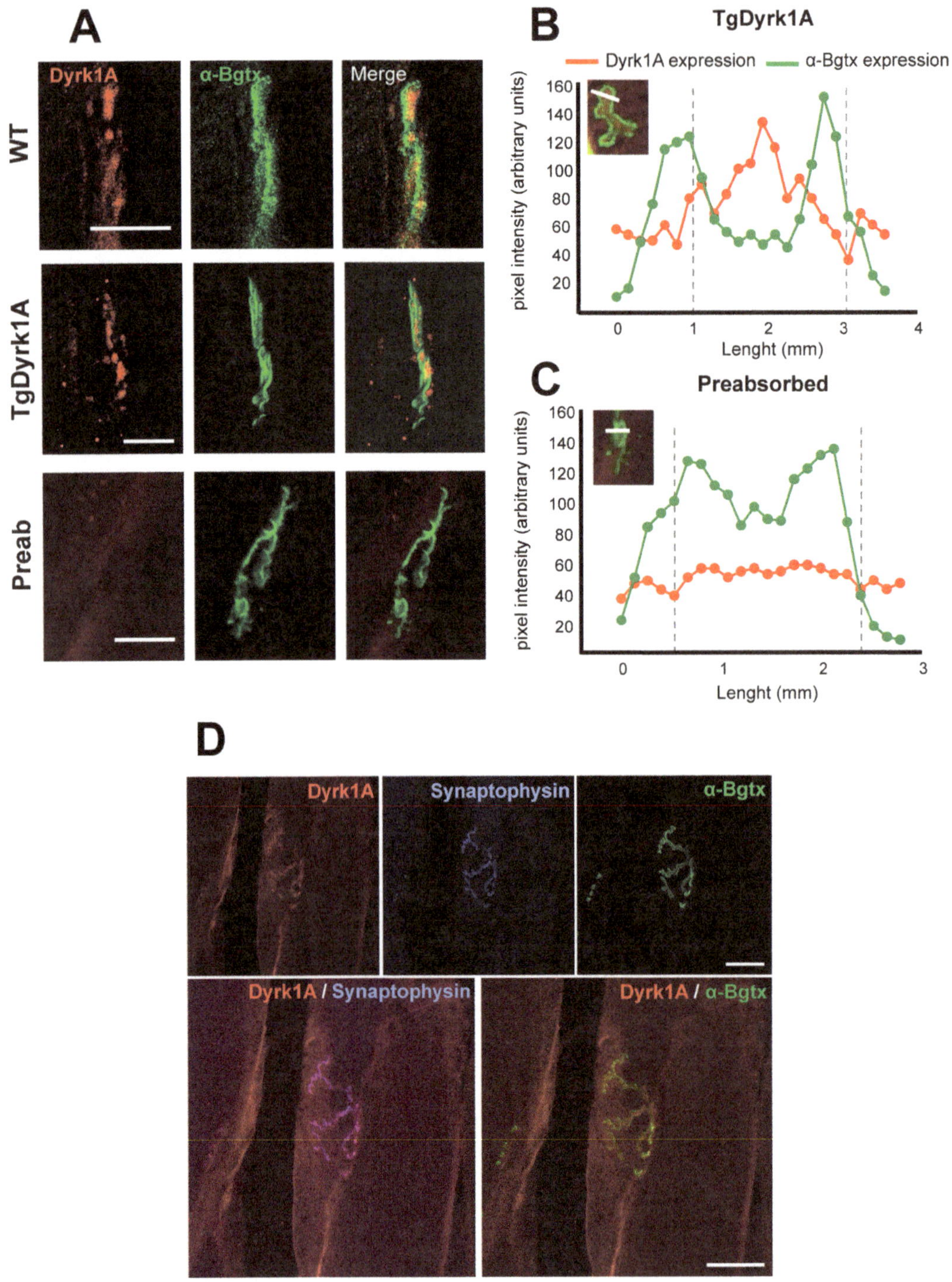

Figure 5. Dyrk1A expression at the neuromuscular junctions. A) Dyrk1A (red) was found in neuromuscular synapses, where it was not co-localized with α-bungarotoxin (αBtx; green) in wild type (upper panel) and TgDyrk1A (middle panel) mice, indicating that Dyrk1A is located in the presynaptic region. Lower panel depicts pre-absorption experiments against mouse anti-Dyrk1A antibody. B-C) Intensity values (arbitrary pixel intensity units) for Dyrk1A (red) and αBtx (green), a marker of acetylcholine receptors, fluorescence were plotted along a line traced over a synaptic fold in individual endplates on (B) TgDyrk1A mice and (C) pre-absorbed antibody. D) Dyrk1A (red, upper left panel) was present at the pre-synaptic site of the neuromuscular junctions, showed by triple fluorescence immunohistochemistry. Synaptophysin (blue, upper central panel) was used as a pre-synaptic marker. α-bungarotoxin (αBtx; green, upper right panel) was used as a post-synpatic marker. Merge images for Dyrk1A and synaptophysin (lower left panel) showed a clear co-localization between both markers. Lower right panel showed only αBtx expression and there was not a co-localization with Dyrk1A. Scale bar: A) 10 μm and D) 25 μm.

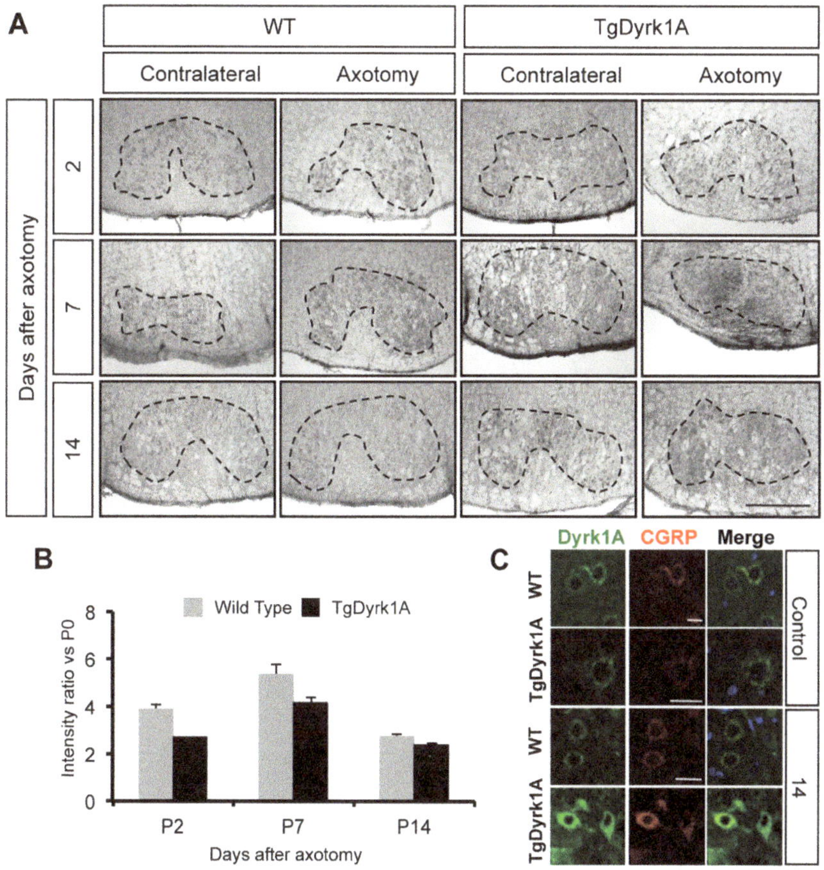

Figure 6. Axonal transport of Dyrk1A in adult mice facial nerve. Axotomies of wild type and TgDyrk1A mice were performed, sacrificing mice at different time points after surgery. A) Expression of Dyrk1A in the facial nucleus was analyzed at different time-points (2, 7, 14 days) post-axotomy in the axotomized and contralateral facial nucleus of wild type (left panel) and TgDyrk1A (right panel) mice. B) The intensity ratio between axotomized and contralateral sides was used to determine Dyrk1A accumulation in the soma as an indicator of the disruption of transport. Expression levels of Dyrk1A in the facial nucleus of wild type and TgDyrk1A mice in non-axotomized conditions (P0) were used for normalizing the ratio at P2, P4 and P14. The expression ratio increased 7 days after surgery as compared to the non-axotomized condition, and was reduced at day 14th post-axotomy in both genotypes. C) To verify Dyrk1A accumulation in the soma of motoneurons after axotomy, we analyzed its co-expression of CGRP. Upper panel shows Dyrk1A (green), CGRP (red) and merge of both in wild type and TgDyrk1A in non-axotomized animals, called basal/control group. 14 days after surgery (lower panel), both genotypes showed an increase of Dyrk1A-CGRP co-expression. Data in the histograms are represented as means +/− SEM. Scale bar for A 15 μm. Scale bar C: upper panel: 55 μm; second upper panel: 60 μm; third upper panel: 50 μm.

Acknowledgments

We like to thank Imma Montoliu for her technical help and Prof. Josep Esquerda, Prof. Jordi Calderó and Dr. María Martínez de Lagrán for their helpful comments and revision of this paper.

Author Contributions

Conceived and designed the experiments: GA MD AC. Performed the experiments: GA MD AC. Analyzed the data: GA MD AC. Contributed reagents/materials/analysis tools: MD AC. Wrote the paper: GA MD AC.

References

1. Dierssen M (2012) Down syndrome: the brain in trisomic mode. Nature reviews Neuroscience 13: 844–858.
2. Latash ML, Anson JG (2006) Synergies in health and disease: relations to adaptive changes in motor coordination. Phys Ther 86: 1151–1160.
3. Latash ML, Corcos DM (1991) Kinematic and electromyographic characteristics of single-joint movements of individuals with Down syndrome. Am J Ment Retard 96: 189–201.
4. Palisano RJ, Walter SD, Russell DJ, Rosenbaum PL, Gemus M, et al. (2001) Gross motor function of children with down syndrome: creation of motor growth curves. Arch Phys Med Rehabil 82: 494–500.
5. Henderson SE, Morris J, Frith U (1981) The motor deficit in Down's syndrome children: a problem of timing? J Child Psychol Psychiatry 22: 233–245.
6. O'Doherty A, Ruf S, Mulligan C, Hildreth V, Errington ML, et al. (2005) An aneuploid mouse strain carrying human chromosome 21 with Down syndrome phenotypes. Science 309: 2033–2037.
7. Galante M, Jani H, Vanes L, Daniel H, Fisher EM, et al. (2009) Impairments in motor coordination without major changes in cerebellar plasticity in the Tc1 mouse model of Down syndrome. Hum Mol Genet 18: 1449–1463.
8. Baxter LL, Moran TH, Richtsmeier JT, Troncoso J, Reeves RH (2000) Discovery and genetic localization of Down syndrome cerebellar phenotypes using the Ts65Dn mouse. Hum Mol Genet 9: 195–202.
9. Olson LE, Roper RJ, Baxter LL, Carlson EJ, Epstein CJ, et al. (2004) Down syndrome mouse models Ts65Dn, Ts1Cje, and Ms1Cje/Ts65Dn exhibit variable severity of cerebellar phenotypes. Dev Dyn 230: 581–589.
10. Guimera J, Casas C, Pucharcos C, Solans A, Domenech A, et al. (1996) A human homologue of Drosophila minibrain (MNB) is expressed in the neuronal regions affected in Down syndrome and maps to the critical region. Hum Mol Genet 5: 1305–1310.
11. Becker L, Mito T, Takashima S, Onodera K (1991) Growth and development of the brain in Down syndrome. Prog Clin Biol Res 373: 133–152.
12. Marti E, Altafaj X, Dierssen M, de la Luna S, Fotaki V, et al. (2003) Dyrk1A expression pattern supports specific roles of this kinase in the adult central nervous system. Brain Res 964: 250–263.
13. Hammerle B, Carnicero A, Elizalde C, Ceron J, Martinez S, et al. (2003) Expression patterns and subcellular localization of the Down syndrome

candidate protein MNB/DYRK1A suggest a role in late neuronal differentiation. Eur J Neurosci 17: 2277–2286.
14. Hammerle B, Elizalde C, Tejedor FJ (2008) The spatio-temporal and subcellular expression of the candidate Down syndrome gene Mnb/Dyrk1A in the developing mouse brain suggests distinct sequential roles in neuronal development. Eur J Neurosci 27: 1061–1074.
15. Altafaj X, Dierssen M, Baamonde C, Marti E, Visa J, et al. (2001) Neurodevelopmental delay, motor abnormalities and cognitive deficits in transgenic mice overexpressing Dyrk1A (minibrain), a murine model of Down's syndrome. Hum Mol Genet 10: 1915–1923.
16. Martinez de Lagran M, Altafaj X, Gallego X, Marti E, Estivill X, et al. (2004) Motor phenotypic alterations in TgDyrk1a transgenic mice implicate DYRK1A in Down syndrome motor dysfunction. Neurobiol Dis 15: 132–142.
17. Ortiz-Abalia J, Sahun I, Altafaj X, Andreu N, Estivill X, et al. (2008) Targeting Dyrk1A with AAVshRNA attenuates motor alterations in TgDyrk1A, a mouse model of Down syndrome. Am J Hum Genet 83: 479–488.
18. Ahn KJ, Jeong HK, Choi HS, Ryoo SR, Kim YJ, et al. (2006) DYRK1A BAC transgenic mice show altered synaptic plasticity with learning and memory defects. Neurobiol Dis 22: 463–472.
19. Fotaki V, Dierssen M, Alcantara S, Martinez S, Marti E, et al. (2002) Dyrk1A haploinsufficiency affects viability and causes developmental delay and abnormal brain morphology in mice. Mol Cell Biol 22: 6636–6647.
20. Martinez de Lagran M, Bortolozzi A, Millan O, Gispert JD, Gonzalez JR, et al. (2007) Dopaminergic deficiency in mice with reduced levels of the dual-specificity tyrosine-phosphorylated and regulated kinase 1A, Dyrk1A(+/−). Genes Brain Behav 6: 569–578.
21. Dierssen M, Fotaki V, Martinez de Lagran M, Gratacos M, Arbones M, et al. (2002) Neurobehavioral development of two mouse lines commonly used in transgenic studies. Pharmacol Biochem Behav 73: 19–25.
22. Casanovas A, Ribera J, Hager G, Kreutzberg GW, Esquerda JE (2001) c-Jun regulation in rat neonatal motoneurons postaxotomy. J Neurosci Res 63: 469–479.
23. Hammerle B, Vera-Samper E, Speicher S, Arencibia R, Martinez S, et al. (2002) Mnb/Dyrk1A is transiently expressed and asymmetrically segregated in neural progenitor cells at the transition to neurogenic divisions. Dev Biol 246: 259–273.
24. Chen-Hwang MC, Chen HR, Elzinga M, Hwang YW (2002) Dynamin is a minibrain kinase/dual specificity Yak1-related kinase 1A substrate. J Biol Chem 277: 17597–17604.
25. Huang Y, Chen-Hwang MC, Dolios G, Murakami N, Padovan JC, et al. (2004) Mnb/Dyrk1A phosphorylation regulates the interaction of dynamin 1 with SH3 domain-containing proteins. Biochemistry 43: 10173–10185.
26. Caldero J, Casanovas A, Sorribas A, Esquerda JE (1992) Calcitonin gene-related peptide in rat spinal cord motoneurons: subcellular distribution and changes induced by axotomy. Neuroscience 48: 449–461.
27. Streit WJ, Dumoulin FL, Raivich G, Kreutzberg GW (1989) Calcitonin gene-related peptide increases in rat facial motoneurons after peripheral nerve transection. Neurosci Lett 101: 143–148.
28. Shapiro BL (2001) Developmental instability of the cerebellum and its relevance to Down syndrome. J Neural Transm Suppl: 11–34.
29. Arque G, de Lagran MM, Arbones ML, Dierssen M (2009) Age-associated motor and visuo-spatial learning phenotype in Dyrk1A heterozygous mutant mice. Neurobiol Dis 36: 312–319.
30. Altafaj X, Ortiz-Abalia J, Fernandez M, Potier MC, Laffaire J, et al. (2008) Increased NR2A expression and prolonged decay of NMDA-induced calcium transient in cerebellum of TgDyrk1A mice, a mouse model of Down syndrome. Neurobiol Dis.
31. Fotaki V, Martinez De Lagran M, Estivill X, Arbones M, Dierssen M (2004) Haploinsufficiency of Dyrk1A in mice leads to specific alterations in the development and regulation of motor activity. Behav Neurosci 118: 815–821.
32. Wegiel J, Kuchna I, Nowicki K, Frackowiak J, Dowjat K, et al. (2004) Cell type- and brain structure-specific patterns of distribution of minibrain kinase in human brain. Brain Res 1010: 69–80.
33. Branchi I, Bichler Z, Minghetti L, Delabar JM, Malchiodi-Albedi F, et al. (2004) Transgenic mouse in vivo library of human Down syndrome critical region 1: association between DYRK1A overexpression, brain development abnormalities, and cell cycle protein alteration. J Neuropathol Exp Neurol 63: 429–440.
34. Sanes JR, Lichtman JW (1999) Development of the vertebrate neuromuscular junction. Annu Rev Neurosci 22: 389–442.
35. Singh DN, Davis K (1982) Development of palm and main-life configurations in Down's syndrome. Prog Clin Biol Res 84: 353–370.
36. Morris AF, Vaughan SE, Vaccaro P (1982) Measurements of neuromuscular tone and strength in Down's syndrome children. J Ment Defic Res 26: 41–46.

11

Whole Genome and Exome Sequencing of Monozygotic Twins with Trisomy 21, Discordant for a Congenital Heart Defect and Epilepsy

Pongsathorn Chaiyasap[1], Supasak Kulawonganunchai[1,2], Chalurmpon Srichomthong[3,4], Sissades Tongsima[2], Kanya Suphapeetiporn[3,4]*, Vorasuk Shotelersuk[3,4]

1 Interdepartment of Biomedical Sciences, Faculty of Graduate School, Chulalongkorn University, Bangkok, Thailand, 2 Genome Institute, National Center for Genetic Engineering and Biotechnology, Khlong Nueng, Khlong Luang, Pathum Thani, Thailand, 3 Center of Excellence for Medical Genetics, Department of Pediatrics, Faculty of Medicine, Chulalongkorn University, Bangkok, Thailand, 4 Excellence Center for Medical Genetics, King Chulalongkorn Memorial Hospital, Thai Red Cross, Bangkok, Thailand

Abstract

Congenital heart defects (CHD) occur in 40% of patients with trisomy 21, while the other 60% have a structurally normal heart. This suggests that the increased dosage of genes on chromosome 21 is a risk factor for abnormal heart development. Interaction of genes on chromosome 21 or their gene products with certain alleles of genes on other chromosomes could contribute to CHD. Here, we identified a pair of monozygotic twins with trisomy 21 but discordant for a ventricular septal defect and epilepsy. Twin-zygosity was confirmed by microsatellite genotyping. We hypothesized that some genetic differences from post-twinning mutations caused the discordant phenotypes. Thus, next generation sequencing (NGS) technologies were applied to sequence both whole genome and exome of their leukocytes. The post-analyses of the sequencing data revealed 21 putative discordant exonic variants between the twins from either genome or exome data. However, of the 15 variants chosen for validation with conventional Sanger sequencing, these candidate variants showed no differences in both twins. The fact that no discordant DNA variants were found suggests that sequence differences of DNA from leukocytes of monozygotic twins might be extremely rare. It also emphasizes the limitation of the current NGS technology in identifying causative genes for discordant phenotypes in monozygotic twins.

Editor: Esteban Ballestar, Bellvitge Biomedical Research Institute (IDIBELL), Spain

Funding: This study was funded through Ratchadapiseksomphot Endowment Fund of Chulalongkorn University (RES560530177-HR) awarded to CS, VS and KS and through the Thailand Research Fund (RTA5680003, RSA5480022). PC is a recipient of Royal Golden Jubilee Ph.D. Program (Grant No. PHD/0071/2552). ST and SK were supported in part by the 2011 Research Chair Grants issued by the National Science and Technology Development Agency (NSTDA) and the Thailand Research Fund (RSA5480026). The funders had no role in study design, data collection and analysis, decision to publish, or preparation of the manuscript.

Competing Interests: The authors have declared that no competing interests exist.

* Email: Kanya.Su@chula.ac.th

Introduction

Down syndrome (DS; OMIM 190685) is a human chromosomal disorder caused by an extra copy of genomic region on chromosome 21. It is one of the most common causes of human genetic disorders occurring at approximately 1 in 750 live births [1]. The extra copy of chromosome 21 is largely resulted from the failure of normal chromosomal segregation in maternal meiosis, which accounts for approximately 87% of DS patients [2]. Common characteristic facial features include oblique eyes, flat nasal bridge, epicanthus, and protruding tongue. Other phenotypes include intellectual deficit, hypotonia and other associated developmental disorders and congenital anomalies [3].

One of the severe phenotypes is congenital heart defect (CHD) occurring in approximately 40% of patients with trisomy 21, albeit about 0.8% occurrence in the general population [1]. This suggests that the increased dosage of genes on chromosome 21 is a risk factor but not sufficient for abnormal heart development [4]. Interaction of genes on chromosome 21 or their gene products with certain alleles of genes on other chromosomes could contribute to CHD.

In view of genetic disorders, phenotypic discordance in monozygotic twins may provide a better understanding of relevant factors that are involved in disease etiology [5]. Although, monozygotic twins are generally considered to be genetically identical, the underlying genetic differences may arise during embryonic development, for example, single nucleotide mutations, deletions, conversion, copy number variation and postzygotic mitotic recombination. These variations have been suggested as possible genetic mechanisms causing discordant monozygotic twins [6]. Some recent studies described single nucleotide polymorphism differences between monozygotic twins [7].

The detection of genetic differences generally relies on genome comparison between a sequence of interest and the reference sequence. However, in the case of monozygotic twins, their sequences can be compared against each other. Identified mismatches could be selected for validation as possible mutations causing the discordant phenotype. For instance, discordance of monozygotic twins with autosomal dominant neurofibromatosis type 1 (NF1) was explained by the presence of a *de novo NF1* mutation in all investigated cells of the affected twin, while the cells from the unaffected twin were mosaic [7].

Table 1. Summary of sequencing results from whole genome and exome sequencing data.

SOLiD 4.0 whole genome sequencing	Twin A	Twin B
Size of genome (UCSC hg18)	2.8 Gb	2.8 Gb
Data mapped to genome (base pair)	78.4 Gb	82.6 Gb
Mean read depth of whole genome	27.22X	28.67X
% Coverage of target regions (>10X)	95.4%	96.3%
HiSeq 2000 whole exome sequencing	**Twin A**	**Twin B**
Size of exome (UCSC hg19)	63 Mb	63 Mb
Total yield (base pair)	10,451 Mb	8,464 Mb
On-target base pair (mapped to target regions)	3,439 Mb	2,812 Mb
Mean read depth of target regions	44.8X	36.7X
% Coverage of target regions (>10X)	83.6%	82.5%

Since only a small number of genetic differences between twins are expected [8], a highly sensitive method with high resolution and whole genome coverage should ideally be applied [9]. With the advent of next generation sequencing (NGS) technology, whole genome single nucleotide differences can efficiently be mapped [10]. Moreover, a genome-wide coverage would allow for a non-biased approach, not restricted to certain pre-selected regions. A conventional Sanger sequencing approach can be used to validate the candidate discordant variants obtained from NGS [11].

Here, we identified a pair of Thai monozygotic twin boys with trisomy 21 discordant for a CHD and epilepsy. We hypothesized that some genetic differences from post-twinning mutations, e.g., Single Nucleotide Variants (SNVs) or small insertions or deletions (Indels) caused the discordant phenotypes. Therefore, NGS was used in order to identify such genetic differences.

Materials and Methods

Ethical statement

The study was approved by the institutional review board of Faculty of Medicine of Chulalongkorn University. Written informed consent was obtained from the parents of patients included in the study.

Patients

Thai twin boys born at the King Chulalongkorn Memorial Hospital, Bangkok, had hypotonia, low-set ears, upslant eyes and flat nasal bridge. A clinical diagnosis of Down syndrome was given and later confirmed by chromosome analysis indicating three copies of chromosome 21 in both twins. Here we assigned twin A as the older brother and twin B as the younger one. Echocardiography revealed that twin A had a ventricular septal defect (VSD), requiring a corrective operation when he was one year and two months old. Although twin B had a normal heart, he developed seizure when he was six months old. Even with several antiepileptics, he continued to seize until he was given vigabatrin when he was one year old; the seizure then stopped. Such seizure was not observed in twin A.

Zygosity analysis

After informed consent, six milliliters of peripheral blood was obtained from both twins and their mother. Genomic DNA was isolated from their white blood cells using QIAamp DNA blood

Table 2. Number of discordant variants after applying different exclusion criteria for WGS and WES experiments.

WGS filtering criteria (using VarScan and GATK to detect variants)	Number of discordant variants
No filtering	5,701
Excluding non-exonic variants (NEV)	11
Excluding NEV and synonymous variants (SV)	8
WES filtering criteria (using in-house variant calling)	**Number of discordant variants**
No filtering	34,226
Excluding NEV	8,640
Excluding NEV with Average depth from both twins ≤30 (AD ≤30)	1,070
Excluding NEV, (AD ≤30) and SV	703
Excluding NEV, (AD ≤30), SV and both twins have depth ≤15 (BD ≤15)	302
Excluding NEV, (AD ≤30), SV, BD ≤15 and variants from <4 reads (V4)	59
Excluding NEV, (AD ≤30), SV, BD ≤15, V4 and false discordant variants eye inspected from IGV visualization (IGV)	13
Excluding NEV, (AD ≤30), SV, BD ≤15, V4, IGV and variants that have frequency <5%	7

Table 3. Details of discordant variants from whole genome and exome sequencing data.

	Gene	Type	Chromosome	Position	Genotype		Depth of coverage Twin A		Variant Frequency Twin A	Depth of coverage Twin B		Variant Frequency Twin B	Sanger sequencing result	
					Reference	Variant	Reference	Variant		Reference	Variant		Twin A	Twin B
Genome data	*ARHGAP11A*	missense	15	30703018	C	A	34	12	26%	27	1	4%	C/C	C/C
	OVGP1	missense	1	111759211	A	G	11	13	54%	22	2	8%	A/G	A/G
	ELK3	deletion	12	95165468	TGTCATCGGG	del	8	2	20%	10	0	0%	TGTCATCGGG	TGTCATCGGG
	NEFL	deletion	8	24866982	C	del	6	0	0%	6	2	25%	C/C	C/C
	NCKAP1L	insertion	12	53211859	ref	TGA	9	0	0%	10	6	38%	ref	ref
	INO80E	deletion	16	29915166	A	del	11	0	0%	7	2	22%	A/A	A/A
	SGK110	insertion	19	60744149	ref	G	5	0	0%	5	5	50%	G/G	G/G
	KRTAP7-1	deletion	21	31123841	T	del	7	0	0%	4	3	43%	del	del
	CAMLG	missense	5	134076812	G	A	14	16	53%	1	18	95%	G/A	G/A
Exome data	*CCT5*	missense	5	10258269	G	T	31	4	11%	30	0	0%	G/G	G/G
	FAF2	missense	5	175913485	C	A	42	4	9%	36	0	0%	C/C	C/C
	ZNF649	missense	19	52394652	C	T	64	6	9%	56	0	0%	T/T	T/T
	RICTOR	missense	5	38958882	G	T	62	5	7%	64	0	0%	G/T	G/T
	TTN	missense	2	179643775	G	T	52	4	7%	49	0	0%	G/G	G/G
	ZNF557	missense	19	7083178	G	A	69	5	7%	61	0	0%	G/G	G/G

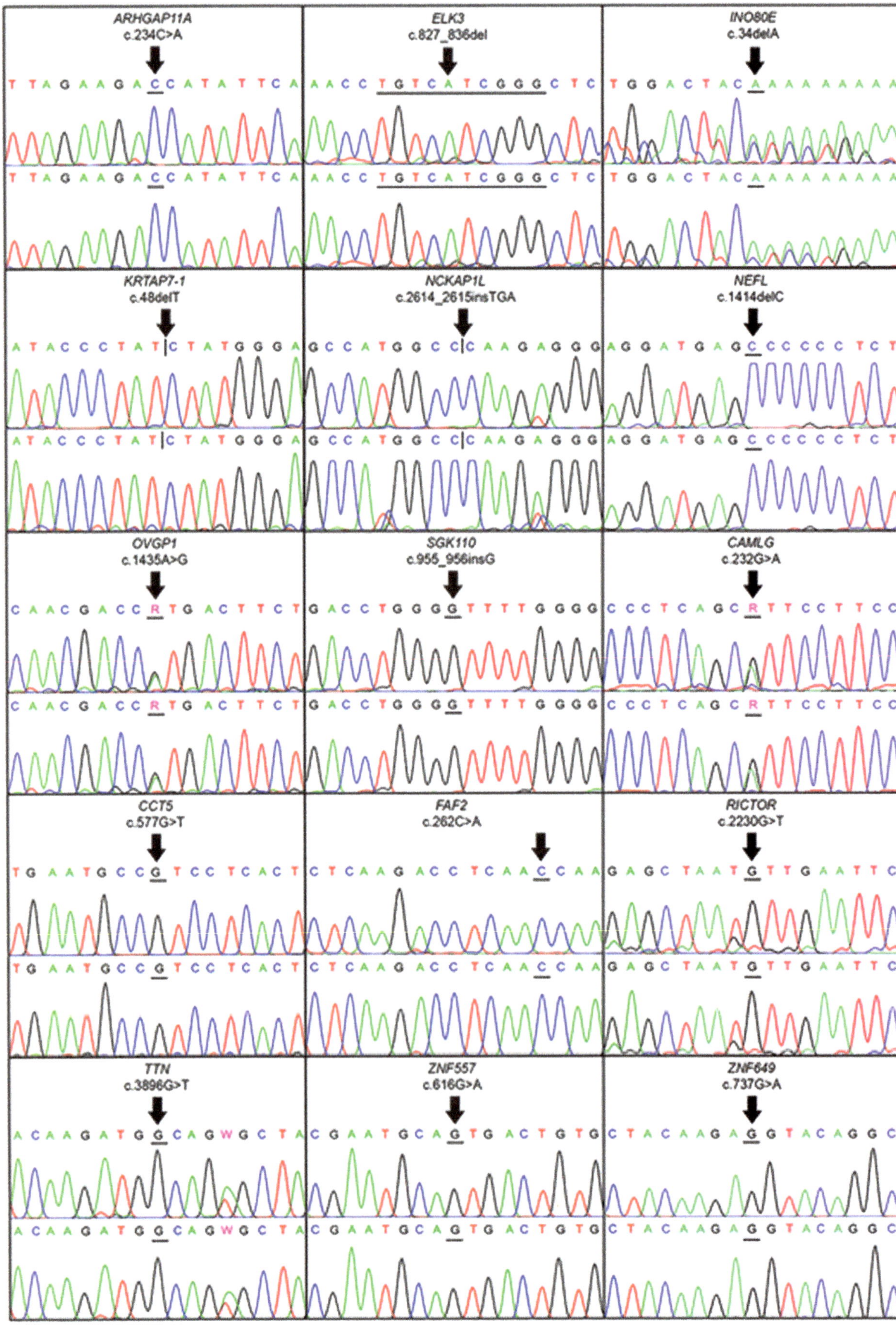
ARHGAP11A
c.234C>A
ELK3
c.827_836del
INO80E
c.34delA
KRTAP7-1
c.48delT
NCKAP1L
c.2614_2615insTGA
NEFL
c.1414delC
OVGP1
c.1435A>G
SGK110
c.955_956insG
CAMLG
c.232G>A
CCT5
c.577G>T
FAF2
c.262C>A
RICTOR
c.2230G>T
TTN
c.3896G>T
ZNF557
c.616G>A
ZNF649
c.737G>A

Figure 1. Electropherograms of Sanger sequencing. Electropherograms of Sanger sequencing of the selected 15 possible discordant variants between the two monozygotic twins identified by either whole genome or exome sequencing experiments. Upper and lower electropherograms of each panel represented twin A and twin B, respectively.

mini kit according to the manufacturer's instruction (Qiagen, Valencia, CA). To confirm that both twins were monozygotic, we used 13 microsatellite markers on 13 different chromosomes, from ABI PRISM Linkage Mapping Set: D1S2785, D2S206, D4S424, D5S408, D7S657, D9S164, D11S1314, D14S74, D15S127, D16S515, D18S1161, D20S117, and D21S1914. In each reaction, we used 1.2 µl of genomic DNA, 9.0 µl of True AllelePCR Premix, 1.0 µl of each primer pair in a total volume of 15 µl and performed PCR following the manufacturer's instruction. Using fluorescently labeled selective primers, DNA analysis was performed on an ABI Prism 3100 genetic analyzer (Applied Biosystems, Foster City) with GeneMapper software (Applied Biosystems).

Genome sequencing and targeted capture exome sequencing

Genomic DNA from both twins was sent for whole genome sequencing (WGS) using the service offered by Beijing Genomic Institute (BGI), China. The sequencing was performed using Applied BiosystemSOLiD4.0 (Sequencing by Oligonucleotide Ligation and Detection) system. The primary sequencing data were analyzed by using standard SOLiD analysis workflow. After that, the sequencing reads were aligned to human genome reference sequence (UCSC hg18) using BioScope software.

Whole exome sequencing (WES) of these genomic DNAs was done using Illumina HiSeq 2000 with the service from Macrogen, Inc., South Korea. Real Time Analysis (RTA) software version 1.7 was used to perform base calling and quality scoring. The reads were then aligned to UCSC hg19 using the Burrows-Wheeler Alignment (BWA) tool [12].

Discordant SNVs/Indels analysis

Both WGS and WES datasets of the twins were deposited to NCBI Sequence Read Archive (SRA) with the sample IDs "SAMN02680286" and "SAMN02688784" for twins A (sample name G3142) and B (G3143), respectively. The experimental IDs for WGS and WES are SRX485008 and SRX522555 for twin A and SRX487546 and SRX522556 for twin B, respectively. These samples can be downloaded from NCBI BioSample database and were registered under a project id "PRJNA240916" in the NCBI BioProject database.

Candidate single nucleotide variants (SNVs) and small insertions or deletions (Indels) were extracted by comparing the twins' alignment data (BAM files). Variant calling was done simultaneously on both alignment data from twins A and B (SAMtools mpileup) in order to avoid false positive variants. If a variant could only be observed in one twin but missing due to no or not enough coverage in the other twin, such a variant would be excluded from the candidate discordant variant set.

VarScan version 2.2.5 was used to identify SNVs from the mpileup alignment data. It compared the read counts, base quality and allele frequency between the twins. Discordant SNVs were called with the sequencing depth greater than or equal to 10X. These SNVs must be present in at least three reads with the minimum variant base quality score >15. Genome Analysis Toolkit (GATK) version 1.0.5974 was used to detect Indels using the Somatic Indel Detector command. The Indel results were compared between the two twins. If Indels were detected in only one twin, the discordant Indels would be called. These resulting discordant variants were filtered again by excluding those variants that were likely to be non-functional, e.g., synonymous variants and/or variants located outside the exonic regions.

For exome sequencing data, the alignment and variant calling were done on each twin data as a standard analysis service from Macrogen using SAMtools. We used in-house variant calling script to call SNVs and Indels. To detect discordant variants, we compared side by side at each locus of the variants. Particularly, the underlying discordance would be detected, only if enough read coverage of the corresponding variant was confirmed on both twins. Nonsynonymous variants with at least 30× coverage would be chosen. Subsequently, we picked variants with variant-supporting reads more than four reads in one twin and did not have variant-supporting reads in the other.

To screen out obvious false positive variants, each of the resulting variants from both whole genome and exome sequencing was visualized along with its alignment data from both twins using Integrative Genomics Viewer (IGV) software version 2.1. The variants that passed the aforementioned criteria would be validated.

Discordant SNVs/Indels validation

Twins' genomic DNA extracted from leukocytes as previously described was amplified by polymerase chain reaction (PCR), using primers specific to the candidate genes that had the resulting discordant SNVs/Indels (Table S1). The PCR products were sent to Macrogen Inc., South Korea for performing Sanger sequencing. Sequences were compared between both twins to verify the discordant variants.

Results

Zygosity analysis

Zygosity analysis showed that both twins had the same alleles of all thirteen microsatellite markers, highly suggesting that they were monozygotic twins.

Discordant SNVs/Indels analysis

Whole genome sequencing of both twins resulted in 27.22× and 28.67× of average coverage (Table 1). The discordant SNVs and Indels from VarScan and GATK resulted in 5,701 variants. After excluding non-exonic and synonymous variants, eight discordant variants (two SNVs and six Indels) were obtained from the whole genome sequencing data (Table 2).

The exome sequencing dataset had higher average coverage at 44.8× and 36.7× for twins A and B, respectively (Table 1). Exome sequencing of both twins resulted in a total of 226,983 variants prior to the discordant analysis. We selected only discordant variants that had average sequencing depths of greater than or equal to 10X, resulting in 34,226 discordant variants. After applying the stringent filtering criteria, 13 putative discordant SNVs with no Indels were chosen to be validated (Table 2). These variants from the exome dataset share no common with the discordant variants from the whole genome sequencing dataset.

Discordant SNVs/Indels validation

We chose 15 variants (all eight of the whole genome and seven out of 13 of the exome sequencing datasets) to be validated by conventional Sanger sequencing (Table 3). The variants from exome datasets were selected by manual observations of each variant's alignment data, using IGV to clarify the mapping result. They were selected when only two haplotypes were found, they were not located at the start or end position of reads and their base quality scores were more than 20 on average. In addition, since CHD occurring in approximately 40% of patients with trisomy 21 and the underlying variants causing discordant CHD should be common variants, we therefore selected the variants with variant frequency of not less than 5% [13]. Of the 13 discordant variants found by exome sequencing, seven met the criteria and were subjected to Sanger sequencing. Electropherograms of all 15 candidate variants showed no differences between the twins (Figure 1).

Discussion

In this study, we used NGS to sequence genome and exome of the monozygotic twins with trisomy 21, discordant for VSD and epilepsy. A rigorous discordant screening revealed 15 SNVs and 6 Indels potentially causing the twin discordance. However, validation of these 15 variants via Sanger sequencing of the corresponding genes showed no differences between the twins.

Because only non-synonymous discordant variants in the coding regions were investigated, it is possible that one of the 5,690 discordant variants in the non-coding regions identified by genome sequencing [14] or one of the 367 synonymous coding variants identified by exome sequencing [15] could have functional consequences and contribute to the discordant phenotype.

Such negative results support the notion that genetic differences between monozygotic twins even with discordant phenotypes are very rare. Several previous studies also failed to map discordant SNVs in monozygotic twins with discordant phenotypes. In particular, Baranzini et al used three platforms—whole genome sequencing (WGS), duplicate array hybridization (DAH) and RNA sequencing (RNA-Seq), to identify discordant SNVs for monozygotic twins discordant for multiple sclerosis. In their study, 3,241, 126, and 322 discordant SNVs were found by WGS, DAH, and RNA-Seq, respectively. Interestingly, they found that no discordant SNVs inferred by one approach were replicated by a second approach, while 98% of concordant SNVs could be replicated by at least two methods. The validation of 15 discordant SNVs via Sanger sequencing showed identical genotypes in the twin pairs [16]. Recent studies of monozygotic twins discordant for VACTERL association, using both WES and high-density microarray approaches, also failed to identify discordant variants that could explain the discordant phenotype [17]. However, discordant variants between monozygotic twins do exist. A study of monozygotic twins discordant for schizophrenia showed two discordant SNVs which were confirmed as actual differences by Sanger sequencing [18].

NGS has successes in finding concordant variants from patients with the same disease. It has been demonstrated in a WGS study of four family members, consisting of two siblings affected with Miller syndrome and primary ciliary dyskinesia and their unaffected parents. They successfully identified the causative gene [19]. Even with a complex disorder like autism, NGS also showed some successes in identification of the causative genes. Whole exome sequencing of 16 probands revealed candidate homozygous recessive mutations in four unrelated families [20].

One possible explanation for a high false positive rate for discordant variants is that NGS technology yields high error rate results. Particularly an overall miscall error rate for Illumina platform is typically around 1% [21]. Given the human genome size of around 3 billion base pairs, it can be assumed that a genome sequencing of a person could have approximately 30 million positions of error calling. This high error rate of genome sequencing process is well illustrated by the study of monozygotic twins discordant for schizophrenia. Of the 846 discordant SNVs identified by genome sequencing, only two SNVs were confirmed as actual differences by Sanger sequencing [18].

We conducted WGS on the twins' DNA in June 2011 and found no discordant variants. Suspecting that the coverage might not be enough on the coding region, we then performed exome sequencing in June 2012, and again found no discordant variants between the two twins. We did not compare variants found by WGS and WES simultaneously. Although the alignment programs and the reference genomes (hg18 vs hg19) used for WGS and WES were different, they should not pose any problems in variant selection as we did not impose the rule that the putative discordant variants must be present in both WGS and WES.

Explanations for a pair of monozygotic twins with identical leukocytes' DNA but discordant phenotype include mosaic genomic alteration. If a somatic mutation occurs before twinning, both twins will have the mutation variant. However, they might show discordant phenotypes because the level of mosaicism in the relevant tissues of the unaffected twin does not reach the necessary level for clinical expression. In addition to mosaic state, epigenetics could be another possible explanation for the different phenotypes in monozygotic twins [22].

Of note, DNA derived from blood may not be suitable for NGS studies of discordant twins [23]. About 70% of all monozygotic twins are monochorionic and share blood circulation in pregnancies. Therefore, the hematopoietic stem cells could be transferred between them and chimeric hematopoietic systems are created. It is therefore possible that post-twinning somatic mutations in one twin could be detected in the co-twin's blood system. This will mask the underlying mutations that cause the disease in the affected twin. Therefore, it is important to sample the tissue with discordant phenotype for DNA extraction. Unfortunately, the tissues with discordant phenotypes (heart and brain) of these twins were unobtainable.

In conclusion, we applied NGS technology in monozygotic twins with trisomy 21 discordant for VSD and epilepsy. Using the stringent filtering criteria, 15 SNVs and 6 Indels were found. However, the validation of those 15 potential discordant variants via Sanger sequencing of the corresponding genes showed no differences. The false positive results emphasized the limitation of current NGS technology in identification of rare genes causing the discordant phenotypes in monozygotic twins.

Supporting Information

Table S1 Primer sequences used for the 15 variant validations.

Author Contributions

Conceived and designed the experiments: PC KS VS. Performed the experiments: PC SK CS. Analyzed the data: PC SK CS ST KS VS. Contributed reagents/materials/analysis tools: PC SK CS ST KS VS. Wrote the paper: PC ST KS VS.

References

1. Antonarakis SE, Lyle R, Dermitzakis ET, Reymond A, Deutsch S (2004) Chromosome 21 and down syndrome: from genomics to pathophysiology. Nat Rev Genet 5: 725–738.
2. Antonarakis SE (1998) 10 years of Genomics, chromosome 21, and Down syndrome. Genomics 51: 1–16.
3. Langdon J, Down H (1966) Observations on an ethnic classification of idiots1. Heredity 21: 695–697.
4. Roizen NJ, Patterson D (2003) Down's syndrome. Lancet 361: 1281–1289.
5. Brickell KL, Leverenz JB, Steinbart EJ, Rumbaugh M, Schellenberg GD, et al. (2007) Clinicopathological concordance and discordance in three monozygotic twin pairs with familial Alzheimer's disease. J Neurol Neurosurg Psychiatry 78: 1050–1055.
6. Ketelaar ME, Hofstra EM, Hayden MR (2012) What monozygotic twins discordant for phenotype illustrate about mechanisms influencing genetic forms of neurodegeneration. Clin Genet 81: 325–333.
7. Maiti S, Kumar KH, Castellani CA, O'Reilly R, Singh SM (2011) Ontogenetic de novo copy number variations (CNVs) as a source of genetic individuality: studies on two families with MZD twins for schizophrenia. PLoS One 6: e17125.
8. Nachman MW, Crowell SL (2000) Estimate of the Mutation Rate per Nucleotide in Humans. Genetics 156: 297–304.
9. Aparicio SA, Huntsman DG (2010) Does massively parallel DNA resequencing signify the end of histopathology as we know it? J Pathol 220: 307–315.
10. Kuhlenbaumer G, Hullmann J, Appenzeller S (2011) Novel genomic techniques open new avenues in the analysis of monogenic disorders. Hum Mutat 32: 144–151.
11. Imelfort M, Batley J, Grimmond S, Edwards D (2009) Genome Sequencing Approaches and Successes Plant Genomics. In: Gustafson JP, Langridge P, Somers DJ, editors: Humana Press. pp. 345–358.
12. Li H, Durbin R (2010) Fast and accurate long-read alignment with Burrows-Wheeler transform. Bioinformatics 26: 589–595.
13. Altshuler DM, Gibbs RA, Peltonen L, Dermitzakis E, Schaffner SF, et al. (2010) Integrating common and rare genetic variation in diverse human populations. Nature 467: 52–58.
14. Makrythanasis P, Antonarakis SE (2013) Pathogenic variants in non-protein-coding sequences. Clin Genet 84: 422–428.
15. Kimchi-Sarfaty C, Oh JM, Kim IW, Sauna ZE, Calcagno AM, et al. (2007) A "silent" polymorphism in the MDR1 gene changes substrate specificity. Science 315: 525–528.
16. Baranzini SE, Mudge J, van Velkinburgh JC, Khankhanian P, Khrebtukova I, et al. (2010) Genome, epigenome and RNA sequences of monozygotic twins discordant for multiple sclerosis. Nature 464: 1351–1356.
17. Solomon BD, Pineda-Alvarez DE, Hadley DW, Hansen NF, Kamat A, et al. (2013) Exome Sequencing and High-Density Microarray Testing in Monozygotic Twin Pairs Discordant for Features of VACTERL Association. Mol Syndromol 4: 27–31.
18. Reumers J, De Rijk P, Zhao H, Liekens A, Smeets D, et al. (2012) Optimized filtering reduces the error rate in detecting genomic variants by short-read sequencing. Nat Biotechnol 30: 61–68.
19. Roach JC, Glusman G, Smit AF, Huff CD, Hubley R, et al. (2010) Analysis of genetic inheritance in a family quartet by whole-genome sequencing. Science 328: 636–639.
20. Chahrour MH, Yu TW, Lim ET, Ataman B, Coulter ME, et al. (2012) Whole-exome sequencing and homozygosity analysis implicate depolarization-regulated neuronal genes in autism. PLoS Genet 8: e1002635.
21. Nielsen R, Paul JS, Albrechtsen A, Song YS (2011) Genotype and SNP calling from next-generation sequencing data. Nat Rev Genet 12: 443–451.
22. Biesecker LG, Spinner NB (2013) A genomic view of mosaicism and human disease. Nat Rev Genet 14: 307–320.
23. Erlich Y (2011) Blood ties: chimerism can mask twin discordance in high-throughput sequencing. Twin Res Hum Genet 14: 137–143.

12

Tracking Subtle Stereotypes of Children with Trisomy 21: From Facial-Feature-Based to Implicit Stereotyping

Claire Enea-Drapeau*, Michèle Carlier, Pascal Huguet

Laboratoire de Psychologie Cognitive, Aix-Marseille University and Centre National de la Recherche Scientifique, Marseille, France

Abstract

Background: Stigmatization is one of the greatest obstacles to the successful integration of people with Trisomy 21 (T21 or Down syndrome), the most frequent genetic disorder associated with intellectual disability. Research on attitudes and stereotypes toward these people still focuses on explicit measures subjected to social-desirability biases, and neglects how variability in facial stigmata influences attitudes and stereotyping.

Methodology/Principal Findings: The participants were 165 adults including 55 young adult students, 55 non-student adults, and 55 professional caregivers working with intellectually disabled persons. They were faced with implicit association tests (IAT), a well-known technique whereby response latency is used to capture the relative strength with which some groups of people—here photographed faces of typically developing children and children with T21—are automatically (without conscious awareness) associated with positive versus negative attributes in memory. Each participant also rated the same photographed faces (consciously accessible evaluations). We provide the first evidence that the positive bias typically found in explicit judgments of children with T21 is smaller for those whose facial features are highly characteristic of this disorder, compared to their counterparts with less distinctive features and to typically developing children. We also show that this bias can coexist with negative evaluations at the implicit level (with large effect sizes), even among professional caregivers.

Conclusion: These findings support recent models of feature-based stereotyping, and more importantly show how crucial it is to go beyond explicit evaluations to estimate the true extent of stigmatization of intellectually disabled people.

Editor: Angela Sirigu, French National Centre for Scientific Research, France

Funding: Support for this research was provided by Aix-Marseille University, the Centre National de la Recherche Scientifique, and the "Fondation Jérôme Lejeune" (France). The funders had no role in study design, data collection and analysis, decision to publish, or preparation of the manuscript.

Competing Interests: The authors have declared that no competing interests exist.

* E-mail: claire.enea-drapeau@univ-amu.fr

Introduction

Trisomy 21 (T21) or Down syndrome is the most frequent genetic disorder associated with intellectual disability, affecting between 1.0 and 2.2 of every 1000 live births according to statistics on prenatal testing and selective abortion [1–4]. Because this chromosomal disorder is also associated with various health problems (e.g., hypotonia, congenital heart defects, gastrointestinal diseases) and distinctive physical stigmata (e.g., round face, epicanthal fold, oblique lid axis, flat nasal bridge), persons with T21 are at high risk of being rejected socially. Not only are the common societal reactions unfavorable in terms of rates of fetal termination and abandonment [2], [5], but those who live with T21 are likely to be stigmatized by other people [6]. This is a critical issue, because stigmatization is one of the greatest obstacles to the successful integration and development of people with intellectual disabilities.

Although research in this area is very limited, it seems that persons with T21, especially children, are typically viewed as "friendly", "affectionate", and "happy" (e.g., [7–9]); with positive personality traits prevailing over the negative ones (e.g., "mentally retarded"). This positive stereotype, however, coexists with ambivalent attitudes about the integration of these children into regular schools (e.g., [8], [10], [11]). Based on a recent survey, Pace et al showed that whereas 45% of adult respondents ($N = 5399$) from the general (U.S.) population agreed with inclusive education for students with T21, 25% disagreed (considering for example that such students are "distracting") and 29% abstained [11]. Likewise, about one-third of adolescent respondents ($N = 1704$) reported they were not willing to work on a class project or spend time outside of school with a student with T21. Although these negative attitudes are not majority rule, and can even be negligible in people who have relationships with persons with T21 [11–13], they may very be the trees that hide the forest.

Of particular interest here, all published studies on the social perception of intellectually disabled people, including those with T21, have measured attitudes and stereotyping solely at the explicit level. This is an important limitation, because social-desirability attitudes may interfere with the measurement of people's responses at this level. We are not suggesting that responses at the explicit level are deliberate lies that people use to cover up their implicit attitudes and convictions, but that it may not be sufficient to focus on consciously-accessible evaluations because people may be unaware of, or unwilling to report, all of their thoughts and feelings. There is ample evidence that attitudes and stereotypes may be used automatically, and thus quickly and effortlessly, without conscious awareness, and yet may influence perception, judgments, or actions even against a person's intentions [14–16]. For example, people who display explicit overt beliefs in the equality of the races may implicitly associate positive attributes (e.g., pleasant words) with White more than with Black persons (or more negative attributes with Black than with White persons). These automatic biases can be found even when pictures of equally unfamiliar Black and White people are used as stimuli, and when differences in stimulus familiarity are statistically controlled (e.g., [17]). There is also evidence that implicit evaluations explain variance in behavior over and above that explained by explicit evaluations (e.g., [18], [19]). Thus, by focusing exclusively on explicit (controlled) evaluations, past research on the social perception of intellectually disabled individuals has most certainly fallen short of revealing the whole picture.

The present study

The present study investigated subtle stereotyping of children with full T21 likely to arise at both levels, i.e., explicit and implicit. First, we looked into whether the explicit evaluations of children's personality can be modulated by the degree to which their facial features are perceived as distinctive of T21. Because facial features can be powerful cues to category membership (e.g., when facial features are associated to racial categories), category-based stereotyping may ensue, as also suggested by standard stereotyping models [20–23]. Feature-based stereotyping may actually operate both between and within categories (e.g., [24–26]), resulting in greater stereotyping of people with a larger number of distinctive features of the category in question. Blair et al found that people with a greater number of Afrocentric facial features were presumed more likely to have traits that are stereotypic of African Americans than people with a smaller number of Afrocentric features [24]. Likewise, Blair et al found that prisoners with a greater number of Afrocentric facial features received more severe sentences than people with a lesser number of Afrocentric features [25]. In subsequent research [26], participants seemed to be able to control some aspects of race-based stereotyping, but appeared unaware of and unable to control (within-race) stereotyping based on Afrocentric features.

Here we suggest that children with T21 may also be subject to stereotyping based on their facial features, resulting in less positive judgments for those with features highly characteristic of this chromosomal disorder, compared to both their counterparts with fewer distinctive features and to typically developing children.

Second, we explored stereotyping of children with T21 using implicit association tests (IAT), a well-known technique whereby response latency is used to capture the relative strength with which some groups of people are associated with positive versus negative attributes in memory [15], [27]. In the current study, participants classified two types of stimuli: children's faces, and positive or negative personality traits, using two designated keys. We predicted faster reaction times when photographed faces of typically developing children (hereafter referred to as TD pictures) and positive traits shared the same key while photographed faces of children with T21 (hereafter referred to as T21 pictures) and negative traits shared the other key. Put differently, we predicted slower reaction times for the opposite combinations of stimuli: TD pictures and negative traits (associated with the same key), and T21 pictures and positive traits (associated with the other key).

Finally, the present research also tested whether the expected effects (of explicit and implicit stereotyping) can be found in people who have relationships with children with T21. There is evidence that relationships with intellectually disabled persons promote positive attitudes toward them (e.g., [11], [28], [29]). Again, however, previous research has left open the question of whether these relationships have any effect beyond mere awareness and reflection. Implicit stereotypes may be so deeply embedded in our culture that they may be activated regardless of whether a person considers them to be valid or invalid, and they have indeed often been described as being difficult to change (e.g., [14], [30]). On this basis, we assumed that even people who have relationships with children with T21 (e.g., professional caregivers) may exhibit subtle forms of negative stereotyping about them.

Thus, here we investigate for the first time subtle stereotyping of children with T21 based on their facial features, using both explicit and implicit levels of investigation, in different social groups ranging from young adult students to professional caregivers working with intellectually disabled persons.

Materials and Methods

Participants

The participants were 165 adults including 55 students (undergraduates and graduates) not enrolled in a psychology course (M_{age} = 20.6 years, range: 18–25; M = 12.9 years of schooling, range: 10–17), 55 persons from the general population (referred to as non-student adults, M_{age} = 38.3 years, range: 18–64; M = 14.0 years of schooling, range: 11–17), and 55 professional caregivers working with intellectually disabled persons, mainly individuals with T21 (M_{age} = 39.1 years, range: 23–62; M = 13.7 years of schooling, range: 11–16). Students were 18 years younger and reported on average less than one year of schooling compare to participants of the two other groups (that did not differ from each other, ps >.28). All gave their written informed consent to participate in the present research, presented as a study on the "face perception of people with trisomy 21". The project obtained approval from the Ethics Committee of Aix-Marseille Univ. (Avis Carlier 18.11.09).

Procedure

All participants started with two counterbalanced T21-IATs created for this study using photographed faces of TD children and children with full T21. All parents of children photographed for the present research gave their written informed consent. Whereas one IAT involved faces weakly typical of T21, the other involved faces strongly typical of T21 (as also determined by a pre-test with another subject sample as described in Text S1). The photographs used in the two IATs were standardized. They showed only a face with a neutral facial expression against a blue background. In each IAT, participants classified 12 pictures, 6 TD pictures (faces of 3 male and 3 female children) and 6 T21 pictures (faces of 3 male and 3 female children with T21), in one of two categories, "trisomy" versus "normal". They also classified 12 traits, 6 positively valenced ones (e.g., affectionate) and 6 negatively valenced ones (e.g., stupid), in one of two trait categories, positive versus negative (see Text S2 for details). In the combined task blocks of each IAT, participants switched between classifying exemplars of one contrast (TD pictures vs. T21 pictures) and exemplars of the other contrast (positive vs. negative traits). In half of the combined task blocks, TD pictures and positive traits were mapped to one response (e.g., right key) and T21 pictures and negative traits were mapped to the other response (e.g., left key). The other half of the combined-task block reversed the response mappings (e.g., TD pictures+negative traits vs. T21 pictures+positive traits). The order of administering combined tasks was randomly counterbalanced across participants. Overall participants performed 312 trials (including practice trials) structured in 7 blocks. The design of the IATs is presented in Table S1. Participants were told that a word or a picture face will occur in the middle of the screen and they have to press a key as quickly as possible to put each of these words or pictures in one of two categories ('Positive' vs. 'Negative' and 'Trisomy' vs. 'Normal', for the words and pictures, respectively). They also learned that these categories would be displayed at the top of the screen along with the associated key. Finally, they were instructed that errors (pressing the wrong key) would be indicated by an 'X' at the center of the screen that would imply to correct their answer to continue. If T21 pictures are more strongly associated to a negative valence than are TD pictures at the implicit level, classification should be faster in the "TD pictures+positive traits vs. T21 pictures+negative traits" blocks than in the "TD pictures+negative traits vs. T21 pictures+positive traits" blocks.

At the end of the two IATs, participants made explicit evaluations of the same pictures (18 in all), via each of the 12 traits used previously, resulting in 216 ratings for each participant. Participants were instructed that pictures would be presented at the center of the computer screen along with a word (bottom of screen). They were asked to indicate spontaneously to what extent the word was appropriate to the picture, using Likert type scale (from 1: "strongly disagree" to 6: "strongly agree"). These evaluations were produced after the two IATs so as not to prime stereotype-related cognition during the implicit tests. Consistent with a myriad of studies on impression formation, most participants agreed willingly to attribute personality traits to unknown persons and none of them stopped the task [31].

Results

Explicit Stereotyping

A mixed ANOVA was conducted with trait valence (positive vs. negative) and target of evaluation (TD pictures, T21 pictures weakly typical of T21, T21 pictures strongly typical of T21) as repeated measures, and source of evaluation (students, non-student adults, and professional caregivers) as between-participant factor. Not surprisingly, this analysis yielded a huge effect of trait valence, $F(1, 162) = 593.23$, $p < .001$, $\eta^2_p = .79$. Participants attributed more positive traits ($M = 4.63$, $SE = .06$) than negative traits ($M = 2.17$, $SE = .05$) to all faces (see Table 1).

This difference favoring positive traits at the explicit level was modulated by both the target and the source of evaluation, $F(4, 324) = 8.49$, $p < .001$, $\eta^2_p = .09$ (See Figure 1). This interaction was examined via two Helmert contrasts for each source of evaluation, with the difference in the trait valence score as the dependent variable. The first contrast compared the TD pictures with the average of the T21 pictures weakly and strongly typical, and thus tested for feature-based stereotyping *between* categories. The second compared the T21 pictures weakly typical with those strongly typical, and thus tested for feature-based stereotyping *within* the T21 category.

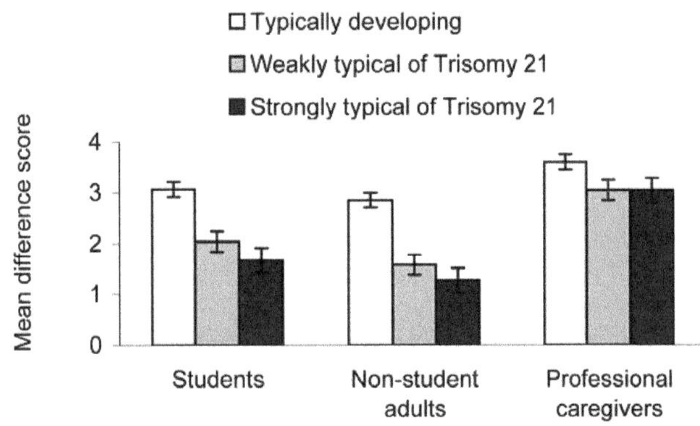

Figure 1. Explicit judgments. Mean difference score (positive traits minus negative traits) on explicit judgments as a function of target of evaluation and source of evaluation. Error bars represent ±1 SEM.

The first contrast revealed a significant difference for each source of evaluation ($ps < .05$), indicating that the difference favoring positive traits at the explicit level was always smaller for T21 pictures than for TD pictures. The second contrast was significant for every source of evaluation ($ps < .05$) except one. Both student and non-student adults made slightly, but significantly, less positive judgments for the pictures strongly typical of T21 than for the weakly typical pictures. This subtle bias was not found among caregivers, for whom the T21 pictures received the most positive ratings. The target by source of evaluation interaction for the positive and negative traits taken separately is described in Text S3.

Implicit Stereotyping (IAT)

IAT scores were calculated following the scoring algorithm recommended by Greenwald et al., including the following features: (a) error trials were removed and replaced with the block mean +600 ms, (b) response latencies >10,000 ms were removed, (c) standard deviations were calculated on all correct response trials, (d) participants who had >10% of trials with responses below 300 ms were removed, and (e) participants who had an error rate of >40% in any of the four combined sorting blocks were also removed [32]. Overall 6 participants were excluded (their inclusion in the statistical analyses did not change the

Table 1. Agreement score to the descriptive traits as a function of source of evaluation and target of evaluation.

	Faces					
	Typically developing		Weakly typical of T21		Strongly typical of T21	
	Traits					
Source of evaluation	Positive	Negative	Positive	Negative	Positive	Negative
Students	4.87 (.58)	1.80 (.56)	4.48 (.76)	2.44 (.81)	4.33 (.88)	2.66 (.99)
Non student adults	4.75 (.70)	1.90 (.65)	4.17 (.87)	2.59 (.90)	4.09 (.91)	2.82 (.94)
Professional caregivers	5.10 (.66)	1.50 (.44)	4.91 (.74)	1.86 (.68)	4.98 (.69)	1.93 (.70)

Note. Standard deviations are shown in parentheses.

results). Likewise, measures of association strength based on the two IATs were computed using the classic *D* measure [32]. *D* was the difference between the mean latencies for the "T21 pictures+positive traits" and "TD pictures+negative traits" block on one hand, and the "T21 pictures+negative traits" and "TD pictures+positive traits" block on the other hand, divided by the inclusive standard deviation of the latencies in the two blocks.

The *D* scores were then analyzed using a mixed ANOVA with the two IATs (based on faces either weakly or strongly typical of T21) as repeated measures, and source of evaluation (students, non-student adults, professionals) as a between-participants factor. This analysis yielded a main effect of source of evaluation, $F(2, 162) = 6.00$, $p = .003$, $\eta^2_p = .07$ (see Figure 2); the target effect, and the source-by-target interaction were not significant ($ps > .40$). The global IAT effect (two IAT-*D* scores averaged) was smaller among the caregivers than among students and non-student adults (Tukey contrast, $p < .05$). As indicated by one-sample t-tests against zero, the global IAT effect was still clearly significant for each source of evaluation: students, $t(54) = 10.44$; non-student adults, $t(54) = 13.08$; and caregivers, $t(54) = 5.91$ (all $ps < .001$). Correlations between implicit and explicit evaluations were rather weak (see Text S4).

Discussion

Research into the social perception of intellectually disabled persons has been largely one-sided, focusing predominantly on thoughts and feelings, which may be distorted by social desirability concerns. In the current research, we found evidence of subtle forms of prejudice toward children with special needs at both the explicit and implicit levels, in this case children with T21.

In line with previous research, students, non-student adults, and professional caregivers all attributed more positive than negative personality traits to children with T21, as they also did for TD children. However, in accordance with standard models of stereotyping operating *between* categories [20–23], this difference in favor of positive traits was lower for children with T21 than for TD children. Perhaps more importantly, as expected from research on feature-based stereotyping operating *within* categories [25], [26], the difference favoring positive traits proved smaller for pictures strongly typical of T21 than for weakly typical ones, at least among students and non-student adults. This is the first evidence that facial features distinctive of a genetic disorder, in this case T21, can lead to stereotyping in two ways, between and within categories. Feature-based stereotyping within the category of T21 pictures did not operate in the professional caregivers, who were also the most positive participants toward those pictures. This is consistent with the idea that relationships with intellectually disabled persons promote positive attitudes toward them (e.g., [11], [29]).

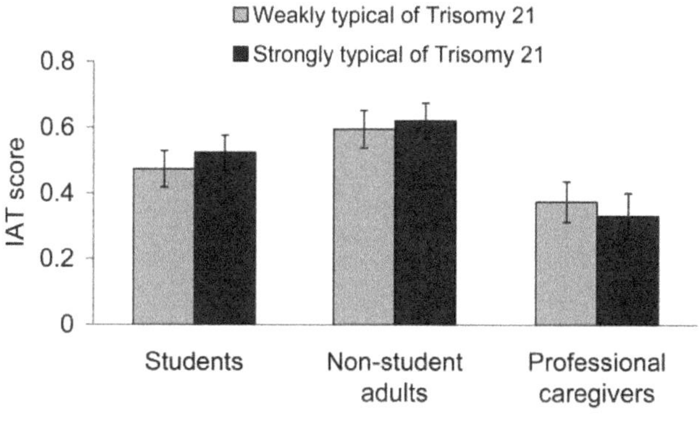

Figure 2. Implicit judgments. Mean IAT scores (±1 SEM) based on pictures weakly and strongly typical of T21, as a function of source of evaluation (students, non-student adults, and professional caregivers).

The IAT findings indicated that, in each group of participants, the T21 pictures were automatically associated with a *negative* valence. Participants, professional caregivers included, were indeed faster at categorizing T21 pictures with negative traits than T21 pictures with positive traits (and faster at categorizing TD pictures with positive traits than TD pictures with negative traits). The IAT effect also occurred regardless of whether the children's faces were strongly or weakly distinctive of T21. Taken together, these findings can be regarded as evidence that negative attitudes about, and stereotyping of, children with T21 in fact prevail at the implicit level.

Finally, the fact that the overall IAT effect was clearly significant in the three groups of participants suggests that professional caregivers' implicit mind-set about children with T21 may not differ from that of non-professionals. One important point must be made here, however. Although each group of participants exhibited a large IAT effect, this effect was significantly smaller in the caregivers than in the students and non-student adults (with equal statistical power). This suggests that caregivers' sustained contact with individuals with T21 may operate somewhat at the implicit level. Consistent with this idea, the caregivers' overall IAT effect decreased significantly with years of professional experience (which ranged from 1 to 34 years), $\beta = -.32$, $t(51) = -2.36$, $p < .03$. This additional finding strengthens the conclusion of a few recent studies indicating a beneficial effect of intergroup contact on implicit evaluations (e.g., [33]). It offers a new reason to believe that even implicit stereotypes (not just explicit ones) can be reduced under the influence of repeated contact with the stigmatized. This critical issue is attracting more and more attention in the struggle against intergroup prejudice (e.g.; [34], [35]). Henry et al. showed that intergroup contact is more likely to have a beneficial impact at the implicit level in low-status groups (e.g., Blacks toward Whites but not Whites toward Blacks) [34]. Our own findings suggest that this impact can also be found in high-status groups, at least when rivalry with the low-status group is not an issue (here non-disabled people with intellectually disabled people).

Thus, the present research reveals that facial features associated with a genetic disorder such as T21 can lead to between- and within-category stereotyping at the explicit level. Although positive evaluations are especially likely at this level, they were reduced when the individuals being rated had facial features highly distinctive of this chromosomal disorder. Our research also reveals that the positive evaluations of children with T21 that can be found at the explicit level can coexist with negative evaluations at the implicit level, which helps explain why the general population is so ambivalent about practical issues such as inclusive education for these children [11], [36]. Taken together, the present findings show how important it is to pay attention to feature-based stereotyping at the explicit level. They also suggest going beyond explicit evaluations when attempting to estimate the true extent of stigmatization of intellectually disabled people. Explaining why implicit stereotyping did not operate within the T21 category is beyond the scope of this paper. However, we suggest that within-category stereotyping cannot be ruled out at this level. As noted earlier, participants in Blair et al research seemed unaware of, and unable to control, stereotyping based on Afrocentric features [26]. Thus, future research is needed to clarify whether feature-based stereotyping can occur at both the explicit and implicit levels.

A limitation of the present study (as well as many other IAT studies) is that the negative associations found at the implicit level do not necessarily mean that children with T21 are the object of implicit prejudice. As suggested earlier in this paper, however, our IAT findings are consistent with the ambivalence of the general population toward inclusive education for students with T21 [11]. Likewise, there is evidence that implicit attitudes can unintentionally lead to discriminatory behaviors such as reducing one's interaction time with the stigmatized [37], [38]. There is also evidence of discriminatory behaviors based on facial features [25]. Additional research, therefore, is also needed to determine whether the implicit attitudes and/or the visibility of the physical stigmata associated with T21 or other disorders influence the way the stigmatized are treated during social interaction. Whether those factors can raise the awareness of the disorder in the stigmatized themselves also merits special attention. People with T21 who have mental ages of about 8 years or more engage in social comparisons with other people, and start to form complex social categories of T21/disability [39–41]. Not only may these individuals be aware of their differences with other people, but their stigmatized identity may actually be chronically accessible, especially when their physical stigmata cannot be easily hidden. Like many other people living with a visible stigmatized identity, persons with salient phenotypic T21 features may also suffer from specific threats, for example, the threat of being judged and treated stereotypically on the basis of their facial features (at least those with mental ages above 7–8 years). This threat may contribute to lowering their performance in test situations, in the same way children and adults may suffer from stereotype threat in test situations due to their gender (e.g., [42–45]), age (e.g., [46]), social or academic background (e.g. [47–49]), or ethnic identities (e.g., [50]). Future research on these issues could help increase our understanding of stigmatization and its related consequences among people with intellectual disabilities.

Finally, one may wonder whether the negative associations found here at the implicit level are specific about T21 or could as well be explained by general implicit attitudes towards disabilities. The very few IAT studies in this area indeed indicate that people tend to associate words or pictures related to various physical disabilities [51–54] and mental illness [53], [55], with negatively connoted words. So far, however, we just did not know whether negative implicit associations could also be found towards people with intellectual disabilities. Here, we offer first evidence that persons (children) with T21, the most representative exemplar of the intellectually disabled, are the target of negative associations at the implicit level despite the positive stereotype that characterize them at the explicit level. As noted by Menolascino, the persons with T21 have long been regarded as "the Prince charming of the mentally retarded population" [56]. This positive view about people with T21 at the explicit level made the capture of negative associations at the implicit level especially informative. In addition, contrary to other exemplars of the intellectually disabled with known aetiology (e.g., Williams syndrome, Fragile X), persons with T21 are the only ones who can easily and automatically be identified as intellectually disabled by the general population, because they share well-known physical stigmata. This additional characteristic offered the possibility (also neglected to date) to test whether intellectually disabled people are subject to stereotyping based on their facial features (i.e., featured-based stereotyping operating within the category of the intellectually disabled). Future research based on direct comparisons between physical and intellectual disabilities might help clarify whether featured-based stereotyping can also be found for people with physical disabilities (using several degrees of physical disability), and whether the type of disability (physical vs. intellectual) makes any difference on the size of explicit and implicit attitudes.

Supporting Information

Text S1 Pictures of children's faces.

Text S2 Positive and negative traits.

Text S3 Target by source-of-evaluation interaction for the positive and negative traits taken separately.

Text S4 Correlations between implicit and explicit evaluations.

Table S1 Design of the two IATs.

Acknowledgments

We are thankful to all participants and especially to families and children who made this work possible. We are indebted to the clinician colleague Catherine Ayoun and heads of the institutions who referred families and/or professional participants.

Author Contributions

Conceived and designed the experiments: CED MC PH. Performed the experiments: CED. Analyzed the data: CED MC PH. Contributed reagents/materials/analysis tools: CED MC PH. Wrote the paper: CED MC PH. Contact with families and institutions: CED MC. Supervised creation of the two T21-IATs: PH.

References

1. Julian-Reynier C, Aurran Y, Dumaret A, Maron A, Chabal F, et al. (1995) Attitudes towards Down's syndrome: follow up of a cohort of 280 cases. J Med Gen 32: 597–599.
2. Olsen CL, Cross PK, Gensburg LJ (2003) Down syndrome: Interaction between culture, demography, and biology in determining the prevalence of a genetic trait. Hum Biol 75: 503–520.
3. Murthy SK, Ashok KM, Mani S, Shara MEA, Al-Rowaished EEM, et al. (2007) Incidence of Down syndrome in Dubai, UAE. Med Princ Pract 16: 25–28. doi:10.1159/000096136.
4. Morris JK, Alberman E (2009) Trends in Down's syndrome live births and antenatal diagnoses in England and Wales from 1989 to 2008: analyses of data from the National Down Syndrome Cytogenetic Register. B Med Jdoi:10.1136/bmj.b3794.
5. Lawson KL, Walls-Ingram SA (2010) Selective abortion for Down syndrome: The relation between the quality of intergroup contact, parenting expectations, and willingness to terminate. J Appl Soc Psychol 40: 554–578.
6. Borthwick C (1996) Racism, IQ and Down's syndrome. Disabil & Society 11: 403–410.
7. Fidler DJ, Hodapp RM (1999) Craniofacial maturity and perceived personality in children with Down syndrome. Am J Ment Retard 104: 410–421. doi:10.1352/0895-8017(1999)104<0410:CMAPPI>2.0.CO;2.
8. Gilmore L, Campbell J, Cuskelly M (2003) Developmental expectations, personality stereotypes, and attitudes towards inclusive education: Community and teacher views of Down syndrome. Int J Disabil Dev Ed 50: 65–76.
9. Mepsted J (1988) Teachers' attitudes. Special Children 17: 14–15.
10. Wishart JG, Manning G (1996) Trainee teachers' attitudes to inclusive education for children with Down's syndrome. J Intell Disabil Res 40: 56–65.
11. Pace JE, Shin M, Rasmussen SA (2010) Understanding attitudes toward people with Down syndrome. Am J Med Gen Part A 152: 2185–2192.
12. Maras P, Brown R (1996) Effects of contact on children's attitudes toward disability: A longitudinal study. J Appl Soc Psychol 26: 2113–2134.
13. Sirlopú D, González R, Bohner G, Siebler F, Ordóñez G, et al. (2008) Promoting positive attitudes toward people with Down syndrome: The benefit of school inclusion programs. J Appl Soc Psychol 38: 2710–2736. doi:10.1111/j.1559-1816.2008.00411.x.

14. Devine PG (1989) Stereotypes and prejudice: Their automatic and controlled components. J Pers Soc Psychol 56: 5–18.
15. Greenwald AG, Banaji MR (1995) Implicit social cognition: Attitudes, self-esteem, and stereotypes. Psychol Rev 102: 4–27. doi:10.1037/0033-295X.102.1.4.
16. Bargh JA, Williams EL (2006) The automaticity of social life. Curr Dir Psychol Sci 15: 1–4.
17. Dasgupta N, McGhee DE, Greenwald AG, Banaji MR (2000) Automatic preference for White Americans: Eliminating the familiarity explanation. J Exp Soc Psychol 36: 316–328. doi:10.1006/jesp.1999.1418.
18. Nosek BA, Smyth FL, Sriram N, Lindner NM, Devos T, et al. (2009) National differences in gender–science stereotypes predict national sex differences in science and math achievement. Proc Nat Acad Sci 106: 10593–10597.
19. Richetin J, Perugini M, Prestwich A, O'Gorman R (2007) The IAT as a predictor of food choice: The case of fruits versus snacks. Int J Psychol 42: 166–173. doi:10.1080/00207590601067078.
20. Brewer MB (1988) A dual process model of impression formation. In: Srull TK, Wyer RS, eds. Memory and cognition in its social context. Advances in social cognition. Hillsdale, NJ, England: Lawrence Erlbaum Associates, Inc. pp 1–36.
21. Fiske ST, Neuberg SL (1990) A continuum of impression formation, from category based to individuating processes: influences of information and motivation on attention and interpretation. Adv Exp Soc Psychol 23: 1–74.
22. Bodenhausen GV, Macrae CN (1997) Stereotype activation and inhibition. In: Wyer RS, ed. The automaticity of everyday life: Advances in social cognition. Mahwah, NJ: Erlbaum. pp 1–52.
23. Mason MF, Cloutier J, Macrae CN (2006) On construing others: Category and stereotype activation from facial cues. Soc Cognition 2: 540–562.
24. Blair IV, Judd CM, Sadler MS, Jenkins C (2002) The role of Afrocentric features in person perception: Judging by features and categories. J Pers Soc Psychol 83: 5–25.
25. Blair IV, Judd CM, Chapleau KM (2004a) The influence of Afrocentric facial features in criminal sentencing. Psychol Sci 15: 674–679.
26. Blair IV, Judd CM, Fallman JL (2004b) The automaticity of race and Afrocentric facial features in social judgments. J Pers Soc Psychol 87: 763–778.
27. Greenwald AG, McGhee DE, Schwartz JLK (1998) Measuring individual differences in implicit cognition: The implicit association test. J Pers Soc Psychol 74: 1464–1480.
28. Levy JM, Jessop DJ, Rimmerman A, Francis F, Levy PH (1993) Determinants of attitudes of New York state employers towards the employment of persons with severe handicaps. J Rehabil 59: 49–54.
29. Unger D (2002) Employers' attitudes toward persons with disabilities in the workforce: Myths or realities? Focus on Autism & Other Developmental Disabilities 17: 2–10.
30. Wilson TD, Lindsey S, Schooler TY (2000) A model of dual attitudes. Psychol Rev 107: 101–126. doi:10.1037/0033-295X.107.1.101.
31. Fiske ST (1993) Social cognition and social perception. Annu Rev Psychol 44: 155–194.
32. Greenwald AG, Nosek BA, Banaji MR (2003) Understanding and using the Implicit Association Test: I. An improved scoring algorithm. J Pers Soc Psychol 85: 197–216.
33. Prestwich A, Kenworthy JB, Wilson M, Kwan-Tat N (2008) Differential relations between two types of contact and implicit and explicit racial attitudes. Brit J Soc Psychol 47: 575–588.
34. Henry PJ, Hardin CD (2006) The contact hypothesis revisited. Psychol Sci 17: 862–868.
35. Turner RN, Crisp RJ (2010) Imagining intergroup contact can reduces implicit prejudice. Br J Soc Psychol 49: 129–142.
36. Carlier M, Ayoun C (2007) Déficiences intellectuelles et intégration sociale. Wavre, Belgique: Editions Mardaga. 221 p.
37. McConnell AR, Leibold JM (2001) Relations among the Implicit Association Test, discriminatory behavior, and explicit measures of racial attitudes. J Exp Soc Psychol 37: 435–442.
38. Greenwald AG, Hamilton Krieger L (2006) Implicit bias: Scientific foundations. California Law Rev 94: 945–967.
39. Finlay WML, Lyons E (2000) Social categorizations, social comparisons and stigma: Presentations of self in people with learning difficulties. Br J Soc Psychol 39: 129–146.
40. Cunningham C, Glenn S (2004) Self-awareness in young adults with Down syndrome: I. Awareness of Down syndrome and disability. Int J Disabil Dev Edu 51: 335–361. doi:10.1080/1034912042000295017.
41. Glenn S, Cunningham C (2004) Self-awareness in young adults with Down syndrome: II. Self-understanding. Int J Disabil Dev Edu 51: 363–381. doi:10.1080/1034912042000295026.
42. Ambady N, Shih M, Kim A, Pittinsky TL (2001) Stereotype susceptibility in children: Effects of identity activation on quantitative performance. Psychol Sci 12: 385–390.
43. Huguet P, Régner I (2007) Stereotype threat among schoolgirls in quasi-ordinary classroom circumstances. J Educ Psychol 99: 545–560.
44. Huguet P, Régner I (2009) Counter-stereotypic beliefs in math do not protect school girls from stereotype threat. J Exp Soc Psychol 45: 1024–1027. doi:10.1016/j.jesp.2009.04.029.
45. Régner I, Smeding A, Gimmig D, Thinus-Blanc C, Monteil JM, et al. (2010) Individual Differences in Working Memory Moderate Stereotype-Threat Effects. Psychol Sci 21: 1646–1648. doi:10.1177/0956797610386619.
46. Mazerolles M, Régner I, Morisset P, Rigalleau F, Huguet P (2012) Stereotype threat strengthens automatic recall and undermines controlled processes in the elderly. Psychol Sci, In press.
47. Croizet J-C, Claire T (1998) Extending the concept of stereotype threat to social class: The intellectual underperformance of students from low socioeconomic backgrounds. Pers Soc Psychol B 24: 588–594.
48. McKown C, Weinstein RS (2003) The development and consequences of stereotype consciousness in middle childhood. Child Dev 74: 498–515. doi:10.1111/1467-8624.7402012.
49. Croizet J-C, Després G, Gauzins M-E, Huguet P, Leyens J-P, et al. (2004) Stereotype threat undermines intellectual performance by triggering a disruptive mental load. Pers Soc Psychol B 30: 721–731. doi:10.1177/0146167204263961.
50. Steele CM, Aronson J (1995) Stereotype threat and the intellectual test performance of African Americans. J Pers Soc Psychol 69: 797–811.
51. Robey KL, Beckley L, Kirschner M (2006) Implicit infantilizing attitudes about disability. J Dev and Physical Disabilities 18: 441–453. doi: 10.1007/s10882-006-9027-3.
52. White MJ, Jackson V, Gordon P (2006) Implicit and explicit attitudes toward athletes with disabilities. J Rehabil 72: 33–40.
53. Thomas A, Doyle A, Vaughn D (2007) Implementation of a computer based implicit association test as a measure of attitudes toward individuals with disabilities. J Rehabil 73: 3–14.
54. Rojahn J, Komelasky KG, Man M (2008) Implicit attitudes and explicit ratings of romantic attraction of college students toward opposite-sex peers with physical disabilities. J Dev Phys Disabil 20: 389–397. doi: 10.1007/s10882-008-9108-6.
55. Peris TS, Teachman BA, Nosek BA (2008) Implicit and explicit stigma of mental illness. J Nerv Ment Dis 196: 752–760. doi: 10.1097/NMD.0b013e3181879dfd.
56. Menolascino FJ (1965) Psychiatric aspects of mongolism. Amer J Ment Def 69: 653–660.

High-Throughput Massively Parallel Sequencing for Fetal Aneuploidy Detection from Maternal Plasma

Taylor J. Jensen[1,9], Tricia Zwiefelhofer[1,9], Roger C. Tim[1,9], Željko Džakula[1], Sung K. Kim[1], Amin R. Mazloom[1], Zhanyang Zhu[1], John Tynan[1], Tim Lu[1], Graham McLennan[2], Glenn E. Palomaki[3], Jacob A. Canick[3], Paul Oeth[1], Cosmin Deciu[1], Dirk van den Boom[2], Mathias Ehrich[2]*

1 Research and Development, Sequenom Center for Molecular Medicine, San Diego, California, United States of America, **2** Research and Development, Sequenom Inc., San Diego, California, United States of America, **3** Women and Infants Hospital, Alpert Medical School of Brown University, Providence, Rhode Island, United States of America

Abstract

Background: Circulating cell-free (ccf) fetal DNA comprises 3–20% of all the cell-free DNA present in maternal plasma. Numerous research and clinical studies have described the analysis of ccf DNA using next generation sequencing for the detection of fetal aneuploidies with high sensitivity and specificity. We sought to extend the utility of this approach by assessing semi-automated library preparation, higher sample multiplexing during sequencing, and improved bioinformatic tools to enable a higher throughput, more efficient assay while maintaining or improving clinical performance.

Methods: Whole blood (10mL) was collected from pregnant female donors and plasma separated using centrifugation. Ccf DNA was extracted using column-based methods. Libraries were prepared using an optimized semi-automated library preparation method and sequenced on an Illumina HiSeq2000 sequencer in a 12-plex format. Z-scores were calculated for affected chromosomes using a robust method after normalization and genomic segment filtering. Classification was based upon a standard normal transformed cutoff value of $z = 3$ for chromosome 21 and $z = 3.95$ for chromosomes 18 and 13.

Results: Two parallel assay development studies using a total of more than 1900 ccf DNA samples were performed to evaluate the technical feasibility of automating library preparation and increasing the sample multiplexing level. These processes were subsequently combined and a study of 1587 samples was completed to verify the stability of the process-optimized assay. Finally, an unblinded clinical evaluation of 1269 euploid and aneuploid samples utilizing this high-throughput assay coupled to improved bioinformatic procedures was performed. We were able to correctly detect all aneuploid cases with extremely low false positive rates of 0.09%, <0.01%, and 0.08% for trisomies 21, 18, and 13, respectively.

Conclusions: These data suggest that the developed laboratory methods in concert with improved bioinformatic approaches enable higher sample throughput while maintaining high classification accuracy.

Editor: Noam Shomron, Tel Aviv University, Israel

Funding: This study was funded by Sequenom, Inc. The funding organization had no further role in study design, data collection and analysis, decision to publish, or preparation of the manuscript.

Competing Interests: TJJ, TZ, RCT, ZD, SKK, ARM, ZZ, JT, TL, GM, PO, CD, DvdB, and ME are all employees of Sequenom, Inc. or Sequenom Center for Molecular Medicine, a wholly owned subsidiary of Sequenom, Inc. Each of these authors are also shareholders of Sequenom, Inc. GEP and JAC were members of the Sequenom Clinical Advisory Board for 6 months and resigned when sample collection for this study was funded. There are no patents, products in development or marketed products to declare.

* E-mail: mehrich@sequenom.com

9 These authors contributed equally to this work.

Introduction

Since the discovery that fetal DNA comprises 3–20% of circulating cell-free (ccf) DNA in maternal plasma [1–3], the utilization of ccf DNA as an analyte for diagnostic purposes has been increasingly recognized as a powerful noninvasive alternative for aneuploidy detection during pregnancy. Multiple research and clinical studies have described the performance of massively parallel sequencing (MPS) to detect fetal aneuploidies, most notably trisomies of chromosomes 21, 18, and 13 [4–8]. To date, the two largest studies in this field have analysed more than 1500 samples each [7–9]. While these studies demonstrated excellent clinical performance with sensitivity and specificity greater than 99%, the underlying sequencing concepts used differ significantly in the depth and width of genomic sampling. One approach uses genome-wide sequencing, while the other uses an approach that limits the analysis to a set of specific genomic regions. The greatest advantage of a whole genome approach is that it enables the impartial analysis of the entire genome, enabling detection of genomic aberrations without *a priori* region selection. Region-specific methods theoretically support higher throughput while still achieving acceptable performance for the two most common trisomies (trisomy 21 and trisomy 18); however, these targeted assays, including those not based on Massively Parallel Sequencing (MPS) [10–12], are restricted by the significant amount of re-development required when additional content, for example less frequent trisomies or sex chromosome aneuploidies, is introduced. Additionally, it remains to be seen how well these targeted methods can identify events such as partial trisomies or other large copy number variations.

An ideal method for noninvasive aneuploidy detection using ccf DNA would combine the breadth of information from genome-wide analysis with the throughput advantages of targeted methods. Next generation sequencing technologies are still rapidly evolving and current developments are already improving genome-wide analysis to the point where throughput advantages of targeted methods may become minimal. Here we present the implementation of a set of recent process enhancements that led to a three-fold increase in throughput and a 4-fold reduction in hands-on time while maintaining clinical accuracy. The three main changes of this modified assay include: automated sequencing library preparation; higher multiplexing levels (from 4-plex to 12-plex); and the implementation of new bioinformatic methods. We outline the development process, which comprised >1500 samples, and show the results from a separate internal study analyzing 1269 samples. The results confirm that the new protocol yields a much simplified workflow amenable to higher throughput while maintaining high sensitivity and specificity for the detection of trisomies 21, 18 and 13.

Materials and Methods

Sample Acquisition and Blood Processing

Clinical samples for the initial evaluation of the high-throughput assay (library preparation development and assay verification) were collected under three separate Investigational Review Board (IRB) approved clinical protocols (BioMed IRB 301-01, Western IRB 20091396, and Compass IRB 00462). All subjects provided written informed consent prior to undergoing any study related procedures including venipuncture for the collection of up to 20 mL of whole blood into EDTA-K2 spray-dried 10 mL Vacutainers (EDTA tubes; Becton Dickinson, Franklin Lakes, NJ) and 30 mL of whole blood into Cell-Free DNA BCT 10 mL tubes (BCT tubes; Streck, Omaha, NE). Samples collected in EDTA tubes were refrigerated or stored on wet ice and were processed to plasma within 6 hours of the blood draw. Samples collected in BCT tubes were stored at ambient temperature and processed to plasma within 72 hours of the blood draw. The maternal whole blood in EDTA tubes was centrifuged (Eppendorf 5810R plus swing out rotor), chilled (4°C) at 2500 g for 10 minutes, and the plasma was collected. The EDTA plasma was centrifuged a second time (Eppendorf 5810R plus fixed angle rotor) at 4°C at 15,500 g for 10 minutes. After the second spin, the EDTA plasma was removed from the pellet that formed at the bottom of the tube and distributed into 4 mL barcoded plasma aliquots and immediately stored frozen at ≤−70°C until DNA extraction. The maternal whole blood in BCT tubes was centrifuged (Eppendorf 5810R plus swing out rotor), warmed (25°C) at 1600 g for 15 minutes and the plasma was collected. The BCT plasma was centrifuged a second time (Eppendorf 5810R plus swing out rotor) at 25°C at 2,500 g for 10 minutes. After the second spin, the BCT plasma was removed from the pellet that formed at the bottom of the tube and distributed into 4 mL barcoded plasma aliquots and immediately stored frozen at ≤−70°C until DNA extraction.

Clinical samples for multiplexing development and clinical evaluation were collected as previously described [7,8]. Briefly, whole blood was collected from enrolled subjects prior to an invasive diagnostic procedure. All samples were collected from pregnant females at increased risk for fetal aneuploidy in their first or second gestational trimester as part of an international collaboration (ClinicalTrials.gov NCT00877292). IRB approval (or equivalent) was obtained for this collaboration at each of 27 collection sites. Some data from this study has been previously published [7,8,13]. Specifically, data generated in 4-plex format and used herein for the 4-plex to 12-plex comparison has been previously published [7,8,13]; however, all data from 12-plex sequencing was generated using the same libraries now sequenced independently in 12-plex format. In addition, for independent confirmation of the high-throughput method, a plasma aliquot from each of the 1269 subjects was processed. Each of these subjects contributed a distinct plasma aliquot to the previously published studies and the fetal karyotype was known. Only samples from singleton pregnancies confirmed to be simple trisomies 21, 18, and 13, or from euploid controls were used.

Nucleic Acid Extraction

ccf DNA was extracted from maternal plasma using the QIAamp Circulating Nucleic Acid Kit (Qiagen) as previously described [5,8].

Fetal Quantifier Assay

The quantity of ccf DNA was assessed for each sample by the Fetal Quantifier Assay (FQA) as previously described [3,5,8].

Semi-Automated Sequencing Library Preparation

Extracted ccf DNA (40 µL) was used as the template for all library preparation. Libraries for the initial increased (12-plex) multiplex experimentation were prepared using previously described methods [7,8,13]. Briefly, ccf DNA was extracted and sequencing libraries prepared using oligonucleotides (Illumina), enzymes (Enzymatics), and manual purification processes between each enzymatic reaction using column-based methods (Qiagen). All newly created libraries used in this study were created in 96-well plate format using a modified version of the manufacturer's protocol for TruSeq library preparation (Illumina) and a semi-automated process that utilized liquid handler instrumentation (Caliper Zephyr; Caliper LifeSciences) with a magnetic bead-based (AMPure XP; Beckman Coulter) cleanup step after the end repair, ligation, and PCR biochemical processes. Since ccf DNA has been well characterized to exist in maternal plasma within a small range of fragment sizes, no size selection was performed upon either the extracted ccf DNA or the prepared libraries [14]. Evaluation of library size distribution and quantification was performed as previously described [8].

Massively Parallel Sequencing

Twelve isomolar sequencing libraries were pooled and sequenced together on the same lane (12-plex) of an Illumina v3 flowcell on an Illumina HiSeq2000 sequencer. Sequencing by synthesis was performed for 36 cycles followed by 7 cycles to read each sample index.

Sequencing Control Samples

Sequencing libraries were prepared from pooled ccf DNA isolated from the plasma of two adult male donors diagnosed with

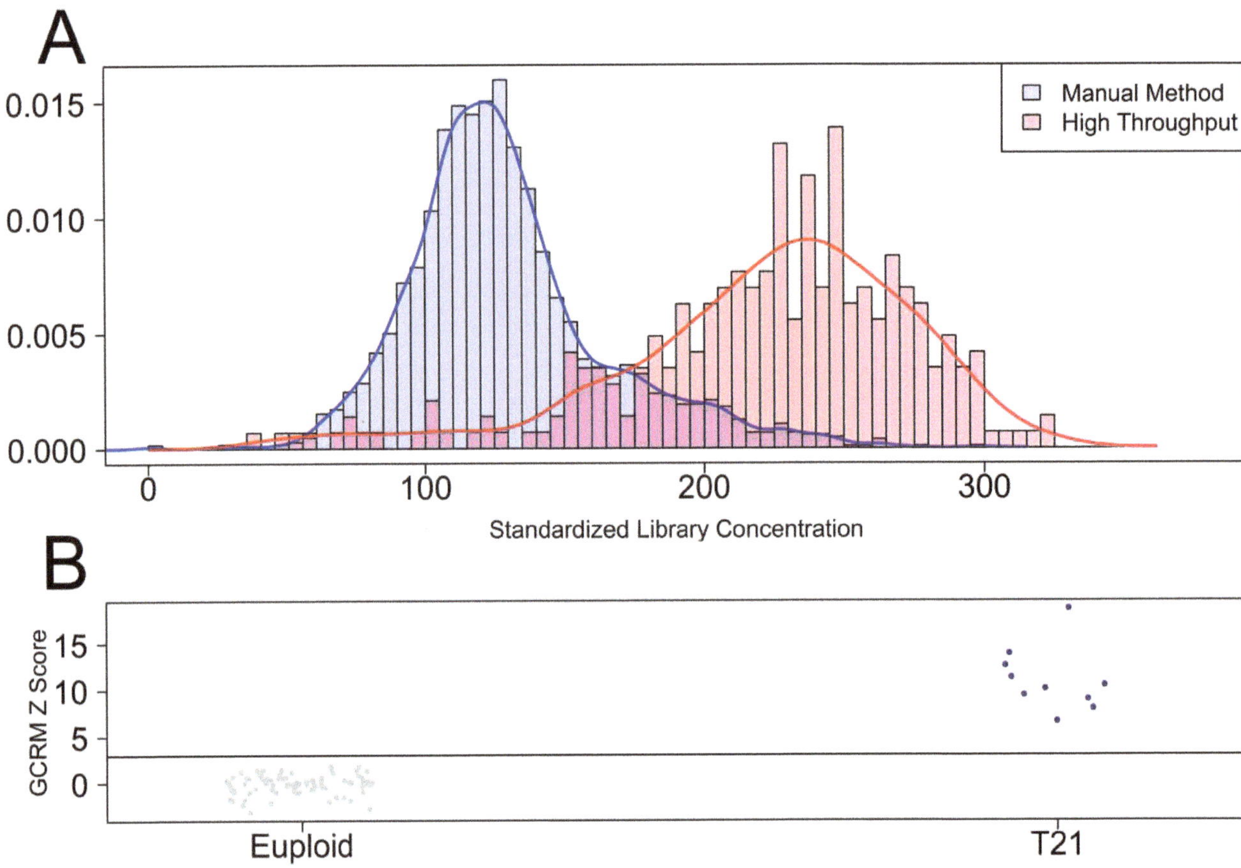

Figure 1. Library preparation optimization. A) The standardized library concentration was compared between semi-automated (n = 287) and manual library preparation methods. B) GCRM based z-scores are shown for each of 93 samples. Confirmed euploid samples (n = 83) are shown in gray; confirmed trisomy 21 samples (n = 10) are shown in blue.

trisomy 21 or non-pregnant euploid female donors. Libraries were quantified and mixed at two concentrations (4% trisomy 21 and 13% trisomy 21) to approximate the contribution of ccf fetal DNA in maternal plasma. Library performance was tested prior to the implementation of these controls in the clinical evaluation study.

Data Analysis

All BCL (base call) output files from the HiSeq2000 were converted to FASTQ format and aligned to the February 2009 build of the human genome (hg19). Since the libraries for multiplex development were prepared manually with the previous version of biochemistry, analysis methods for these data and the GCRM analysis of the 1269 sample evaluation study were applied as previously described [7]. For the high-throughput assay configuration, reads were aligned to hg19 allowing for only perfect matches within the seed sequence using Bowtie 2 [15]. For analysis purposes, the reads mapped to each chromosome were quantified using standard histograms comprising adjacent, non-overlapping 50 kbp long genomic segments. After binning, selection of included 50 kbp genomic segments was determined using a previously described cross validation method [16]. Regions were excluded from further analysis based upon exhibiting high inter-sample variance, low mappability [17], or high percentage of repetitive elements (Repeat Library 20090604; http://www.repeatmasker.org). Finally, aligned reads corresponding to the remaining 50 kbp genomic segments were normalized to account for GC bias [18] and used to calculate the fraction of aligned reads derived from each chromosome. A robust z-score was calculated as previously described using the formula $Z_{Chromosome} = (\text{Chromosome Fraction}_{Sample} - \text{Median Chromosome Fraction}_{Flowcell}) / \text{Median Absolute Deviation}_{Population}$. The median chromosome fraction was calculated specific to each flowcell while the Median Absolute Deviation (MAD) was a constant value derived from a static MAD.

Table 1. Summary of sample types utilized for each of the studies performed.

	Number of Samples By Karyotype				
Study Description	**Unknown**	**Euploid**	**Trisomy 21**	**Trisomy 13**	**Trisomy 18**
Library Optimization	0	83	10	0	0
12-plex Sequencing	0	1629	205	12	54
Verification	1587	1093	134	6	36

Results

Previous clinical studies using genome-wide MPS for non-invasive fetal aneuploidy detection have shown a range of 92–

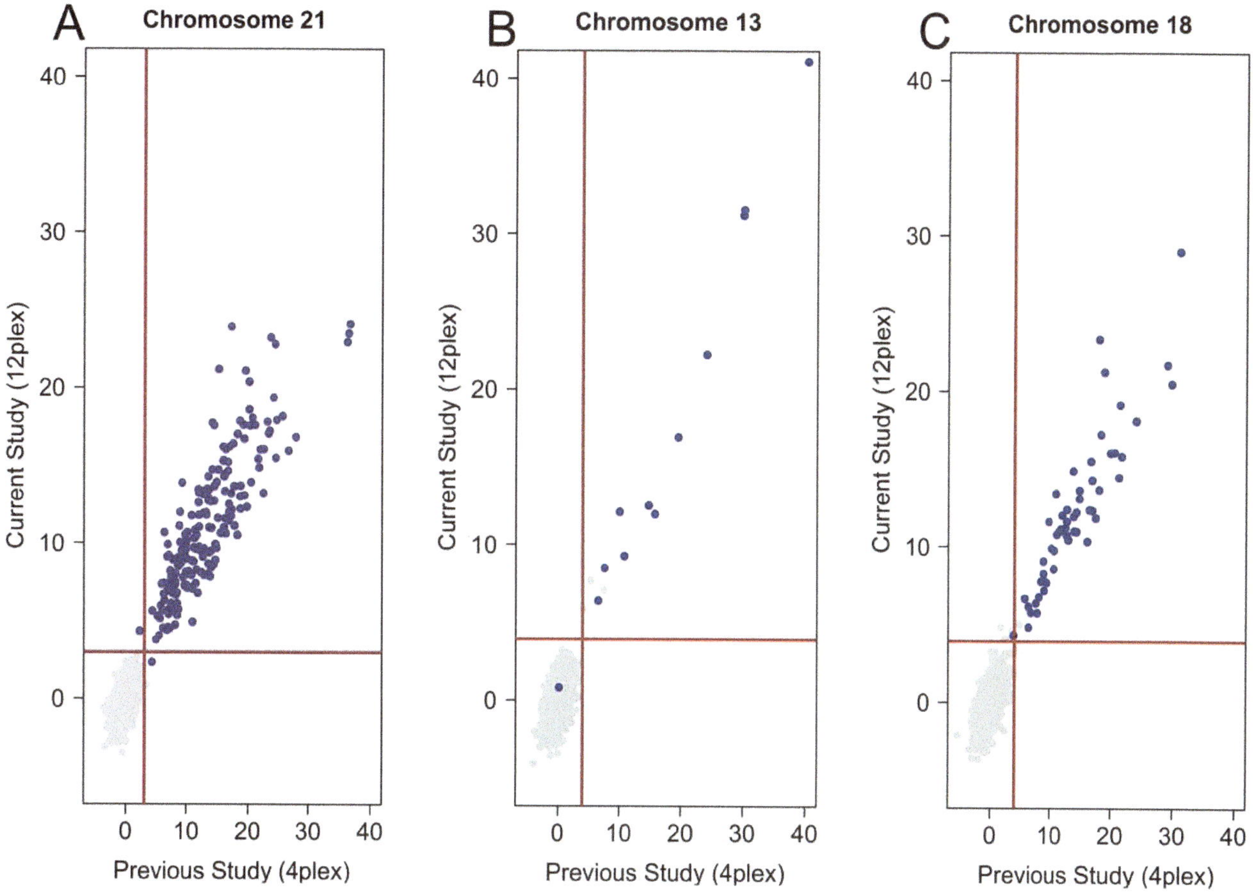

Figure 2. Paired comparison of z-scores. Z-scores were calculated for paired samples with previously described GC normalized, repeat masked z-scores on the x-axis [7] and z-scores from the same libraries sequenced in 12-plex on the y-axis. Samples classified by karyotype analysis as trisomies for A) Chromosome 21, B) Chromosome 13, or C) Chromosome 18 are shown in blue; unaffected samples for each aneuploidy condition are shown in gray. Red horizontal and vertical lines in each plot represent the respective classification cutoff for that chromosome (z = 3 for chromosome 21, z = 3.95 for chromosomes 13 and 18).

100% detection rate while maintaining a false positive rate of less than 1%. Our goal was to maintain or improve upon this performance while streamlining the protocol and increasing sample throughput [5,7,8]. Improvements focused on three aspects: I) optimizing library preparation to enable robust yield and increased throughput; II) increasing the number of individually molecularly indexed samples pooled together in a single flowcell lane (multiplex level); and III) improving analytical methods for aneuploidy classification.

Traditional sequencing library preparation is labor intensive, time consuming and sensitive to operator-to-operator variability. To alleviate these issues, we developed a semi-automated process utilizing a 96-channel liquid handling platform. TruSeq library preparation biochemistry was optimized for the low abundance of ccf DNA recovered from 4 mL of plasma (10–20 ng), which was a 50-fold reduction from the 1 µg recommended input quantity for the TruSeq library preparation kit. In addition, manual purification procedures were replaced with an automated AMPure XP bead purification process optimized for speed, reproducibility and ccf DNA recovery. Comparison of a set of 287 libraries prepared using this method to libraries produced using the manual method [7,8] revealed an increase in median library concentration

Table 2. Summary of analysis results for each of the studies performed. Sens = sensitivity.

	Analysis Results By Chromosome						
Study Description	**Spec Chr21**	**Sens Chr21**	**Spec Chr13**	**Sens Chr13**	**Spec Chr 18**	**Sens Chr18**	**Analysis Method**
Library Optimization	100	100	NA	NA	NA	NA	GCRM
12-plex Sequencing	100	99.5	99.84	91.7	99.73	100	GCRM
Verification	99.91	100	99.92	100	100	100	New

Spec = specificity; NA = Not applicable.

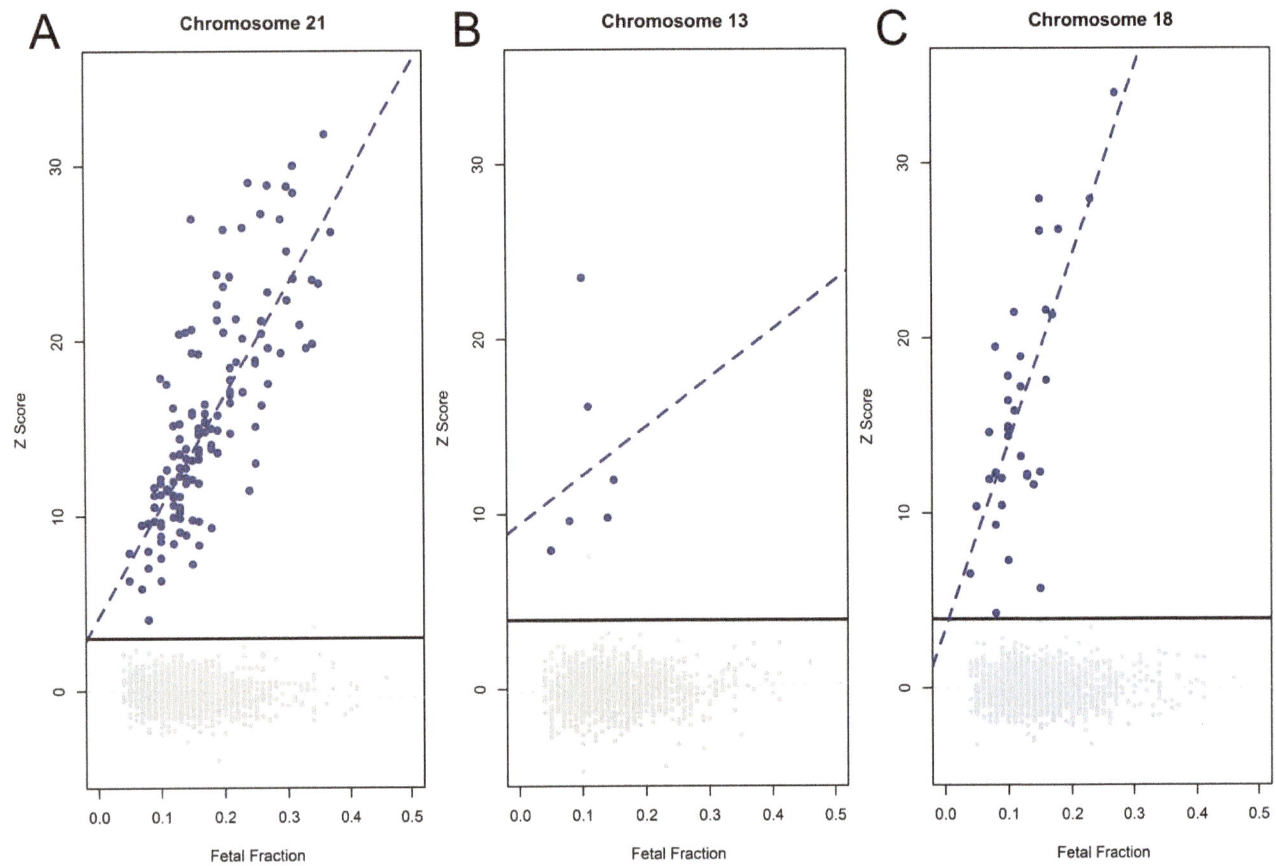

Figure 3. Z-score is linked to fetal fraction. The chromosome specific z-score for each aneuploid chromosome is plotted against the proportion of fetal DNA (fetal fraction). Samples classified by karyotype analysis as trisomies for A) Chromosome 21, B) Chromosome 13, or C) Chromosome 18 are shown in blue; unaffected samples for each aneuploidy condition are shown in gray. Black horizontal line in each plot represents the respective classification cutoff for each chromosome (z = 3 for chromosome 21, z = 3.95 for chromosomes 13 and 18). Dashed blue line in each panel represents a robust linear fit of aneuploid samples. Dashed gray line in each panel represents a robust linear fit of all unaffected samples.

from 124 to 225 nM after standardization for elution volume (Figure 1A). The combined semi-automated process produced 96 libraries in 5 hours, requiring only a single technician and 1.5 hours of hands-on labor time. This resulted in a 4-fold increase in throughput coincident with a 4-fold decrease in labor without sacrificing library yield or quality [7,8]. We sequenced and analyzed 93 libraries (83 confirmed euploid samples and 10 confirmed trisomy 21 samples; Table 1) prepared using this method and found accurate classification performance in this small data set (Figure 1B; Table 2).

Libraries prepared and sequenced in 4-plex during a previous study were sequenced in 12-plex to determine the feasibility of increased multiplexing [7,8]. Illumina v3 flowcells and sequencing biochemistry, in combination with HCS software improvements, produced a 2.23-fold increase (from 72 to 161 million) in total read counts per lane. We sequenced and analyzed 1900 libraries in 12-plex including 1629 euploid samples, 205 trisomy 21 samples, 54 trisomy 18 samples, and 12 trisomy 13 samples (Table 1) and compared the z-scores for chromosomes 21, 18, and 13 to 4-plex results (Figure 2). Since previous studies had indicated an increase in assay performance using an elevated z-score cutoff, classification was based upon z = 3.95 for chromosomes 18 and 13 [7]. The classification for chromosome 21 remained at z = 3. Using these classification cutoffs, there were a total of 7 discordant classification results between 4-plex and 12-plex sequencing. For chromosome 21, 2 samples previously misclassified (1 false positive, 1 false negative) were correctly classified while a previously noted true positive was not detected. Four samples were misclassified as false positive samples for chromosome 18 whereas they had previously been correctly classified; each of these libraries was highly GC biased. All samples were concordant for trisomy 13 classification. When sequencing in 12-plex, 99.3% of aneuploid samples (204/205 trisomy 21, 54/54 trisomy 18, and 11/12 trisomy 13) were detected with a false-positive rate of 0% (0/1695), 0.27% (5/1846) and 0.16% (3/1888) for trisomies 21, 18 and 13, respectively (Table 2). Overall, these data suggest that the performance of the assay when executed with 12-plex multiplexing is similar to previously published results [7,8].

Next, a verification study was performed using the optimized library preparation method coupled to 12-plex sequencing (high-throughput assay configuration) to ensure process integrity. We analyzed sequencing results from a total of 2856 samples, 1269 of which had a known karyotype. These 1269 clinical samples were comprised of 1093 euploid, 134 trisomy 21, 36 trisomy 18 and 6 trisomy 13 samples (Table 1). Metrics found previously to be critical to assay success were measured (Figure S1). The median fetal DNA fraction for samples was 0.14 (range: 0.04–0.46), similar to that reported in previous studies (Figure S1A) [5,7,8]. The median library concentration was 28.21 nM (range: 7.53–42.19 nM), resulting in a total yield similar to previous methods

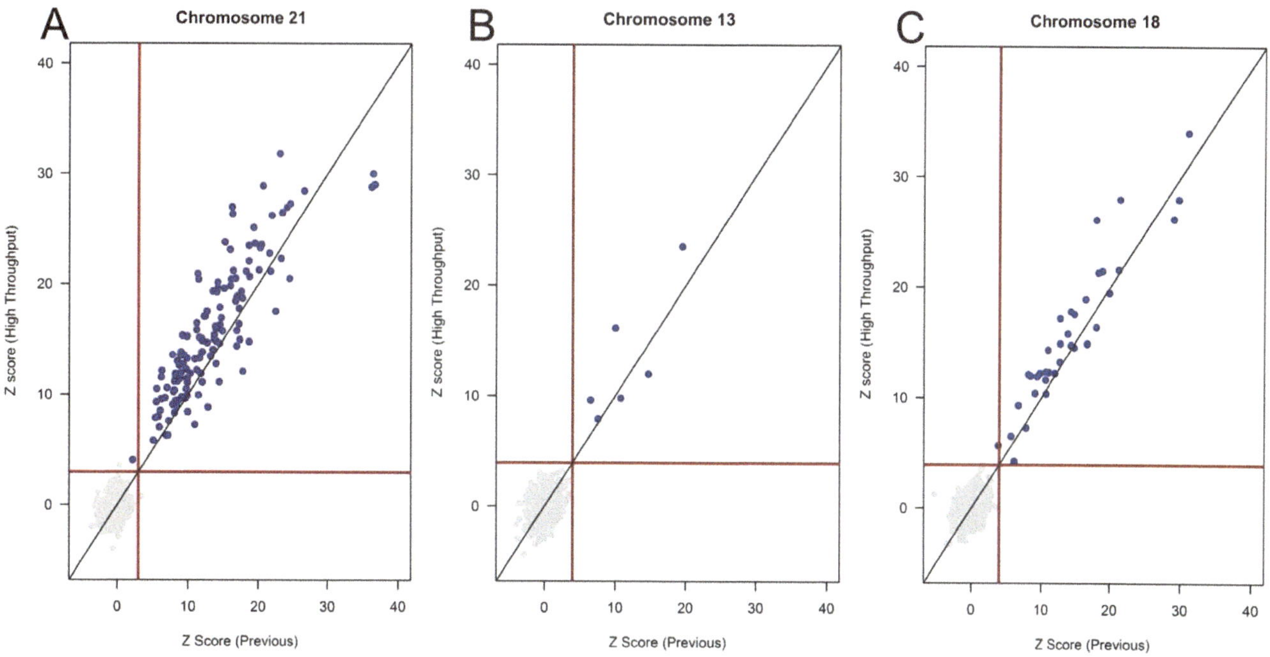

Figure 4. Paired comparison of z-scores. Z-scores were calculated for 1269 paired samples with previously described GC normalized, repeat masked z-scores on the x-axis [7] and z-scores from the high-throughput assay on the y-axis. Samples classified by karyotype analysis as trisomies for A) Chromsome 21, B) Chromosome 13, or C) Chromosome 18 are shown in blue; unaffected samples for each aneuploidy condition are shown in gray. Red horizontal and vertical lines in each plot represent the respective classification cutoff for that chromosome (z = 3 for chromosome 21, z = 3.95 for chromosomes 13 and 18). Black line in plot represents y = x.

(Figure S1B) [5]. Finally, the median number of aligned autosomal reads per sample was 16,291,390 (range: 8,825,886–35,259,563) (Figure S1C).

Initial comparison of the data generated from the 1269 samples with known fetal karyotype to a distinct plasma aliquot previously sequenced from the same subject revealed a decrease in the discriminatory distance (difference between the 95th percentile of euploid samples and the 5th percentile of trisomy 21 samples) from 4.9 to 3.09 when analyzed using previously established methods which normalized for GC content and removed reads overlapping with repeat regions (GCRM; Figure S2). To mitigate this effect concomitant with decreasing overall analysis time, a new bioinformatic algorithm specific to the high-throughput assay data was developed. This method based calculations for classification upon only those 50 kbp genomic segments with stable representation across individuals. When applied to the same high-throughput data set, the discriminatory distance between euploid and trisomy 21 samples increased to 6.49 (Figure S2). Overall, new bioinformatic approaches result in an increase in discriminatory distance between euploid and trisomy 21 samples relative to previously described methods.

The results from the high-throughput assay were analyzed using the new analysis methods for 67 control and 1269 subject samples. We sequenced 33 libraries prepared from pooled euploid plasma (0% T21 library), 17 control libraries containing 4% trisomy 21 DNA, and 17 control libraries containing 13% trisomy 21 DNA. In all cases, the pooled euploid samples had a z-score less than 3 while the 4% and 13% trisomy 21 control samples had a z-score greater than 3 (Figure S3). We then compared the classification accuracy of the 1269 subject samples with known karyotype information. Based upon these classification limits described above (z-score = 3 for chromosome 21, z-score = 3.95 for chromosomes 18 and 13), all confirmed fetal aneuploidies (134 trisomy 21, 36 trisomy 18, 6 trisomy 13) were detected with a false positive rate of 0.09% (1/1135), <0.01% (0/1233), and 0.08% (1/1263) for trisomies 21, 18, and 13, respectively (Figure 3; Table 2). As previously demonstrated [7,8,19], there is a positive correlation between fetal fraction and the magnitude of the z-score while there is no correlation between these metrics for euploid samples.

Distinct plasma samples from each of the 1269 subjects were previously sequenced and thus serve as a comparison for performance [7,8]. To ensure a comparable evaluation, z-scores from the previously published studies were calculated using GCRM values and a population size (for median and MAD calculations) of 96 samples, equivalent to the sample number used for median calculations using high-throughput analysis. Comparison of the two studies revealed the correct classification of a previously reported false negative trisomy 21 sample and a previously reported false positive trisomy 21 sample; however, there was one additional false positive during this study (Figure 4). There were no discordant samples when comparing trisomy 13 classification and the correct classification of a single trisomy 18 sample with a previous z-score slightly below 3.95. Evaluation of paired z-scores for aneuploid samples revealed a mean difference of 2.19 for trisomy 21, 1.56 for trisomy 18, and 1.64 for trisomy 13, reflecting an increase in z-score for aneuploid samples using the high-throughput methods. There was a statistically significant increase in z-score for confirmed trisomy 21 and trisomy 18 samples using the high-throughput assay ($p = 4.24\ e^{-12}$ and $p = 0.0002$, respectively; paired wilcox test) relative to the previous study, but no significant difference in z-scores for confirmed trisomy 13 samples ($p = 0.31$; paired wilcox test). There were no statistically significant differences in chromosome 21, chromosome 18, or chromosome 13 z-scores for euploid samples ($p = 0.06$, $p = 0.90$, $p = 0.82$, respectively; paired wilcox test). This significant increase in aneuploid z-scores without significantly impacting euploid samples further indicates an expansion of the analytical distance between euploid and aneuploid samples for chromosomes 21 and 18 when using the high-throughput assay configuration and new bioinformatic methods.

Discussion

Several studies, both small and large, have shown the extremely high sensitivity and specificity of fetal aneuploidy detection using MPS-based analysis of ccf DNA [4–9,19–25]. Consequently, it is imperative that each new modification to this concept is tested in a sufficiently powered study. The development presented here was preceeded by research activities and followed by additional verification and validation studies conducted in a CLIA-certified laboratory. In total, the entire process of bringing a new laboratory-developed test from research through validation was supported by data from over 5000 tested samples. In this study, we sequenced more than 3400 samples during research, optimization and development. We then performed a clinical evaluation study utilizing 1269 samples, of which we detected all 176 aneuploid samples while maintaining a false positive rate of 0.09% or less for each trisomy.

Next generation sequencing and its implementation into clinical practice is still a rapidly evolving field. In less than one year our throughput per sequencer has more than doubled and the hands-on time required was reduced by 4-fold. Genome-wide analysis methods of ccf DNA will benefit most from this trend. Each advancement in sequencing translates directly into the ability to provide more information to the physician. It has already been shown that the detection of sub-chromosomal alterations as small as 3 MB (such as 22q11.2) is enabled by an approximately 20-fold increase in sequencing [26,27]. At the current rate of progress, genome-wide analysis of ccf DNA is likely to provide detection of subchromosomal alterrations >10 MB within a year and potentially achieve results comparable to karyotyping within 3 to 5 years.

We have developed an assay which enables a 4-fold increase in library preparation throughput and coupled that to a 3-fold increase in sample multiplexing to allow for high-throughput ccf DNA sample processing. Using these methods in combination with improved analytics, we have shown improved sensitivity and specificity for noninvasive aneuploidy detection while decreasing technician and instrument requirements. Overall, these data suggest that the developed high-throughput assay is technically robust and clinically accurate, enabling detection of all tested fetal aneuploidies (176/176) with a low false positive rate (≤0.09% for each chromosome).

Supporting Information

Figure S1 Summary of sequencing paramaters. A) Proportion of ccf DNA derived from the fetus in 1269 patient samples quantified using methylation-based discriminitory analysis. B) Distribution of the concentration (nM) of prepared sequencing libraries. C) Total number of aligned reads for each of 1269 libraries.

Figure S2 New bioinformatic methods increase discriminatory distance. Libraries from two distinct plasma aliquots from the same donor were created, sequenced, and analyzed. Z-scores were calculated as previously described (GCRM) or using the new bioinformatic method (New Method). Blue samples = Trisomy 21, Gray samples = Non-Trisomy 21 (Includes trisomy 13 and trisomy 18 samples). The gap was calculated as the difference in chromosome 21 z-scores from the 95th percentile of non-trisomy 21 samples to the 5th percentile of trisomy 21 samples. GCRM = GC normalized, Repeat Masked.

Figure S3 Chromosome 21 z-scores of control samples. Chromosome 21 z-scores of each of three control samples are shown. Euploid pool = distinct library created from pooled euploid plasma; Low Pos = low positive control comprised of mixing 96% non-pregnant female library with 4% trisomy 21 library; High Pos = high positive control comprised of mixing 87% non-pregnant female library with 13% trisomy 21 library. Red line at z = 3 represents classification cutoff for chromosome 21.

Acknowledgments

The authors would like to thank Vach Angkachatchai, Lesley Cagasan, Julia Clemens, Farnaz Ehya, Jessica Hsieh, Daniella Hubbard, Rochelle Jean-Jacques, Yabo Jin, Stephanie Lin, Haiping Lu, Vivian Lu, Erin McCarthy, Christine Safanayong, Bright Sagoe, Helen Tao, Jack Wang, Wen Wu, and Marc Wycoco for performing the laboratory work; Pat Liu for performing the data processing; Dr. Allan Bombard and Jill Harris for sample collection and coordination; and Dr. Charles Cantor and Dr. Ron Lindsay for critical review of the manuscript.

Author Contributions

Conceived and designed the experiments: PO CD DvdB ME GEP JAC. Performed the experiments: TJJ TZ RCT JT. Analyzed the data: TJJ ZD SKK ARM ZZ TL CD ME. Contributed reagents/materials/analysis tools: GEP JAC. Wrote the paper: TJJ TZ GM ME.

References

1. Lo YM, Corbetta N, Chamberlain PF, Rai V, Sargent IL, et al. (1997) Presence of fetal DNA in maternal plasma and serum. Lancet 350: 485–487.
2. Lo YM, Tein MS, Lau TK, Haines CJ, Leung TN, et al. (1998) Quantitative analysis of fetal DNA in maternal plasma and serum: implications for noninvasive prenatal diagnosis. Am J Hum Genet 62: 768–775.
3. Nygren AO, Dean J, Jensen TJ, Kruse S, Kwong W, et al. (2010) Quantification of fetal DNA by use of methylation-based DNA discrimination. Clin Chem 56: 1627–1635.
4. Chiu RW, Chan KC, Gao Y, Lau VY, Zheng W, et al. (2008) Noninvasive prenatal diagnosis of fetal chromosomal aneuploidy by massively parallel genomic sequencing of DNA in maternal plasma. Proc Natl Acad Sci U S A 105: 20458–20463.
5. Ehrich M, Deciu C, Zwiefelhofer T, Tynan JA, Cagasan L, et al. (2011) Noninvasive detection of fetal trisomy 21 by sequencing of DNA in maternal blood: a study in a clinical setting. Am J Obstet Gynecol 204: 205 e1–11.
6. Fan HC, Blumenfeld YJ, Chitkara U, Hudgins L, Quake SR (2008) Noninvasive diagnosis of fetal aneuploidy by shotgun sequencing DNA from maternal blood. Proc Natl Acad Sci U S A 105: 16266–16271.
7. Palomaki GE, Deciu C, Kloza EM, Lambert-Messerlian GM, Haddow JE, et al. (2012) DNA sequencing of maternal plasma reliably identifies trisomy 18 and trisomy 13 as well as Down syndrome: an international collaborative study. Genet Med 14: 296–305.
8. Palomaki GE, Kloza EM, Lambert-Messerlian GM, Haddow JE, Neveux LM, et al. (2011) DNA sequencing of maternal plasma to detect Down syndrome: An international clinical validation study. Genet Med 13: 913–920.
9. Norton ME, Brar H, Weiss J, Karimi A, Laurent LC, et al. (2012) Non-Invasive Chromosomal Evaluation (NICE) Study: results of a multicenter prospective cohort study for detection of fetal trisomy 21 and trisomy 18. Am J Obstet Gynecol 207: 137 e1–8.
10. Della Ragione F, Mastrovito P, Campanile C, Conti A, Papageorgiou EA, et al. (2010) Differential DNA methylation as a tool for noninvasive prenatal diagnosis (NIPD) of X chromosome aneuploidies. J Mol Diagn 12: 797–807.
11. Papageorgiou EA, Karagrigoriou A, Tsaliki E, Velissariou V, Carter NP, et al. (2011) Fetal-specific DNA methylation ratio permits noninvasive prenatal diagnosis of trisomy 21. Nat Med 17: 510–513.
12. Patsalis PC, Tsaliki E, Koumbaris G, Karagrigoriou A, Velissariou V, et al. (2012) A new non-invasive prenatal diagnosis of Down syndrome through

epigenetic markers and real-time qPCR. Expert Opin Biol Ther 12 Suppl 1: S155–161.
13. Canick JA, Kloza EM, Lambert-Messerlian GM, Haddow JE, Ehrich M, et al. (2012) DNA sequencing of maternal plasma to identify Down syndrome and other trisomies in multiple gestations. Prenat Diagn 32: 730–734.
14. Lo YM, Chan KC, Sun H, Chen EZ, Jiang P, et al. (2010) Maternal plasma DNA sequencing reveals the genome-wide genetic and mutational profile of the fetus. Sci Transl Med 2: 61ra91.
15. Langmead B, Salzberg SL (2012) Fast gapped-read alignment with Bowtie 2. Nat Methods 9: 357–359.
16. Brunger AT (1992) Free R value: a novel statistical quantity for assessing the accuracy of crystal structures. Nature 355: 472–475.
17. Derrien T, Estelle J, Marco Sola S, Knowles DG, Raineri E, et al. (2012) Fast computation and applications of genome mappability. PLoS One 7: e30377.
18. Alkan C, Kidd JM, Marques-Bonet T, Aksay G, Antonacci F, et al. (2009) Personalized copy number and segmental duplication maps using next-generation sequencing. Nat Genet 41: 1061–1067.
19. Sparks AB, Struble CA, Wang ET, Song K, Oliphant A (2012) Noninvasive prenatal detection and selective analysis of cell-free DNA obtained from maternal blood: evaluation for trisomy 21 and trisomy 18. Am J Obstet Gynecol 206: 319 e1–9.
20. Ashoor G, Syngelaki A, Wagner M, Birdir C, Nicolaides KH (2012) Chromosome-selective sequencing of maternal plasma cell-free DNA for first-trimester detection of trisomy 21 and trisomy 18. Am J Obstet Gynecol 206: 322 e1–5.
21. Chen EZ, Chiu RW, Sun H, Akolekar R, Chan KC, et al. (2011) Noninvasive prenatal diagnosis of fetal trisomy 18 and trisomy 13 by maternal plasma DNA sequencing. PLoS One 6: e21791.
22. Chiu RW, Akolekar R, Zheng YW, Leung TY, Sun H, et al. (2011) Non-invasive prenatal assessment of trisomy 21 by multiplexed maternal plasma DNA sequencing: large scale validity study. BMJ 342: c7401.
23. Chiu RW, Sun H, Akolekar R, Clouser C, Lee C, et al. (2010) Maternal plasma DNA analysis with massively parallel sequencing by ligation for noninvasive prenatal diagnosis of trisomy 21. Clin Chem 56: 459–463.
24. Faas BH, de Ligt J, Janssen I, Eggink AJ, Wijnberger LD, et al. (2012) Non-invasive prenatal diagnosis of fetal aneuploidies using massively parallel sequencing-by-ligation and evidence that cell-free fetal DNA in the maternal plasma originates from cytotrophoblastic cells. Expert Opin Biol Ther 12 Suppl 1: S19–26.
25. Sparks AB, Wang ET, Struble CA, Barrett W, Stokowski R, et al. (2012) Selective analysis of cell-free DNA in maternal blood for evaluation of fetal trisomy. Prenat Diagn 32: 3–9.
26. Jensen TJ, Džakula Ž, Deciu C, van den Boom D, Ehrich M (2012) Detection of Microdeletion 22q11.2 in a Fetus by Next-Generation Sequencing of Maternal Plasma. Clin Chem 58: 1148–1151.
27. Peters D, Chu T, Yatsenko SA, Hendrix N, Hogge WA, et al. (2011) Noninvasive prenatal diagnosis of a fetal microdeletion syndrome. N Engl J Med 365: 1847–1848.

14

Massive-Scale RNA-Seq Analysis of Non Ribosomal Transcriptome in Human Trisomy 21

Valerio Costa[1], Claudia Angelini[2], Luciana D'Apice[3], Margherita Mutarelli[4], Amelia Casamassimi[5], Linda Sommese[6], Maria Assunta Gallo[7], Marianna Aprile[1], Roberta Esposito[1], Luigi Leone[1], Aldo Donizetti[1], Stefania Crispi[1], Monica Rienzo[5], Berardo Sarubbi[8], Raffaele Calabrò[8], Marco Picardi[9], Paola Salvatore[10], Teresa Infante[11], Piergiuseppe De Berardinis[3], Claudio Napoli[5,11], Alfredo Ciccodicola[1]*

1 Institute of Genetics and Biophysics "A. Buzzati-Traverso", CNR, Naples, Italy, **2** Istituto per le Applicazioni del Calcolo, Mauro Picone, CNR, Naples, Italy, **3** Institute of Protein Biochemistry, CNR, Naples, Italy, **4** Telethon Institute of Genetics and Medicine (TIGEM), Naples, Italy, **5** Department of General Pathology and Excellence Research Centre on Cardiovascular Diseases, 1st School of Medicine, Second University of Naples, Naples, Italy, **6** Section of Microbiology, Department of Experimental Medicine, 1st School of Medicine, Second University of Naples, Naples, Italy, **7** Centro Diagnostico San Ciro, Portici, Italy, **8** Cardiology Department of Second University of Naples, "Monaldi Hospital", Naples, Italy, **9** Department of Biochemistry and Medical Biotechnology, University of Naples "Federico II", Naples, Italy, **10** Department of Cellular and Molecular Biology and Pathology "L. Califano", University of Naples "Federico II" and Ceinge Biotecnologie Avanzate s.c.a.r.l., Naples, Italy, **11** Fondazione-SDN (Institute of Diagnostic and Nuclear Development), IRCCS, Naples, Italy

Abstract

Hybridization- and tag-based technologies have been successfully used in Down syndrome to identify genes involved in various aspects of the pathogenesis. However, these technologies suffer from several limits and drawbacks and, to date, information about rare, even though relevant, RNA species such as long and small non-coding RNAs, is completely missing. Indeed, none of published works has still described the whole transcriptional landscape of Down syndrome. Although the recent advances in high-throughput RNA sequencing have revealed the complexity of transcriptomes, most of them rely on polyA enrichment protocols, able to detect only a small fraction of total RNA content. On the opposite end, massive-scale RNA sequencing on rRNA-depleted samples allows the survey of the complete set of coding and non-coding RNA species, now emerging as novel contributors to pathogenic mechanisms. Hence, in this work we analysed for the first time the complete transcriptome of human trisomic endothelial progenitor cells to an unprecedented level of resolution and sensitivity by RNA-sequencing. Our analysis allowed us to detect differential expression of even low expressed genes crucial for the pathogenesis, to disclose novel regions of active transcription outside yet annotated *loci*, and to investigate a plethora of non-polyadenilated long as well as short non coding RNAs. Novel splice isoforms for a large subset of crucial genes, and novel extended untranslated regions for known genes—possibly novel miRNA targets or regulatory sites for gene transcription—were also identified in this study. Coupling the rRNA depletion of samples, followed by high-throughput RNA-sequencing, to the easy availability of these cells renders this approach very feasible for transcriptome studies, offering the possibility of investigating in-depth blood-related pathological features of Down syndrome, as well as other genetic disorders.

Editor: Diego Di Bernardo, Fondazione Telethon, Italy

Funding: This project was supported by COST Action BM1006: "Next Generation Sequencing Data Analysis Network" (NGS) from European Cooperation in the field of Scientific and Technical Research (C. Angelini and A. Ciccodicola); Legge 5, Regione Campania (A. Ciccodicola); Progetto di Rilevante Interesse Nazionale Ministero Italiano Università e Ricerca 2006 and 2008 (Code0622153_002) "Meccanismi fisiopatologici di danno vascolare/trombotico ed angiogenesi" and (Code2008T85HLH_002) "Regolazione dell'espressione genica della via SIRT1/FoxO1- dipendente in cellule endoteliali progenitrici della nicchia vascolare" (C. Napoli); and Regione Campania 2008–2010 to the II University of Naples (C. Napoli). The funders had no role in study design, data collection and analysis, decision to publish, or preparation of the manuscript.

Competing Interests: The authors have declared that no competing interests exist.

* E-mail: ciccodic@igb.cnr.it

Introduction

Expression profiles of thousands of genes in various organs and cell lines have been successfully determined by using different methods and approaches such as microarray, serial and cap analysis of gene expression, and massively parallel signature sequencing [1–11]. These approaches have led to the identification of differentially expressed genes in physiological and pathological conditions, such as Down syndrome (DS) [12–15], Alzheimer, Parkinson [16–18] and cardiovascular diseases [2,8,19,20].

In Down syndrome the dosage imbalance of human chromosome 21 (HSA21) genes, and the subsequent global gene deregulation observed overall the genome [12,21,22], have long been associated to different aspects of DS pathogenesis. Expression analyses of DS tissues and mouse models have reported conflicting results [23,24], showing that HSA21 gene expression greatly varies across trisomic tissues [14,22]. However, most of published works has focused on hybridization-based technologies - suffering from hybridization and cross-hybridization artefacts and offering a limited dynamic range - or tag-based approaches, suffering for the ambiguous mapping of their short reads. Hence, to date we completely lack information about other rare, even though physiologically relevant, RNA classes such as small coding and (long-) non-coding RNAs. In addition, there is not yet evidence of DS-specific splice isoforms for genes crucial in the pathogenesis and, to date, none of published works has described, in a single experiment, the complete transcriptional networks in Down syndrome.

The introduction of next generation sequencing (NGS) technologies has revealed the complexity of mammalian transcriptomes, enabling to effectively explore - with an unprecedented throughput capacity - simple and complex genomes [25–31]. NGS have shown that most of nucleotides are expressed, highlighting that only a small fraction of all transcribed sequences (less than 2%) is represented by mRNA [32,33], and that not yet well-characterized RNA species, such as microRNA recently described in DS [34] as well as small nucleolar RNA (snoRNA), are emerging as potential factors contributing to pathological phenotypes [35,36].

In the last years, in order to identify genes contributing to DS phenotype and to its phenotypic variability, the above-mentioned standard approaches for gene expression profiling have been applied to several mouse models with segmental duplications of DNA segments orthologous to human chromosome 21. Alternatively, transcriptome studies on human DS subjects have been so far performed on *post-mortem* tissues and/or fetuses, and few studies have focused on RNAs isolated from human adult whole blood samples [12,37–39]. Thus, it would be clinically relevant to investigate, with an innovative and high-throughput approach, early gene regulatory mechanisms linked to cardiovascular disease, cancer and immune disorders linked to DS.

To this purpose, we analysed for the first time the global transcriptome of human trisomic and euploid endothelial progenitor cells (EPCs) to an unprecedented level of resolution and sensitivity by RNA-Seq on a next generation sequencing platform. By using a selective depletion of abundant rRNA molecules from samples - followed by the sequencing of strand-specific cDNA libraries - we were able to measure the effects of trisomy 21 in a specific cell type affected in DS, and also to quantify the defect during postnatal development, possibly correlating gene expression changes to the observed phenotype. Indeed, literature data and our recent findings strongly indicate that circulating EPCs, whose levels are linked to tissue regeneration, are impaired in DS [12,40–42]. These cells play pivotal role in the maintenance of endothelium integrity, repair after injury and postnatal neovascularization and several studies suggest their use in the clinical setting [43–47]. Moreover, accumulating evidences indicate a reduced availability, and/or impaired EPC function in cardiovascular and metabolic diseases [12,45,48–50]. Endothelial dysfunction, angiogenesis suppression and infection recurrence are hallmarks of DS, and the impairment in the number and function of circulating progenitors may promote a wide number of diseases. The massive-scale RNA-Seq and the easy availability of these cells from affected individuals allow to shed light on endothelium-related pathological features of DS, rendering this analysis feasible on a large number of samples.

Results

Strand-oriented libraries preparation and sequencing

The ability, and the power, to measure gene expression in RNA-Seq experiments is strictly correlated to the number of sequence reads mapped to transcribed regions in a particular cell/tissue/organism. In the light of this, for a whole-transcriptome (WT) analysis we planned both our sequencing strategy and platform usage (Figure S1).

To this aim, a systematic depletion - from total RNA samples - of very abundant rRNA molecules (consisting of about 95% of cellular RNA), was performed. This procedure, coupled with the massive sequencing on NGS platform, allows to investigate the entire transcriptional landscape of an organism, offering the possibility to analyse - within the same experiment - polyA$^+$ mRNAs, long as well as small coding and non-coding RNA species. It clearly represents a great opportunity, and a challenge, compared to the commonly used approaches relying on polyA$^+$ enrichment of the samples [30–32,51–57].

In addition, since preserving the strandedness is fundamental for further data analysis and interpretation, we created strand-oriented libraries (SOLs) for each sample. Indeed, SOLs usage allows to determine the correct directionality of transcription and gene orientation (for both annotated and unannotated expressed regions), thus facilitating the detection of opposing and overlapping transcripts.

In this study, we generated SOLs from rRNA-depleted total RNAs isolated from human EPCs [7,58] of a female affected from trisomy 21 and one age- and sex-matched euploid, and sequenced them to a depth of about 100 million of 50 nt reads per library on a SOLiD v3 platform (Applied Biosystems).

Mapping strategy and visualization

The sequenced reads were mapped on human genome (hg19) using RNA-MATE [30]. Mapping strategy and results are illustrated in Figure S2 and Table S1. Details of the mapping strategy are given in "Materials and Methods" and File S1.

We noted that filtering reads derived from very abundant rRNAs molecules (5.8S, 18S, 28S) has a great impact on rRNA-depleted WT experiments since they still constitute a significant fraction of total sequenced reads, whereas adapter-filtered reads represent a negligible amount. However, at least for the purpose of this work, they can be used as a measure of ribodepletion efficiency rather than a real measure of interest.

The cyclic alignment implemented in RNA-MATE ensured the detection of expressed regions from both annotated exons and junctions from a custom library, also giving the possibility to detect the expression of previously unannotated regions and to identify novel combinatorial exon usage for every known *locus*. The low extent of antisense mapping of reads (about 0.07% for both libraries) to splice junctions' libraries, was used to assess SOLs' directionality and to tune the mapping parameters. In addition, most of reads (about 90%) that mapped to the genome and to junction library were 50 nt in length with few sequence mismatches. Such results are comparable to those obtained in analogous studies and constitute an overall measure of the quality the produced data.

At the end of the alignment strategy three types of reads were distinguished: uniquely assignable reads (UARs), multiple reads (MRs) and reads without a specific mapping location (denoted as unmatched reads; see "Materials and Methods", Figure S2 and Figure S3). For the sake of simplicity we considered only UARs and reads mapping on junction library for further analyses. We noted that discarding MRs - which mainly derive from conserved domains of gene families and/or common repeats - is likely to introduce an experimental bias, decreasing the coverage and reducing the possibility to investigate expressed retrotransposons and most of highly conserved gene families [26]. However, since a significant fraction of multiple reads was assigned to UARs category using a rescue procedure, we reduced the above-mentioned mapping bias ("Materials and Methods" and File S1) [59].

We also noted that the sequenced reads mapped at 50 nt length (with few mismatches) contribute to about 91% of DS and 86% of euploid unique reads, and to about 76% and 71% of finally assigned UARs for DS and euploid, respectively.

We observed, as expected due to the presence of an extra copy of HSA21 for DS sample, a higher amount of sequenced reads mapping to this chromosome, with the highest (1.33) DS/euploid mapped reads ratio than observed for the other chromosomes (mean ratio 0.99±0.05). A similar unbalancing in reads' mapping was also observed for the mitochondrial chromosome (chr M) (ratio = 1.23) mainly due to the highly variable number of mitochondria in a cell, organism and tissue type.

To better elucidate the landscape of gene expression in both states we classified all mapped reads in the following categories: reads mapping to 1) annotated RefSeq gene models, 2) intronic regions, 3) intergenic regions, 4) known RefSeq splice junctions and 5) novel combinatorial junctions and 6) mitochondrial genome. The mapping of the categories from 1) to 3) and 6) is depicted in Figure S4. The analysis of each category is described in the following sections.

Gene expression quantification

Since we previously described in EPCs isolated from DS individuals a global deregualtion of gene expression compared to euploid cells [14], we used RNA-Seq to have a better quantitative estimate of gene expression from both known genes and previously uncharacterized expressed regions. To this aim we scored each *locus* activity in both trisomic and euploid cells by counting the number of reads mapping to annotated RefSeq transcripts (release 38) [60]. In particular, for gene *loci* with a single transcript we estimated gene expression as the number of UARs mapping to the entire length of the transcript, whilst for genes with multiple splice isoforms a measure of global *locus* activity was obtained summing the reads mapped to any independent exon (or part of exon) of each possible transcript (details in File S1). In both cases, the reads count deriving from reads mapped to the junctions library were added to each corresponding *locus*.

The representative RefSeq categories (Human Gene Nomenclature Committee, HGNC) [61] comprising all the genes detected and analyzed in the WT experiment are shown in Figure 1A. In DS as well as euploid sample, about 92% of detected *loci* with evidence of active transcription in circulating progenitors fall in the mRNA category. Surprisingly, the distribution of mapped reads per category revealed a 2- to 10-fold enrichment of non-coding RNAs, particularly snoRNA, in both analyzed samples (Figure 1B and 1C). Moreover, the distribution of mapped reads (in terms of genomic positions) showed, as expected, a strong bias toward regions already annotated as genes in RefSeq: on average, about 50% of mapped reads fell in such regions. However, we noted that such percentage is significantly smaller than observed using polyA$^+$ enrichment protocols.

The gene expression values of already annotated genes were measured and expressed as reads per kilobase of transcript (or gene model) per million mapped reads (RPKM) [55]. Using a threshold of 0.1 RPKM, we detected a total of 17474 and 16800 RefSeq genes for DS and euploid EPCs respectively with at least one mapped read, and 13144 RefSeq genes with evidence of active transcription common for both trisomic and euploid EPCs.

In particular, due to our interest in investigating gene expression in the context of DS, we also focused on HSA21 genes. Hence, on a total of 260 RefSeq annotated HSA21 genes, we detected 148 and 141 genes expressed at levels below the threshold for DS and euploid EPCs samples, respectively.

All RefSeq genes, whose expression was detected within the experiment, were further classified according to RPKM values in 5 categories of expression: 1) very low, 2) low, 3) intermediate, 4) high and 5) very high (Figure 2; see "Materials and Methods"). This categorization revealed us, for both trisomic and euploid samples, a strong enrichment of snoRNAs in the highest RPKM categories (these RNAs were about 15% of total genes in category 4, and about 90% in category 5), clearly showing these molecules are below mRNAs – and if we exclude rRNAs - the second RNA group for abundance, and they also represent the more expressed RNA fraction in rRNA-depleted WT experiment.

To visualize in a user-friendly way the gene expression data derived from reads mapping, we prepared genome-wide, strand-specific, nucleotide-resolution files for each library corresponding to the trisomic and euploid states. In particular, these files contain information about reads mapping to the entire human genome, to splice junctions and RPKM categories for each analyzed RefSeq gene (see File S1). These resources represent a very powerful tool for genetics and genomics studies as they allow to easily investigate the entire landscape of gene expression alongside public genome annotations within UCSC Genome Browser [62] as "custom tracks" (Supplementary files available upon request).

Evidence and quantification of intronic and intergenic transcription

An intriguing finding of this study was the observation that, in both DS and euploid libraries, about 50% of all mapped reads occurred outside the annotated *loci*, outside the furthest 5′ and 3′ exons of already known genes, strongly indicating that many RefSeq genes may require extension or revision. This finding also suggests that this relevant extent of extra-genic transcription may possibly account for some of the pathological features observed in Down syndrome, as well as it is likely to occur for other human inherited disorders.

Thus, to address the extent of intronic and intergenic transcription, reads mapping to hg19 in non-RefSeq regions were divided into three categories: 1) intronic (inR) and 2) intergenic (igR) regions, and 3) chr M.

In particular, in the trisomic sample, about 8.7 M of sequenced reads mapped to inRs, 5.9 M into igRs and 2.0 M to chrM, for a total of 16.6 M of reads mapped to non-RefSeq regions. For the euploid sample, about 7.3 M of reads mapped to inRs, 5.6 M into igRs and 1.4 M to chrM for a total of 14.3 M of reads mapped to non-RefSeq regions (Figure S4).

To identify yet unannotated transcribed regions, potentially representing novel disease-specific expressed regions, and to better elucidate the still uncharacterized landscape of gene expression in trisomic EPCs compared to euploid cells, reads were further filtered with combined annotations from UCSC "known genes" and Ensembl databases (File S1) [63,64]. We found that in DS sample about 4.6 M of reads (of which 2 M from chr M and 2.6 M from both intergenic and intronic) were supporting either UCSC or Ensembl annotation, whilst more interestingly 12 M of reads were still mapped to unannotated regions. In the euploid sample, about 3.9 M (of which 1.4 M from chr M and 2.5 M from both intergenic and intronic) supported either the annotations, whilst 10.4 M of reads still mapped to unannotated regions. We also observed that most UCSC and Ensembl annotations covered about 98% of the reads mapping on chr M, about 30% of intergenic and about 10% of intronic regions, for both samples.

Finally, the reads mapping to yet unannotated regions, from both DS and euploid samples were pooled together and used to predict candidate novel intronic and intergenic transcriptionally active regions (inTARs and igTARs, respectively) - possibly

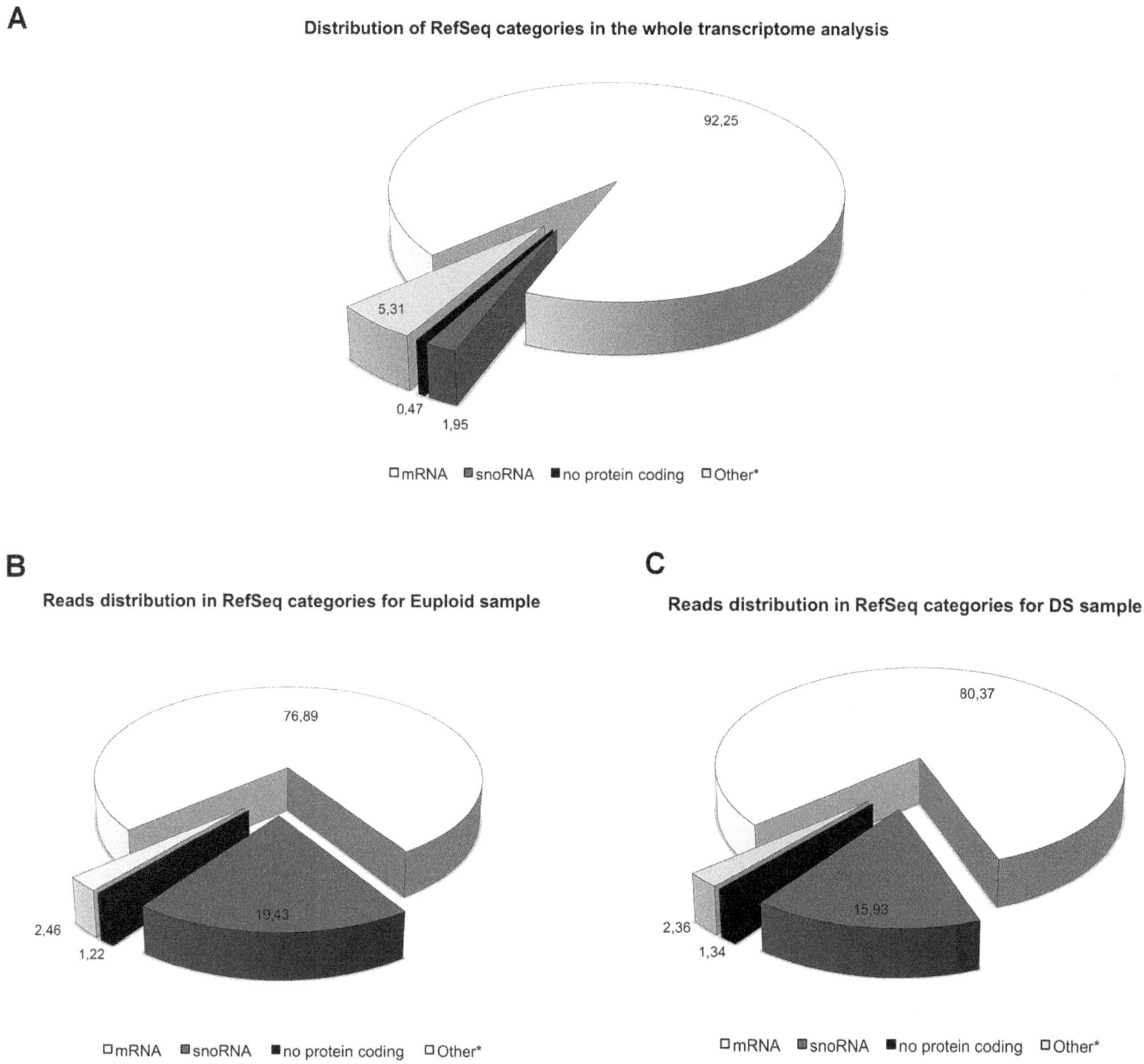

Figure 1. RefSeq categories and reads distribution. Distribution of the abundance of the RefSeq categories (HGNC) in the observed actively transcribed loci of the two states (A); Distribution of the UARs across the distinct RefSeq categories. DS (B) and euploid (C). The "other" category, marked with asterisk, include less represented RNAs (pseudogenes, microRNA, snRNA, scRNA, antisense, vault and RNAse) according to HGNC. Percentages are shown in the pie chart.

representing new genes - or to revise previously annotated gene models (definitions are given in File S1).

To this purpose, we noticed that 4.2 M of mapped reads in DS and 3.9 M in euploid - assigned to intergenic unannotated regions - spanned across 4.9×10^{9} bp (considering both strands), and 7.8 M of mapped reads in DS and 6.5 M in euploid - assigned to unannotated intronic regions - spanned across 1×10^{9} bp (considering both strands). The size of, such huge, unannotated regions do not allow to easily identify the presence of significant signal (i.e density of reads mapping together) from the background noise, resembling the search of a needle in a haystack. Therefore, *ad hoc* refinement procedure with $\mathbf{W}=500$ and $\mathbf{T}=30$ (described in "Refinement of non-RefSeq loci") was used to automatically extract reads' dense transcriptionally active regions in a computationally fast way. The refinement procedure, applied on the pooled samples, allowed us to define 21804 igTARs (spanning across about 17 Mb) in which for both samples mapped about 1.8 M of sequenced reads (about 45% of unannotated intergenic reads). In a similar way, we defined 99030 inTARs (spanning across about 80 Mb) in which were mapped about 4.1 M and 3.7 M of reads for DS and euploid, respectively (more than 55% of unannotated intronic reads for both samples). All regions were annotated in a BED format and the expression levels of both inTARs and igTARs were then measured for each sample.

Since not yet annotated TARs may be relevant for DS pathogenesis, we focused on the quantitative evaluation of these regions. The analysis revealed that 21648 igTARS and 98156 inTARs were transcriptionally active in DS progenitor cells, whereas 21608 igTARS and 97709 inTARs were active in the euploid state. Of these, 21460 igTARs were regions of active

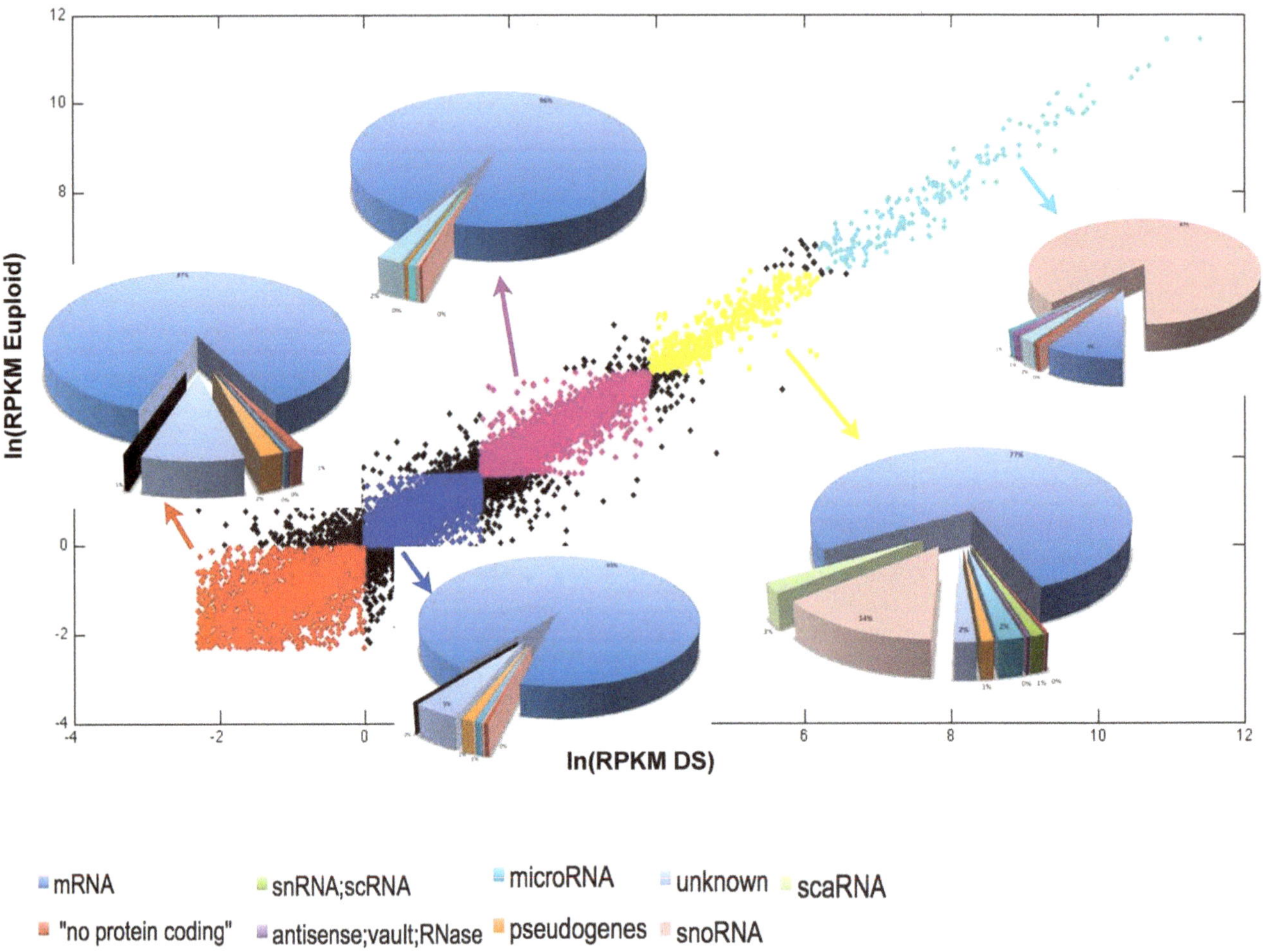

Figure 2. Comparison of RPKM content for RefSeq genes. Distribution of RefSeq categories (according to HGNC) within each class of RPKM.

transcription common to both states, whilst 187 and 148 were respectively DS and euploid specific. Similarly, we identified 96864 inTARs common to both samples, with 1092 and 745 regions DS and euploid specific, respectively.

A random selection of a small subset of newly identified TARs underwent manual curation for further analysis. Particularly, we noted that many highly expressed unannotated regions felt in large repeats family (RepeatMasker based on RepBase library), comprising short - which include *Alu* family - and long interspersed nuclear elements (SINE and LINE), spanning overall the human genome, and also RNA repeats (such as SSU-rRNA family). However, an accurate estimate of the expression within such regions is strongly biased in both samples due to the multiple localization of these regions alongside the human genome, and thus further focused studies are needed in order to better address the extent of expression of such repeats families.

In addition, we also scanned a subset of inTARs and igTARs for the presence of putative open reading frames (ORFs). The analysis revealed that a high fraction of these newly identified TARs, both intronic and intergenic contain ORFs longest than 200 bp. In particular, some inTARs conserved the correct frame of the gene they are located within, suggesting these are likely to represent alternative exons. On the other hand, it has been observed that a subset of analyzed igTARs (150–250 bp in length) did not show any ORF, suggesting they may represent novel small and long non-coding RNAs.

However, these preliminary findings strongly suggest these newly identified regions of active transcription require both further experimental validations - and also computational efforts - in order to address in a genome-wide fashion whether they represent novel genes - and/or exons of already known genes- and novel short (or long) intergenic transcripts, and whether the differential expression of these expressed extragenic regions may be linked at some extent to observed DS phenotypes.

Independently, we also studied the transcriptional activity in close proximity to 3′ and 5′ UTRs of RefSeq loci, in order to understand whether these regions could possibly represent extensions of already annotated genes. Particularly, we focused on expressed regions using a user-defined window 150 bp in length, located both upstream 5′ UTRs and downstream 3′ UTRs. We found 3600 and 2948 candidate genes showing a clear evidence of an extended 3′ UTR in DS and euploid samples, respectively (example in Figure 3A). Of these, 1868 extended regions were common to both samples, giving a strongest evidence for the refinement of untranslated regions of these RefSeq loci. We believe that state-specific extended UTRs (specifically those expressed in DS progenitor cells) may be important for gene expression regulation and/or for mRNA

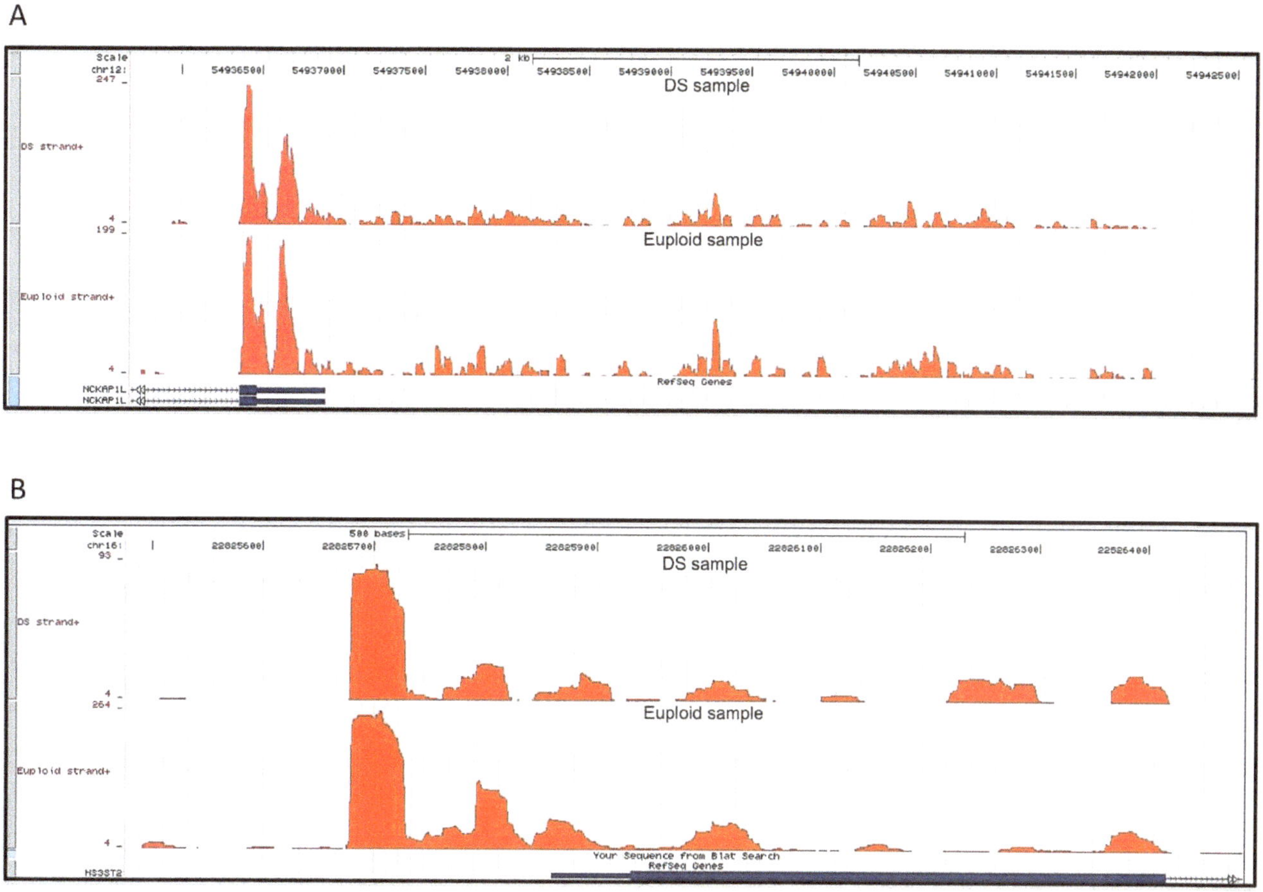

Figure 3. Evidence of 3′ and 5′ UTRs gene extensions. Illustration of 3′ (A) and 5′ (B) extended UTRs that are present in both samples.

stability and processing, possibly accounting for some DS pathological features. More interestingly, we observed that most of newly-defined or extended 3′UTRs contain putative novel miRNA binding sites (data not shown), characteristic of 3′UTRs of annotated transcripts, suggesting these regions may potentially contribute to microRNA-mediated regulation of these transcripts. This finding is crucial for understanding putative novel mechanisms of regulation for genes already known to be involved in DS pathogenesis, and may also be helpful to identify novel candidates in the trisomy 21.

Finally, for 5′ UTRs we found a lower number of candidate genes (1491 and 1280 for DS and euploid, respectively) possibly needing annotation revision, which indicates that current annotations are more biased toward the 3′ UTRs of expressed transcripts (example in Figure 3B).

Survey on the alternative splicing

Massive-scale RNA sequencing data, other than identifying differential expression of genes in a disease, are useful to human genetics in what they can be used to investigate alternative splicing, also discovering novel splice isoforms for crucial genes. For instance, identifying sequence reads that span exon-exon junctions could help to define exon usage and alternative splicing (although reconstructing entire transcripts will be challenging, particularly with short reads and it will require a very high coverage and the use of paired-end reads to achieve a good accuracy).

However, to illustrate the great potential of these data for studying both canonical and alternative splicing in the context of Down syndrome, we performed a preliminary analysis to identify reads that span exon-exon junctions. We detected a total of 92939 splice junctions in DS sample and 80200 in euploid; of these, 64115 and 56621 (DS and euploid, respectively) mapped with at least 3 sequenced reads, whilst 48604 and 43308 (DS and euploid, respectively) mapped with at least 5 sequenced reads (Table S2).

In addition, as expected for large-scale RNA-Seq data, we found evidence of several alternative splicing events (ASEs) in known RefSeq genes with a user-defined threshold of 3 and 5 mapped reads. To achieve a highest reliability of these data, we considered a user-defined threshold of at least 5 mapped reads as informative for ASEs (Figure S5). By using this approach, we found that 1621 splice junctions in DS and 1783 in euploid were representative of ASEs (i.e either multiple donor or multiple acceptor junctions; details in "Materials and Methods").

In order to identify ASEs specific of DS progenitor cells, avoiding a "threshold-dependent" exclusion of any given junction (i.e of junctions with a number of mapped reads slightly below the chosen threshold), we marked as "sample-specific" only junctions without any mapping in the euploid state (and *viceversa*). By using this procedure, we found that about 18% of all ASEs detected in each sample were sample specific. Indeed, we identified 294 DS-specific and 323 euploid-specific alternative splice events (Figure S5 and Table S2). Of these, 135 junctions for DS and 229 for euploid (45.9% and 70.9% of total state-specific ASEs, respectively) were completely unannotated (i.e. non-RefSeq, -UCSC, or -Ensembl), thus representing good candidates for further analyses aimed to fully characterize novel disease-specific isoforms within DS isolated EPCs. Examples of genes with evidence of sample specific splicing are depicted in Figure 4.

Interestingly, this analysis showed evidence of a DS-specific splice junction (transcript variant NM_130436.2; proteinID Q13627-2) in a crucial HSA21 gene involved in DS pathogenesis, namely *DYRK1A* [65]. For all mentioned cases, sequence reads supporting evidence of alternative splicing will be helpful for further detailed analyses aimed to resolve, if any, possible exon-annotation conflicts.

In the context of the syndrome, we also observed that some interesting genes, involved in the immune response and angiogenesis pathways - and previously shown to be deregulated in DS EPCs [12] - had evidence of yet unannotated sample-specific isoforms. Further analyses are needed to address whether these isoforms may play a role in DS pathogenesis.

The transcriptome complexity of DS beyond the rRNA

NGS has revealed the evidence of previously not well, characterized - or completely uncharacterized - RNA molecules, emerging as crucial regulators of many biological processes and for their potential link to human diseases. Small RNAs, including miRNAs, regulators of gene expression involved in various cellular processes, as well as small nucleolar RNAs (snoRNAs) - central to ribosome maturation and guides for site-specific modification of rRNAs - are acquiring greater attention for their involvement in human inherited disorders [35,36]. In addition, long as well as short non coding RNAs, whose functional significance is still debated, and other classes of coding and non coding RNAs have been also described at transcriptional start sites, splice sites or in large intergenic regions [66–68].

In our experiment, not limited to the annotated polyA$^+$ mRNA fraction, we detected and quantified active transcription in both human trisomic and euploid isolated EPCs from snoRNAs, small nuclear RNA (snRNA), miRNAs and other non-coding RNA, including lincRNAs.

In particular, we focused on UARs mapping to annotated snoRNAs, for which, as above described for the RefSeq genes, we measured gene expression as RPKM. Evidence of active transcription from 289 snoRNA (171 C/D box snoRNAs alias SNORD genes, 95 H/ACA box snoRNAs alias SNORA genes and 23 Cajal body-specific scaRNAs) was observed for DS cells, and the expression of 289 snoRNAs (173 C/D box, 93 H/ACA box and 23 Cajal body-specific scaRNAs) was detected in the euploid state. For both analysed samples, we observed a significantly strong increase (about 170-fold) in mean RPKM values for this class of RNAs compared to ploy-A$^+$ transcripts (Figure 2).

In addition, we independently selected snoRNA belonging to "Very high" and "High" RPKM categories, which represent almost the totality of snoRNAs, and observed that the vast majority of these localize within the introns of RefSeq genes (namely host genes). Then, we analyzed the expression level, in terms of RPKM, of their related host genes. Table S3 shows the occurrence of each RPKM category of the host genes for two classes of snoRNAs, both in DS and euploid samples. We noted that 221 highly-expressed snoRNAs common to both states (76% of the total), preferentially - if not exclusively - mapped within intronic regions of highly-expressed genes (Figure 5A). More interestingly, none of highly-expressed snoRNA localized within

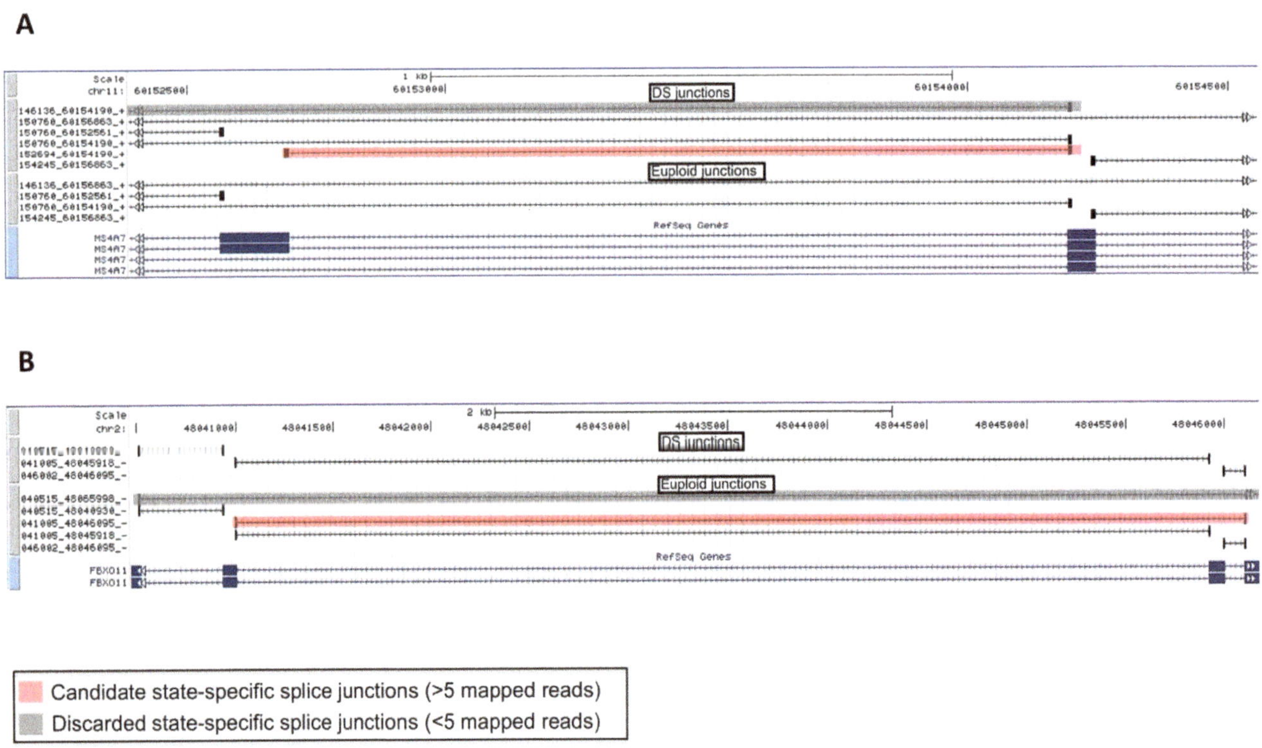

Figure 4. State-specific alternative splicing. Example of sample-specific alternative splicing events with T1 = 5. Reliable junctions are highlighted in light red for both cases (DS in panel A and euploid in panel B). Junctions highlighted in light grey are below the threshold. State-specific junctions are those not showing any hit in the other sample.

A

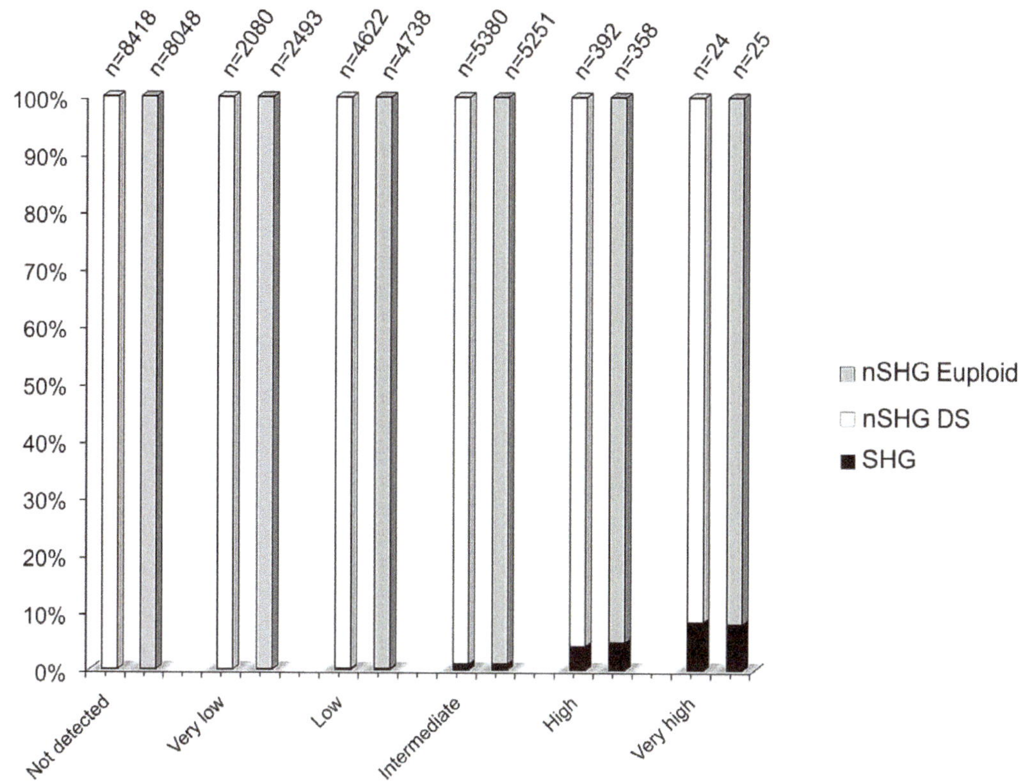
n=8418
n=8048
n=2080
n=2493
n=4622
n=4738
n=5380
n=5251
n=392
n=358
n=24
n=25
100%
90%
80%
70%
60%
50%
40%
30%
20%
10%
0%
Not detected
Very low
Low
Intermediate
High
Very high
nSHG Euploid
nSHG DS
SHG

B

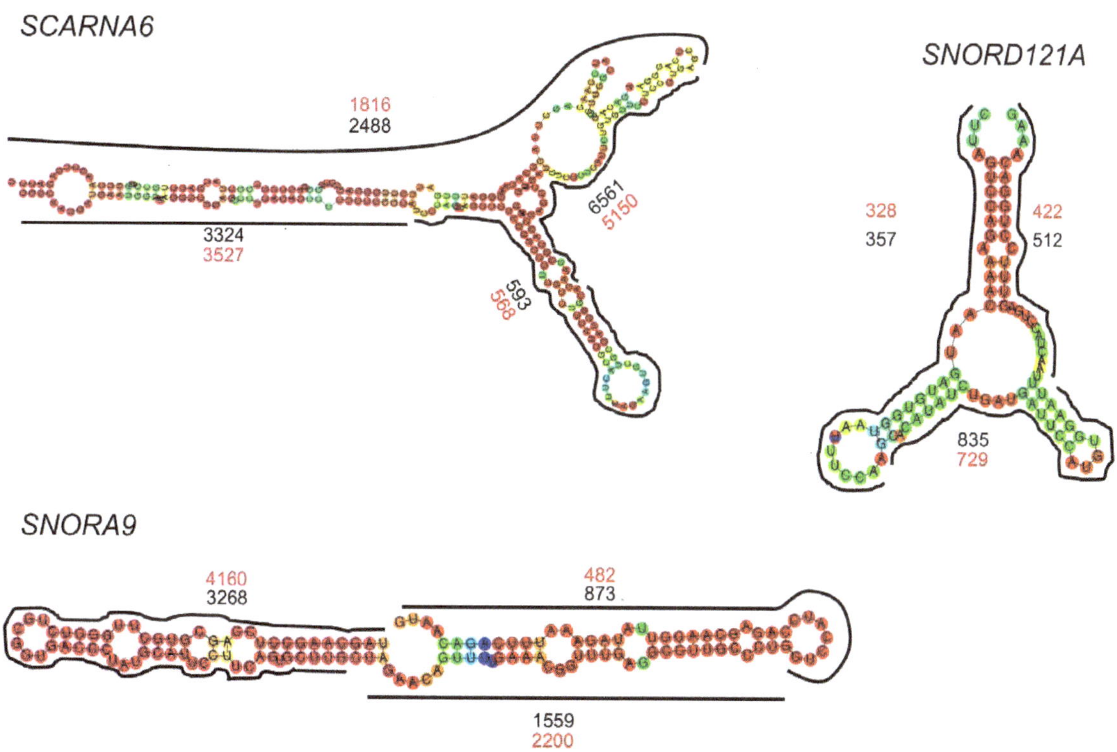
SCARNA6
1816
2488
3324
3527
6561
5150
593
568
SNORD121A
328
357
422
512
835
729
SNORA9
4160
3268
482
873
1559
2200

Figure 5. snoRNAs expression and mapping block patterns. (A) illustrates the percentage of snoRNAs host genes (SHG) vs non host genes (nSHG) within each RPKM category for both DS and euploid samples. (B) is a schematic representation of maximum coverage of few examples of snoRNAs, showing a characteristic mapping block pattern. Black and red numbers refer to DS and euploid maximum coverage, respectively.

introns or in close proximity of RefSeq genes with low or without any evidence of expression (Table S3), suggesting this class of small RNAs is preferentially located within euchromatic regions of very active transcription.

Moreover, since it has been recently shown that snoRNAs can be processed into snoRNA-derived RNAs (sdRNAs) [67], we analysed our WT data to address these specific features. Hence, we interestingly observed, as recently shown by Langenberger and colleagues [69], a correlation between reads' mapping pattern and snoRNAs processing steps, and possibly with their structural - and thus functional - properties (Figure 5B). As there depicted, snoRNAs clearly show specific block patterns with a characteristic reads coverage distribution. The particular enrichment of reads mapping to specific snoRNA sites is very likely to be correlated to its processing steps. A similar correlation with the secondary structure processing of non coding RNAs, even though at a lower extent due to RNA extraction protocol and library construction, was also observed for miRNAs (data not shown). However, these findings highlight the great potential of RNA-Seq data, deriving from ribosomal RNA-depleted samples rather than polyA$^+$ enrichment procedure, for a better functional classification and the identification of novel non-coding RNAs.

Furthermore, a significant differential expression (DE) of snoRNAs in human trisomic EPCs (compared to euploid) was also observed (Table S4). In particular, 46 C/D box snoRNAs (3 up- and 43 down-regulated), 31 H/ACA box (9 up- and 22 down-regulated) and 9 Cajal body-specific scaRNAs (2 up- and 7 down-regulated) were differentially expressed in DS compared to euploid cells. Interestingly, we noted that the gene with the highest expression of HSA21 was a member of H/ACA box, *SNORA80*, which showed a strong evidence of DE in the trisomic cells.

Similarly, the expression of annotated RefSeq miRNA encoding genes was also measured. Expression from about 180 of them was detected, although about 20% of them had a small number of mapped reads in both samples. A significant DE in DS isolated progenitors compared to euploid, was also observed for a small subset of them (15 miRNA with a significant number of mapped reads; data not shown).

Finally, we also measured the expression from annotated lincRNAs (*Homo sapiens* GRCh37, Ensembl 58). Since the average length of these regions was significantly higher than RefSeq genes, on average RPKM values were smaller. However, a significant expression was detected for 1335 and 1269 regions for DS and euploid sample respectively, even though a subset of them completely or partially overlapped with RefSeq genes or repeated regions. After removing them from further analyses, we observed a significant differential expression in the trisomic state for 45 lincRNAs (Figure S6).

Differentially expressed genes in human trisomy 21

Given the quantitative nature of our analysis, we used UARs and reads mapping to junction library to detect DE genes between the trisomic and euploid states.

In particular, we observed 1629 DE genes marked as "good" (about 12% of total detected genes in both samples), 158 as "strong", 54 "acceptable", whilst a large fraction (1827 genes) showed weak evidence of DE in the trisomic state since it did not pass the 1.5 fold-change cut-off. We selected only DE genes marked "strong" and "good" for further analyses (definitions are given in "Materials and Methods").

Of these 1787 genes showing evidence of differential expression between samples, 956 were up-regulated and 831 down-regulated in DS endothelial progenitors (Figure 6A). In contrast, about 75% of RefSeq annotated genes did not show any evidence of DE in the syndrome (Figure 6B). We also observed that 55 HSA21 genes - out of the 132 expressed in both DS and euploid cells - were DE in the trisomic state and, more interestingly, most of them (50 genes out of 55 HSA21 genes differentially expressed in DS) were up-regulated. Quantitative Real-Time PCR was used to validate the expression values in 24 actively transcribed *loci* per sample, confirming the evidence of DE also for genes marked as "weak" or "no change" (Figure S7 and Table S5).

The list of DE genes was then analyzed by using PANTHER (Protein ANalysis THrough Evolutionary Relationships) Classification System [70] in order to establish the occurrence of more representative deregulated pathways in the syndrome. The analysis revealed a particular enrichment for inflammation, angiogenesis, integrin and Wnt signaling pathways (Figure 7A). In addition, to highlight the most relevant biological processes possibly contributing to DS phenotypes previously observed in EPCs [12], we used a newly developed application for Gene Ontology (GO) analysis on RNA-seq data, namely GO-Seq [71]. By using the selection of genes DE within DS progenitor cells, we observed a particular enrichment for GO terms related to immune and inflammatory responses, cell adhesion and chemokine/ cytokine receptor activities (Figure 7B). These GO terms are in agreement with the independent analysis of enriched gene pathways performed with PANTHER. Taken together these findings, which confirm independent results deriving from a genome-wide microarray analysis on EPCs isolated from young DS [12], strongly suggest that these biological processes, and the related genes, require much attention to further address their involvement in DS vascular and immune-related phenotypes.

Furthermore, in order to understand whether the newly identified igTARs and inTARs were differentially expressed within the syndrome, a similar approach was also used. In particular, we found that 44, out of the total 21804 igTARs identified in DS cells, were classified as strong DE regions, 1792 showed good evidence of DE, and 130 were classified as acceptable DE. For what concerns the inTARs, among the 99030 defined regions, we found 48 of them with strong evidences of DE in DS sample, 3173 with good and 720 defined as acceptable evidence of DE. In both cases, we noticed that the observed fold changes were sufficiently large, hence the threshold effect was negligible. Results are shown in Figure S8. These results suggest a possible involvement of such expressed regions in the pathogenesis of this syndrome, indicating that some yet unknown genetic determinants may be responsible of, or contribute to, the wide spectrum of DS pathological phenotypes.

Discussion

RNA-Seq experiments revealed that the transcriptional landscape in higher eukaryotes is much more complex than previously anticipated, with a high proportion of transcripts originating from intergenic regions, referred to as "dark matter" [72,73], thought to be transcriptionally silent or antisense to genes [33]. Previously

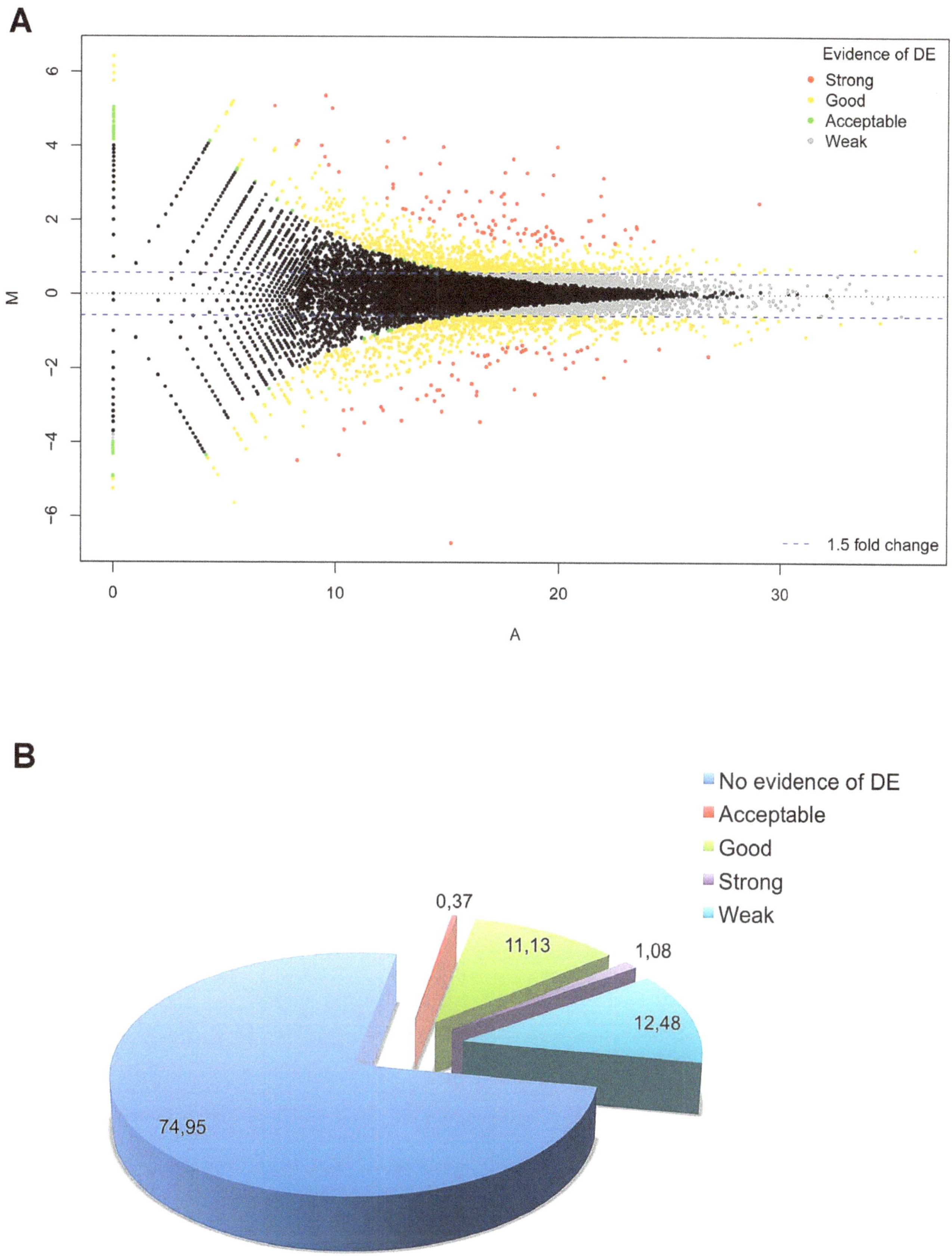

Figure 6. Differentially expressed RefSeq genes in human trisomy 21. (A) Standard MA-plot of the normalized global observed counts per each RefSeq gene. (B) shows the percentage of RefSeq genes classified as strong, good, acceptable evidence of DE with respect to those not showing any statistical evidence.

A

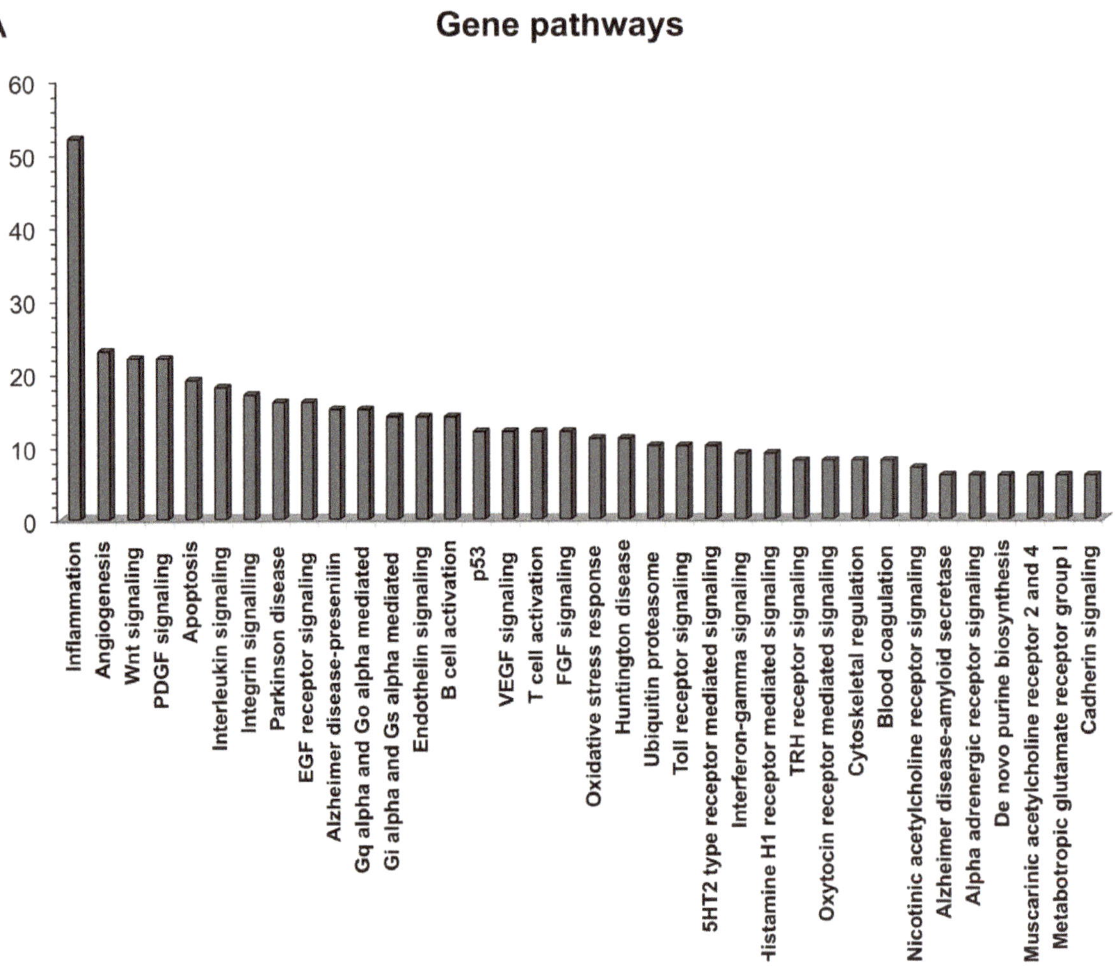
Gene pathways
60
50
40
30
20
10
0
Inflammation
Angiogenesis
Wnt signaling
PDGF signaling
Apoptosis
Interleukin signaling
Integrin signalling
Parkinson disease
EGF receptor signaling
Alzheimer disease-presenilin
Gq alpha and Go alpha mediated
Gi alpha and Gs alpha mediated
Endothelin signaling
B cell activation
p53
VEGF signaling
T cell activation
FGF signaling
Oxidative stress response
Huntington disease
Ubiquitin proteasome
Toll receptor signaling
5HT2 type receptor mediated signaling
Interferon-gamma signaling
istamine H1 receptor mediated signaling
TRH receptor signaling
Oxytocin receptor mediated signaling
Cytoskeletal regulation
Blood coagulation
Nicotinic acetylcholine receptor signaling
Alzheimer disease-amyloid secretase
Alpha adrenergic receptor signaling
De novo purine biosynthesis
Muscarinic acetylcholine receptor 2 and 4
Metabotropic glutamate receptor group I
Cadherin signaling

B

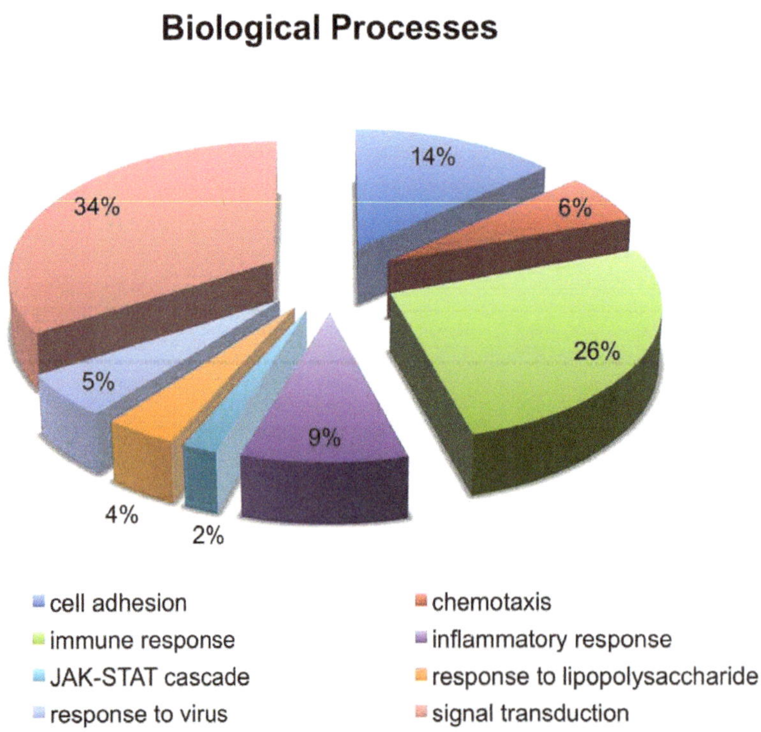
Biological Processes
14%
6%
26%
9%
2%
4%
5%
34%
cell adhesion
chemotaxis
immune response
inflammatory response
JAK-STAT cascade
response to lipopolysaccharide
response to virus
signal transduction

Figure 7. Pathway of differentially expressed RefSeq genes in DS sample. Bar graph representation of differentially expressed genes in DS vs euploid samples. (A) More enriched gene pathways are represented. The number of total DE RefSeq genes is also depicted. (B) Pie chart showing the percentages of representative GO terms (biological processes) enriched in DE genes in the DS sample compared to euploid.

published transcriptome sequencing data based on the polyA$^+$ enrichment started to shed light on the transcriptional complexity in humans and other organisms [27–31]. Nonetheless, the information revealed by using this approach could only detect a fraction of the total RNA content, representing the tip of the iceberg. In contrast, in our study we show the clear advantage of the whole trasncriptome analysis of rRNA-depleted samples for studying Down syndrome. Hence, our approach offers the possibility to detect previously not well-characterised - or completely uncharacterized - non-coding RNA, such as snoRNAs, miRNAs and others, emerging as novel candidates for their possible contribution to the pathogenesis of different human disorders [34–36]. Coupling the ribodepletion procedure of samples followed by massive-scale RNA sequencing provides new intriguing opportunities to better understand the underlying molecular bases of complex phenotypes, such as herein described for Down syndrome.

In contrast, in the last years, most of studies mainly focused on hybridization- and tag-based expression profiling on *post-mortem* DS tissues and fetuses, with only few of them considering adult whole blood samples as a good source of RNA to address these aspects [37–39]. Since angiogenesis' suppression, endothelial dysfunction and infection recurrence are hallmarks of DS, and several studies suggest the use of endothelial progenitors - previously shown to be impaired in DS [12] - in the clinical setting [43–47], these cells represent an optimal source for studying blood-related DS pathological features. Therefore, the possibility to investigate in a genome-wide scale and easy-accessible non-invasive manner - early gene regulatory mechanisms responsible of cardiovascular disease, cancer and immune disorders in DS, would be of great clinical interest. Hence, our study was accurately designed to investigate these issues.

The analysis of the whole transcriptome of DS-isolated EPCs allowed us to detect differential expression - compared to the euploid sample - of even low expressed genes in immune and inflammatory pathways, crucial for DS pathogenesis, showing the great potential of RNA-Seq to detect even subtle changes in gene expression. Clearly, we are aware that we cannot conclusively attribute to trisomy 21 all the changes in transcript levels found within this single case-control study since RNA-Seq decreases the experimental noise, but cannot reduce the individual variability. In order to separate the confounding effect due to the individual variability from the effect related to DS condition, a larger number of biological replicates - for each condition - should be considered. However, in this case, most of gene expression changes identified in the present work confirmed other data derived from previous independent studies performed on the same specific cell type in more DS and euploid samples [12].

At the same time we also disclosed novel regions of active transcription falling outside annotated *loci*, with strong evidence of DE within DS progenitor cells. In addition, our work revealed a wide *spectrum* of not yet well-characterized non-coding RNAs (particularly snoRNAs) with evidence of differential expression, some of them localized on HSA21 and shown to be over-expressed in DS cells, possibly accounting for some of the observed angiogenesis- and immune-related DS phenotypes.

Moreover, our approach allowed us to identify novel DS-specific splicing isoforms for a large subset of genes, even belonging to crucial pathways involved in DS pathogenesis (i.e. *DYRK1A*) [65]. Alternative splicing is currently known to generate either novel transcripts – possibly encoding novel domains – or to have regulatory roles through balancing levels of those mRNAs encoding functional proteins [74] and, very recently, it has been highlighted the power of RNA-Seq in detecting splicing differences in brain regions of individuals affected by Alzheimer's disease [75].

In addition, low-expressed transcripts, subtle changes in the expression of both known and, more interestingly, yet unannotated transcripts, were also investigated. It should be noted that a fundamental aspect of gene expression regulation, emerging as a crucial issue for inherited disorders and cancer in humans, is the identification of *cis*- and *trans*-acting regulatory regions within 5′ and 3′ UTRs of genes. To this aim, the present study shows the great potential of RNA-seq towards the identification of novel putative extended UTRs for already known genes, possibly representing novel miRNA targets or regulatory sites for gene transcription, and to our knowledge this is the first paper describing the complete transcriptome of HSA21 trisomic endothelial progenitor cells.

On the other hand, it is clear that the high extent of complexity, not completely detected by commonly used approaches, opens several new challenges either from computational and experimental point of view, not easily solvable within a single study. For instance, the much higher level of mapping disclosed, and then measured, into unannotated TARs, requires suitable procedures to build appropriate novel gene models. Further studies will be then required to combine information from annotated genes, extended 3′ and 5′ - and exon boundaries - with those arising from igTARs and inTARs. A possible way to cope with this problem could be to build-up putative gene models and assess them by using data-driven library of junctions and iteratively repeat the mapping in a similar way as proposed by TopHat [76]. Another challenge to face is the reconstruction, and thus the further quantification, of multiple isoforms of a transcript, including those arising unannotated TARs or coming from revised gene models, in a statistical rigorous way.

Clearly, as occurs for any data-driven procedure, such approaches are likely to require very high coverage, a large number of samples and the integration with different type of biological information and data in order to be robust.

In conclusion, although with the limitation for the number of analyzed samples, we have shown the great potential of performing whole transcriptome RNA sequencing using ribosomal-depleted samples from a technical, technological and bioinformatics point of view. We believe the above-described procedures may represent a useful guideline even for larger, and more statistically significant, case-control studies based on RNA-Seq.

Since transcriptome profiling represents a powerful tool for the functional analysis of EPCs in health and disease [77], coupling this innovative technological approach, as shown herein within the context of Down syndrome, to the easy availability of circulating progenitor cells from blood samples, render this kind of analysis very feasible for large-scale studies of transcriptome in both physiological and pathological states.

Materials and Methods

Total RNA isolation and ribodepletion

Cells were isolated as described in [7] from peripheral blood samples of DS and euploid donors recruited at the Second

University of Naples, and an approval statement was obtained by the ethics' review board of the "Monaldi Hospital", Second University of Naples. Written informed consent was obtained from individuals involved in this study according to the principles expressed in the Declaration of Helsinki.

Briefly, total mononuclear cells were isolated by density gradient centrifugation of peripheral blood samples on Histopaque-1077 (Sigma). Cells were washed twice with PBS, plated on culture dishes pre-coated with gelatin and fibronectin and maintained in endothelial growth medium-2 (EGM2; Cell Systems). Cells were cultured at 37°C with 5% CO2 in a humidified atmosphere. After four days, non-adherent cells were removed and adherent cells were collected for RNA isolation.

Total RNA was isolated from endothelial progenitor cells as described [7]. Integrity and quantity of RNA was evaluated by Experion (Biorad), following the manufacturer's instructions. Ribosomal RNA depletion was performed on 10 µg of isolated total RNA by using magnetic beads (RiboMinus™ Eukaryote Kit for RNA-Seq, Invitrogen) according to the manufacturer's protocol (see for technical details File S1). 10 µg of total RNA were incubated at 72°C for 5 min to allow a complete denaturation for efficient hybridization to single-stranded eukaryote rRNA sequence-specific 5′-biotin labeled oligonucleotide probes (targeted against 5S, 5.8S, 18S and 28S human rRNAs) containing locked nucleic acids (LNA) at specific positions. Then, streptavidin-coated RiboMinus™ Magnetic Beads were used to capture rRNA-probes complexes to be further discarded form total RNA samples. The efficiency of rRNA depletion was evaluated on the Experion. Resulting RNA was successfully fragmented with RNase III and, after cleanup with RiboMinus™ Concentration Module (Invitrogen) according to the manufacturer's protocol, resulting fragmented samples were quantified on the Qubit Fluorometer (Invitrogen). The appropriate size distribution of fragmented RNA was finally evaluated on the Experion. The experimental procedure used in this work is illustrated in Figure S1.

Stand-oriented cDNA library preparation

100 ng of the fragmented RNA samples were hybridized and ligated to double stranded oligonucleotides adapter suited for the 5′ SOLiD System sequencing (details in File S1). Reverse transcription was performed using ArrayScript™ Reverse Transcriptase. Purified cDNA samples were denatured on 6% TBE-Urea gel, and size selection (150–250 bp) was performed. PCR amplification on gel slices was then performed using AmpliTaq® DNA Polymerase, and yield of purified PCR products was assessed on the Qubit Fluorometer and NanoDrop spectrophotometer (Invitrogen). Size distribution of cDNA libraries was evaluated on the Experion.

SOLiD sequencing

We drove 500 pg of each library onto 1-µm-diameter beads using emulsion PCR, according to the SOLiD™ Whole Transcriptome Analysis Kit (Applied Biosystems). Libraries were sequenced using the Applied Biosystems SOLiD sequencing, as 50-mers. We sequenced ~200,000,000 (100 M for each sample, euploid and DS) beads using 'sequencing by ligation' chemistry on a SOLiD sequencer version 3 (Applied Biosystems). Approximately 97% of beads deposited onto the slice generated good-quality sequence reads 50 nt in length (Figure S2 and Table S1).

SOLiD processed files have been submitted to the Gene Expression Omnibus (GEO; http://www.ncbi.nlm.nih.gov/geo/) repository (accession n. GSE27443).

Quantitative Real-Time for RNA-Seq validation

Quantitive Real-Time PCRs were performed on the same euploid and DS rRNA-depleted samples that underwent library construction and further sequencing on the SOLiD platform. Amplification reaction mix contained 1× SYBR Green PCR master mix (Applied Biosystems), 160 nM of each primer and about 50 ng of cDNA (RNA equivalent) as template. PCR conditions were 95°C for 10 min followed by 40 cycles of 95°C 30 sec, 60°C 30 sec and 72°C 30 sec. Melting curves were generated after amplification. Data were collected using the 7900HT Fast real time PCR system (Applied Biosystems); each assay for each of the 24 analysed genes (Figure S7) was performed in duplicate in both rRNA-depleted samples. Primers were designed using Oligo 4.0-s. The relative gene expression was calculated using the $2^{-\Delta\Delta Ct}$ method [78].

Mapping strategy and data visualization

The whole mapping strategy is illustrated in Figure S2 and consists in several steps. First, the total reads produced were filtered out accordingly to quality values, secondly, those reads that mapped to the adapters and to the ribosomal sequences were further removed, thirdly RNA-MATE software [59] version 1.1 was used to map the usable reads either to the genome and to a custom-designed library of exon-junction sequences, (see File S1).

RNA-MATE is an open source software specifically designed to map RNA-Seq data generated from the SOLiD system. It works cyclically. At each cycle it attempts to map usable reads first to the reference genome and subsequently to the junctions' library. At the end of each cycle, reads failed to map to the genome or to the junctions library were left-end trimmed using a pre-defined lengths schema.

RNA-MATE allows a user to control the number of mismatches tolerated for each cycle, however it does not incorporate the possibility of mapping gaps, reducing the possibility of locating reads with small indel. Moreover, it requires the pre-construction of a junctions library limiting the possibility of identifying de-novo junctions. However, the assessment and the correct interpretation of mapping strategies that are junctions model free has not been completely elucidated and good performance are obtained only at the price of a much higher coverage. Moreover, tail-end trimming the reads at each cycle allows either to cope with the behaviour of the quality values (that are usually worst in last bases of the reads) and to partially handle the presence of novel splicing junctions allowing to map the right side of the read.

By default, RNA-MATE allows to directly assign multiple reads with a single "best hit" to that specific position. In our pipeline, all remaining multiple reads (with at most 10 mapping positions) underwent the rescue procedure with default parameters.

At the end of the alignment procedure three types of reads were identified: UARs, MRs and unmapped reads (see File S1 for definitions).

Annotation and quantification of RefSeq transcriptional events

Given the results of the alignment, first we performed a within sample analysis aimed to extract and characterize the activity of both states independently, then we provided a cross-comparison between trisomic and euploid cells aimed to detect differences in term of gene expression.

In order to provide a quantitative estimate of gene expressions in both trisomic and euploid cells, we considered genes in the ReqSeq annotation. However we suitably revised the annotation to remove ambiguities due to overlapping genes, see File S1 for technical details. The annotation contains 215952 annotated elements (i.e., exons or part of them) in a BED format corresponding to 21122 uniquely identified (and non redundant) RefSeq genes or group/family of RefSeq genes.

For each gene in the RefSeq annotation a preliminary estimate of the global expression was obtained by computing the number of UARs starting in all the annotated elements (i.e., exons or part of exons) corresponding to the same gene. Then, the final expression value was corrected by adding to each specific *locus* the read counts derived from the splice junctions. Additionally, an exon by exon usage map and the corresponding reads counts was provided in order to facilitate isoforms identification.

To account for transcripts of different lengths when selecting active genes, the gene expression counts values of annotated loci were converted in RPKM [55]. For each sample, only loci with RMKM>0.1 were considered detected.

Expressed genes in both samples were further classified according to RPKM distributions in 5 categories: 1) very low expression, 2) low expression, 3) intermediate, 4) high and 5) very high expression (Figure 2 and details in File S1).

The analysis of RefSeq loci was also aimed to detect a particular enrichment in 3′ (or 5′) UTRs (see File S1).

Identification of alternative splicing events

We inferred the evidence of multiple isoforms within each annotated gene on the basis of the reads that mapped to the splicing junctions and we suggested the presence of novel isoforms from the type of junction mapped (i.e., junctions annotated in some database such that RefSeq, UCSC or Ensembl or novel combinatorial junctions). In particular, we considered as alternative splicing marks either the multiple donors or the multiple acceptor (or both) junctions (see File S1 for definition).

For the sake of simplicity to reduce the effect of the random matching, a junction was considered reliable if there were at least T1 reads mapped on it. Then the identification proceeded as follows. First, for each sample, we retrieved all the reliable junctions and, among them we selected those containing either multiple donors or multiple acceptors. Then, RefSeq genes containing such junctions were detected. Such genes constitute an initial list of candidates to the presence of multiple splicing isoforms. The lists can be further filtered using information arising from exon by exon map usage to remove mapping artefacts. Secondly, the two samples were cross-compared as follows: the spliced junctions common to both samples were identified then, for each sample, a list of candidate sample specific junctions was obtained. To remove the effect of the user specific threshold T1, each list was subsequently filtered, by removing those junctions that received any number of hits in the other sample.

Finally, since each junction was also classified as RefSeq junction, UCSC, Ensembl junction or as putative new junction accordingly to if it was annotated in the corresponding database or it was a results of a pure combinatorial process, we use such information to detect those genes containing putative new junctions that are candidate to show novel (unannotated) isoforms.

Refinement of non-RefSeq *loci*

Given the RefSeq annotation we defined and annotated on each strand on the genome igRs and inRs (File S1) to cover all the genome. The annotation was performed independently on each strand and regions were labelled, enumerated and described in a BED file. The regions were quantified in each sample to provide a measure of the overall mapping in non RefSeq regions. In order to quantify the strength of the signal in the truly unannotated regions, both igR and inR were filtered on the basis of the UCSC and Ensembl Annotation (see File S1).

Remaining regions were re-labelled and enumerated. The reads count was repeated on both samples. For comparative purposes and to assess the consistency of UCSC and Ensembl databases, the reads count was also performed on the UCSC and Ensembl Annotation filtered by the RefSeq annotation.

Subsequently, to more precisely determine novel active regions, each unannotated genomic region (either igR and inR) that showed presence of signal (i.e., mapped reads) underwent an ad-hoc refinement procedure. The refinement procedure is aimed to more precisely define the approximate location of the active regions within the unannotated regions (i.e., to identify igTARs and inTARs, where there is a concentration of reads, removing those regions or part of regions which showed sparse or no signal at all).

The refinement procedure was performed either on each samples independently - to determine sample specific annotations (data not shown) - and by pooling together the two samples in order to determine a set of unannotated active regions, igTARs and inTARs, on which trisomic and euploid cells can be compared. The reads count was finally repeated for each sample.

Statistical tests for differential expression

In order to detect DE between trisomic and euploid states, we first compared the two samples at RefSeq level, then we compared the previously identified un-annotated intergenics and intronic regions.

Statistical significance has been inferred from the total observed reads count in each locus combining together a bunch of tests, namely DEGseq [79], DESeq [80] and edgeR [81] for which R-packages are available under Bioconductor (www.bioconductor.org/packages/2.7). Such tests are based on slightly different assumptions that usually produce a different level of stringency - and sometime different results - when applied to small sample experiments. However, all of them are particularly suited for RNA-Seq data, hence they were independently applied to the dataset. For each locus we compute a p-value and its corresponding adjusted p-value or q-value to detect significant change in the expression (i.e., DE loci).

A cut-off of 0.1 was used for DESeq (that was found very conservative for small sample), while a cut off of 0.0001 was used for both edgeR and DEGseq (both of them resulted to be more permissive. Additionally, a threshold of 1.5 on the fold change between the normalized samples was imposed to filter out those genes whose significance appeared marginal (see File S1 for details).

Finally, the results of each selection were cross-compared either to compromise with their assumptions and to illustrate their impact in the final choice.

DE evidence was finally classified as "strong", "good", and "acceptable". All DE genes below the fold-change threshold, but found significant in at least one test, were classified as "weak" evidence. Figure 6A shows the scattered plot of the normalized log intensities vs the normalized log ratio between the two samples for RefSeq loci.

Supporting Information

Figure S1 Experimental procedure. Schematic representation of the whole RNA-Seq experiment. Depicted are: Total RNA isolation (1) and ribo-depletion (2). Ribo-depleted total RNA is fragmented (3), then ligated to specific adaptors (4) and retro-transcribed (5). The resulting cDNA is size selected by gel electrophoresis (6), and cDNAs are PCR amplified (7). Then size distribution is evaluated on Experion (8). Emulsion PCR is finally used for the clonal amplification of SOLs (9). Enriched beads are deposited onto glass slides (10), and sequenced by ligation on the SOLiD v3 platform.

Figure S2 Data analysis pipeline. Schematic representation of the data analysis workflow described in detail in "Materials and Methods".

Figure S3 Summary of mapping results. Distribution of the sequenced reads according to the mapping procedure. DS sample (A) and Euploid (B).

Figure S4 Distribution of the UARs in the human genome. Distribution of the UARs according to RefSeq genes, intronic intergenic regions and mitochondrial chromosome. DS sample (A) and Euploid (B).

Figure S5 Detection of alternative splicing events. Schematic representation of the computational analysis used to detect sample-specific ASEs both canonical and unannotated. Reliability of the junction was measured with T1 = 3 (A) and with T1 = 5 (B).

Figure S6 Differential expression of lincRNAs. Standard MA-plot of the normalized global observed counts per each lincRNA.

Figure S7 Quantitative Real-Time PCR validation. A random selection of "no change" (A) and weak DE (B) RefSeq genes between the analyzed samples confirmed by qRT-PCR. Relative expression levels for a selection of DE RefSeq genes in DS state (C).

Figure S8 Differential expression of igTARs and inTARs. Standard MA-plot of the normalized global observed counts per each identified igTAR (A) and inTAR (B). Venn diagrams showing the number of regions with evidence of DE according to each statistical method used (igTARs in panel C and inTARs in panel D).

Table S1 Mapping summary.

Table S2 Summary of mapping on the junctions.

Table S3 Distribution of RPKM expression level of snoRNA host genes.

Table S4 List of differentially expressed snoRNAs in human trisomy 21.

Table S5 Primer pairs used for quantitative RT-PCR.

File S1 Supporting Materials and Methods.

Acknowledgments

We thank the patients and individuals recruited as controls for their participation. We thank Drs. Fabio Raffaldi and Raimo Tanzi, Applied Biosystems by Life Technologies, for experimental help and Prof. Antonio Baldini for insightful discussions and comments on the manuscript.

Author Contributions

Conceived and designed the experiments: VC CA LD'A CN A. Ciccodicola. Performed the experiments: VC CA LD'A MM A. Casamassimi MR LS MAG MA RE LL AD SC. Analyzed the data: VC CA LD'A MM A. Casamassimi MAG MA RE BS RC PS TI PDB CN A. Ciccodicola. Contributed reagents/materials/analysis tools: CA MM LS MAG AD SC BS RC MP PS PDB CN A. Ciccodicola. Wrote the paper: VC CA LD'A MM A. Casamassimi SC CN A. Ciccodicola.

References

1. Okoniewski MJ, Miller CJ (2006) Hybridization interactions between probesets in short oligo microarrays lead to spurious correlations. BMC Bioinformatics 7: 276.
2. Napoli C, Lerman LO, Sica V, Lerman A, Tajana G, et al. (2003) Microarray analysis: a novel research tool for cardiovascular scientists and physicians. Heart 89: 597–604.
3. Harbers M, Carninci P (2005) Tag-based approaches for transcriptome research and genome annotation. Nat Methods 2: 495–502.
4. Velculescu VE, Zhang L, Vogelstein B, Kinzler KW (1995) Serial analysis of gene expression. Science 270: 484–487.
5. Brenner S, Johnson M, Bridgham J, Golda G, Lloyd DH, et al. (2000) Gene expression analysis by massively parallel signature sequencing (MPSS) on microbead arrays. Nat Biotechnol 18: 630–634.
6. Shiraki T, Kondo S, Katayama S, Waki K, Kasukawa T, et al. (2003) Cap analysis gene expression for high-throughput analysis of transcriptional starting point and identification of promoter usage. Proc Natl Acad Sci U S A 100: 15776–15781.
7. Salvatore P, Casamassimi A, Sommese L, Fiorito C, Ciccodicola A, et al. (2008) Detrimental effects of Bartonella henselae are counteracted by L-arginine and nitric oxide in human endothelial progenitor cells. Proc Natl Acad Sci U S A 105: 9427–9432.
8. Napoli C, de Nigris F, Welch JS, Calara FB, Stuart RO, et al. (2002) Maternal hypercholesterolemia during pregnancy promotes early atherogenesis in LDL receptor-deficient mice and alters aortic gene expression determined by microarray. Circulation 105: 1360–1367.
9. El-Meanawy MA, Schelling JR, Pozuelo F, Churpek MM, Ficker EK, et al. (2000) Use of serial analysis of gene expression to generate kidney expression libraries. Am J Physiol Renal Physiol 279: F383–392.
10. Yamashita T, Hashimoto S, Kaneko S, Nagai S, Toyoda N, et al. (2000) Comprehensive gene expression profile of a normal human liver. Biochem Biophys Res Commun 269: 110–116.
11. Pauws E, Moreno JC, Tijssen M, Baas F, de Vijlder JJ, et al. (2000) Serial analysis of gene expression as a tool to assess the human thyroid expression profile and to identify novel thyroidal genes. J Clin Endocrinol Metab 85: 1923–1927.
12. Costa V, Sommese L, Casamassimi A, Colicchio R, Angelini C, et al. (2010) Impairment of circulating endothelial progenitors in Down syndrome. BMC Med Genomics 3: 40.
13. Korbel JO, Tirosh-Wagner T, Urban AE, Chen XN, Kasowski M, et al. (2009) The genetic architecture of Down syndrome phenotypes revealed by high-resolution analysis of human segmental trisomies. Proc Natl Acad Sci U S A 106: 12031–12036.
14. Sommer CA, Pavarino-Bertelli EC, Goloni-Bertollo EM, Henrique-Silva F (2008) Identification of dysregulated genes in lymphocytes from children with Down syndrome. Genome 51: 19–29.
15. Malagó W, Jr., Sommer CA, Del Cistia Andrade C, Soares-Costa A, Abrao Possik P, et al. (2005) Gene expression profile of human Down syndrome leukocytes. Croat Med J 46: 647–656.
16. Brochier C, Gaillard MC, Diguet E, Caudy N, Dossat C, et al. (2008) Quantitative gene expression profiling of mouse brain regions reveals differential transcripts conserved in human and affected in disease models. Physiol Genomics 33: 170–179.
17. Grünblatt E, Zander N, Bartl J, Jie L, Monoranu CM, et al. (2007) Comparison analysis of gene expression patterns between sporadic Alzheimer's and Parkinson's disease. J Alzheimers Dis 12: 291–311.
18. Xu PT, Li YJ, Qin XJ, Kroner C, Green-Odlum A, et al. (2007) A SAGE study of apolipoprotein E3/3 E3/4 and E4/4 allele-speciWc gene expression in hippocampus in Alzheimer disease. Mol Cell Neurosci 36: 313–331.
19. Yang Z, Gagarin D, St Laurent G, 3rd, Hammell N, Toma I, et al. (2009) Cardiovascular inflammation and lesion cell apoptosis: a novel connection via the interferon-inducible immunoproteasome. Arterioscler Thromb Vasc Biol 29: 1213–1219.

20. Gnatenko DV, Dunn JJ, McCorkle SR, Weissmann D, Perrotta PL, et al. (2003) Transcript profiling of human platelets using microarray and serial analysis of gene expression. Blood 101: 2285–2293.
21. Esposito G, Imitola J, Lu J, De Filippis D, Scuderi C, et al. (2008) Genomic and functional profiling of human Down syndrome neural progenitors implicates S100B and aquaporin 4 in cell injury. Hum Mol Genet 17: 440–457.
22. Li CM, Guo M, Salas M, Schupf N, Silverman W, et al. (2006) Cell type-specific over-expression of chromosome 21 genes in fibroblasts and fetal hearts with trisomy 21. BMC Med Genet 7: 24.
23. Mao R, Zielke CL, Zielke HR, Pevsner J (2003) Global up-regulation of chromosome 21 gene expression in the developing Down syndrome brain. Genomics 81: 457–467.
24. FitzPatrick DR, Ramsay J, McGill NI, Shade M, Carothers AD, et al. (2002) Transcriptome analysis of human autosomal trisomy. Hum Mol Genet 11: 3249–3256.
25. ENCODE Project Consortium (2007) Identification and analysis of functional elements in 1% of the human genome by the ENCODE pilot project. Nature 447: 799–816.
26. Costa V, Angelini C, De Feis I, Ciccodicola A (2010) Uncovering the complexity of transcriptomes with RNA-Seq. J Biomed Biotechnol 2010: 853916.
27. Tang F, Barbacioru C, Wang Y, Nordman E, Lee C, et al. (2009) mRNA-Seq wholetranscriptome analysis of a single cell. Nat Methods 6: 377–382.
28. Hashimoto S, Qu W, Ahsan B, Ogoshi K, Sasaki A, et al. (2009) High-resolution analysis of the 5 -end transcriptome using a next generation DNA sequencer. PLoS ONE 4: e4108.
29. Sultan M, Schulz MH, Richard H, Magen A, Klingenhoff A, et al. (2008) A global view of gene activity and alternative splicing by deep sequencing of the human transcriptome. Science 321: 956–960.
30. Cloonan N, Forrest AR, Kolle G, Gardiner BB, Faulkner GJ, et al. (2008) Stem cell transcriptome profiling via massive-scale mRNA sequencing. Nat Methods 5: 613–619.
31. Marioni JC, Mason CE, Mane SM, Stephens M, Gilad Y (2008) RNA-Seq: an assessment of technical reproducibility and comparison with gene expression arrays. Genome Res 18: 1509–1517.
32. Lindberg J, Lundeberg J (2010) The plasticity of the mammalian transcriptome. Genomics 95: 1–6.
33. Jacquier A (2009) The complex eukaryotic transcriptome: unexpected pervasive transcription and novel small RNAs. Nat Rev Genetics 10: 833–844.
34. Kuhn DE, Nuovo GJ, Martin MM, Malana GE, Pleister AP, et al. (2008) Human chromosome 21-derived miRNAs are overexpressed in down syndrome brains and hearts. Biochem Biophys Res Commun 370: 473–477.
35. Takumi T (2010) A humanoid mouse model of autism. Brain Dev 32: 753–758.
36. Duker AL, Ballif BC, Bawle EV, Person RE, Mahadevan S, et al. (2010) Paternally inherited microdeletion at 15q11.2 confirms a significant role for the SNORD116 C/D box snoRNA cluster in Prader-Willi syndrome. Eur J Hum Genet Jun 30.
37. Lin AE, Basson CT, Goldmuntz E, Magoulas PL, McDermott DA, et al. (2008) Adults with genetic syndromes and cardiovascular abnormalities: clinical history and management. Genet Med 10: 469–494.
38. Abildgaard L, Ellebaek E, Gustafsson G, Abrahamsson J, Hovi L, et al. (2006) Optimal treatment intensity in children with Down syndrome and myeloid leukaemia: data from 56 children treated on NOPHO-AML protocols and a review of the literature. Ann Hematol 85: 275–280.
39. Hasle H (2001) Pattern of malignant disorders in individuals with Down's syndrome. Lancet Oncol 2: 429–436.
40. Diller GP, van Eijl S, Okonko DO, Howard LS, Ali O, et al. (2008) Circulating endothelial progenitor cells in patients with Eisenmenger syndrome and idiopathic pulmonary arterial hypertension. Circulation 117: 3020–3030.
41. Holmes DK, Bates N, Murray M, Ladusans EJ, Morabito A, et al. (2006) Hematopoietic progenitor cell deficiency in fetuses and children affected by Down's syndrome. Exp Hematol 34: 1611–1615.
42. Jablonska B, Ford D, Trisler D, Pessac B (2006) The growth capacity of bone marrow CD34 positive cells in culture is drastically reduced in a murine model of Down syndrome. C R Biol 329: 726–732.
43. Krenning G, van Luyn MJ, Harmsen MC (2009) Endothelial progenitor cell-based neovascularization: implications for therapy. Trends Mol Med 15: 180–189.
44. Hirschi KK, Ingram DA, Yoder MC (2008) Assessing identity phenotype and fate of endothelial progenitor cells. Arterioscler Thromb Vasc Biol 28: 1584–1595.
45. Zampetaki A, Kirton JP, Xu Q (2008) Vascular Repair by Endothelial Progenitor Cells Cardiovasc Res 78: 413–421.
46. Shantsila E, Watson T, Lip GY (2007) Endothelial progenitor cells in cardiovascular disorders. J Am Coll Cardiol 49: 741–752.
47. Yoder MC, Mead LE, Prater D, Krier TR, Mroueh KN, et al. (2007) Redefining endothelial progenitor cells via clonal analysis and hematopoietic stem/progenitor cell principals. Blood 109: 1801–1809.
48. Sabatier F, Camoin-Jau L, Anfosso F, Sampol J, Dignat-George F (2009) Circulating endothelial cells microparticles and progenitors: key players towards the definition of vascular competence. J Cell Mol Med 13: 454–471.
49. Napoli C, Balestrieri A, Ignarro LJ (2007) Therapeutic approaches in vascular repair induced by adult bone marrow cells and circulating progenitor endothelial cells. Curr Pharm Des 13: 3245–3251.
50. Vasa M, Fichtlscherer S, Aicher A, Adler K, Urbich C, et al. (2001) Number and migratory activity of circulating andothelial progenitor cells inversely correlate with risk factors for coronary artery disease. Circ Res 89: E1–7.
51. Mangone M, Manoharan AP, Thierry-Mieg D, Thierry-Mieg J, Han T, et al. (2010) The landscape of C. elegans 3′UTRs. Science 329: 432–435.
52. Nagalakshmi U, Wang Z, Waern K, Shou C, Raha D, et al. (2008) The transcriptional landscape of the yeast genome defined by RNA sequencing. Science 320: 1344–1349.
53. Core LJ, Waterfall J, Lis JT (2008) Nascent RNA sequencing reveals widespread pausing and divergent initiation at human promoters. Science 322: 1845–1848.
54. Morin R, Bainbridge M, Fejes A, Hirst M, Krzywinski M, et al. (2008) Profiling the HeLa S3 transcriptome using randomly primed cDNA and massively parallel short-read sequencing. BioTechniques 45: 81–94.
55. Mortazavi A, Williams BA, McCue K, Schaeffer L, Wold B (2008) Mapping and quantifying mammalian transcriptomes by RNA-Seq. Nat Methods 5: 621–628.
56. Rosenkranz R, Borodina T, Lehrach H, Himmelbauer H (2008) Characterizing the mouse ES cell transcriptome with Illumina sequencing. Genomics 92: 187–194.
57. Bainbridge MN, Warren RL, Hirst M, Romanuik T, Zeng T, et al. (2006) Analysis of the prostate cancer cell line LNCaP transcriptome using a sequencing-by-synthesis approach. BMC Genomics 7: 246.
58. Casamassimi A, Balestrieri ML, Fiorito C, Schiano C, Maione C, et al. (2007) Comparison between total endothelial progenitor cell isolation versus enriched CD133+ culture. J Biochem 141: 503–511.
59. Cloonan N, Xu Q, Faulkner GJ, Taylor DF, Tang DT, et al. (2009) RNA-MATE: a recursive mapping strategy for high-throughput RNAsequencing data. Bioinformatics 25: 2615–2616.
60. Pruitt KD, Tatusova T, Maglott DR (2007) NCBI reference sequences (RefSeq): a curated non-redundant sequence database of genomes transcripts and proteins. Nucleic Acids Res 35(Database issue): D61–65.
61. Bruford EA, Lush MJ, Wright MW, Sneddon TP, Povey S, et al. (2008) The HGNC Database in 2008: a resource for the human genome. Nucleic Acids Res 36(Database issue): D445–448.
62. Kuhn RM, Karolchik D, Zweig AS, Wang T, Smith KE, et al. (2009) The UCSC Genome Browser Database: update 2009. Nucleic Acids Res 37(Database issue): D755–761.
63. Hsu F, Kent WJ, Clawson H, Kuhn RM, Diekhans M, et al. (2006) The UCSC Known Genes. Bioinformatics 22: 1036–1046.
64. Hubbard TJ, Aken BL, Ayling S, Ballester B, Beal K, et al. (2009) Ensembl 2009. Nucleic Acids Res 37(Database issue): D690–697.
65. Baek KH, Zaslavsky A, Lynch RC, Britt C, Okada Y, et al. (2009) Down's syndrome suppression of tumour growth and the role of the calcineurin inhibitor DSCR1. Nature 459: 1126–1130.
66. Taft RJ, Simons C, Nahkuri S, Oey H, Korbie DJ, et al. (2010) Nuclear-localized tiny RNAs are associated with transcription initiation and splice sites in metazoans. Nat Struct Mol Biol 17: 1030–1034.
67. Taft RJ, Glazov EA, Lassmann T, Hayashizaki Y, Carninci P, et al. (2009) Small RNAs derived from snoRNAs. RNA 15: 1233–1240.
68. Guttman M, Amit I, Garber M, French C, Lin MF, et al. (2009) Chromatin signature reveals over a thousand highly conserved large non-coding RNAs in mammals. Nature 458: 223–227.
69. Langenberger D, Bermudez-Santana CI, Stadler PF, Hoffmann S (2010) Identification and classification of small rnas in transcriptome sequence data. Pac Symp Biocomput 2010: 80–87.
70. Mi H, Dong Q, Muruganujan A, Gaudet P, Lewis S, et al. (2010) PANTHER version 7: improved phylogenetic trees orthologs and collaboration with the Gene Ontology Consortium. Nucleic Acids Res 38(Database issue): D204–210.
71. Young MD, Wakefield MJ, Smyth GK, Oshlack A (2010) Gene ontology analysis for RNA-seq: accounting for selection bias. Genome Biol 11: R14.
72. Ponting CP, Belgard TG (2010) Transcribed dark matter: meaning or myth? Hum Mol Genet Sep 20.
73. van Bakel H, Nislow C, Blencowe BJ, Hughes TR (2010) Most "dark matter" transcripts are associated with known genes. PLoS Biol 8: e1000371.
74. Keren H, Lev-Maor G, Ast G (2010) Alternative splicing and evolution: diversification, exon definition and function. Nat Rev Genet 11: 345–355.
75. Twine NA, Janitz K, Wilkins MR, Janitz M (2011) Whole transcriptome sequencing reveals gene expression and splicing differences in brain regions affected by Alzheimer's disease. PLoS One 6: e16266.
76. Trapnell C, Pachter L, Salzberg SL (2009) TopHat: discovering splice junctions with RNA-Seq. Bioinformatics 25: 1105–1111.
77. Gremmels H, Fledderus JO, Balkom BW, Verhaar MC (2011) Transcriptome Analysis in Endothelial Progenitor Cell Biology. Antioxid Redox Signal Feb 14.
78. Livak KJ, Schmittgen TD (2001) Analysis of relative gene expression data using real-time quantitative PCR and the 2(-Delta Delta C(T)) Method. Methods 25: 402–408.
79. Wang L, Feng Z, Wang X, Wang X, Zhang X (2010) DEGseq: an R package for identifying differentially expressed genes from RNA-seq data. Bioinformatics 26: 136–138.
80. Anders S, Huber W (2010) Differential expression analysis for sequence count data. Nature Proceedings http://precedings.nature.com/documents/4282/version/2.
81. Robinson MD, McCarthy DJ, Smyth GK (2010) edgeR: a Bioconductor package for differential expression analysis of digital gene expression data. Bioinformatics 26: 139–140.

15

Age-Related Decrease of Meiotic Cohesins in Human Oocytes

Makiko Tsutsumi[1], Reiko Fujiwara[1], Haruki Nishizawa[2], Mayuko Ito[1,2], Hiroshi Kogo[3], Hidehito Inagaki[1], Tamae Ohye[1], Takema Kato[1], Takuma Fujii[2], Hiroki Kurahashi[1]*

1 Division of Molecular Genetics, Institute for Comprehensive Medical Science, Fujita Health University, Toyoake, Aichi, Japan, **2** Department of Obstetrics and Gynecology, Fujita Health University, Toyoake, Aichi, Japan, **3** Department of Anatomy and Cell Biology, Gunma University Graduate School of Medicine, Maebashi, Gunma, Japan

Abstract

Aneuploidy in fetal chromosomes is one of the causes of pregnancy loss and of congenital birth defects. It is known that the frequency of oocyte aneuploidy increases with the human maternal age. Recent data have highlighted the contribution of cohesin complexes in the correct segregation of meiotic chromosomes. In mammalian oocytes, cohesion is established during the fetal stages and meiosis-specific cohesin subunits are not replenished after birth, raising the possibility that the long meiotic arrest of oocytes facilitates a deterioration of cohesion that leads to age-related increases in aneuploidy. We here examined the cohesin levels in dictyate oocytes from different age groups of humans and mice by immunofluorescence analyses of ovarian sections. The meiosis-specific cohesin subunits, REC8 and SMC1B, were found to be decreased in women aged 40 and over compared with those aged around 20 years ($P<0.01$). Age-related decreases in meiotic cohesins were also evident in mice. Interestingly, SMC1A, the mitotic counterpart of SMC1B, was substantially detectable in human oocytes, but little expressed in mice. Further, the amount of mitotic cohesins of mice slightly increased with age. These results suggest that, mitotic and meiotic cohesins may operate in a coordinated way to maintain cohesions over a sustained period in humans and that age-related decreases in meiotic cohesin subunits impair sister chromatid cohesion leading to increased segregation errors.

Editor: Qinghua Shi, University of Science and Technology of China, China

Funding: This work was supported by grants from JSPS KAKENHI (22790334 and 25860255 to MT and 21028020 and 23013019 to HK, URL: http://www.jsps.go.jp/j-grantsinaid/). The funders had no role in study design, data collection and analysis, decision to publish, or preparation of the manuscript.

Competing Interests: The authors have declared that no competing interests exist.

* E-mail: kura@fujita-hu.ac.jp

Introduction

Chromosomal segregation errors that arise during meiotic cell division produce aneuploid gametes with an incorrect number of chromosomes. Aneuploidy of fetal chromosomes causes miscarriage or results in newborns with congenital birth defects such as Down syndrome (DS). It is well known that the extra chromosome in trisomy 21 in DS mainly originates from segregation errors during maternal meiosis I, and that the risk of DS increases with maternal age [1,2]. The frequency of DS is 1/1400 births in 20–24 year-old women. This rises to 1/350 in 35-year-old and 1/25 in 45-year-old and older women [3]. In addition, age-related oocyte aneuploidy causes an elevated risk of pregnancy loss in older women i.e. the rate of chromosomal anomalies among clinically diagnosed miscarriages is about 50% in women younger than 35 but is 75% in women above this age. The incidence of miscarriage is 9% in women in their early 20 s and rises to 75% in women aged 45 and over [4,5]. These also indicate significant increase of aneuploidy in older women. However, the etiology of maternal age-related increases in chromosomal segregation errors remains unclear.

Meiotic cohesins have a key role in correct segregation of chromosomes in meiosis [6–8]. The ring-shaped cohesin complex is required for sister chromatid cohesion during meiosis and also in mitotic cell division. In mammalian oocytes, the establishment of cohesions during pre-meiotic DNA replication is followed by entry into prophase of meiosis I. After homologous chromosomes are connected at the crossover site via homologous recombination, the oocytes become arrested at the diplotene stage of prophase I for a prolonged period (dictyate stage) during the fetal stage. After sexual maturation, meiosis resumes and the first cell division occurs before ovulation. During this prolonged period, the homologous chromosomes are kept together until the onset of anaphase I by sister chromatid cohesion distal to the chiasma. However, it has been shown that SMC1B and REC8, meiosis-specific components of the cohesin complex, do not undergo turnover after birth in female mice [9,10]. It is possible that this might cause the gradual decrease in the cohesin levels. The deterioration of cohesion in the chromosome arm leads to meiosis I nondisjunction via the premature dissociation of chiasma between homologous chromosomes. This deterioration in the centromere induces predivision of sister chromatids. These events result increase the risk of age-related segregation error in humans [11–14].

To verify this hypothesis, the levels of the meiotic cohesin subunits, SMC1B and REC8, as well as the mitotic cohesin subunits, RAD21 and SMC1A, and the SMC3 subunit used in common between meiotic and mitotic cohesin complexes, was examined in dictyate oocytes from humans and mice. The immunofluorescence signal intensities on ovarian tissue sections were quantified and demonstrated an age-related decrease in the meiosis-specific cohesins in both humans and mice. These results lend support to the hypothesis that a decrease in the cohesins with age induces chromosomal segregation errors. Moreover, these results highlight a novel hypothesis underlying the maintenance mechanism of cohesions in humans in which the life span is much longer than that of mice.

Materials and Methods

Ethics statement

This study was approved by the Ethical Review Board for Clinical Research at Fujita Health University. All of the patients gave written informed consent. All animal experiments were approved by the Animal Care and Use Committee at Fujita Health University (I0501).

Human ovarian tissue

Human ovarian tissues were obtained from 8 women (age range: 19–49 years) who were undergoing surgery for ovarian tumors at Fujita Health University Hospital. Samples were derived from the normal region within the dissected tumor. Ovarian tissues were immediately embedded in Tissue-Tek OCT compound (Sakura Finetek), snap-frozen in liquid nitrogen in the operating room and stored at −70°C within 1 hour of dissection.

Mice

C57BL/6NCr mice were obtained from Japan SLC. Ovaries from female mice were embedded, snap-frozen and stored at −70°C as described above.

Antibodies

Rabbit polyclonal anti-human REC8 antibodies were raised against amino acid residues 427–443 of the human REC8 protein. Rabbit polyclonal anti-human SMC1B antibodies were raised against amino acid residues 1219–1235 of the human SMC1B protein. Guinea pig polyclonal anti-mouse SMC1B antibodies were raised against amino acid residues 1215–1248 of mouse SMC1B. Guinea pig polyclonal anti-mouse REC8 antibodies were raised as described previously [15]. The resulting antisera were affinity purified on columns coupled to the peptide. The specificities of the antibodies described above were confirmed as shown in Figure S1. All antibodies used in this study are listed in Table S1.

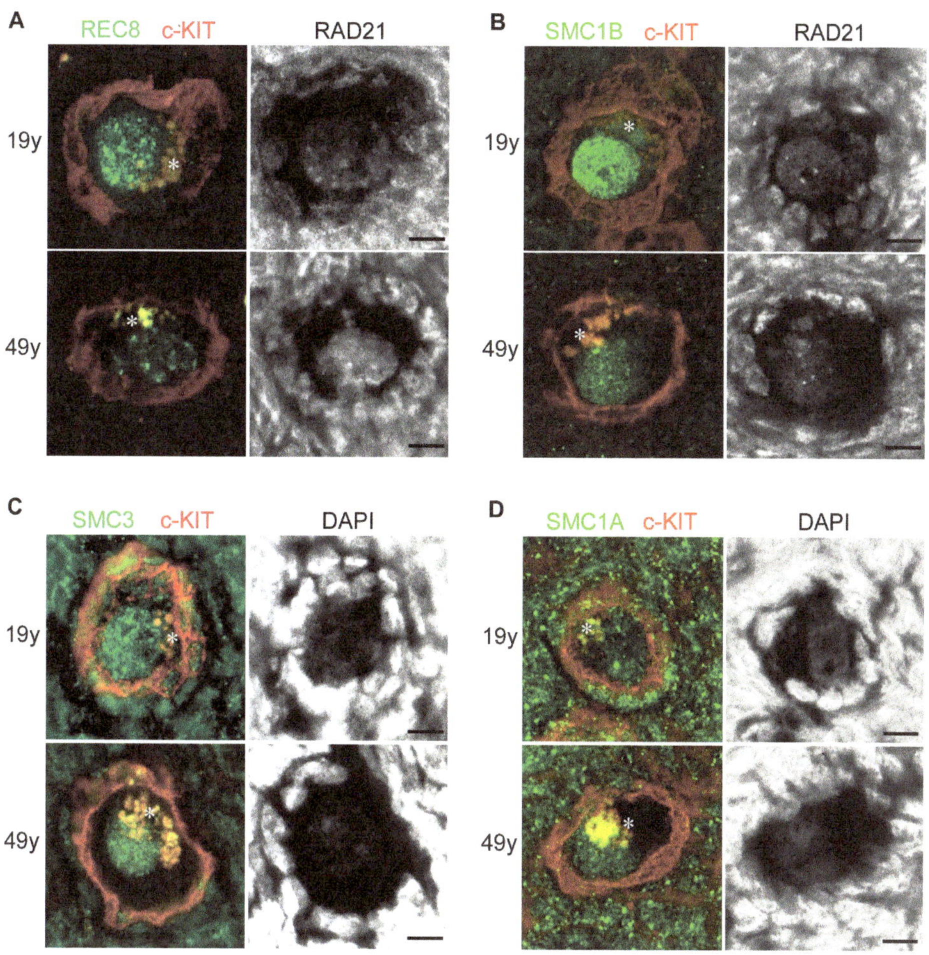

Figure 1. Immunofluorescent staining of human oocytes in ovarian sections from 19- and 49-year-old women. (A, B) REC8 or SMC1B (green) proteins co-immunostained with RAD21. (C, D) SMC3 or SMC1A (green) signals counterstained with DAPI. C-KIT (red) was used as a marker of oocytes. Asterisks indicate autofluorescence in the cytoplasmic region of the oocytes. Bar, 10 μm.

Immunofluorescent staining

Ovarian frozen tissue sections were prepared and fixed as described previously [16]. Briefly, sections were fixed in methanol:acetone:chloroform (1:1:1) for 10 min on ice and then washed three times in PBS. After blocking with 10% normal donkey serum in PBS for 30 min at room temperature, staining with primary and secondary antibodies were performed as described [17]. The exception was when using biotin-conjugated secondary antibodies where the slides were incubated with Alexa Fluor 350-conjugaed streptavidin (Life Technologies) for 15 min and then washed three times after washing of the secondary antibodies.

Image analysis

Slides were observed under a fluorescence microscope (Axio Imager M1 or Axio Imager Z2, Carl Zeiss) equipped with a digital camera (AxioCam HRc, Carl Zeiss). Images were captured using the same settings controlled by Axiovision 4.8 software (Carl Zeiss). Densitometric analysis of the immunofluorescence signals from oocyte and somatic cell nuclei was performed using Axiovision 4.8 software. Schematic drawings explaining the method to determine the relative cohesin concentrations are described in Figure S2. Data analysis was performed using Excel software.

Results

Age-related decrease of meiosis-specific cohesins in human dictyate oocytes

To compare the cohesin levels in oocytes from women of different ages, we employed an immunofluorescence technique using ovarian tissue sections (Fig. 1). Cohesin complexes in oocytes consist of REC8, SMC1B and SMC3 subunits, whilst in somatic cells comprise RAD21, SMC1A and SMC3 subunits. By immunofluorescence staining, meiosis-specific cohesin subunits, REC8 and SMC1B, were detectable in the nuclei of dictyate oocytes and exhibited a threadlike distribution with dense aggregates as previously reported [18]. but not in somatic cells on ovarian tissue sections (Fig. 1A, B). SMC3, a shared cohesin subunit both meiotic and mitotic cells, could be detected in the nuclei of both oocytes and somatic cells (Fig. 1C). The mitotic cohesin subunits RAD21 and SMC1A, which are substituted in meiosis with meiosis-specific cohesins REC8 and SMC1B, respectively, were also detectable both in somatic cells and oocytes (Fig. 1A, B, D).

To determine the relative oocyte cohesin concentration, the immunofluorescent signals corresponding to mitotic cohesins in the nuclei of somatic cells were used to normalize the signal intensities among samples. REC8 or SMC1B proteins were immunostained along with RAD21 as an internal control

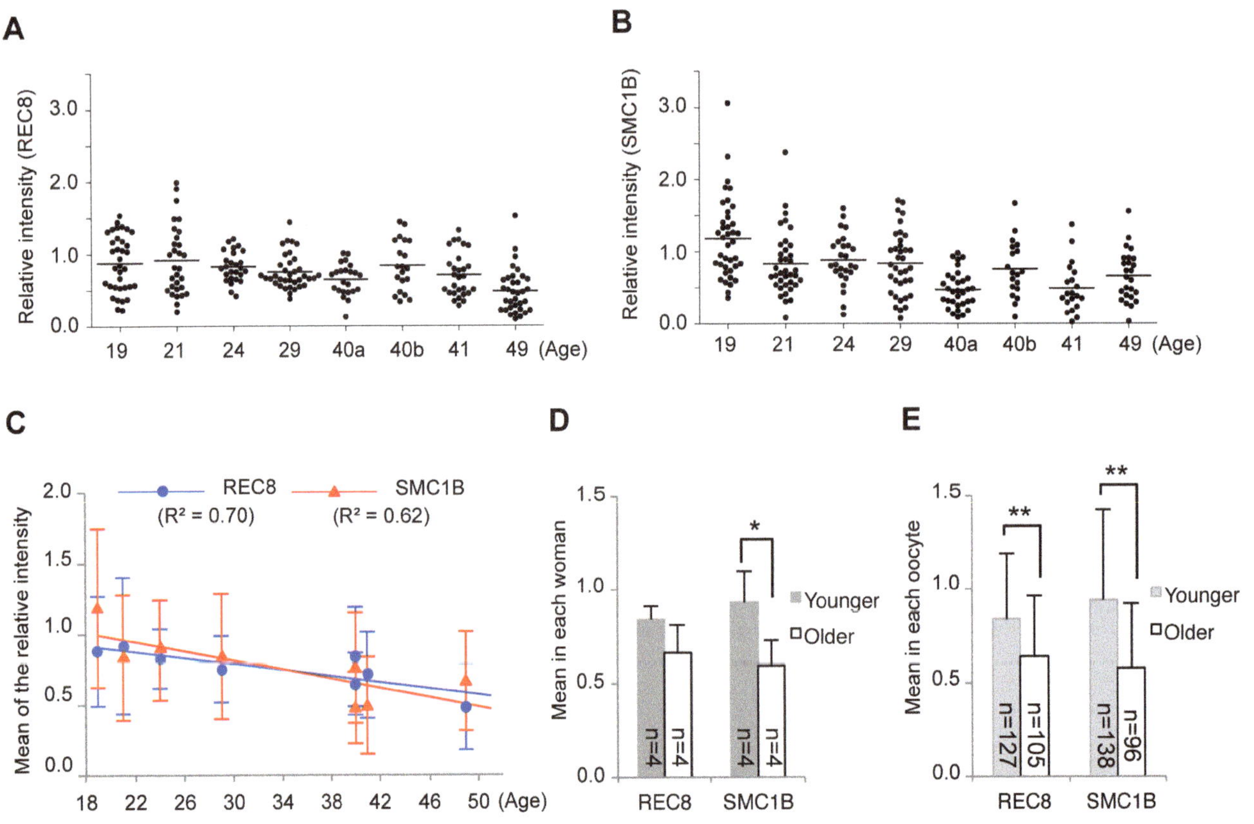

Figure 2. Quantitative results for meiosis-specific cohesins in human oocytes. (A, B) Relative signal intensity of REC8 or SMC1B. Intensities were determined as described in Figure S2. Specimens were obtained from two 40 year old female subjects (40a and 40b). Horizontal bars indicate the mean cohesin levels for each subject. (C) Regression analyses of the mean cohesin signal intensities shown in (A) and (B) (mean ± SD). The regression lines are indicated by solid lines. The coefficients of determination are indicated in parentheses. (D, E) Comparisons of the signal intensity means between grouped samples. Women were grouped as younger (≤29-year-old) or older (≥40-year-old). (D) The cohesin signal intensity means shown in (A–C) were compared between groups (mean ± SD). (E) The cohesin signal intensity means in single oocytes were compared between groups (mean ± SD). *$P<0.05$, **$P<0.01$, Student's *t*-test.

(Fig. 1A, B). The relative amounts of cohesins in oocytes were estimated as a ratio of the signal intensity in oocytes to that of mitotic cohesins in somatic cells (Fig. S2).

We examined the signal intensity of meiosis-specific cohesins in oocytes from 8 women aged 19 to 49 years (Fig. 2A, B). Immunofluorescent signals for the meiosis-specific cohesins, REC8 and SMC1B, were detected in the oocytes of all samples examined (Fig. 1A, B). These signal intensities showed a wide distribution, which was partly due to the variability between each oocyte and also due to the position of the sections since the thicknesses of these sections are smaller than the diameter of the oocyte nuclei (Fig. 1A, B). We found that the mean REC8 and SMC1B signal intensities among individual women showed a negative correlation with age (Fig. 2C). We further analyzed these signal intensities by dividing our female subject into younger (≤29-year-old; mean ± SD: 23.3±4.3 year-old) and older (≥40-year-old; mean ± SD: 42.5±4.4 year-old) groups. The decrease observed in the SMC1B levels in the older group was significant although REC8 did not show a significant decrease (Fig. 2D). However, when the signal intensities of each oocyte were compared, the REC8 and SMC1B levels in the older group were significantly decreased by 24% and 38%, respectively, compared with the younger women (Fig. 2E). Similar results were obtained when REC8 was co-immunostained with pan-histone as another internal control (Fig. S3).

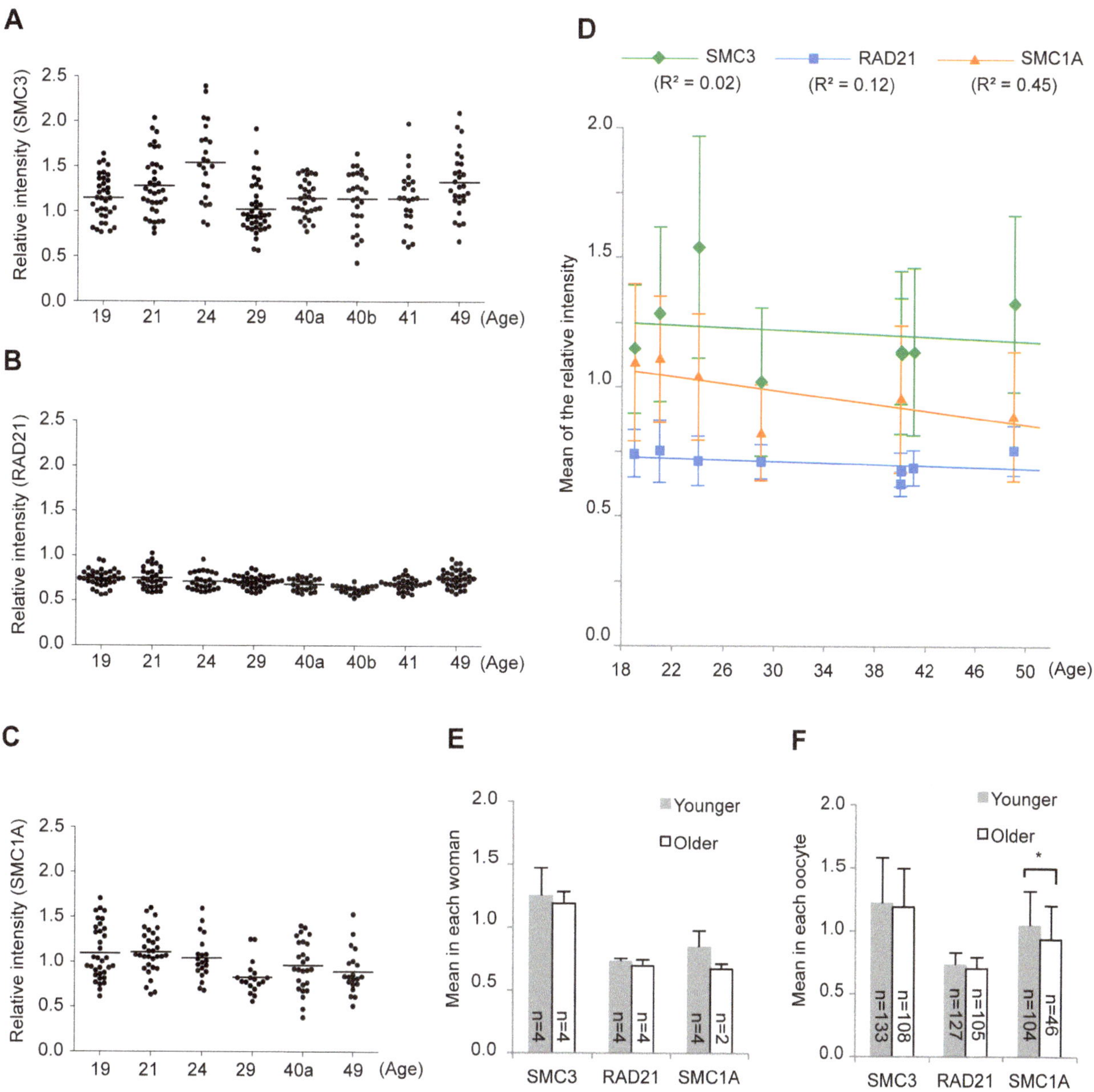

Figure 3. Quantitative results for the mitotic cohesin levels in human oocytes. (A–C) Relative signal intensities for SMC3, RAD21 or SMC1A. (D) Regression analyses of the cohesin signal intensity means shown in (A–C) (mean ± SD). Lines are the regression lines. The coefficients of determination are in parentheses. (E, F) Comparisons of the signal intensity means between grouped samples. Women were grouped as indicated in Figure 2. (E) The cohesin signal intensity means shown in (A–D) were compared between groups (mean ± SD). (F) The cohesin signal intensity means in single oocytes were compared between groups (mean ± SD). *$P<0.05$, Student's *t*-test.

We also examined the relative SMC3, RAD21 and SMC1A levels in human oocytes (Figs. 1 and 3A–C). In contrast to the meiosis-specific cohesins, the signal intensities of these proteins did not significantly change with age, although a slight decrease in the SMC1A level was evident in oocytes of older women (Fig. 3D–F).

Cohesins in the dictyate oocytes of the mouse

To evaluate whether our above findings are unique to humans in which a long life span leads to years of dictyate arrest, we performed similar immunofluorescence experiments in the mouse. Two-month-old and 10-month-old wild-type B6 mice, which have just become sexually matured and have reached the late reproductive age, respectively, were examined (Fig. 4). In each age group, samples were derived from 3 mice. The signal intensity of REC8 in the older mice was significantly lower than that of younger mice (Fig. 5A, C, D) as demonstrated in our human analyses (Fig. 2). Likewise, the signal intensity of SMC1B in older mice was also low relative to that of younger mice (Fig. 5B, C, D). Thus, meiosis-specific cohesins in mouse oocytes decrease in an age-related manner as with humans.

We found from our immunofluorescence analyses that the signal intensity of SMC3 in older mice was not significantly different from that of younger mice. This result is similar to that found in humans, although the signal intensities of oocytes to somatic cells in mice were found to be slightly lower than those in humans (Fig. 6A, D, E). In contrast, the signal intensity of RAD21 in older mice showed a slight increase compared with younger mice (Fig. 6B, D, E). Interestingly, and in contrast to humans, the immunofluorescent signal intensity of SMC1A in the nuclei of mouse oocytes was barely detectable relative to that in somatic cells (Figs. 1D and 4C). Although the mean signal intensity of SMC1A in each older mouse was almost similar to that in each younger mouse (Fig. 6C, D), the mean signal intensity in each oocyte was increased slightly in older mice, as was observed for RAD21 (Fig. 6E).

Discussion

Age-related decrease in meiosis-specific cohesin subunits

In our present study, we demonstrate an age-related decrease of meiosis- specific cohesin subunits, REC8 and SMC1B, in dictyate oocytes both in humans and mice. In contrast, the signal levels of the cohesin subunits common to mitotic cells, SMC3, RAD21 and SMC1A, did not change. To our knowledge, this is the first report to demonstrate an age-related decrease in the cohesin concentrations in human oocytes at the protein level. Although it has been reported that cohesin staining in MI and MII oocytes from women of different ages (age range: 18–34) indicated no decrease in the older women [18], this may be possibly attributed to the samples derived from relatively young women compared to our present study.

It has been long accepted that age-related increases in oocyte aneuploidy do not occur in mice. Long dictyate arrest in humans due to a long life span is likely to underlie this difference. However, age-related aneuploidy has been detected in certain mouse strains such as C57BL/6 [19,20]. Indeed, age-related decreases in REC8 have been reported previously in the C57BL-related strains [11,12]. It is therefore currently believed that this phenomenon is strain-dependent. These findings are consistent with the linkage between the age–related increase of aneuploidy and decrease in cohesin levels seen also in humans.

The mechanism of reduction in cohesin levels on the chromatin in dictyate oocytes remains to be clarified. Oxidative damage or spontaneous hydrolysis of peptide bonds that are generally involved in protein aging are one possible cause of this degradation [13]. It has also been suggested that leaky separase activity may cause a loss of cohesins [13,21]. Although separase intrinsically cleaves the cohesin ring at anaphase onset [22], the expression

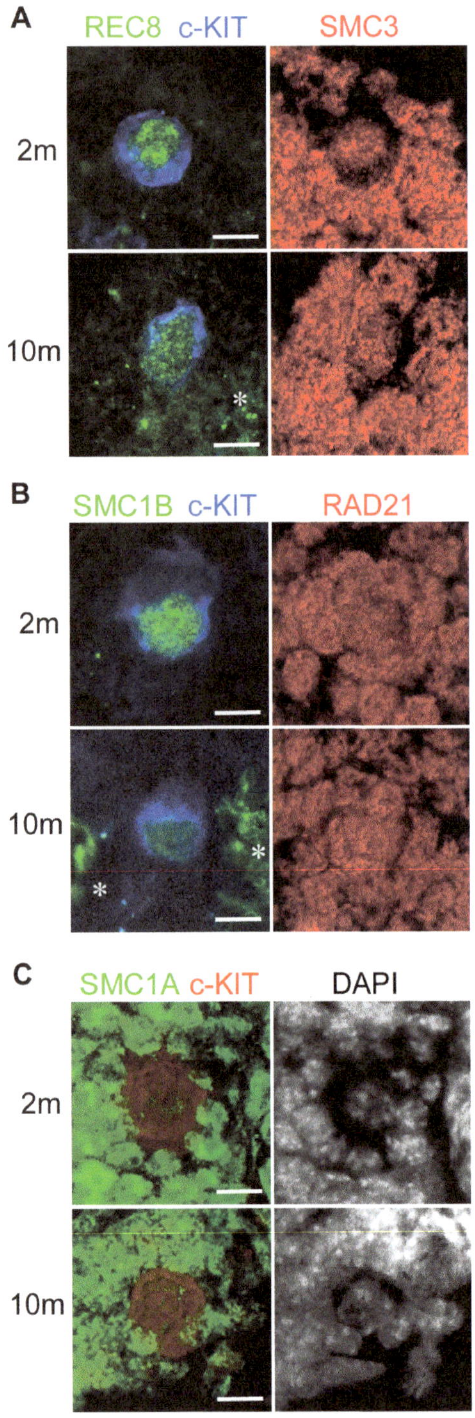

Figure 4. Immunofluorescent staining of mouse oocytes in ovarian sections from 2- and 10-month-old female mice. (A) Slides were co-immunostained with REC8 (green) and SMC3 (red). (B) Slides were co-immunostained with SMC1B (green) and RAD21 (red). (C) SMC1A (green) signals with DAPI nuclear counterstaining. Asterisks indicate autofluorescence. Bar, 10 μm.

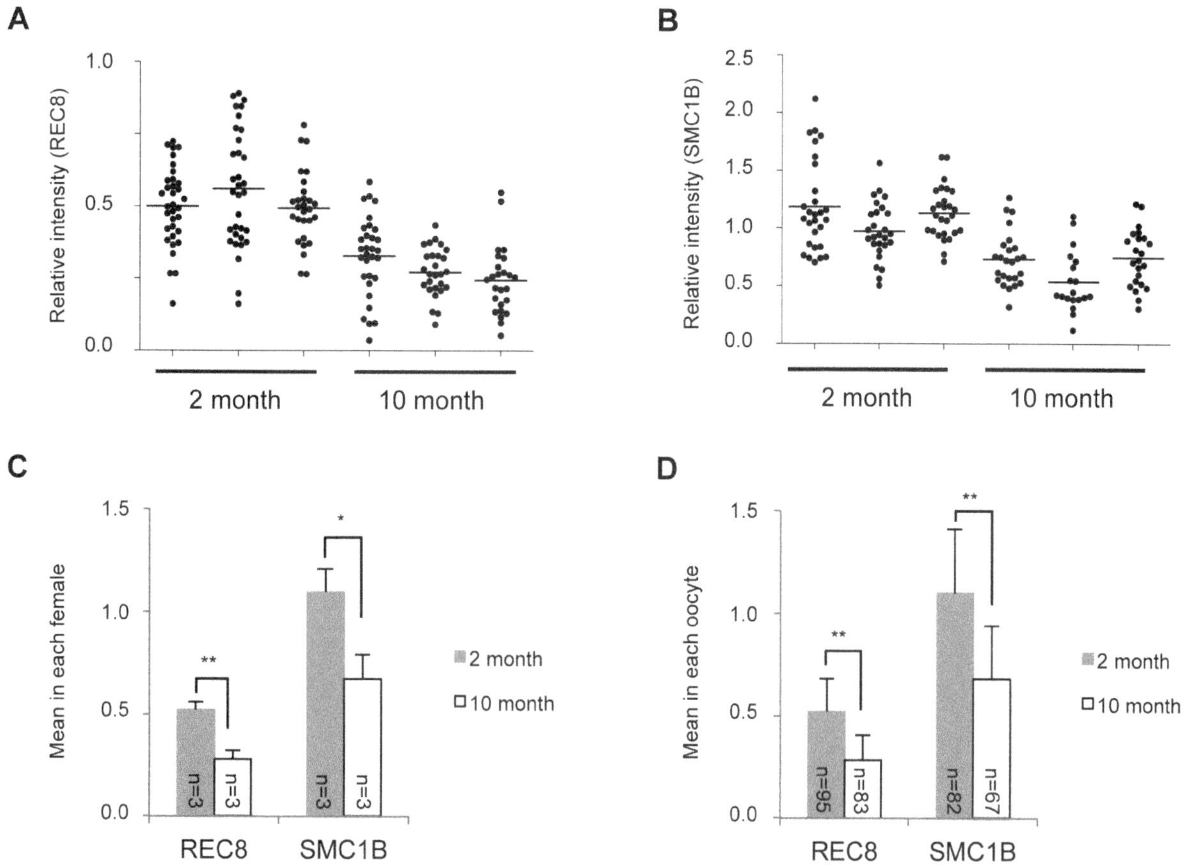

Figure 5. Quantitative results for meiosis-specific cohesin levels in 2- and 10-month-old mouse oocytes. (A, B) Relative signal intensity of REC8 or SMC1B. Intensities were determined as indicated in Figure S2. Three mice were used at each age. Horizontal bars are the mean cohesin levels within each female. (C) Cohesin signal intensity means in each female (mean ± SD). (D) Cohesin signal intensity means in each oocyte (mean ± SD). *$P<0.05$, **$P<0.01$, Student's t-test.

level of this enzyme was previously found to be up-regulated in metaphase II oocytes in older women compared with younger [23].

The expression patterns of cohesin mRNAs in human oocytes determined by microarray analyses were reported previously [23,24]. Whilst SMC3, RAD21 and SMC1A mRNAs are substantially expressed in oocytes, REC8 and SMC1B transcripts were only weakly detectable in these experiments. Thus, once meiosis-specific cohesin subunits undergo degradation, they would not undergo turnover in human or mouse, which facilitates the age-related decrease in the meiotic cohesin levels [9,10].

Coordination of meiotic and mitotic cohesins

Whilst the meiotic cohesins in mouse oocytes of a certain strain decrease within a few months, the cohesins are retained for decades in humans. It is tempting to imagine that special safeguarding mechanism had to be evolved in the long-living humans, and those mechanisms are absent in mice. We speculate that mitotic and meiotic cohesins may coordinately contribute maintaining the cohesion levels for long periods in humans. In our current study, we show that the SMC1A level was comparable between oocytes and somatic cells in humans, but only marginally detectable in mice. Based on the amino acid sequence of its epitope, the anti-SMC1A antibody used for detection of human SMC1A will not cross react with human SMC1B which is present in oocytes. It is suggested that both SMC1A-RAD21 and SMC1B-REC8 cohesins are present in human oocytes, and that SMC1A-RAD21 undergoes turnover even during dictyate arrest. This might partly contribute to maintaining the cohesin levels for a prolonged period in humans. In addition, the signal intensities of RAD21 and SMC1A were found to be slightly increased in aged mice in our present experiments. We suggest that this is supportive evidence for the upregulation of the mitotic cohesins in mouse oocytes to compensate for the loss of meiosis-specific cohesins. However, it has been shown that the SMC1A level is too marginal to compensate for the reduction in SMC1B in the mouse [25]. Nonetheless, no increase in SMC1A or RAD21 has been observed in human in accordance with the decrease in their meiotic counterparts, SMC1B and REC8. Even the baseline levels of SMC1A and RAD21 in human are still not sufficient to completely compensate for the loss of meiosis-specific cohesins. It is possible in this regard that the newly synthesized cohesins may be less able to hold sister chromatids together during meiosis since the cohesion establishment factors are not recruited without the DNA replication machinery [26,27].

Age-related decrease in cohesin and increase in aneuploidy

The frequency of trisomy in conceptuses is 2–3% in women aged in their twenties, but it rises exponentially in women in their mid-thirties to reach 35% in women aged over 40 [1]. However, the meiosis-specific cohesin levels in our current experiments

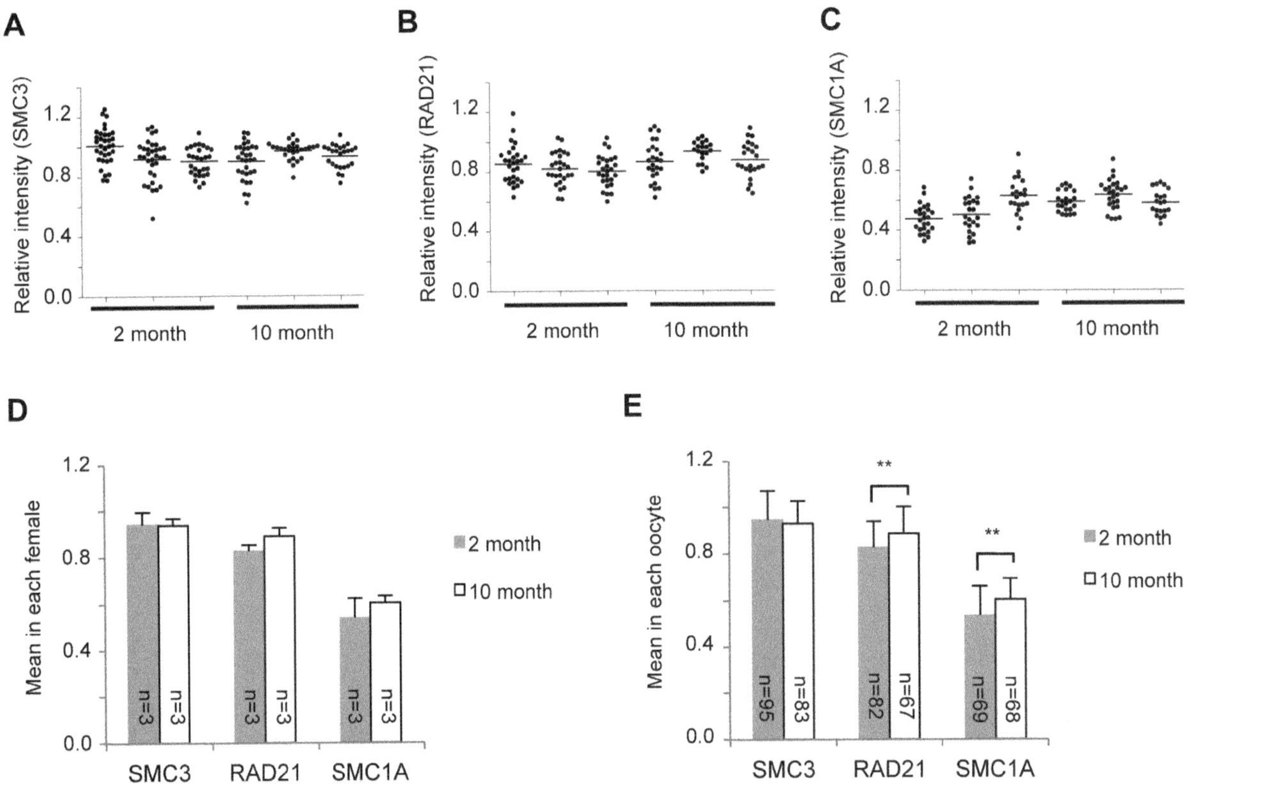

Figure 6. Quantitative results for mitotic cohesin levels in mouse oocytes. (A–C) Signal intensities for SMC3, RAD21 or SMC1A determined as described in Figure S2. (D) Cohesin signal intensity means in each female (mean ± SD). (E) Cohesin signal intensity means in each oocyte (mean ± SD). $^{**}P<0.01$, Student's *t*-test.

showed a linear negative correlation with the age of the sample donors. As a cause of this disparity, one possibility is a threshold effect of the cohesin level with regard to segregation error susceptibility i.e. there may be a threshold level of cohesins that can hold sister chromatids together against physical force. We thus speculate that the meiotic chromosomes may undergo malsegregation until these levels reach this threshold.

An alternative possibility is that the cohesins, in regulating gene expression, are involved in the exponential increase in aneuploidy. Cohesin depletion may cause a substantial effect on gene expression through defects in transcriptional regulatory functions [8,28,29]. Indeed, the expression of various genes in mature oocytes has been shown to change with age [23,30,31]. Thus, the chromosomes with impaired cohesions would be more susceptible to segregation error possibly because of spindle checkpoint defects caused by altered gene expression [23,32].

In accordance with the results of our present study, the age-related increase of interkinetochore distance between sister chromatids has been observed in the metaphase II oocytes of humans, suggesting a deterioration of chromosome cohesion with advancing age [33]. Without replenishment of meiosis-specific cohesins, cohesion between sister chromatids gradually deteriorates over time. This causes premature resolution of the chiasma between homologs or the premature separation of sister chromatids during the dictyate stage. Since these pre-separated chromosomes are distributed into daughter cells randomly, they are prone to malsegregation leading to gametes with aneuploidy. In our present study, besides the age-effect, we observed a variation among individuals in the rate of cohesin decrease. This might be due to the differences in genetic background and/or lifestyle. In future studies, a determination of the genetic variation affecting cohesin robustness will help to predict the susceptibility of individuals. A further elucidation of the mechanism underlying the decrease or maintenance of meiotic cohesins will contribute to the development of novel strategies to prevent age-related aneuploidy.

Supporting Information

Figure S1 Specificity of the antibodies. (A) Western blot analysis using affinity-purified antibodies. Testes lysates from human or mouse were loaded on the same gel. After electrophoresis and blotting, blots were stained with Ponceau S, and the each lane was cut into strips. SMC1B and REC8 were detected as 145-kDa and 75- to 82-kDa bands, respectively. Asterisks and dots indicate nonspecific bands reacted with the secondary antibodies. (B) Negative control of cohesin-immunostaining using IgGs and the secondary antibodies. (C) Negative control of cohesin-immunostaining using preimmune sera. (D) Negative control of cohesin-immunostaining using antibodies absorbed by preincubation with the peptide immunogens.

Figure S2 Representative immunofluorescent staining pattern of human oocytes. Green and blue signal intensities within the circled areas, indicating the oocyte nucleus, were respectively determined, as well as 5 randomly chosen somatic nuclei in the vicinity of the oocyte. The signal intensity of REC8 (green) was defined as: (area density of green signal in oocyte nucleus - mean area density of green signal in 5 somatic nuclei)/ mean area density of blue staining in 5 somatic nuclei. Because the green signals detected in somatic nuclei are background, these were subtracted from the signals in the oocytes. The signals in the oocytes were adjusted using the blue signal corresponding to the RAD21 cohesin subunit that is constitutively expressed in somatic cells. The signal intensity for RAD21 was defined as: area density of blue signal in the oocyte nucleus/mean area density of blue signal in 5 somatic nuclei.

Figure S3 Quantitative results for REC8 in human oocytes adjusted for the histone signals of somatic nuclei. (A) Immunofluorescent staining of human oocytes in ovarian sections from 19- and 49- year-old women. REC8 (green) proteins co-immunostained with histone (red) using anti-histone antibody (1:400; H11-4; Millipore). C-KIT (blue) was used as a marker of oocytes. Asterisks indicate autofluorescence in the cytoplasmic region of the oocytes. Bar, 10 μm. (B) Relative signal intensity of REC8. Intensities were determined as described in Figure S2, more specifically, histone signal in somatic nuclei was used to adjust the REC8 signal intensity. Specimens were obtained from 4 women (age range: 19–49 years). (C) Regression analysis of the REC8 signal intensity means shown in (B) (mean ± SD). Line indicates the regression line. The coefficient of determination is in parenthesis. (D) Comparisons of the signal intensity means between grouped samples. Women were grouped as indicated in Figure 2. The REC8 signal intensity means in single oocytes were compared between groups (mean ± SD). $^{**}P<0.01$, Student's *t*-test.

Table S1 Antibodies used in this study.

Acknowledgments

We thank S. Ikeda and S. Hamada-Tsutsumi for technical assistance.

Author Contributions

Conceived and designed the experiments: MT RF HN HK HI TO TK HK. Performed the experiments: MT RF MI. Analyzed the data: MT RF HK MI HI TO TK HK. Wrote the paper: MT HN HK HI TO TK HK. Provided human tissues: HN TF.

References

1. Hassold T, Hunt P (2001) To err (meiotically) is human: the genesis of human aneuploidy. Nat Rev Genet 2: 280–291.
2. Hassold T, Hall H, Hunt P (2007) The origin of human aneuploidy: where we have been, where we are going. Hum Mol Genet 16: R203–208.
3. Yoon PW, Freeman SB, Sherman SL, Taft LF, Gu Y, et al. (1996) Advanced maternal age and the risk of Down syndrome characterized by the meiotic stage of chromosomal error: a population-based study. Am J Hum Genet 58: 628–633.
4. Grande M, Borrell A, Garcia-Posada R, Borobio V, Muñoz M, et al (2012). The effect of maternal age on chromosomal anomaly rate and spectrum in recurrent miscarriage. Hum Reprod 27: 3109–3117.
5. Nybo Andersen AM, Wohlfahrt J, Christens P, Olsen J, Melbye M (2000) Maternal age and fetal loss: population based register linkage study. BMJ 320: 1708–1712.
6. Revenkova E, Eijpe M, Heyting C, Hodges CA, Hunt PA, et al. (2004) Cohesin SMC1 beta is required for meiotic chromosome dynamics, sister chromatid cohesion and DNA recombination. Nat Cell Biol 6: 555–562.
7. Lee J, Okada K, Ogushi S, Miyano T, Miyake M, et al. (2006) Loss of Rec8 from chromosome arm and centromere region is required for homologous chromosome separation and sister chromatid separation, respectively, in mammalian meiosis. Cell Cycle 5: 1448–1455.
8. Wood AJ, Severson AF, Meyer BJ (2010) Condensin and cohesin complexity: the expanding repertoire of functions. Nat Rev Genet 11: 391–404.
9. Revenkova E, Herrmann K, Adelfalk C, Jessberger R (2010) Oocyte cohesin expression restricted to predictyate stages provides full fertility and prevents aneuploidy. Curr Biol 20: 1529–1533.
10. Tachibana-Konwalski K, Godwin J, van der Weyden L, Champion L, Kudo NR, et al. (2010) Rec8-containing cohesin maintains bivalents without turnover during the growing phase of mouse oocytes. Genes Dev 24: 2505–2516.
11. Chiang T, Duncan FE, Schindler K, Schultz RM, Lampson MA (2010) Evidence that weakened centromere cohesion is a leading cause of age-related aneuploidy in oocytes. Curr Biol 20: 1522–1528.
12. Lister LM, Kouznetsova A, Hyslop LA, Kalleas D, Pace SL, et al. (2010) Age-related meiotic segregation errors in mammalian oocytes are preceded by depletion of cohesin and Sgo2. Curr Biol 20: 1511–1521.
13. Jessberger R (2012) Age-related aneuploidy through cohesion exhaustion. EMBO Rep 13: 539–546.
14. Kurahashi H, Tsutsumi M, Nishiyama S, Kogo H, Inagaki H, et al. (2012) Molecular basis of maternal age-related increase in oocyte aneuploidy. Congenit Anom (Kyoto) 52: 8–15.
15. Kouznetsova A, Novak I, Jessberger R, Höög C (2005) SYCP2 and SYCP3 are required for cohesin core integrity at diplotene but not for centromere cohesion at the first meiotic division. J Cell Sci 118: 2271–2278.
16. Eijpe M, Heyting C, Gross B, Jessberger R (2000) Association of mammalian SMC1 and SMC3 proteins with meiotic chromosomes and synaptonemal complexes. J Cell Sci 113: 673–682.
17. Tsutsumi M, Kowa-Sugiyama H, Bolor H, Kogo H, Inagaki H, et al. (2012) Screening of genes involved in chromosome segregation during meiosis I: in vitro gene transfer to mouse fetal oocytes. J Hum Genet 57: 515–522.
18. Garcia-Cruz R, Brieño MA, Roig I, Grossmann M, Velilla E, et al. (2010) Dynamics of cohesin proteins REC8, STAG3, SMC1 beta and SMC3 are consistent with a role in sister chromatid cohesion during meiosis in human oocytes. Hum Reprod 25: 2316–2327.
19. Koehler KE, Schrump SE, Cherry JP, Hassold TJ, Hunt PA (2006) Near-human aneuploidy levels in female mice with homeologous chromosomes. Curr Biol 16: R579–580.
20. Selesniemi K, Lee HJ, Muhlhauser A, Tilly JL (2011) Prevention of maternal aging-associated oocyte aneuploidy and meiotic spindle defects in mice by dietary and genetic strategies. Proc Natl Acad Sci U S A 108: 12319–12324.
21. Chiang T, Schultz RM, Lampson MA (2011) Age-dependent susceptibility of chromosome cohesion to premature separase activation in mouse oocytes. Biol Reprod 85: 1279–1283.
22. Hauf S, Waizenegger IC, Peters JM (2001) Cohesin cleavage by separase required for anaphase and cytokinesis in human cells. Science 293: 1320–1323.
23. Grøndahl ML, Yding Andersen C, Bogstad J, Nielsen FC, Meinertz H, et al. (2010) Gene expression profiles of single human mature oocytes in relation to age. Hum Reprod 25: 957–968.
24. Markholt S, Grøndahl ML, Ernst EH, Andersen CY, Ernst E, et al. (2012) Global gene analysis of oocytes from early stages in human folliculogenesis shows high expression of novel genes in reproduction. Mol Hum Reprod 18: 96–110.
25. Bickel SE (2005) Aging (not so) gracefully. Nat Genet 37: 1303–1304.
26. Lengronne A, McIntyre J, Katou Y, Kanoh Y, Hopfner KP, et al. (2006) Establishment of sister chromatid cohesion at the S. cerevisiae replication fork. Mol Cell 23: 787–799.
27. Skibbens RV (2000) Holding your own: establishing sister chromatid cohesion. Genome Res 10: 1664–1671.
28. Nasmyth K, Haering CH (2009) Cohesin: its roles and mechanisms. Annu Rev Genet 43: 525–558.
29. Rudra S, Skibbens RV (2013) Cohesin codes - interpreting chromatin architecture and the many facets of cohesin function. J Cell Sci 126: 31–41.
30. Fragouli E, Bianchi V, Patrizio P, Obradors A, Huang Z, et al. (2010) Transcriptomic profiling of human oocytes: association of meiotic aneuploidy and altered oocyte gene expression. Mol Hum Reprod 16: 570–582.
31. Titus S, Li F, Stobezki R, Akula K, Unsal E, et al. (2013) Impairment of BRCA1-related DNA double-strand break repair leads to ovarian aging in mice and humans. Sci Transl Med 5: 172ra21.
32. Steuerwald N, Cohen J, Herrera RJ, Sandalinas M, Brenner CA (2001) Association between spindle assembly checkpoint expression and maternal age in human oocytes. Mol Hum Reprod 7: 49–55.
33. Duncan FE, Hornick JE, Lampson MA, Schultz RM, Shea LD, et al. (2012) Chromosome cohesion decreases in human eggs with advanced maternal age. Aging Cell 11: 1121–1124.

16

Genome-Wide Expression Analysis in Down Syndrome: Insight into Immunodeficiency

Chong Li[1,2], Lei Jin[2], Yun Bai[2], Qimin Chen[3], Lijun Fu[3], Minjun Yang[2], Huasheng Xiao[4], Guoping Zhao[1,2], Shengyue Wang[1,2]*

1 School of Life Science, Fudan University, Shanghai, China, **2** Shanghai-MOST Key Laboratory of Health and Disease Genomics, Chinese National Human Genome Center at Shanghai, Shanghai, China, **3** Shanghai Children's Medical Center, Shanghai Jiao Tong University School of Medicine, Shanghai, China, **4** National Engineering Center for Biochip at Shanghai, Shanghai, China

Abstract

Down syndrome (DS) is caused by triplication of Human chromosome 21 (Hsa21) and associated with an array of deleterious phenotypes, including mental retardation, heart defects and immunodeficiency. Genome-wide expression patterns of uncultured peripheral blood cells are useful to understanding of DS-associated immune dysfunction. We used a Human Exon microarray to characterize gene expression in uncultured peripheral blood cells derived from DS individuals and age-matched controls from two age groups: neonate (N) and child (C). A total of 174 transcript clusters (gene-level) with eight located on Hsa21 in N group and 383 transcript clusters including 56 on Hsa21 in C group were significantly dysregulated in DS individuals. Microarray data were validated by quantitative polymerase chain reaction. Functional analysis revealed that the dysregulated genes in DS were significantly enriched in two and six KEGG pathways in N and C group, respectively. These pathways included leukocyte trans-endothelial migration, B cell receptor signaling pathway and primary immunodeficiency, etc., which causally implicated dysfunctional immunity in DS. Our results provided a comprehensive picture of gene expression patterns in DS at the two developmental stages and pointed towards candidate genes and molecular pathways potentially associated with the immune dysfunction in DS.

Editor: Lynette Kay Rogers, The Ohio State Unversity, United States of America

Funding: This work was supported by the Chinese National Key Program on Basic Research (973 Project) (2005CB522407). URL:http://program.most.gov.cn/. The funders had no role in study design, data collection and analysis, decision to publish, or preparation of the manuscript.

Competing Interests: Huasheng Xiao is a full-time employee of National Engineering Center for Biochip at Shanghai.

* E-mail: wangsy@chgc.sh.cn

Introduction

Down syndrome (DS; trisomy 21) is characterized by a complete, or occasionally partial, triplication of Hsa21. With an incidence of about one in 750 births [1], DS is the most common autosomal abnormality affecting live-born infants. More than 80 clinical features with variation in number and in severity are reported in DS [2].

DS patients are clinically associated with multiple blood cell-related phenotypes, including increased risk to develop leukemia, decreased lymphocyte counts, markedly enhanced incidence of autoimmune disorders as well as vulnerability to recurrent bacterial and viral infections [3,4,5,6]. Moreover, pneumonia and other types of respiratory infections are the most common causes of death in DS children and early adults [7]. The abnormalities highlight that DS individuals are very likely associated with intrinsic defects of the immune system [8]. However, the molecular mechanisms by which trisomy 21 leads to the immune system disorders in DS remain poorly investigated. Transcriptome of peripheral blood cells from DS would provide a unique molecular window into immunodeficiency relevant to DS. Several gene-expression studies in T lymphocytes [9] and blood cells [10] from DS patients reported dysregulated expression of some immune-associated genes, yet very small sample size or age-unmatched controls restricted statistical analysis.

Here, we characterized gene-expression in uncultured blood cells from DS and age-matched control samples in neonate and child group. The dysregulated genes in DS at the two developmental stages were identified and showed a comprehensive picture of gene expression patterns. Furthermore, classification of dysregulated genes based on their known functions provided insight into immunodeficiency in DS patients.

Results

Identification of differentially expressed genes between DS and control samples

Using the Affymetrix GeneChip Human Exon 1.0 ST Array containing ~20,000 known human genes, we performed gene expression analysis in DS peripheral blood cells and age-matched controls from N and C group. Of 17,626 core transcript clusters with RefSeq-supported annotation, 13,027 in C group and 13,168 in N group (corresponding to 12,876 and 13,017 well-characterized genes, respectively) were reliably expressed. In RNA-Seq analysis of endothelial progenitor cells from DS and control, 13,144 active RefSeq genes were shared by both the cells [11]. This suggests that the number of the expressed genes in DS and control cells was comparable in the two studies.

To identify differentially expressed genes between DS and controls in each group, we used ANOVA in combination with fold change in gene expression. Consistent with the observations of Prandini et al. [12], gender and DS×gender effects were not significant for expressed Hsa21 genes in DS individuals; however, expression of some non-Hsa21 genes were significantly affected by the two effects in each group. Therefore, the two effects were kept in our analysis. In N group, 174 (1.3%) of the 13,168 transcript clusters, containing 113 (64.9%) up-regulated genes and 61 (35.1%) down-regulated genes, were differentially expressed between DS and controls (Figure 1A, Table S1). In C group, 383 (2.9%) transcript clusters displayed differential expression between DS and controls. Pearson's correlation test showed no significant results between the child age and expression of the genes (smallest q value was 0.99). Among the 383 transcript clusters, 312 (81.5%) were up-regulated and 71 (18.5%) were down-regulated in DS children (Figure 1B, Table S2). The higher percentage of up-regulated genes in N and C group was similar to prior report [13]. In the two groups, only 22 dysregulated genes, including six transcript clusters on Hsa21, were shared (Table 1). Elevated expression of the six transcript clusters was also implicated in other DS cells or tissue (Table 1). For the 22 transcript clusters, the extent of fold change between the two groups was significantly correlated (Pearson's cor = 0.92, $P = 1.28\times10^{-9}$), suggesting their importance in DS phenotypes at the two developmental stages.

Furthermore, the dysregulated genes in each group were divided into four intervals according to fold change (Figure 2). The genes that were mildly altered in expression, with fold change between 0.5~0.77 or 1.3~2.0, accounted for the majority of the dysregulated genes in each group. The genes whose expression was intensively varied (fold change <0.5 or >2) were in the minority.

Expression variation of Hsa21 genes in DS

Given trisomy of Hsa21, we assessed expression variation of genes on this chromosome. There are 237 transcript clusters on the array, corresponding to 234 known genes on Hsa21. Of the transcript clusters, 157 (66%) and 146 (62%) were expressed in N and C group, respectively. There were 5.1% (8/157) in N group and 38.3% (56/146) in C group with significant expression difference between DS and age-matched controls (Figure 1C, D). Of the expressed Hsa21 genes in the two groups, no significantly down-regulated genes was detected in DS samples (Figure 1C and D), which is consistent with other reports [12,14] and reflects the dosage effects of trisomy. The average expression ratios (DS/control) of expressed Hsa21 genes were 1.29±0.43 (mean ± sd) in N group and 1.40±0.35 in C group, revealing an overall up-regulation of Hsa21 genes which is also observed in previous data [12,15,16,17].

QPCR validation

To confirm changes in gene-expression levels detected by the arrays and assess our statistical methods, we conducted approximately 2,500 QPCRs of all 37 cDNA samples from DS and control individuals. We first checked our definitions about a reliably expressed gene. To this end, several genes, whose normalized expression signals on the array in some individuals were close to the threshold according to our definition, were analyzed in the assay. These genes included *VAV2* in N group and *BTG3*, *PDGFD* and *PDGFRB* in C group. Their signals, albeit very weak relative to the endogenous genes, were detected by QPCR in all samples, thereby indicating the reasonable threshold defined by our criterions. We next selected a subset of the genes from each group and measured their expression levels. These genes included Hsa21 and non-Hsa21 genes that were statistically up-regulated, unaltered or down-regulated in analysis of the array. DS/control ratio for each gene was calculated and was very consistent with fold change obtained from the array (Table S3, Figure S1), with a Pearson correlation coefficient of 0.91 ($P = 2.2\times10^{-14}$) (Figure 3).

Chromosomal distribution of the dysregulated genes

We analyzed chromosomal distribution of the dysregulated genes in N and C group to evaluate effects of trisomy 21 on the whole genome. Of the dysregulated transcript clusters, 326 and 166 were mapped to non-Hsa21 in N and C group, respectively. These data are in agreement with the prior data [13,15,18], providing further evidence for the idea that both expression changes of Hsa21 and non-Hsa21 genes contribute to the etiology of DS. Chromosomal distribution of these dysregulated genes in N group and C group were showed in Figure 4. Figure 5 illustrated the percentage of the dysregulated genes in the expressed genes at individual chromosome and the whole genome level (corresponding to "all"). Through binomial tests, chromosome 21 in each group was significantly overrepresented with $Pc = 0.027$ in N group and $Pc < 10^{-6}$ in C group after Benjamini-Hochberg (BH) correction [19]. None of the remaining chromosomes was significantly overrepresented or underrepresented at $Pc < 0.05$.

Hierarchical cluster analysis of the dysregulated genes

In Figure 6, we illustrated the results of hierarchical clustering on the dysregulated transcript clusters in DS. Cluster analysis clearly separated the DS neonates from controls (Figure 6A). The child samples were divided into two major distinguishable groups, leaving one DS exception (D6) grouped into the control group (Figure 6B). This exception is not surprising, because although some phenotypes frequently occur in DS patients, the degree to which individual is affected varies. It is likely that the misclassification of the DS child is a reflection of mild phenotypic abnormalities caused by a combination of environmental and genetic variation.

We further asked whether hierarchical clustering could distinguish DS from control individuals based on the dysregulated non-Hsa21 genes. DS neonates were also separated from the matched controls (Figure S2A), which is similar to the observation that hierarchical clustering distinguishes DS from control fetuses based on the non-Hsa21 altered genes in amniotic fluid cell-free mRNA [18]. Unlike N group, DS and control children were clearly divided into three groups (Figure S2B). The first group included 11 controls and sample D6 that showed different expression patterns from the other DS samples in Figure 6B. The second group included the remaining 9 DS samples. The third group, including control C1, 3, 5 and 8, seemed to display intermediate patterns between the other two groups. The four controls were also grouped together as shown in Figure 6B, showing less well-defined expression patterns in these samples.

Effects of transcription factors on disruption of non-Hsa21 genes in DS

The dysregulated non-Hsa21 genes in each group demonstrated the pervasive effects of trisomy 21 on the whole genome. One hypothesis suggests that disruption of non-Hsa21 genes in DS is through modulation of transcription factors (TFs) [20]. Therefore, we searched the dysregulated genes in each group for TFs. Expectedly, ten TFs in C group and two in N group were deregulated (Table 2). We next asked whether targets of the TFs were accordingly altered in expression. We first checked *Pax5* which was down-regulated in both of the groups. Six genes, *CD19*,

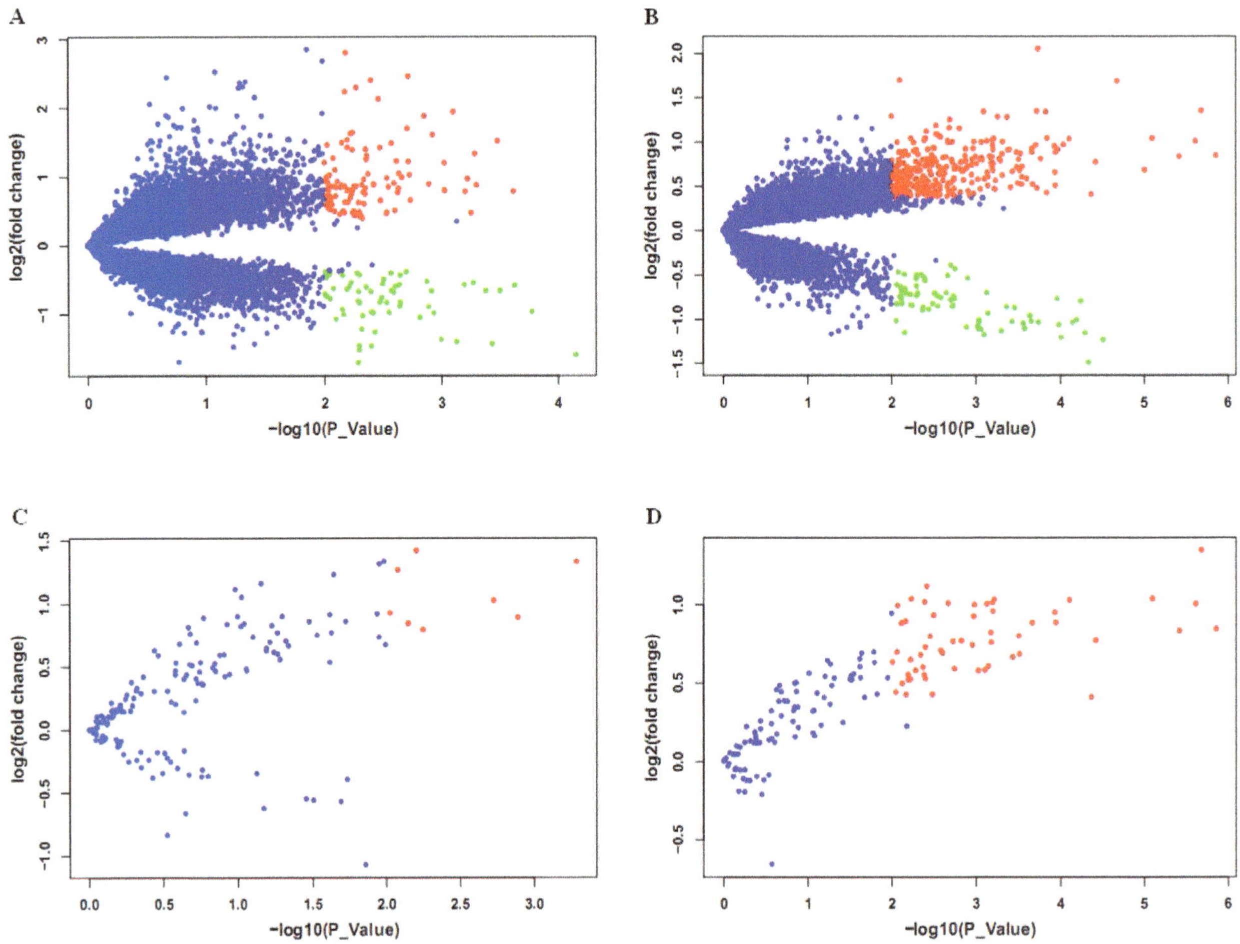

Figure 1. A global and local view of expression patterns in DS in the two age groups. Each dot represents a gene. Red and green dots indicate genes significantly up- and down-regulated in the DS samples, respectively. Blue dots indicate genes without change. (A) and (B) represent the expressed transcript clusters on whole genome in N and C group, respectively. (C) and (D) represent the expressed transcript clusters located on Hsa21 in N and C group, respectively.

CD79A, *BLNK*, *EBF1*, *FCER2* and *SPIB*, are activated by *Pax5* [21,22,23]. Expression of these targets was down-regulated in DS children and neonates, however, only *CD79A*, *BLNK*, *FCER2* and *SPIB* were expressed with significant alteration in DS children (Table S6). We further examined expression pattern of the known targets of the other TFs in our array data. A total of 31 genes can be activated or repressed by the TFs (Table S6); nonetheless, expression of the targets was not significantly altered accordingly. The reason for this could be that dysregulation of target gene expression also depends on other deregulated TFs or coactivators. These data indicate that deregulation of these TFs plays limited roles in massive disruption of non-Hsa21 gene expression in DS.

Functional analysis of the dysregulated genes

To explore biological functions of the dysregulated genes in each group, we analyzed the biological process and KEGG pathways through Onto-tools. The significantly enriched GO biological processes and KEGG pathways (Pc<0.05 after BH correction) were showed in Table 3. One GO biological process and two KEGG pathways were found to be enriched in N group. Likewise, one GO biological process and six KEGG pathways were enriched in C group.

Discussion

In present study, we analyzed gene expression difference between uncultured blood cells from DS and controls at the two age stages. A total of 383 and 174 dysregulated transcripts were identified in DS children and neonates, respectively and the array data were validated by approximately 2,500 QPCRs. Using functional profiling analysis, we identified significantly disrupted biological pathways which were relevant to immunodeficiency observed in DS.

The frequency (35.1%) of the down-regulated genes in DS neonates was higher than that (18.5%) in DS children. In amniotic fluid cell-free mRNA [18] and heart tissue [24] from DS fetuses, 46% and 59% of the dysregulated genes showed down-regulation, respectively. However, the reason for these observations is unclear. Given that TFs usually can activate or repress multiple targets, we postulated that the deregulated TFs exclusively in N or C group could contribute to the frequency difference observed in our study. *GRHL1* expression was up-regulated exclusively in DS neonates, however, its target, *P450scc* [25], showed normal expression. Similarly, the known targets of the altered TFs only in DS children were normally expressed (Table S6). The data point to limited contribution of TFs to the frequency difference between N and C

Table 1. The common dysregulated genes in the two age groups.

Gene symbol	Gene description	N group		C group		Chr.	Reference[b]
		Ratio	P	Ratio	P		
NAV1	neuron navigator 1	1.45	9.1E-03	1.35	4.7E-03	chr1	no
RALGPS2	Ral GEF with PH domain and SH3 binding motif 2	0.42	3.7E-03	0.43	9.9E-05	chr1	no
AFF3	AF4/FMR2 family, member 3	0.39	1.0E-03	0.61	6.6E-03	chr2	no
OSBPL10	oxysterol binding protein-like 10	0.33	1.0E-04	0.43	3.1E-05	chr3	no
TLR10	toll-like receptor 10	0.36	5.0E-03	0.46	9.0E-04	chr4	no
HLA-DOA	major histocompatibility complex, class II, DO alpha	0.50	1.2E-03	0.61	7.0E-04	chr6	no
HLA-DOB	major histocompatibility complex, class II, DO beta	0.43	4.7E-03	0.49	1.0E-04	chr6	no
PLXNA4	plexin A4	1.77	9.3E-03	1.60	6.0E-04	chr7	no
NPDC1	neural proliferation, differentiation and control, 1	1.50	9.6E-03	1.60	3.0E-04	chr9	no
PAX5	paired box 5	0.36	3.9E-03	0.55	1.9E-03	chr9	no
C13orf18	chromosome 13 open reading frame 18	0.49	4.7E-03	0.47	1.3E-03	chr13	no
P2RX5	purinergic receptor P2X, ligand-gated ion channel, 5	0.50	3.8E-03	0.63	6.9E-03	chr17	no
CD22	CD22 molecule	0.30	5.1E-03	0.49	2.0E-04	chr19	no
CLEC17A	C-type lectin domain family 17, member A	0.38	7.0E-04	0.55	4.0E-04	chr19	no
CST7	cystatin F (leukocystatin)	2.74	9.4E-03	1.80	6.3E-03	chr20	no
ATGAT3[a]	1-acylglycerol-3-phosphate O-acyltransferase 3	1.73	5.7E-03	2.05	8.1E-06	chr21	[12]
ATGAT3[a]	1-acylglycerol-3-phosphate O-acyltransferase 3	1.90	9.4E-03	1.79	1.4E-06	chr21	[12]
ITGB2	integrin, beta 2	2.03	1.9E-03	1.73	3.5E-03	chr21	[12,13,14,16,30]
PDXK	pyridoxal (pyridoxine, vitamin B6) kinase	2.51	5.0E-04	1.93	1.0E-04	chr21	[14,16]
PTTG1IP	pituitary tumor-transforming 1 interacting protein	1.79	7.1E-03	1.46	6.4E-03	chr21	[13,14,16]
TRPM2	transient receptor potential cation channel, subfamily M, member 2	2.67	6.3E-03	1.51	4.3E-03	chr21	[12]
SLC9A7	solute carrier family 9 (sodium/hydrogen exchanger), member 7	0.52	6.9E-03	0.69	5.1E-03	chrX	no

[a]Different transcript clusters of the same gene.
[b]Reference detecting dysregulation of the gene in DS studies.

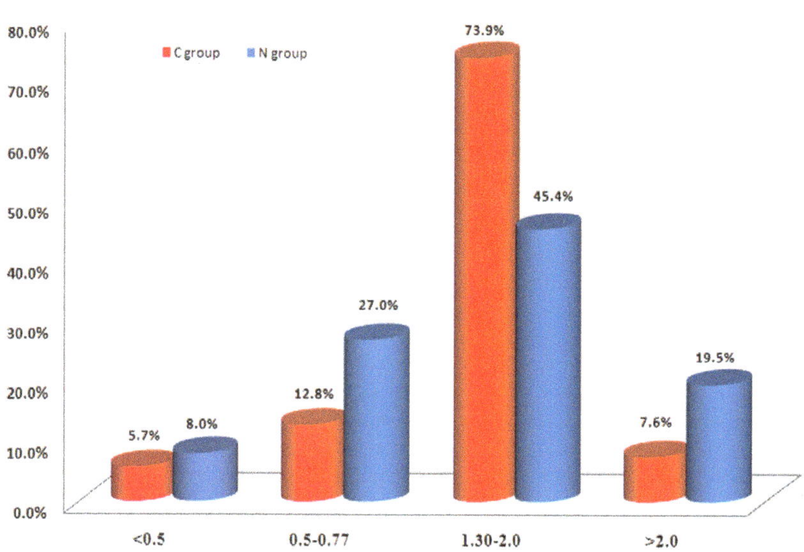

Figure 2. Fold change (DS/control) distribution of the dysregulated genes in DS. The x-axis indicates fold changes which are divided into four intervals and the y-axis represents percentage of the genes in one interval in all the dysregulated genes in one group.

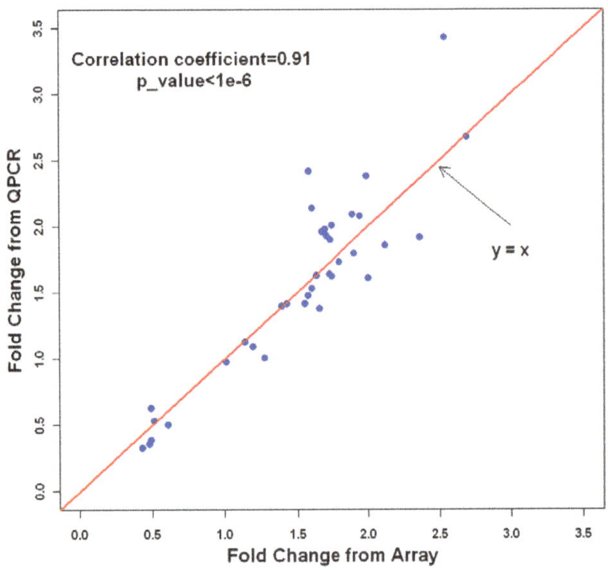

Figure 3. Comparison of fold change between array and QPCR.
A blue dot represents a gene.

group. Other mechanism responsible for the observations remains further postulated.

In DS neonates, only eight transcript clusters on Hsa21 were significantly up-regulated in expression. The finding is compatible with the previous data that a quite small number of Hsa21 genes are dysregulated in DS fetus samples [16,18,26]. We thus hypothesize that triplication of Hsa21 *per se* induces a modest dysregulation of Hsa21 genes during early developmental stages. The modest dysregulation might partially account for the phenotypes of DS individuals and mouse models at early stages. It has been reported that the basal forebrain cholinergic system is apparently normal in DS fetuses and infants, based on both neuronal numbers and choline acetyltransferase activity [27,28]. In Ts65Dn mice, the cerebellum has normal size at birth as compared to wild type littermates [29].

We analyzed functions of the 22 common dysregulated genes in both age groups. Among the 22 genes, *ITGB2, HLA-DOA, HLA-DOB, Pax5* and *CD22* are more associated with the immune system based on published data. *ITGB2* encodes β chain of the integrin lymphocyte functional antigen-1 (*LFA-1*) and its overexpression increases aggregation of DS lymphoblastoid cell lines (LCLs) [30]. *HLA-DOA* and *HLA-DOB* form HLA-DO which functions as a modulator of Ag presentation [31]. Their down-regulation in DS might affect efficiency of Ag presentation. Both *Pax5* and *CD22* were down-regulated in DS children and neonates. *Pax5* plays an essential role in B-lineage commitment [32]. Strikingly, *Pax5*(−/−) cells show slower growth, decreased surface IgM expression, and total loss of B cell receptor signaling [33]. *CD22*-deficient mice exhibits a reduced number of mature B cells in circulation and a significant diminution of surface Ig levels in these B cell subpopulations [34,35]. Deregulation of the five genes suggests their critical roles in immunodeficiency in DS patients.

We further explored biological functions of the dysregulated genes in the two age groups at a genome-wide level. In N group, innate immune response and two KEGG pathways, systemic lupus erythematosus (SLE) and leukocyte trans-endothelial migration, were enriched. The process or pathways are directly linked to the immune system, thereby supporting the hypothesis that the immune system in DS is intrinsically deficient from the very beginning [8]. Leukocyte trans-endothelial migration is vital for immune surveillance and inflammation [36]. In this pathway, *Vav2* expression in DS neonates was down-regulated (Table S3). The gene is an activator of *Cdc42*, *Rac1* and *RhoA* [37] which regulate actin dynamics and gene expression. Down-regulation of *Vav2* could disturb leukocyte migration, for knockdown of *Vav2* prevents *Rac* activation in some cells [38].

In C group, one biological process and six pathways were significantly deregulated in PBMCs of DS patients. In the process of leukocyte adhesion, overexpression of *ITGB2* and *ITGAL* whose products form integrin LAF-1 has been reported in LCLs from DS patients and increase adhesiveness of these cells [30]. It is worthy of note that product of *ITGB1* can form 11 heterodimeric integrins through pairing with alpha chain of integrins [39]. Up-regulated expression of the gene could have an impact on balance of the associated integrins. The first three pathways are focal adhesion, cell adhesion molecules (CAMs) and regulation of actin cytoskeleton which are implicated in cell growth, survival and mobility [40,41,42]. It has been shown that absolute total lymphocytes are significantly lower in DS children than controls [43,44,45]. Also, T lymphocyte maturation is impaired in DS individuals [46]. Our findings could be used to evaluate these observations associated with DS. The three remaining pathways are B cell receptor signaling pathway, primary immunodeficiency and natural killer cell mediated cytotoxicity. Individuals with DS display increased susceptibility to recurrent infections [4] and significantly reduced IgG2 levels [45]. Moreover, lower NK cytotoxic activity compared to controls has been observed in DS children and adults [47,48]. Disturbance of the three pathways could contribute to immune dysfunction observed in DS.

There are several potential limitations in this work. One limitation is that total RNA was isolated from distinct cell types and cell composition between N and C group. Another is smaller sample size in N group which could reduce statistical power. For a more comprehensive analysis of gene expression in DS, one would need to consider cell type difference and sample size.

Materials and Methods

Ethics statement

The Ethical Committee of the Chinese National Human Genome Center at Shanghai approved this project for the involvement of human subjects (approval ID: 201201) and parents of all the individuals provided written informed consent.

Samples and groups

All samples, including 15 DS patients and 22 controls, were collected at the Shanghai Children's Medical Centre from peripheral blood of the participants. All DS patients were confirmed by karyotyping. The samples were divided into two groups: N group (5 DS versus 7 control individuals, age: 3 days to 38 days) and C group (10 DS versus 15 control individuals, age: 1 year to 13 years). In each group, age and cell type were matched between DS and controls. Although the mean age of all the DS individuals was less than that of all control individuals, the difference was not statistically significant ($p = 0.27$ and $p = 0.20$ for C and N group, respectively, Student's t test) (Table S4).

Total RNA isolation

From the 25 child samples (C group), peripheral blood mononuclear cells (PBMCs) were isolated from peripheral blood using Lympholyte ®-H (CEDARLANE), and total RNA was extracted using the mirVana^{TM} miRNA Isolation Kit (Invitrogen)

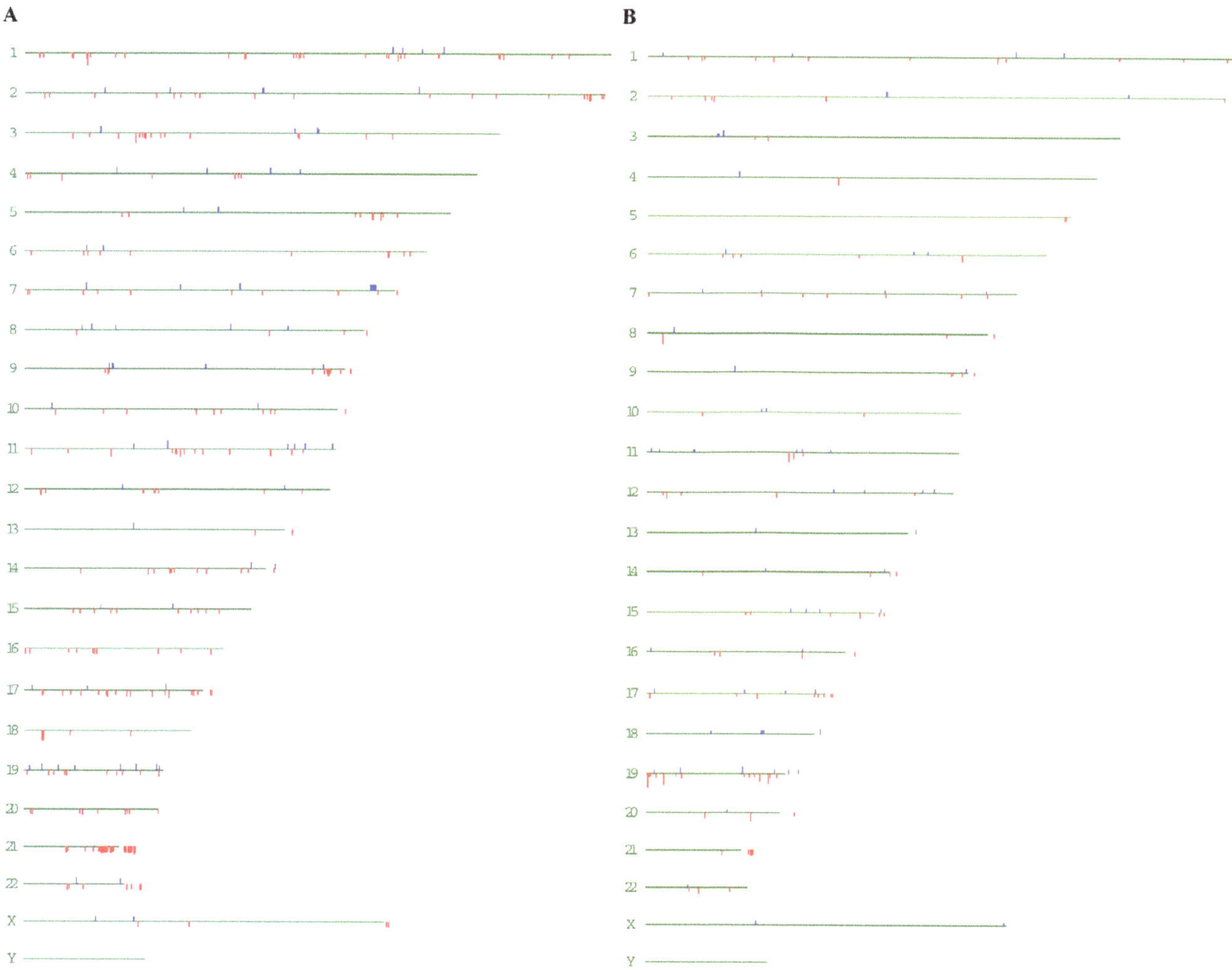

Figure 4. Chromosomal distribution of the differentially expressed genes. (A) and (B) indicate the chromosomal distribution of the 174 and 383 differentially expressed transcript clusters in N and C group between DS and age-matched controls, respectively. Blue bars represent lower expressed genes and red bars represent higher expressed genes in DS individuals.

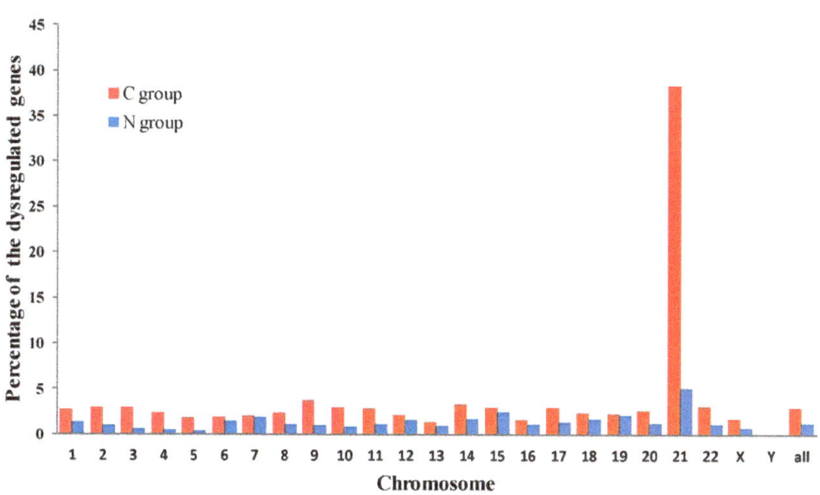

Figure 5. Percentage of dysregulated genes in expressed genes. Each bar indicates the percentage of the dysregulated genes in the expressed genes on each chromosome. "all" represents the percentage of total dysregulated genes in all expressed genes in each group.

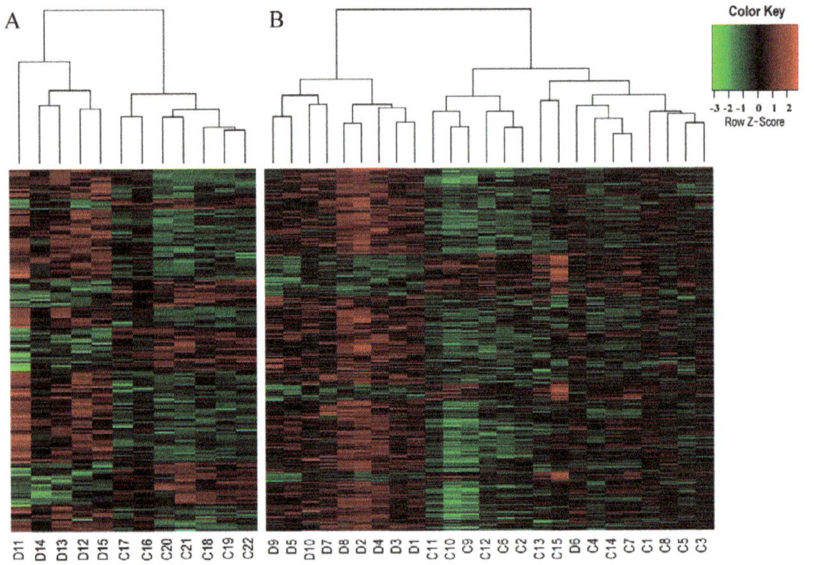

Figure 6. Hierarchical clustering of the differentially expressed genes. (A) hierarchical clustering of N group (DS: D11–D15 versus control: C16–C22) based on the 174 dysregulated transcript clusters (rows). (B) hierarchical clustering of C group (DS: D1–D10 versus control: C1–C15) based on the 383 differentially expressed transcript clusters. Red indicates higher expression and green indicates lower expression.

according to the manufacturer's protocol. The remaining 12 neonate samples (N group) had limited blood volume; therefore, total RNA was extracted from peripheral blood cells (PBCs). RNA concentration and purity was tested using a Nanodrop 2000c spectrophotometer (Thermo Scientific). RNA quality was further assessed with the Agilent 2100 Bioanalyzer using RNA 6000 Nanochips (Agilent Technologies). None of the 37 RNA samples had DNA contamination or RNA degradation. RNA samples were stored at −80°C for hybridization.

Screening of *GATA1* mutation in DS samples

DS neonates are at an increased risk of transient leukemia (TL) [49] and as many as 10% of them are affected by transient myeloid disorder [50]. Somatic mutations of *GATA1* exon 2 including insertions, deletions, and point mutations are found in almost all cases of DS-associated TL [51,52]. *GATA1* encodes hematopoietic transcription factor [52,53] and its mutation in DS samples could affect transcriptomes and lead to an unfair comparison between DS and controls. Therefore, we checked for the presence of *GATA1* mutation in DS neonates and children. Genomic DNAs from the DS samples were isolated with QIAamp Blood DNA Mini kits (Qiagen) according to the manufacturer's protocol.

Table 2. The dysregulated transcription factors in DS.

Accession number	Gene symbol	Gene description	Ratio (DS/control)	P_value (ANOVA)	Chromosome	Group
NM_005263	*GFT1*	growth factor independent 1 transcription repressor	1.82	2.9E-04	chr1	C
NM_001040667	*HSF4*	heat shock transcription factor 4	1.38	6.0E-04	chr16	C
NM_003121	*SPIB*	Spi-B transcription factor (Spi-1/PU.1 related)	0.49	9.1E-04	chr19	C
NM_001001890	*RUNX1*	runt-related transcription factor 1	1.50	1.8E-03	chr21	C
NM_002040	*GABPA*	GA binding protein transcription factor, alpha subunit 60 kDa	1.55	9.8E-03	chr21	C
NM_001951	*E2F5*	E2F transcription factor 5, p130-binding	0.49	8.7E-03	chr8	C
NM_016734	*PAX5*	paired box 5	0.55	1.9E-03	chr9	C
NM_022465	*IKZF4*	IKAROS family zinc finger 4 (Eos)	1.34	8.3E-03	chr12	C
NM_015995	*KLF13*	Kruppel-like factor 13	1.51	7.2E-03	chr15	C
NM_001031804	*MAF*	v-maf musculoaponeurotic fibrosarcoma oncogene homolog (avian)	1.99	8.6E-04	chr16	C
NM_198182	*GRHL1*	grainyhead-like 1 (Drosophila)	1.39	2.9E-03	chr2	N
NM_016734	*PAX5*	paired box 5	0.36	3.9E-03	chr9	N

Table 3. Enriched GO biological processes and KEGG pathways in the dysregulated genes in DS.

Age group	GO/KEGG ID	Biological Process/KEGG Pathway	Gene Symbol	P[a]	Pc[b]
Neonate group	GO: 45087	innate immune respones	*C1QC; FCGR1A; PGLYRP1; C1R; TLR10; CYBA; AKIRIN2*	<1.0E-04	9.3E-04
	KEGG: 05322	Systemic lupus erythematosus	*HLA-DOA; HLA-DOB; C1R; C1QC; FCGR1A; ELA2*	2.0E-04	9.0E-03
	KEGG: 04670	Leukocyte transendothelial migration	*CYBA; ITGB2; MAPK14; VAV2; MMP9*	1.1E-03	2.4E-02
Child group	GO: 7159	leukocyte adhesion	*CERCAM; ITGAL; ITGB2; ITGB1; EZR*	<1.0E-05	6.5E-03
	KEGG: 04510	Focal adhesion	*PDGFRB; MAP2K1; FYN; ITGA10; DIAPH1; COL6A2; PDGFD; CAPN2; SHC1; LAMB2; PPP1CA; ITGAV; ERBB2; ITGB1*	1.6E-06	6.9E-05
	KEGG: 04514	Cell adhesion molecules (CAMs)	*ITGB1; ITGB2; ITGAV; NCAM1; ITGAL; CD22; HLA-DOA; PTPRM; SPN; HLA-DOB; CNTAP2*	2.0E-06	6.9E-05
	KEGG: 04810	Regulation of actin cytoskeleton	*ITGB1; ITGB2; ITGAV; ITGAL; TIAM1; PPP1CA; PDGFRB; PDGFD; EZR; MAP2K1; DIAPH1; ITGA10*	6.6E-05	1.6E-03
	KEGG: 04662	B cell receptor signaling pathway	*CD79A; RASGRP3; BLNK; CD22B; CD78B; CD72*	4.0E-04	6.2E-03
	KEGG: 05340	Primary immunodeficiency	*BLNK; CD79A; TNFRSF13C; ADA*	1.6E-03	2.2E-02
	KEGG: 04650	Natural killer cell mediated cytotoxicity	*PRF1; MAP2K1; SHC1; CD244; FYN; ITGB2; ITGAL*	2.4E-03	2.8E-02

[a]Nominal p values.
[b]Adjusted p values after BH correction.

Amplicons including the whole *GATA1* exon 2 were obtained by PCR using forward (5′-TGTCTGAGGACCCCTTCTGT-3′) and reverse (5′-AAGCTTCCAGCCATTTCTGA-3′) primer and then sequenced. Sequence comparisons were performed by use of programs available from NCBI. However, no mutation of *GATA1* exon 2 was found in the DS samples used in this study (Files S 1).

Array hybridization

For each sample, ribosomal RNA was removed from 1 μg of total RNA with the RiboMinus Human/Mouse Transcriptome Isolation kit (Invitrogen) [54,55]. A similar approach for the depletion of abundant rRNA molecules was used in RNA-seq analysis [11,56], which could investigate a plethora of non-polyadenilated mRNA. cDNA was synthesized using the GeneChip WT (Whole Transcripts) cDNA Synthesis and Amplification Kit (Affymetrix) according to manufacturer's instructions. The sense cDNA was fragmented and end labeled by use of the GeneChip WT Terminal Labeling Kit (Affymetrix). Approximately 5.5 mg of biotin-labeled DNA target was hybridized to the Affymetrix GeneChip Human Exon 1.0 ST Array at 45°C for 16 hr following manufacturer's protocol (Affymetrix). Arrays were washed after hybridization, stained on a GeneChip Fluidics Station 450 and scanned on a GCS3000 Scanner (Affymetrix). Raw data were extracted from the scanned images and the Expression Console software (Affymetrix) was used for data analysis.

Normalization and summarization of array hybridization data

Expression Console software (Affymetrix) was used to quantile-normalize the probe fluorescence intensities over all 37 samples with PM-GCBG background correction. An iterative probe logarithmic intensity error (IterPlier) model (http://www.affymetrix.com/support/technical/technotes/plier_technote.pdf) was used to summarize the meta-probe set (representing gene expression) intensities. To stabilize variance, a constant of 16 was added to all probe set intensities, and then the signal values were $\log_2$ transformed. Removing the transcript clusters without any RefSeq-supported annotation, we generated the expression signals of 17,626 transcript clusters with core sets. A transcript cluster was considered to be reliably expressed when the $\log_2$-transformed expression signal was larger than 6.0 in at least 90% of the all samples in each group [54]. The remaining transcript clusters in each group, which met this criterion as determined by using R software (http://www.r-project.org/), were utilized for further analysis.

Raw microarray data have been deposited with GEO (Accession No. GSE35665).

Identifying differentially expressed genes in each age group

In this study, gender was less well matched between DS and controls in each group. Gender and interaction of DS and gender effects could have an impact on gene expression variation. To identify differentially expressed genes between DS and control individuals in each group which are independent of the two effects, we used analysis of variance (ANOVA) at an individual gene level.

For each gene, the following linear model was used:

$$y_{ijk} = \mu + D_i + G_j + DG_{ij} + \varepsilon_{ijk}$$

Where y_{ijk} is the normalized expression of the gene in log2 for *i*th disease type (DS or control), *j*th gender (male or female), and *k*th sample in each group; the symbols D, G and DG represent the fixed effects due to the disease, gender as well as interaction of disease×gender, respectively; the error for each gene for sample ijk is designated as εijk. ANOVA was performed using R software.

Multiple testing (BH correction) was performed on P values after ANOVA, no gene in DS neonates and only eight genes in DS children were significantly dysregulated ($q<0.05$). Thus, we referred to the method of Conti et al. [15] and applied P value after ANOVA and fold change (DS/control) for differentially expressed genes between DS and controls in each group. Specifically, genes with significantly different expression between DS and control individuals met following criteria: P value<0.01 and fold change (DS/control)>1.30 (up-regulated) or <0.77 (down-regulated). Here, fold change is equal to 2 ^ delta mean value, which is the error of the mean of $\log_2$ (DS) and mean of $\log_2$ (control).

Due to broad age range (from 1 year to 13 years) in C group, we determined correlation of differentially expressed genes with age and assessed whether the variable had effects on gene expression. Pearson's correlation test was performed for age, as described by Lockstone et al [13] and P values were adjusted by use of BH correction.

Quantitative real-time PCR

For validation of expression ratios between DS and control samples obtained from the array, total RNA was reverse transcribed into cDNA using PrimeScript™ RT reagent Kit (TaKaRa). Quantitative real-time PCR (QPCR) was performed on 11 genes from N group and 25 genes from C group using the LightCycler 480 (Roche Diagnostics) or the StepOne Plus (Applied Biosystems) systems with SYBR® Premix Ex Taq™ II (Perfect Real Time) (TaKaRa). Each gene was amplified in replicates of three. The genes and their primer sequences, designed by Primer 3 software [57], were described in Table S5. *UBA7* (NCBI Gene ID 7318) and *RNF4* (NCBI Gene ID 6047) were used as endogenous control genes [14]. For each sample, we normalized the mean cycle threshold value (C_t) by subtracting the mean of the C_t generated from the two reference genes. The same ANOVA as the array analysis above was used to test statistical significance of difference in gene expression between DS and controls.

Chromosomal distribution of significantly dysregulated genes in DS

Distribution of significantly dysregulated genes in DS individuals was tested against the null chromosomal distribution of the expressed transcript clusters in N and C group, respectively. Significant chromosomes were identified with binomial test ($Pc<0.05$ after BH correction), as described by Zhang et al [54]. STRIPE software was used to plot the chromosomal distribution of the dysregulated transcript clusters in each group [58].

Cluster analysis

For the transcript clusters in each group that were differentially expressed between DS and control samples, Euclidean distance of expression levels was computed and hierarchical clustering was performed using complete-linkage method (the hclust function in the stats package) in R software. Heatmaps were plotted using the heatmap.2 function in the gplots package with the "scale = 'row'" option set to "z-score normalize the rows".

GO and KEGG pathway analysis

Onto-Express and Pathway-Express in Onto-tools [59] were used to identify enriched Gene Ontology (GO) [60] terms and Kyoto Encyclopedia of Genes and Genomes (KEGG) [61] pathways, respectively. Among the differentially expressed genes in each group, GO terms or KEGG pathways that were over-represented relative to the gene set on the Affymetrix Human Exon 1.0 ST Array were selected (four or more hits [54], hypergeomatric test $Pc<0.05$ after BH correction).

Supporting Information

Figure S1 Box plots of normalized expression levels of 36 genes from QPCR. The Y-axis is normalized expression values and the x-axis is sample (D: DS versus C: control). Each panel represents a gene. DS and control in each panel is represented by red and green box in N group and by red and blue box in C group, respectively.

Figure S2 Hierarchical clustering of the differentially expressed non-Hsa21 genes. (A) hierarchical clustering of N group (DS: D11–D15 versus control: C16–C22) based on the non-Hsa21 dysregulated transcript clusters (rows). (B) hierarchical clustering of C group (DS: D1–D10 versus control: C1–C15) based on the non-Hsa21 differentially expressed transcript clusters.

Table S1 List of the dysregulated genes in neonate group.

Table S2 List of the dysregulated genes in child group.

Table S3 Comparison between microarray data and QPCR.

Table S4 Characteristics of samples.

Table S5 List of oligonucleotide primers used in the QPCR.

Table S6 Expression pattern of known targets of the transcription factors.

File S1 Sequences of *GATA1* exon 2 in DS samples.

Acknowledgments

We thank Jiong Tao (Shanghai Jiaotong University Xinhua Hospital, Shanghai, China) for karyotyping of all DS samples.

Author Contributions

Conceived and designed the experiments: SW GZ. Performed the experiments: CL LJ YB HX. Analyzed the data: CL SW LJ YB MY. Contributed reagents/materials/analysis tools: QC LF . Wrote the paper: CL SW.

References

1. Roper RJ, Reeves RH (2006) Understanding the basis for Down syndrome phenotypes. PLoS Genet 2: e50.
2. Epstein CJ, Korenberg JR, Anneren G, Antonarakis SE, Ayme S, et al. (1991) Protocols to establish genotype-phenotype correlations in Down syndrome. Am J Hum Genet 49: 207–235.

3. Hitzler JK, Zipursky A (2005) Origins of leukaemia in children with Down syndrome. Nat Rev Cancer 5: 11–20.
4. Ram G, Chinen J (2011) Infections and immunodeficiency in Down syndrome. Clin Exp Immunol 164: 9–16.
5. Lintas C, Sacco R, Persico AM (2012) Genome-wide expression studies in autism spectrum disorder, Rett syndrome, and Down syndrome. Neurobiol Dis 45: 57–68.
6. Bloemers BL, van Bleek GM, Kimpen JL, Bont L (2010) Distinct abnormalities in the innate immune system of children with Down syndrome. J Pediatr 156: 804–809, 809 e801–809 e805.
7. Bittles AH, Bower C, Hussain R, Glasson EJ (2007) The four ages of Down syndrome. Eur J Public Health 17: 221–225.
8. Kusters MA, Verstegen RH, Gemen EF, de Vries E (2009) Intrinsic defect of the immune system in children with Down syndrome: a review. Clin Exp Immunol 156: 189–193.
9. Giannone S, Strippoli P, Vitale L, Casadei R, Canaider S, et al. (2004) Gene expression profile analysis in human T lymphocytes from patients with Down Syndrome. Ann Hum Genet 68: 546–554.
10. Tang Y, Schapiro MB, Franz DN, Patterson BJ, Hickey FJ, et al. (2004) Blood expression profiles for tuberous sclerosis complex 2, neurofibromatosis type 1, and Down's syndrome. Ann Neurol 56: 808–814.
11. Costa V, Angelini C, D'Apice L, Mutarelli M, Casamassimi A, et al. (2011) Massive-scale RNA-Seq analysis of non ribosomal transcriptome in human trisomy 21. PLoS One 6: e18493.
12. Prandini P, Deutsch S, Lyle R, Gagnebin M, Delucinge Vivier C, et al. (2007) Natural gene-expression variation in Down syndrome modulates the outcome of gene-dosage imbalance. Am J Hum Genet 81: 252–263.
13. Lockstone HE, Harris LW, Swatton JE, Wayland MT, Holland AJ, et al. (2007) Gene expression profiling in the adult Down syndrome brain. Genomics 90: 647–660.
14. Ait Yahya-Graison E, Aubert J, Dauphinot L, Rivals I, Prieur M, et al. (2007) Classification of human chromosome 21 gene-expression variations in Down syndrome: impact on disease phenotypes. Am J Hum Genet 81: 475–491.
15. Conti A, Fabbrini F, D'Agostino P, Negri R, Greco D, et al. (2007) Altered expression of mitochondrial and extracellular matrix genes in the heart of human fetuses with chromosome 21 trisomy. BMC Genomics 8: 268.
16. Mao R, Wang X, Spitznagel EL Jr, Frelin LP, Ting JC, et al. (2005) Primary and secondary transcriptional effects in the developing human Down syndrome brain and heart. Genome Biol 6: R107.
17. Kahlem P, Sultan M, Herwig R, Steinfath M, Balzereit D, et al. (2004) Transcript level alterations reflect gene dosage effects across multiple tissues in a mouse model of down syndrome. Genome Res 14: 1258–1267.
18. Slonim DK, Koide K, Johnson KL, Tantravahi U, Cowan JM, et al. (2009) Functional genomic analysis of amniotic fluid cell-free mRNA suggests that oxidative stress is significant in Down syndrome fetuses. Proc Natl Acad Sci U S A 106: 9425–9429.
19. Benjamini Y, Hochberg Y (1995) Controlling the false discovery rate: A practical and powerful approach to multiple testing. Journal of the Royal Statistical Society B 57: 289–230.
20. FitzPatrick DR (2005) Transcriptional consequences of autosomal trisomy: primary gene dosage with complex downstream effects. Trends Genet 21: 249–253.
21. Schebesta A, McManus S, Salvagiotto G, Delogu A, Busslinger GA, et al. (2007) Transcription factor Pax5 activates the chromatin of key genes involved in B cell signaling, adhesion, migration, and immune function. Immunity 27: 49–63.
22. Pridans C, Holmes ML, Polli M, Wettenhall JM, Dakic A, et al. (2008) Identification of Pax5 target genes in early B cell differentiation. J Immunol 180: 1719–1728.
23. Visan I, Goller M, Berberich I, Kneitz C, Tony HP (2003) Pax-5 is a key regulator of the B cell-restricted expression of the CD23a isoform. Eur J Immunol 33: 1163–1173.
24. Bruce KD, Cagampang FR, Argenton M, Zhang J, Ethirajan PL, et al. (2009) Maternal high-fat feeding primes steatohepatitis in adult mice offspring, involving mitochondrial dysfunction and altered lipogenesis gene expression. Hepatology 50: 1796–1808.
25. Henderson YC, Frederick MJ, Jayakumar A, Choi Y, Wang MT, et al. (2007) Human LBP-32/MGR is a repressor of the P450scc in human choriocarcinoma cell line JEG-3. Placenta 28: 152–160.
26. Li CM, Guo M, Salas M, Schupf N, Silverman W, et al. (2006) Cell type-specific over-expression of chromosome 21 genes in fibroblasts and fetal hearts with trisomy 21. BMC Med Genet 7: 24.
27. Kish S, Karlinsky H, Becker L, Gilbert J, Rebbetoy M, et al. (1989) Down's syndrome individuals begin life with normal levels of brain cholinergic markers. J Neurochem 52: 1183–1187.
28. Lubec B, Yoo BC, Dierssen M, Balic N, Lubec G (2001) Down syndrome patients start early prenatal life with normal cholinergic, monoaminergic and serotoninergic innervation. J Neural Transm Suppl: 303–310.
29. Roper RJ, Baxter LL, Saran NG, Klinedinst DK, Beachy PA, et al. (2006) Defective cerebellar response to mitogenic Hedgehog signaling in Down [corrected] syndrome mice. Proc Natl Acad Sci U S A 103: 1452–1456.
30. Taylor GM, Haigh H, Williams A, D'Souza SW, Harris R (1988) Down's syndrome lymphoid cell lines exhibit increased adhesion due to the over-expression of lymphocyte function-associated antigen (LFA-1). Immunology 64: 451–456.
31. Nagarajan UM, Lochamy J, Chen X, Beresford GW, Nilsen R, et al. (2002) Class II transactivator is required for maximal expression of HLA-DOB in B cells. J Immunol 168: 1780–1786.
32. Nutt SL, Heavey B, Rolink AG, Busslinger M (1999) Commitment to the B-lymphoid lineage depends on the transcription factor Pax5. Nature 401: 556–562.
33. Nera KP, Kohonen P, Narvi E, Peippo A, Mustonen L, et al. (2006) Loss of Pax5 promotes plasma cell differentiation. Immunity 24: 283–293.
34. Tedder TF, Tuscano J, Sato S, Kehrl JH (1997) CD22, a B lymphocyte-specific adhesion molecule that regulates antigen receptor signaling. Annu Rev Immunol 15: 481–504.
35. Cesano A, Gayko U (2003) CD22 as a target of passive immunotherapy. Semin Oncol 30: 253–257.
36. van Buul JD, Hordijk PL (2004) Signaling in leukocyte transendothelial migration. Arterioscler Thromb Vasc Biol 24: 824–833.
37. Abe K, Rossman KL, Liu B, Ritola KD, Chiang D, et al. (2000) Vav2 is an activator of Cdc42, Rac1, and RhoA. J Biol Chem 275: 10141–10149.
38. Arora PD, Marignani PA, McCulloch CA (2008) Collagen phagocytosis is regulated by the guanine nucleotide exchange factor Vav2. Am J Physiol Cell Physiol 295: C130–137.
39. Takada Y, Ye X, Simon S (2007) The integrins. Genome Biol 8: 215.
40. Wozniak MA, Modzelewska K, Kwong L, Keely PJ (2004) Focal adhesion regulation of cell behavior. Biochim Biophys Acta 1692: 103–119.
41. Mammoto A, Ingber DE (2009) Cytoskeletal control of growth and cell fate switching. Curr Opin Cell Biol 21: 864–870.
42. Montoya MC, Sancho D, Vicente-Manzanares M, Sanchez-Madrid F (2002) Cell adhesion and polarity during immune interactions. Immunol Rev 186: 68–82.
43. Bloemers BL, Broers CJ, Bont L, Weijerman ME, Gemke RJ, et al. (2010) Increased risk of respiratory tract infections in children with Down syndrome: the consequence of an altered immune system. Microbes Infect 12: 799–808.
44. de Hingh YC, van der Vossen PW, Gemen EF, Mulder AB, Hop WC, et al. (2005) Intrinsic abnormalities of lymphocyte counts in children with down syndrome. J Pediatr 147: 744–747.
45. Broers CJ, Gemke RJ, Weijerman ME, Kuik DJ, van Hoogstraten IM, et al. (2012) Frequency of lower respiratory tract infections in relation to adaptive immunity in children with Down syndrome compared to their healthy siblings. Acta Paediatr 101: 862–867.
46. Guazzarotti L, Trabattoni D, Castelletti E, Boldrighini B, Piacentini L, et al. (2009) T lymphocyte maturation is impaired in healthy young individuals carrying trisomy 21 (Down syndrome). Am J Intellect Dev Disabil 114: 100–109.
47. Cossarizza A, Ortolani C, Forti E, Montagnani G, Paganelli R, et al. (1991) Age-related expansion of functionally inefficient cells with markers of natural killer activity in Down's syndrome. Blood 77: 1263–1270.
48. Montagna D, Maccario R, Ugazio AG, Nespoli L, Pedroni E, et al. (1988) Cell-mediated cytotoxicity in Down syndrome: impairment of allogeneic mixed lymphocyte reaction, NK and NK-like activities. Eur J Pediatr 148: 53–57.
49. Pine SR, Guo Q, Yin C, Jayabose S, Druschel CM, et al. (2007) Incidence and clinical implications of GATA1 mutations in newborns with Down syndrome. Blood 110: 2128–2131.
50. Groet J, McElwaine S, Spinelli M, Rinaldi A, Burtscher I, et al. (2003) Acquired mutations in GATA1 in neonates with Down's syndrome with transient myeloid disorder. Lancet 361: 1617–1620.
51. Vyas P, Crispino JD (2007) Molecular insights into Down syndrome-associated leukemia. Curr Opin Pediatr 19: 9–14.
52. Alford KA, Reinhardt K, Garnett C, Norton A, Bohmer K, et al. (2011) Analysis of GATA1 mutations in Down syndrome transient myeloproliferative disorder and myeloid leukemia. Blood 118: 2222–2238.
53. Wechsler J, Greene M, McDevitt MA, Anastasi J, Karp JE, et al. (2002) Acquired mutations in GATA1 in the megakaryoblastic leukemia of Down syndrome. Nat Genet 32: 148–152.
54. Zhang W, Duan S, Kistner EO, Bleibel WK, Huang RS, et al. (2008) Evaluation of genetic variation contributing to differences in gene expression between populations. Am J Hum Genet 82: 631–640.
55. Kwan T, Benovoy D, Dias C, Gurd S, Provencher C, et al. (2008) Genome-wide analysis of transcript isoform variation in humans. Nat Genet 40: 225–231.
56. Huber-Keener KJ, Liu X, Wang Z, Wang Y, Freeman W, et al. (2012) Differential Gene Expression in Tamoxifen-Resistant Breast Cancer Cells Revealed by a New Analytical Model of RNA-Seq Data. PLoS One 7: e41333.
57. Rozen S, Skaletsky H (2000) Primer3 on the WWW for general users and for biologist programmers. Methods Mol Biol 132: 365–386.
58. Ghai R, Lindemann H, Chakraborty T (2006) Integrated functional visualization of eukaryotic genomes. BMC Bioinformatics 7: 348.
59. Khatri P, Bhavsar P, Bawa G, Draghici S (2004) Onto-Tools: an ensemble of web-accessible, ontology-based tools for the functional design and interpretation of high-throughput gene expression experiments. Nucleic Acids Res 32: W449–456.
60. Ashburner M, Ball CA, Blake JA, Botstein D, Butler H, et al. (2000) Gene ontology: tool for the unification of biology. The Gene Ontology Consortium. Nat Genet 25: 25–29.
61. Kanehisa M, Goto S, Kawashima S, Okuno Y, Hattori M (2004) The KEGG resource for deciphering the genome. Nucleic Acids Res 32: D277–280.

17

Genetic Variation Is the Major Determinant of Individual Differences in Leukocyte Endothelial Adhesion

Michael A. Grassi[1]*, Vidhya Rao[1], Kathryn P. Winkler[1], Wei Zhang[2], Joseph D. Bogaard[1], Siquan Chen[3], Bonnie LaCroix[6], Divya Lenkala[6], Jalees Rehman[4], Asrar B. Malik[4], Nancy J. Cox[5], R. Stephanie Huang[6]

1 Department of Ophthalmology & Visual Sciences, University of Illinois at Chicago, Chicago, Illinois, United States of America, **2** Department of Pediatrics, University of Illinois at Chicago, Chicago, Illinois, United States of America, **3** Cellular Screening Center, Institute for Genomics and Systems Biology, University of Chicago, Chicago, Illinois, United States of America, **4** Department of Pharmacology, University of Illinois at Chicago, Chicago, Illinois, United States of America, **5** Section of Genetic Medicine, University of Chicago, Chicago, Illinois, United States of America, **6** Section of Hematology/Oncology, University of Chicago, Chicago, Illinois, United States of America

Abstract

Objective: To determine the genetic contribution to leukocyte endothelial adhesion.

Methods: Leukocyte endothelial adhesion was assessed through a novel cell-based assay using human lymphoblastoid cell lines. A high-throughput screening method was developed to evaluate the inter-individual variability in leukocyte endothelial adhesion using lymphoblastoid cell lines derived from different donors. To assess heritability, ninety-two lymphoblastoid cell lines derived from twenty-three monozygotic twin pairs and twenty-three sibling pairs were compared. These lymphoblastoid cell lines were plated with the endothelial cell line EA.hy926 and labeled with Calcein AM dye. Fluorescence was assessed to determine endothelial cell adhesion to each lymphoblastoid cell line. Intra-pair similarity was determined for monozygotic twins and siblings using Pearson pairwise correlation coefficients.

Results: A leukocyte endothelial adhesion assay for lymphoblastoid cell lines was developed and optimized (CV = 8.68, Z′-factor = 0.67, SNR = 18.41). A higher adhesion correlation was found between the twins than that between the siblings. Intra-pair similarity for leukocyte endothelial adhesion in monozygotic twins was 0.60 compared to 0.25 in the siblings. The extent to which these differences are attributable to underlying genetic factors was quantified and the heritability of leukocyte endothelial adhesion was calculated to be 69.66% (p-value<0.0001).

Conclusions: There is a heritable component to leukocyte endothelial adhesion. Underlying genetic predisposition plays a significant role in inter-individual variability of leukocyte endothelial adhesion.

Editor: Gerard Pasterkamp, University Medical Center Utrecht, Netherlands

Funding: We gratefully acknowledge support from the following organizations for this research: NIH K08 EY019089-02, National Eye Institute Core Grant EY001792 for Vision Research and an unrestricted grant from Research to Prevent Blindness, Inc., New York, NY. RSH received support from NIH/NIGMS grant K08GM089941, NIH/NCI Grant R21 CA139278, NIH/NIGMS Pharmacogenomics of Anticancer Agents grant U01GM61393, the University of Chicago Breast Cancer SPORE Career Development Award, the University of Chicago Cancer Center Support Grant (#P30 CA14599) and the National Center for Advancing Translational Sciences of the NIH [UL1RR024999]. The funders had no role in study design, data collection and analysis, decision to publish, or preparation of the manuscript.

Competing Interests: The authors have declared that no competing interests exist.

* E-mail: grassim@uic.edu

Introduction

Leukocyte endothelial adhesion has been implicated as a key disease process in many conditions of major public health import such as multiple sclerosis, atherosclerosis, inflammatory bowel disease, diabetic retinopathy, malignancy, pulmonary edema, rheumatoid arthritis, and stroke [1,2]. Attempts to target leukocyte trafficking as a treatment for these conditions have been successful, but often have serious complications given the multiple off-target effects of many of these drugs e.g. prednisone [2,3]. Leukocyte–endothelial interactions are primarily attributed to cell-surface adhesion molecules including the integrins, members of the IgG superfamily, and selectins. There remain many other, yet undefined, molecules and signaling pathways that mediate leukocyte endothelial adhesion [4]. Improved characterization of the molecular underpinnings of leukocyte endothelial adhesion could have far reaching biomedical impact as it may improve therapeutic targeting and specificity for many common diseases. Genomic studies may have the capability of accomplishing this goal, but require there to be an underlying genetic basis for leukocyte endothelial adhesion.

Corroborating lines of evidence suggest that genetic variability contributes to differences in leukocyte endothelial adhesion. For instance, it has been shown that the expression of cell surface adhesion molecules on endothelial cells varies between individuals [5] and is highly heritable. Rainwater et al. demonstrated that in the setting of TNF-α there is a significant genetic contribution to the expression of E-selectin, VCAM, and ICAM-1 [6]. Moreover, hematologic malignancies like leukemia caused by underlying chromosomal re-arrangements reveal differential gene expression of adhesion molecules resulting in altered endothelial adhesion [7]. For instance, in Burkitt lymphoma endothelial adhesion is significantly decreased [8]. Findings in a rare Mendelian condition, leukocyte adhesion deficiency, also suggest that there is a genetic component to leukocyte endothelial adhesion. Leukocyte adhesion deficiency is an immunodeficiency characterized by severe recurrent bacterial infections [9]. The condition is caused by a lack of leukocyte β-2 integrins that produce an impairment of leukocyte interactions necessary to fight infection. A broad clinical range of leukocyte adhesion deficiency exists that correlates with the severity of the pathogenic mutation. Similarly, individuals with Down's syndrome (Trisomy 21) have a genetic basis for their enhanced adhesive characteristics in comparison to normal subjects [10]. Trisomy 21 leukocytes demonstrate increased expression of CD18 integrin, which is found on chromosome 21 [10]. Taken together these findings suggest that there may be a significant underlying genetic component that contributes to differences in leukocyte endothelial adhesion.

To explore the hypothesis that inter-individual genetic variability contributes to differences in leukocyte endothelial adhesion we assessed adhesion in monozygotic twins and compared them to matched sibling pairs. We quantified the extent to which these differences are attributable to underlying genetic factors [11,12] to determine the heritability of leukocyte endothelial adhesion.

Materials and Methods

Ethics

Participants gave written informed consent. The University of Illinois at Chicago Institutional Review Board approved all protocols and informed consent documents in accordance with federal regulations and the principles expressed in the Declaration of Helsinki.

Cell lines and Cell culture

Ninety–two lymphoblastoid cell lines (twenty-three monozygotic twin pairs and twenty-three sibling pairs) were purchased from Coriell Institute for Medical Research (http://ccr.coriell.org/) (Table S1). The minimum number of lymphoblastoid cell lines pairs required for the study was estimated as previously described [13]. Monozygotic twin cell lines used in the study were GM14381, GM14382, GM14405, GM14406, GM14414, GM14417, GM14432, GM14433, GM14452, GM14453, GM14467, GM14468, GM14478, GM14479, GM14506, GM14507, GM14520, GM14521, GM14568, GM14569, GM14581, GM14582, GM14408, GM14409, GM14447, GM14448, GM14592, GM14593, GM14474, GM14475, GM14503, GM14504, GM14532, GM14533, GM14535, GM14536, GM14583, GM14584, GM14476, GM14477, GM14480, GM14481, GM14495, GM14496, GM14501, GM14502. The sibling cell lines used in the study were GM7004, GM07012, GM07044, GM7052, GM07343, GM07344, GM11922, GM11923, GM11982, GM11983, GM11985, GM11986, GM11997, GM11999, GM12036, GM12038, GM12104, GM12105, GM12147, GM12149, GM12150, GM12157, GM11834, GM11841, GM12047, GM12048, GM07351, GM07352, GM14666, GM14672, GM14661, GM14662, GM14682, GM14704, GM12328, GM12265, GM11871, GM11872, GM13117, GM13118, GM12276, GM12277, GM07023, GM07059, GM07062, GM07053. Sibling pairs were all comprised of full siblings. Ramos, a Burkitt Lymphoma cell line obtained from ATCC (CRL-1596, ATCC, Manassas, VA) was a kind gift from Dr. Chandran (Rosalind Franklin University, North Chicago, IL). A Trisomy 21 lymphoblastoid cell line, GM03716, was purchased from Coriell cell repositories (Camden, New Jersey). U937, a monocytic cell line, and EA.hy926, a transformed endothelial cell line, were obtained from ATCC (American Type Culture Collection, Manassas, VA). Peripheral blood mononuclear cells were obtained from a healthy control donor.

Leukocyte-Endothelial Cell Adhesion Assay

Lymphoblastoid cell lines were plated on the endothelial cell line EA.hy926 to test their adhesion. EA.hy926 cells were counted using the Beckman coulter counter, plated at a density of 12,000 cells/well in flat clear bottom black 96-well plates (Corning, Acton, MA), and cultured to confluency for 48 hours. On the day of the assay, lymphoblastoid cell lines or peripheral blood mononuclear cells were suspended in RPMI 1640 with 10% FBS at a concentration of 8×10^5 cells/mL and incubated with 2 μM Calcein AM for 30 min at 37°C. The cells were collected and subjected to three washes with PBS (1X, Gibco, Life technologies, Grand Island, NY) to remove the free Calcein AM. Calcein AM labeled cells were added at a density of 50,000 cells/well on top of confluent monolayer cultures of EA.hy926 cells in 96-well plates and incubated for 30 min at 37°C. Nonadherant cells were removed by an optimized automated wash protocol adapted using the EP3 liquid handling system. Calcein AM fluorescence in the labeled cells was assessed by the high content imager Acumen at an excitation and emission wavelength of 485/535 nm before and after each wash. Endothelial adhesion for each cell line was determined by measuring the total area of fluorescence in relative fluorescence units (RFU) of each well following the third wash. The (%) remaining RFU/Input was determined by the following formula: [Total area of fluorescence (RFU) following third wash / Total area of fluorescence (RFU) before wash] ×100. A standard curve for lymphoblastoid cell lines, peripheral blood mononuclear cells, and the control cell lines (Trisomy lymphoblastoid cell line, U937, and Ramos) was generated using known concentrations of respective cell lines and fitting to a four parametric logistic curve (Figure S1). The % adherent cells were derived from the standard curve. The leukocyte endothelial adhesion (LEA) of each lymphoblastoid cell line was represented as either (%) of input relative fluorescent units (RFU) or (%) of input cell number.

Statistical Analysis

A mean, standard deviation, and coefficient of variation (CV) of leukocyte endothelial adhesion for each lymphoblastoid cell line was calculated. Plates included positive and negative controls for quality control. Positive controls were a Trisomy 21 lymphoblastoid cell line that also provided a reference for the control of inter-plate variability. Ramos, a Burkitt lymphoma cell line, served as an additional positive control. The negative controls were EA.hy926 cells alone. A Z′-factor and CV for each plate was determined. A composite Z′-factor was determined to assess the overall robustness of the assay using the equation $[Z'=1-\frac{(3*\sigma_p+3*\sigma_n)}{(3*\mu_p-3*\mu_n)}]$with Trisomy 21 as the positive control and Ramos as the negative control. A Z′-factor of >0.5 is equivalent to a separation of 12 standard deviations between μ_p and μ_n.

Intra-pair similarity was determined for monozygotic twins and siblings using the interclass correlation coefficient (ICC). Heritability was estimated by using the twinan90 function in the R package [14]. Sibling pairs were treated as dizygotic twins and heritability $(h^2)$was estimated using the equation, $[h^2 = 2x(_{ICC}MZ - _{ICC}SIB)]$, where r corresponds to the interclass correlation coefficient of twin and sibling pairs respectively [15].

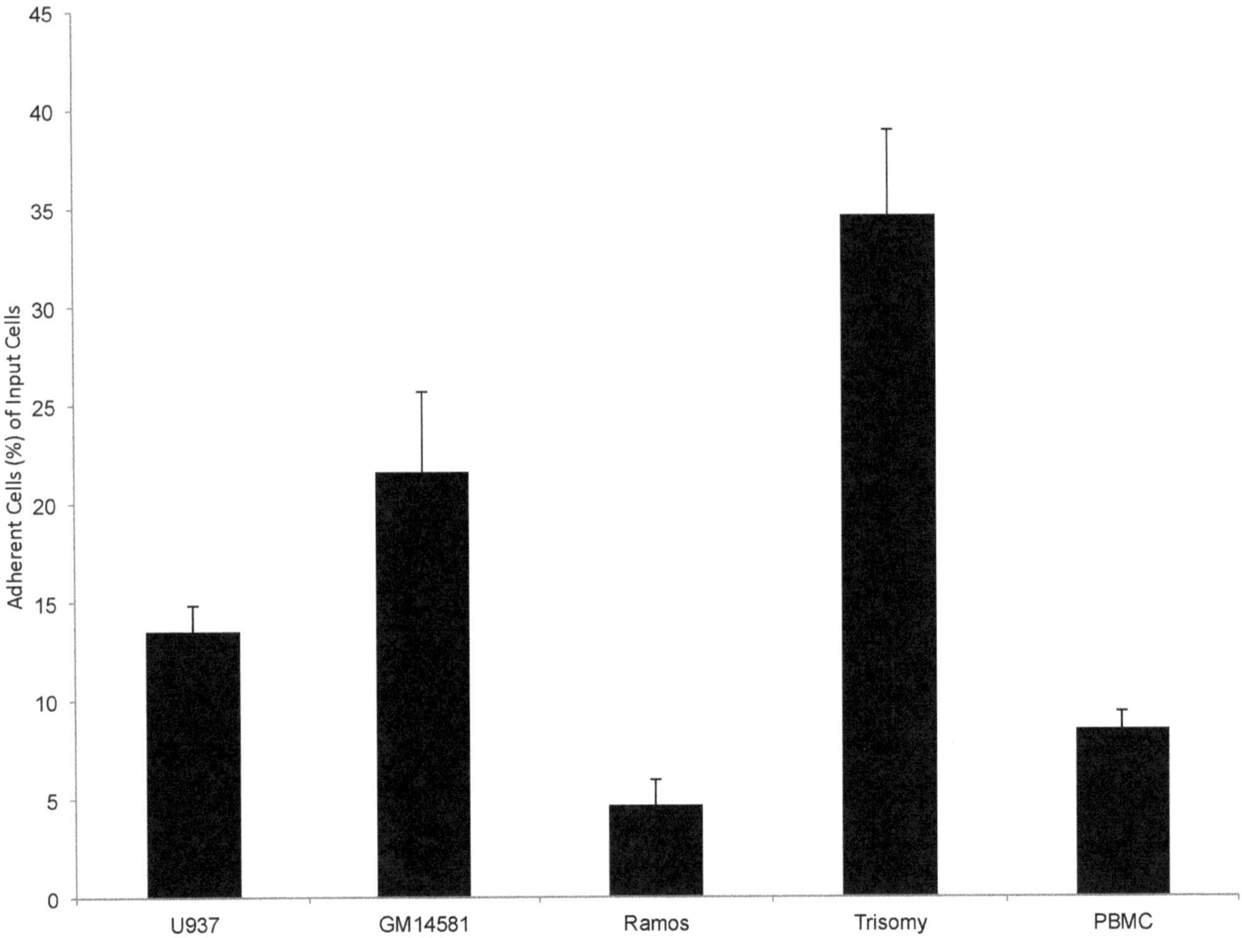

Figure 1. Percentage of adherent cells by sample type. Number of cells is the percentage remaining after three washes. The assay reveals a large dynamic range between the Burkitt lymphoma Ramos cell line (negative control) and the Trisomy 21 lymphoblastoid cell line (positive control). Consistent with other reports, peripheral blood mononuclear cells demonstrated approximately 5–10% adhesion. Percentages were derived based on conversion of relative fluorescent units from a standardized curve.

We performed 10,000 simulations by randomizing the samples to generate a null distribution. We estimated an empirical p-value for the heritability. Linear Pearson's correlation coefficient (r) was used to determine the contributions of potential confounders e.g., subject age, gender, cell growth rate, ethnicity and transformation time. Statistical calculations and graphing were performed using Intercooled Stata 8 (Stata Corp., College Station, TX).

Results

Adhesion assay development, optimization and validation

We developed and optimized a leukocyte endothelial adhesion assay for lymphoblastoid cell lines (CV = 8.68, Z′-factor = 0.67, SNR = 18.41). Specifically, we have successfully converted this assay onto a 96-well plate platform amenable to robotic screening. The advantage of this format is that it affords a high degree of consistency and repeatability between runs (Figure 1). A 96-well plate platform is particularly advantageous for this experiment given the large numbers of samples that were utilized. A total of 8 technical replicates were performed to determine the leukocyte endothelial adhesion of each lymphoblastoid cell line. For a given plate, standard deviations and coefficients of variation significantly less than 10% suggest that there is little variability between replicates of a given cell line. In addition, we calculated a Z′-factor of 0.67 for the assay, suggesting that the assay is excellent from the standpoint of quality control. The Z′-factor is a measure of the statistical effect that assesses the suitability of a particular assay for use in a full-scale high-throughput screen by essentially comparing the range between the positive vs. the negative control samples. In order to control for plate to plate variability, samples were standardized based on the adhesion of the Trisomy 21 lymphoblastoid cell line and the adhesion of the U937 monocytic cell line on each plate. For instance, the leukocyte endothelial adhesion of lymphoblastoid cell line GM14581 was tested in three different plates and its ratio of adhesion relative to the Trisomy 21 cell line was 0.64, 0.67 and 0.68 respectively. Standardized coefficients for the same cells (GM14581, Ramos and U937) on different plates did not demonstrate a statistically significant difference (p-value = 0.62).

The assay demonstrates a large dynamic range, with close to a 7-fold difference, evident between the control cell lines, namely the low adhesive Burkitt lymphoma Ramos line and the highly adhesive Trisomy 21 lymphoblastoid cell lines (Figure 1). Specifically, in terms of leukocyte endothelial adhesion the Ramos line revealed 5% of cells remaining whereas over 35% of the Trisomy

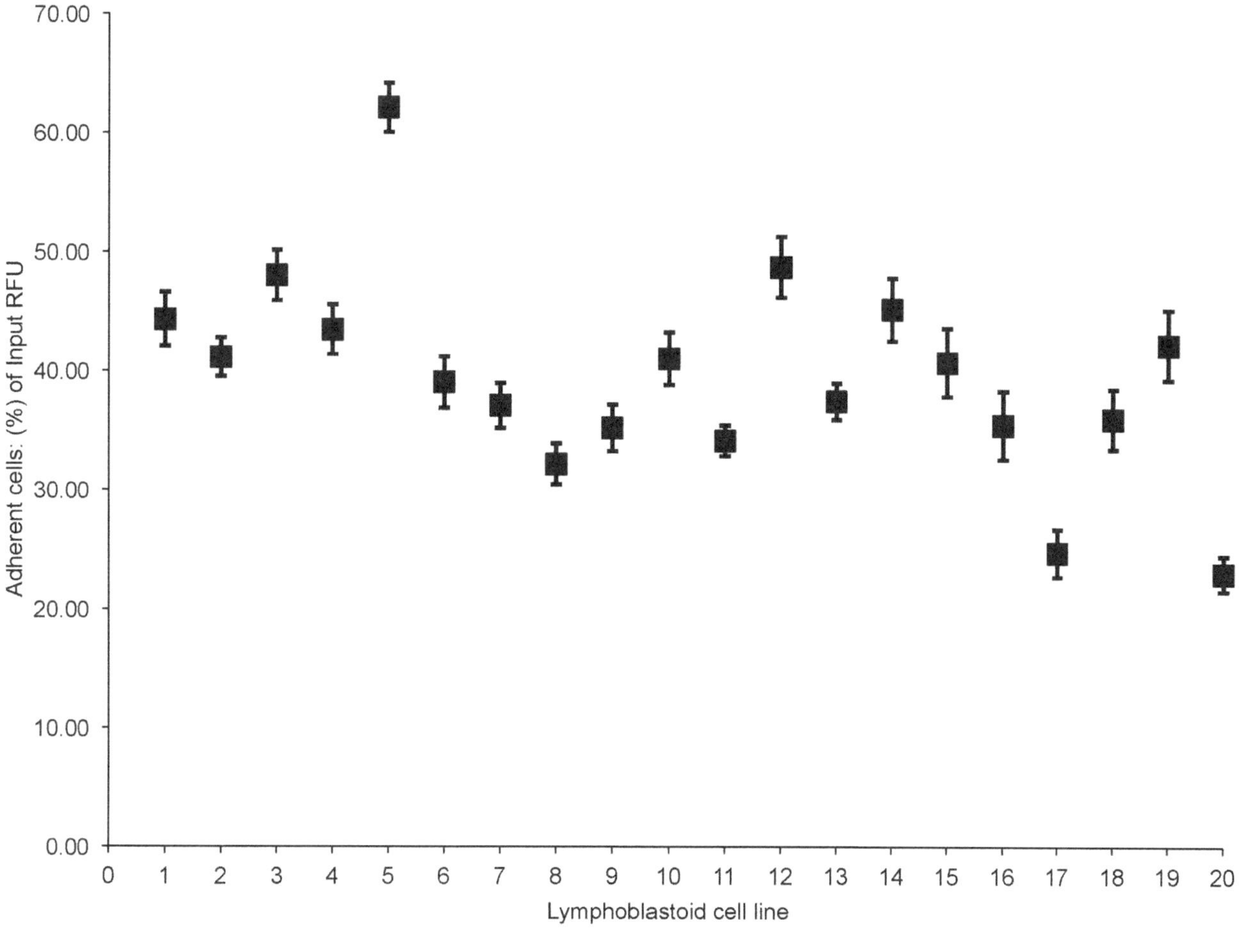

Figure 2. Variations in leukocyte endothelial adhesion among 20 selected unrelated lymphoblastoid cell lines. Leukocyte endothelial adhesion was assessed in 20 unrelated lymphoblastoid cell lines. For each cell line, 8 technical replicates were obtained per plate. The figure reveals inter-lymphoblastoid cell line differences in leukocyte endothelial adhesion with a range from 22.42–61.12% input RFU, a mean of 40.25% (std. dev. ±10.37), and a median of 39.80%. Minimal variability is evident in the assay with a CV of less than 10% (CV = 8.68, Z′-factor = 0.67, SNR = 18.41).

21 cells were remaining following three washes. Normal lymphoblastoid cell lines fell in the middle of this range. Peripheral blood mononuclear cells revealed 5–10% adhesion, consistent with prior reports [10,16,17].

Inter-individual Variation in Leukocyte Endothelial Adhesion

Using twenty unrelated lymphoblastoid cell lines generated from normal subjects, we measured their leukocyte endothelial adhesion in order to estimate the inter-individual variability obtained through our high-throughput assay. Figure 2 reveals the range of adhesion in normal lymphoblastoid cell lines. Specifically the range was from 22.42–62.12% input RFU with a mean of 40.25% (std. dev. ±10.37), and a median of 39.80%.

Heritability of Leukocyte Endothelial Adhesion

We were interested to assess the extent to which genetic factors contributed to inter-individual differences in leukocyte endothelial adhesion. We performed a heritability study for leukocyte endothelial adhesion utilizing lymphoblastoid cell lines derived from identical twins and those derived from matching sibling pairs. The hypothesis was that there would be greater correlation between the adhesion of the identical twins than that of the sibling pairs. Summarized subject data are reported in Table S1. Figure 3 reveals that this was indeed the case. Figure 3 demonstrates the leukocyte endothelial adhesion for each pair of lymphoblastoid cell lines. A higher correlation in adhesion was observed between the twins (Fig. 3A) than in the siblings (Fig. 3B) with an intra-pair similarity for leukocyte endothelial adhesion in monozygotic twins of 0.60 compared to 0.25 in the sibling pairs. The extent of heritability is essentially an extension of the excess correlation seen in monozygotic twins versus sibling pairs. We quantified the extent to which these differences are attributable to underlying genetic factors [11,12] and found the heritability of leukocyte endothelial adhesion to be 69.66% (p-value$<$0.0001) (Fig. 3C), meaning that essentially 70% of the variability in leukocyte endothelial adhesion between individuals can be attributed to genetic factors.

Role of confounding factors

It is certainly possible, though, that confounding factors contribute to differences in leukocyte endothelial adhesion between lymphoblastoid cell lines. In Figure 4, we sought to identify non-genetic factors that could potentially confound our analysis. We assessed whether or not there was any correlation of leukocyte endothelial adhesion for 20 unrelated individuals with subject age (Figure 4A), gender (Figure 4B), cell growth rate

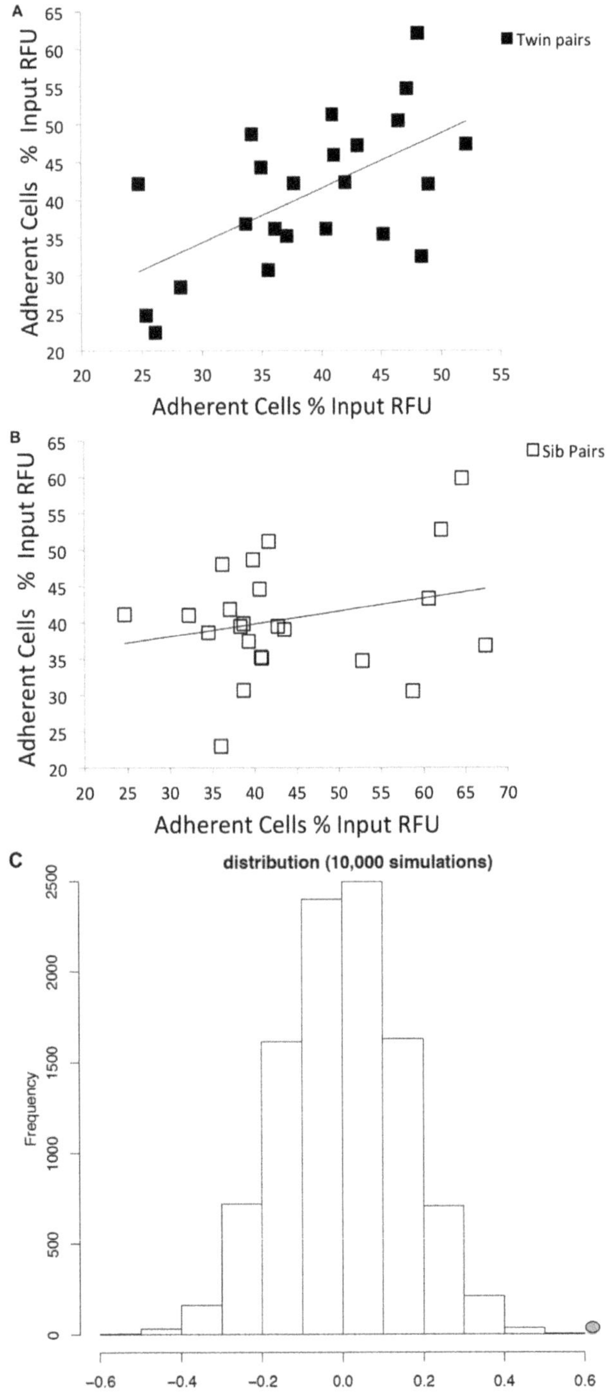

Figure 3. Intra-pair similarity for leukocyte endothelial adhesion is greater in monozygotic twins than sibling pairs. Figure 3A shows the correlation in adhesion of 23 monozygotic twin pairs compared to 23 matched sibling pairs (Figure 3B). Axes represent the % of adherent cells based on RFU, with each axis corresponding to one of the two subjects for a given pair. A higher mean correlation is seen in the identical twins ($_{ICC}$MZ 0.60) as compared to the siblings ($_{ICC}$SIB 0.25). The resultant heritability had an empirical p-value$<$0.0001 based on 10,000 simulations by randomizing the samples to generate a null distribution (Figure 3C). The round dot represents the observed heritability value from our study.

(Figure 4C) transformation time (Figure 4D) and ethnicity (Figure 4E). Subject age (p-value = 0.71), gender (p-value = 0.23), transformation time (p-value = 0.49), cell growth rate (p-value = 0.94) and ethnicity (p-value = 0.49) all had no correlation with endothelial adhesion. Sample constraints prevented matching the two groups exactly based ethnicity. There is a suggestion in the literature that there may be some variation in adhesion based on ethnicity [18,19]. In hindsight, this observation is not surprising in light of our heritability analysis as ethnicity is a crude measure of genetic background. In this study we observed no difference in mean adhesion between white and Black subjects. More importantly, from the standpoint of confounding there was also no ethnic based difference in the variance of adhesion (p-value = 0.57). A literature search did not reveal any other covariates known to influence leukocyte endothelial adhesion.

Discussion

The leukocyte endothelial adhesion assay we developed is able to sensitively and reproducibly detect differences in leukocyte adhesion to endothelial cell monolayers. This novel high-throughput assay was able for the first time to reveal the extent to which the important biological property of leukocyte endothelial adhesion is impacted by genetic variation.

Lymphoblastoid cell lines have evolved into a powerful model system for functional population-based studies in humans. Lymphoblastoid cell lines are transformed cell lines derived from a subject's circulating B-lymphocytes. They were originally generated as a perpetual resource of a specific subject's DNA. Given the associated difficulties with maintenance, storage, collection, and the control of confounding variables in clinical samples, they have evolved into a popular model system [20,21]. In large part this trend is due to the fact that lymphoblastoid cell lines to date are the only feasible and cost-effective method to conduct functional, cellular or molecular assays in large population-based human studies. As a cell line, environmental factors can be controlled between lines, which removes many confounders that are routinely found in clinical samples. Hence, transformation of clinical samples into lymphoblastoid cell lines provides convenience, replicability, and environmental uniformity.

In this study, we sought to explore the feasibility of using lymphoblastoid cell lines to assess the heritability of leukocyte endothelial adhesion. It was first necessary to create a high-throughput assay for leukocyte endothelial adhesion that would enable us to compare the adhesion of multiple different cell lines. We developed a robust assay (Z'-factor = 0.67). The excellent Z'-factor suggests that the variability introduced by the washing step in other high-throughput assays was not an issue in our assay [22].

To our knowledge the present paper is the first study to determine the heritability of leukocyte endothelial adhesion. Current approaches have the power to reveal the genetic network underlying this trait. For these genetic tools to work, though, there must be a heritable basis to leukocyte endothelial adhesion. A substantial body of literature implicates genetic variation as a basis for differential leukocyte adhesion [7,8] in conditions that include chromosomal alterations [10], Mendelian conditions [9], and complex disease [23]. In this study, we quantitate the extent that genetic factors contribute to inter-individual variability in leukocyte endothelial adhesion. By comparing leukocyte endothelial adhesion between monozygotic twins and matched sibling pairs, we found that 70% of the variation in leukocyte endothelial adhesion is due to underlying genetic factors.

The use of lymphoblastoid cell lines is a potential limitation of this study, though. An issue regarding the use of lymphoblastoid

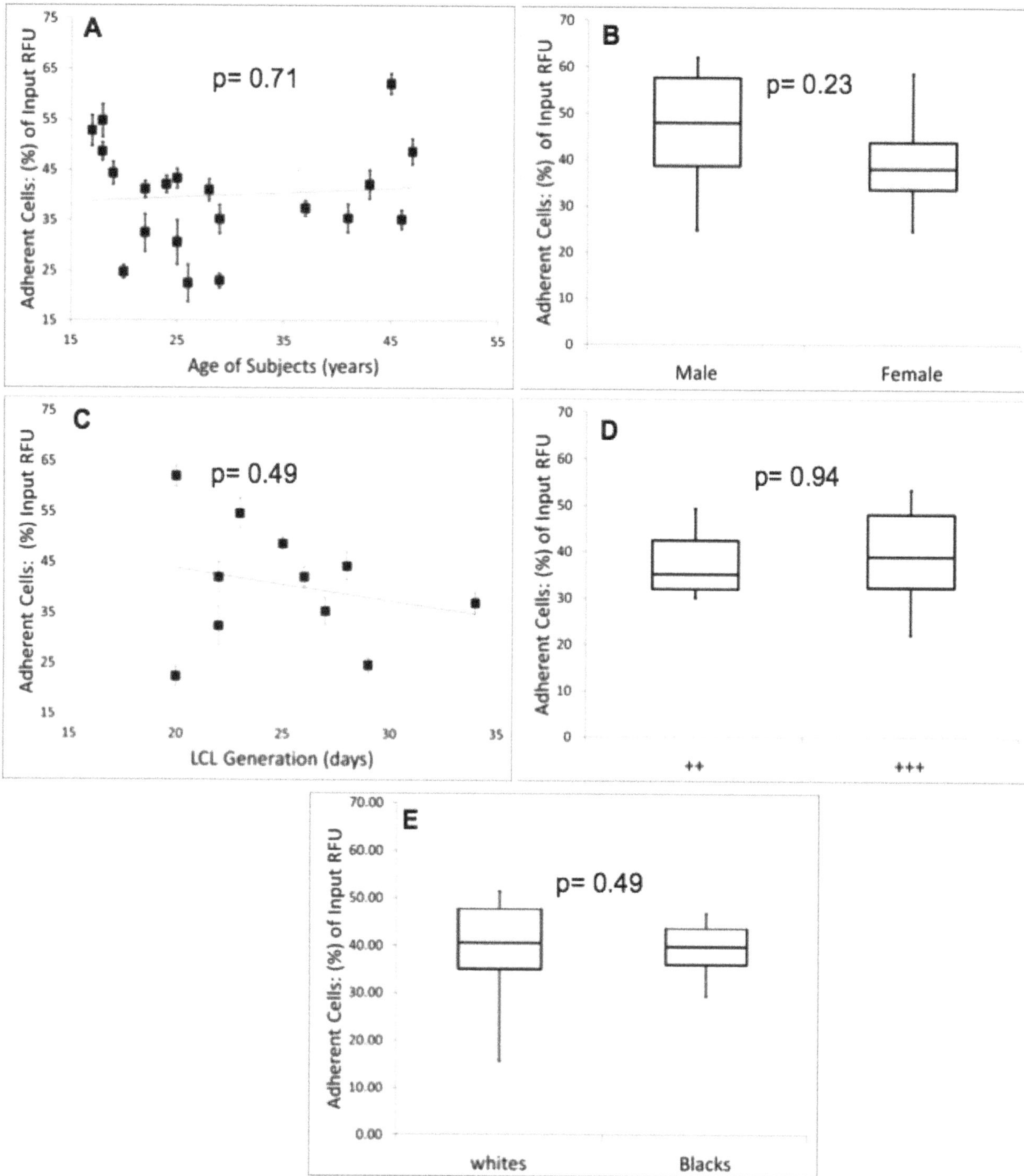

Figure 4. Impact of confounding factors on leukocyte endothelial adhesion among 20 unrelated lymphoblastoid cell lines. In 4A, we explored the role of subject age on leukocyte endothelial adhesion. No correlation was observed (p-value = 0.77). Figure 4B stratifies adhesion by gender. As found in prior studies leukocyte endothelial adhesion is slightly decreased in women, although this was not statistically significant in our cohort (p-value = 0.23). In figure 4C we determined if the duration of lymphoblastoid cell line generation from peripheral blood mononuclear cell affected the adhesion and found no correlation. In 4D we assessed the impact of cell culture growth on adherence. Lymphoblastoid cell line slow culture growers with a doubling time of seven days are represented by ++ and fast culture growers with a doubling time of 3 days are represented by +++. We found that cell cutlure growth conditions did not affect adhesion (p-value = 0.85). In figure 4E we assesed the effect of ethnicity on LEA and observed that ethnicity had no effect on LEA (p-value = 0.49).

cell lines is the extent to which they serve as relevant surrogates for different primary tissues. Previous work has demonstrated the broad translatability of studies with lymphoblastoid cell lines [24], in particular for complex traits in which white blood cells are the most relevant human tissue as in leukocyte endothelial adhesion or the diseases of type 1 diabetes, Crohn's disease, and multiple sclerosis [25,26]. While endothelial cells are important in mediating leukocyte endothelial adhesion and there are unique molecular features specific to endothelial cells [27,28], it is their interaction with white blood cells that results in the leukocyte endothelial adhesion phenotype [29]. Hence, it is likely that many of the genetic factors influencing leukocyte endothelial adhesion can be identified with lymphoblastoid cell lines alone.

A persistent concern about the usefulness of lymphoblastoid cell lines is that changes associated with the Epstein-Barr virus transformation reduce their value and relevance as a model. The virus transformation of primary white blood cells does change some of the cellular properties within the lymphoblastoid cell lines [30]. The Epstein-Barr virus transformation induces a shift in white blood cells to an activated state [31,32]. Caliskan et al. [30] identified an enrichment of gene expression for the pathways of transcription regulation, cell cycle control, and immune response in the lymphoblastoid cell lines. A standard component of leukocyte endothelial adhesion assays is the external activation of endothelial cells with agents such as interleukin-1β or TNF-α to facilitate leukocyte adhesion. In our studies, exogenous addition of these agents did not improve lymphoblastoid cell line adhesion, likely due to the activated state of the lymphoblastoid cell lines [33]. There is also concern that over time lymphoblastoid cell lines may change cellular properties. In studies by Im et al. of 540 HapMap lymphoblastoid cell lines, differences in cellular growth rate were observed when lymphoblastoid cell line populations that were obtained at different times were compared [34]. It is possible that there may be age and generation dependent effects on activity or expression of cellular mediators with lymphoblastoid cell lines. We did not find adhesion to be confounded by lymphoblastoid cell line-specific factors.

Adhesion in lymphoblastoid cell lines demonstrates similar variation observed in primary leukocytes. In our experiments, we observed, that the Burkitt lymphoma cell lines show the least endothelial adhesion while Trisomy 21 lymphoblastoid cells bind the highest compared to the lymphoblastoid cell lines derived from 92 normal subjects. A study comparing the expression of adhesion molecules as determined by flow cytometry in lymphoblastoid cell lines generated from normal peripheral blood mononuclear cells and Burkitt lymphoma cell lines demonstrated that the normal lymphoblastoid cell lines express higher levels of integrins, including integrin alpha 4 beta 1, leukocyte function associated antigen LFA-1, and integrin alpha 5 beta 3 as well as enhanced expression of the IgG superfamily adhesion molecules, like ICAM-1, and leukocyte function associated antigen type 3, and, glycoproteins like L-selectin and CD34 [8]. This is consistent with our observation of less adhesion of Burkitt lymphoma cell lines than the normal lymphoblastoid cell lines. The increased adhesion seen in Down's syndrome is thought to be due to over-expression of the CD18 integrin found on chromosome 21 [10]. Thus, lymphoblastoid cell lines appear to maintain the majority of factors that influence the unique endothelial adhesion of their primary leukocytes.

Another potential limitation is the use of an immortalized endothelial cell line. EA.hy926 is one of the best-characterized and most frequently used endothelial cell lines [35]. It is a product of the fusion of human umbilical vein endothelial cells and human lung carcinoma line A549. It is contact inhibited in growth and expresses von Willebrand factor. It is a transformed endothelial cell line that expresses intercellular adhesion molecule 1, vascular cell adhesion molecule 1, and E-selectin [36]. Given its similar leukocyte binding properties to human umbilical vein endothelial cells, EA.hy926 is frequently used in adhesion assays [37]. EA.hy926 has the distinct advantage for this study of homogeneity unlike human umbilical vein endothelial cells, or other primary cell lines, which are harvested from multiple donors [37] and suffer from lot to lot variability. The introduction of such variability would be problematic for a genetic study of this nature.

There are several strengths of this study. The assay was implemented on a high- throughput platform with very little intra-individual or inter-plate variability. Access to a large cohort of monozygotic twin and sibling pair lines enabled us to confidently identify leukocyte endothelial adhesion as a heritable trait. Heritability is the best statistic for the representation of the genetic contribution to phenotypic variance [38]. In particular, the use of identical twins and sibling pairs allows one to assume that the total variation introduced by the common environment shared by family members is equal [38]. We were able to exclude systematic underlying confounding factors including age, gender [39], ethnicity [18,19] and cell culture conditions [31,40]. Finally, while there have been many other studies that have obliquely suggested the heritability of this trait, this is the first one to our knowledge that was designed to directly assess and quantify it.

In summary, there is a major heritable component to leukocyte endothelial adhesion. Genetic predisposition appears to play a significant role in inter-individual variability of leukocyte endothelial adhesion. As such, future genetic studies should be able to identify those key molecular elements that regulate this important cellular trait.

Supporting Information

Figure S1 Standard curves for cell lines. Four parametric logistic curves of (A) Trisomy 21 lymphoblastoid cell line (B) Ramos Burkitt lymphoma (C) GM14581 a reperesentative twin lymphoblastoid cell line (D) U937 a monocytic leukemic cell line (E) and peripheral blood mononuclear cells (PBMC) were generated using known concentration Calcein AM labeled cells. On the x-axis is the known concentration of cells lines and on the Y- Axis are the relative fluorescence units. The standard curve generated was used to deduce the adherent cells that remained following washes.

Table S1 Subject Characteristics.

Acknowledgments

The authors would like to thank Dr. Graeme Bell for many helpful discussions; the Pharmacogenetics of Anticancer Agents Research Group for providing lymphoblastoid cell lines; Dr. Chandran of Rosalind Franklin University in North Chicago, IL for providing the Burkitt lymphoma cell lines; Sam Bettis and Rita Grantner of the Institute for Genomics and Systems Biology for assistance in running the assay; and Dr. Qing Chang, PhD, for assistance in designing the assay.

Author Contributions

Conceived and designed the experiments: MAG. Performed the experiments: MAG VR KPW SC BL DL. Analyzed the data: WZ JDB. Contributed reagents/materials/analysis tools: WZ RSH. Wrote the paper: MAG. Contributed to discussion and interpretation of results: NJC ABM JR RSH.

References

1. Pate M, Damarla V, Chi DS, Negi S, Krishnaswamy G (2010) Endothelial cell biology: role in the inflammatory response. Advances in clinical chemistry 52: 109–130.
2. Ulbrich H, Eriksson EE, Lindbom L (2003) Leukocyte and endothelial cell adhesion molecules as targets for therapeutic interventions in inflammatory disease. Trends in pharmacological sciences 24: 640–647.
3. Luster AD, Alon R, von Andrian UH (2005) Immune cell migration in inflammation: present and future therapeutic targets. Nature immunology 6: 1182–1190.
4. Carlos TM, Harlan JM (1994) Leukocyte-endothelial adhesion molecules. Blood 84: 2068–2101.
5. Bharadwaj A, Appukuttan B, Wilmarth PA, Pan Y, Stempel AJ, et al. (2012) Role of the retinal vascular endothelial cell in ocular disease. Progress in retinal and eye research.
6. Rainwater DL, Shi Q, Mahaney MC, Hodara V, Vandeberg JL, et al. (2010) Genetic regulation of endothelial inflammatory responses in baboons. Arteriosclerosis, thrombosis, and vascular biology 30: 1628–1633.
7. Lucio PJ, Faria MT, Pinto AM, da Silva MR, Correia Junior ME, et al. (1998) Expression of adhesion molecules in chronic B-cell lymphoproliferative disorders. Haematologica 83: 104–111.
8. Rincon J, Prieto J, Patarroyo M (1992) Expression of integrins and other adhesion molecules in Epstein-Barr virus-transformed B lymphoblastoid cells and Burkitt's lymphoma cells. International journal of cancer Journal international du cancer 51: 452–458.
9. el Habbal MH, Strobel S (1993) Leucocyte adhesion deficiency. Archives of disease in childhood 69: 463–466.
10. Taylor GM, Haigh H, Williams A, D'Souza SW, Harris R (1988) Down's syndrome lymphoid cell lines exhibit increased adhesion due to the over-expression of lymphocyte function-associated antigen (LFA-1). Immunology 64: 451–456.
11. Wen Y, Gorsic LK, Wheeler HE, Ziliak DM, Huang RS, et al. (2011) Chemotherapeutic-induced apoptosis: a phenotype for pharmacogenomics studies. Pharmacogenetics and genomics 21: 476–488.
12. Vanscoy LL, Blackman SM, Collaco JM, Bowers A, Lai T, et al. (2007) Heritability of lung disease severity in cystic fibrosis. American journal of respiratory and critical care medicine 175: 1036–1043.
13. Visscher PM (2004) Power of the classical twin design revisited. Twin Res 7: 505–512.
14. Williams CJ, Christian JC, Norton JA Jr. (1992) TWINAN90: a FORTRAN program for conducting ANOVA-based and likelihood-based analyses of twin data. Comput Methods Programs Biomed 38: 167–176.
15. Falconer DS, Mackay TFC (1996) Introduction to quantitative genetics. Essex, England: Longman. xiii, 464 p. p.
16. Zhang DH, Marconi A, Xu LM, Yang CX, Sun GW, et al. (2006) Tripterine inhibits the expression of adhesion molecules in activated endothelial cells. Journal of leukocyte biology 80: 309–319.
17. Murphy JF, Bordet JC, Wyler B, Rissoan MC, Chomarat P, et al. (1994) The vitronectin receptor (alpha v beta 3) is implicated, in cooperation with P-selectin and platelet-activating factor, in the adhesion of monocytes to activated endothelial cells. The Biochemical journal 304 (Pt 2): 537–542.
18. Lutsey PL, Cushman M, Steffen LM, Green D, Barr RG, et al. (2006) Plasma hemostatic factors and endothelial markers in four racial/ethnic groups: the MESA study. Journal of thrombosis and haemostasis : JTH 4: 2629–2635.
19. Miller MA, Sagnella GA, Kerry SM, Strazzullo P, Cook DG, et al. (2003) Ethnic differences in circulating soluble adhesion molecules: the Wandsworth Heart and Stroke Study. Clinical science 104: 591–598.
20. Niu N, Qin Y, Fridley BL, Hou J, Kalari KR, et al. (2010) Radiation pharmacogenomics: a genome-wide association approach to identify radiation response biomarkers using human lymphoblastoid cell lines. Genome research 20: 1482–1492.
21. Welsh M, Mangravite L, Medina MW, Tantisira K, Zhang W, et al. (2009) Pharmacogenomic discovery using cell-based models. Pharmacological reviews 61: 413–429.
22. Park JY, Arnaout MA, Gupta V (2007) A simple, no-wash cell adhesion-based high-throughput assay for the discovery of small-molecule regulators of the integrin CD11b/CD18. Journal of biomolecular screening 12: 406–417.
23. Miyamoto K, Khosrof S, Bursell SE, Moromizato Y, Aiello LP, et al. (2000) Vascular endothelial growth factor (VEGF)-induced retinal vascular permeability is mediated by intercellular adhesion molecule-1 (ICAM-1). The American journal of pathology 156: 1733–1739.
24. Bullaughey K, Chavarria CI, Coop G, Gilad Y (2009) Expression quantitative trait loci detected in cell lines are often present in primary tissues. Human molecular genetics 18: 4296–4303.
25. Nicolae DL, Gamazon E, Zhang W, Duan S, Dolan ME, et al. (2010) Trait-associated SNPs are more likely to be eQTLs: annotation to enhance discovery from GWAS. PLoS Genet 6: e1000888.
26. Grundberg E, Small KS, Hedman AK, Nica AC, Buil A, et al. (2012) Mapping cis- and trans-regulatory effects across multiple tissues in twins. Nature Genetics 44: 1084–1089.
27. Browning AC, Halligan EP, Stewart EA, Swan DC, Dove R, et al. (2012) Comparative gene expression profiling of human umbilical vein endothelial cells and ocular vascular endothelial cells. The British journal of ophthalmology 96: 128–132.
28. Smith JR, Chipps TJ, Ilias H, Pan Y, Appukuttan B (2012) Expression and regulation of activated leukocyte cell adhesion molecule in human retinal vascular endothelial cells. Exp Eye Res 104: 89–93.
29. Serra AM, Waddell J, Manivannan A, Xu H, Cotter M, et al. (2012) CD11b+ bone marrow-derived monocytes are the major leukocyte subset responsible for retinal capillary leukostasis in experimental diabetes in mouse and express high levels of CCR5 in the circulation. Am J Pathol 181: 719–727.
30. Caliskan M, Cusanovich DA, Ober C, Gilad Y (2011) The effects of EBV transformation on gene expression levels and methylation profiles. Human molecular genetics 20: 1643–1652.
31. Choy E, Yelensky R, Bonakdar S, Plenge RM, Saxena R, et al. (2008) Genetic analysis of human traits in vitro: drug response and gene expression in lymphoblastoid cell lines. PLoS genetics 4: e1000287.
32. Rochford R, Cannon MJ, Sabbe RE, Adusumilli K, Picchio G, et al. (1997) Common and idiosyncratic patterns of cytokine gene expression by Epstein-Barr virus transformed human B cell lines. Viral immunology 10: 183–195.
33. Olson JA, Whitelaw CM, McHardy KC, Pearson DW, Forrester JV (1997) Soluble leucocyte adhesion molecules in diabetic retinopathy stimulate retinal capillary endothelial cell migration. Diabetologia 40: 1166–1171.
34. Im HK, Gamazon ER, Stark AL, Huang RS, Cox NJ, et al. (2012) Mixed effects modeling of proliferation rates in cell-based models: consequence for pharmacogenomics and cancer. PLoS genetics 8: e1002525.
35. Bouis D, Hospers GA, Meijer C, Molema G, Mulder NH (2001) Endothelium in vitro: a review of human vascular endothelial cell lines for blood vessel-related research. Angiogenesis 4: 91–102.
36. Brown KA, Vora A, Biggerstaff J, Edgell CJ, Oikle S, et al. (1993) Application of an immortalized human endothelial cell line to the leucocyte:endothelial adherence assay. Journal of immunological methods 163: 13–22.
37. Thornhill MH, Li J, Haskard DO (1993) Leucocyte endothelial cell adhesion: a study comparing human umbilical vein endothelial cells and the endothelial cell line EA-hy-926. Scandinavian journal of immunology 38: 279–286.
38. Tenesa A, Haley CS (2013) The heritability of human disease: estimation, uses and abuses. Nature reviews Genetics 14: 139–149.
39. Nathan L, Pervin S, Singh R, Rosenfeld M, Chaudhuri G (1999) Estradiol inhibits leukocyte adhesion and transendothelial migration in rabbits in vivo : possible mechanisms for gender differences in atherosclerosis. Circulation research 85: 377–385.
40. Stark AL, Zhang W, Mi S, Duan S, O'Donnell PH, et al. (2010) Heritable and non-genetic factors as variables of pharmacologic phenotypes in lymphoblastoid cell lines. The pharmacogenomics journal 10: 505–512.

18

Low Bone Turnover and Low BMD in Down Syndrome: Effect of Intermittent PTH Treatment

Tristan W. Fowler[1,2]⁹, Kent D. McKelvey[3]⁹, Nisreen S. Akel[1,2], Jaclyn Vander Schilden[2], Anthony W. Bacon[2], John W. Bracey[2], Timothy Sowder[2], Robert A. Skinner[2], Frances L. Swain[2], William R. Hogue[2], Donna B. Leblanc[3], Dana Gaddy[1,2], Galen R. Wenger[4], Larry J. Suva[1,2]*

1 Department of Physiology & Biophysics, University of Arkansas for Medical Sciences, Little Rock, Arkansas, United States of America, **2** Department of Orthopaedic Surgery, Center for Orthopaedic Research, University of Arkansas for Medical Sciences, Little Rock, Arkansas, United States of America, **3** Department of Genetics, University of Arkansas for Medical Sciences, Little Rock, Arkansas, United States of America, **4** Department of Pharmacology, University of Arkansas for Medical Sciences, Little Rock, Arkansas, United States of America

Abstract

Trisomy 21 affects virtually every organ system and results in the complex clinical presentation of Down syndrome (DS). Patterns of differences are now being recognized as patients' age and these patterns bring about new opportunities for disease prevention and treatment. Low bone mineral density (BMD) has been reported in many studies of males and females with DS yet the specific effects of trisomy 21 on the skeleton remain poorly defined. Therefore we determined the bone phenotype and measured bone turnover markers in the murine DS model Ts65Dn. Male Ts65Dn DS mice are infertile and display a profound low bone mass phenotype that deteriorates with age. The low bone mass was correlated with significantly decreased osteoblast and osteoclast development, decreased bone biochemical markers, a diminished bone formation rate and reduced mechanical strength. The low bone mass observed in 3 month old Ts65Dn mice was significantly increased after 4 weeks of intermittent PTH treatment. These studies provide novel insight into the cause of the profound bone fragility in DS and identify PTH as a potential anabolic agent in the adult low bone mass DS population.

Editor: Pierre J. Marie, Inserm U606 and University Paris Diderot, France

Funding: This work was supported by NIH R01-DK54044 and R21-74024 (DG), NIH R01 HD047656 (GRW), UAMS Translational Research Institute (TRI) clinical award (KGM), UAMS TRI UL1RR029884, the Winthrop P Rockefeller Chair in Clinical Genetics (KDM) and the Carl L. Nelson Endowed Chair in Orthopaedic Creativity (LJS). The funders had no role in study design, data collection and analysis, decision to publish, or preparation of the manuscript.

Competing Interests: The authors have declared that no competing interests exist.

* E-mail: suvalarryj@uams.edu

⁹ These authors contributed equally to this work.

Introduction

Although Down syndrome (DS) was initially described in 1866 [1], the pathophysiology of many clinical aspects of the DS phenotype have not been elucidated. Low bone mass and the associated increased fracture rates are clinical features that complicate DS [2]. As the life expectancy of individuals with DS has increased to greater than age 50 [3,4], the bone health of adolescent and adult DS patients has become an important medical issue. With the increasing life expectancy, many concerns regarding the risk of osteoporosis have been raised [5,6,7]. In fact, the accrual of bone mass during childhood and adolescence may reduce osteoporosis risk later in life and low bone mass in young adulthood is a strong risk factor for later osteoporosis and fracture [8,9].

Several investigators, including ourselves have reported that adults (and children) with DS have lower bone mass, expressed as BMD, especially in the lumbar spine, compared with their peers without mental retardation or with mental retardation but without DS [5,10,11,12,13]. Known secondary causes for low BMD include dietary insufficiency (vitamin D and calcium intake), endocrine (hypothyroidism, hyperparathyroidism, hypogonadism), and autoimmune disorders (celiac disease) which lead to inadequate nutrition. Low activity levels, low sunlight exposure and anti-convulsant use have also been associated with decreased bone mass but these are not consistent risk factors in DS, leaving the underlying pathophysiology unknown [2]. In addition, despite numerous reports in the literature of BMD measurements in DS, the measurement of bone biochemical markers in community dwelling DS patients compared to the normal population or the detailed analysis of the skeletons of DS mouse models are scarce; [7,14]. Finally, no bone anabolic therapies have been evaluated in DS.

The Ts65Dn mouse is one of several mouse models of DS that has been developed to investigate the pathology of DS phenotypes [15]. The Ts65Dn mouse strain is a DS model characterized by segmental trisomy for the region of mouse chromosome (Mmu) 16 that contains approximately 75% of the human chromosome (Hsa) 21-homologous genes. Approximately 324 genes recognized on human chromosome 21 (Hsa21) are split over three mouse chromosomes: Mmu10, Mmu16 and Mmu17 [16].

To investigate bone health in DS, we determined the skeletal phenotype of the Ts(17^{16})65Dn (Ts65Dn) mouse model of DS at both 3 and 24 months of age [17,18] and evaluated the efficacy of an anabolic regimen of human PTH in these animals. We hypothesized that in addition to the characteristic behavioral and craniofacial features of DS exhibited by Ts65Dn mice, the skeletons of these mice would model the bone phenotype of the human condition. In this study, the skeletal phenotype of young and aged Ts65Dn mice was determined. When compared with low BMD and bone turnover measurements in adult male DS patients [13], male Ts65Dn mice phenocopy the bone phenotype of the patients with striking consistency.

The studies revealed that just as in people with DS, the Ts65Dn mice have low bone mass that is the result of an intrinsic cellular defect resulting in low bone turnover and decreased bone formation. The low bone turnover state is present despite the profound hypogonadism and the low bone mass was increased by 4 weeks of intermittent PTH therapy. As such, anabolic treatment options should be considered in the management of the low bone mass that is prevalent in DS.

Results

Skeletal Phenotype of Trabecular and Cortical Bone in Ts65Dn Mice

Three-dimensional analysis of trabecular microarchitecture by μCT was performed on the proximal tibia and distal femur. Ts65Dn mice had a significantly decreased bone volume/total volume (BV/TV) at both 3 months and 24 months of age (Figure 1A; Figure S1). There was also a significant decrease in the trabecular number (Tb.N.) in 3 month and 24 month old Ts65Dn mice (Figure 1B) and a corresponding significant increase in the trabecular spacing (Tb.Sp.) (Figure 1B). However, although Tb.N. was significantly decreased, trabecular thickness (Tb.Th.) was not altered in Ts65Dn mice at either age, suggesting that although bone turnover is decreased, the molecular regulation of trabecular thickness is maintained in these animals.

In addition to examining the effects of aneuploidy on trabecular bone, we also examined cortical bone from Ts65Dn mice (Figure 1C). Transverse CT slices were acquired at the femoral midshaft to assess total cross sectional area, cortical bone area, and medullary area (TA, BA, and MA, (mm^2)); bone area fraction (BA/TA, %); cortical thickness (mm); anteroposterior and mediolateral diameters (mm). Sub-region analysis of the mid-shaft of the femur revealed that trisomy significantly decreased cortical thickness in both 3-month old (Figure S2) and 24-month Ts65Dn mice (Figure 1C). Cortical cross-sectional area (CSA), periosteal perimeter, and total cross-sectional area were also significantly decreased in the 24-month Ts65Dn mice compared to age-matched WT control mice (Figure S2), while cortical porosity was unchanged (Data not shown). The decrease in the cortical bone geometric parameters of 24-month old Ts65Dn mice was associated with significantly decreased mechanical strength. The peak load and stiffness of 24 month old Ts65Dn femurs was significantly decreased compared with age-matched littermate controls (Figure S2). Thus, the skeletal effects of trisomy in Ts65Dn mice are decreased trabecular bone volume and architecture, as well as changes in cortical parameters that result in decreased overall bone stiffness and bone strength.

Decreased Bone Turnover is Responsible for the Low Bone Mass in Ts65Dn Mice

Several quantitative analyses were performed to determine whether the decreased bone mass and strength in Ts65Dn mice were mediated by decreased bone turnover despite hypogonadism, as we have observed in people with DS [13]. Static histomorphometric analysis of the secondary spongiosa of paraffin-embedded sections of the decalcified proximal tibia (as well as femur; data not shown) of 3-month old mice (Figure 2) demonstrated that Ts65Dn mice have significant decreases in osteoblast surface per bone surface and osteoclast surface per bone surface, and significantly decreased numbers of osteoclasts on the bone surface. To determine if the observed decreases in osteoblast and osteoclasts were associated with decreased bone remodeling bone formation rate was measured using dynamic histomorphometry in non-decalcified methyl methacrylate-embedded sections as we have described [19,20]. The analysis in 3-month old Ts65Dn mice demonstrated significantly decreased bone formation rate (BFR) per bone surface (Figure 2). The significantly decreased BFR resulted in significant changes in the serum concentration of markers for bone resorption and bone formation in 24-month, but not 3-month, old Ts65Dn mice. Serum TRAP 5b levels were significantly decreased indicating a decrease in overall bone resorption (Figure 2). Furthermore, there was a significant decrease in the serum P1NP levels, indicating a decrease in the amount of bone formation (Figure 2). These results demonstrate that the significantly decreased numbers of osteoblasts and osteoclasts on the bone surface resulting in decreased bone formation and bone resorption are responsible for the observed low bone mass phenotype in Ts65Dn mice. These observations recapitulate the low bone turnover phenotype in people with DS [13], confirm the reported low bone mass of Ts65Dn [14], and support the notion that DS patients with low BMD are candidates for anabolic but not anti-resorptive bone-targeted therapy.

Cellular Defect in Ts65Dn Mice Involves Both Decreased Osteoblast and Osteoclast Differentiation

In an effort to determine the cellular mechanism responsible for the low bone mass phenotype in Ts65Dn mice, *ex vivo* bone marrow cultures were initiated and stimulated towards either osteoblastogenesis or osteoclastogenesis [19,21]. Bone marrow derived from Ts65Dn mice had a significantly decreased capacity for osteoblast recruitment compared to control littermates, as measured by the number of alkaline phosphatase (AP+) colonies per well after 10 days of culture in osteoblastogenic media (Figure 3A) [22]. Furthermore, the ability of these cells to undergo maturation to mineralizing osteoblasts was also significantly decreased when compared to littermate controls, as measured by the number of mineralized nodules per well (Figure 3B). Collectively, these results demonstrate that Ts65Dn mice have an intrinsic cell deficit in the mesenchymal lineage, leading to a decreased pool of cells that are capable of being recruited into the osteoblastic lineage.

Ex vivo bone marrow cultures from Ts65Dn and wild-type littermates were also cultured towards osteoclasts as described [19,21]. After 14 days in culture, cells from the Ts65Dn bone marrow produced significantly fewer mature tartrate resistant acid phosphatase positive (TRAP+), multinucleated cells per well than wild type controls (Figure 3C). These data demonstrate that the hematopoietic lineage is also significantly affected in Ts65Dn mice, with a resulting decrease in osteoclastogenesis, paralleling the observed decrease in osteoclast surface/bone surface and activity observed *in vivo*. Therefore, the low bone mass observed in Ts65Dn is the result of a decrease in bone turnover, due to an intrinsic defect in the production of normal numbers of mature bone forming osteoblasts and bone resorbing osteoclasts. This cellular defect is occurring in the face of the hypogonadism and infertility that characterizes male Ts65Dn mice [2,23].

Intermittent PTH Increases BMD in Ts65Dn Mice

Given the low bone mass phenotype and low bone turnover states of both humans with DS and Ts65Dn mice, the effect of intermittent anabolic PTH therapy in 3 month old WT and

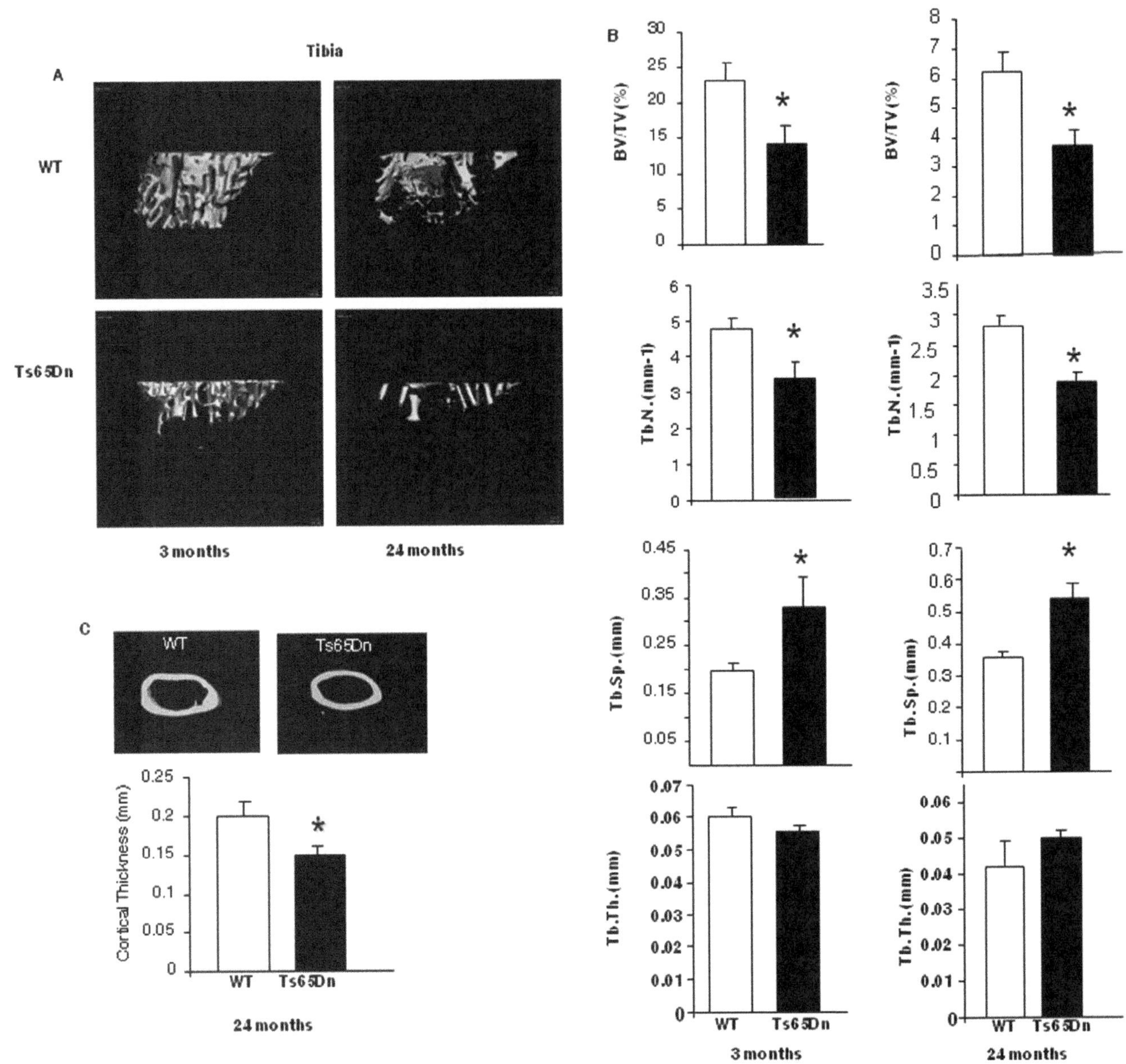

Figure 1. Trisomy effects on the proximal tibia and femur or 3-month and 24-month Ts65Dn mice. (**A**) Micro CT reconstructions of metaphyseal tibial cancellous bone in 3-month (left column) and 24-month (right column) old WT (top) and Ts65Dn (bottom) mice. The low bone volume is evident at 3-months in the Ts65Dn mice vs. WT. (**B**). Micro CT analysis of % bone volume/tissue volume (BV/TV), trabecular number (Tb.N.), trabecular thickness (Tb.Th.), trabecular separation (Tb.Sp) in Ts65Dn 3-month and 24-month old WT and Ts65Dn proximal tibia. (**C**). Decreased cortical thickness at the femoral midshaft by micro CT in 24 month old WT and Ts65Dn mice. Representative MicroCT reconstructions of the midshaft and measurement of cortical thickness in both WT and Ts65Dn are shown. *, $p<0.05$ vs. WT.

Ts65Dn mice was determined. Intermittent PTH is the only FDA-approved bone anabolic therapy. Since the effects of PTH for the stimulation of bone mass in situations of low bone turnover are not well documented, two different doses of PTH(1–34) were used.

Mice were treated with daily i.p. injections of 30 or 80 ug/kg PTH(1–34), or vehicle control, for 28 days. PTH increased whole-body BMD in both 3 month old WT and Ts65Dn mice as determined by DXA (Figure 4A). In WT mice, both PTH treatment doses significantly increased whole-body BMD compared with untreated mice. In contrast in Ts65Dn mice, although both PTH doses increased whole body BMD only the 80 ug/kg dose reached statistical significance (Figure 4A). The magnitude of the increase in BMD in Ts65Dn mice was similar to the magnitude of the response in WT mice (Figure 4A). Bone volume fraction (BV/TV) in the tibia was lower in Ts65Dn than age-matched WT mice (Figure 4B). The effect of PTH on the trabecular bone compartment of the tibia (Figure 4B) showed that the effect of PTH on trabecular BMD and BV/TV was similar in both WT and Ts65Dn mice (Figure 4B). As with the whole-body DXA measurements, the PTH effect was significant only at the 80 ug/kg dose in Ts65Dn mice. In both treatment groups, the PTH-stimulated increase in trabecular BV/TV (Figure 5B) was associated with significantly increased

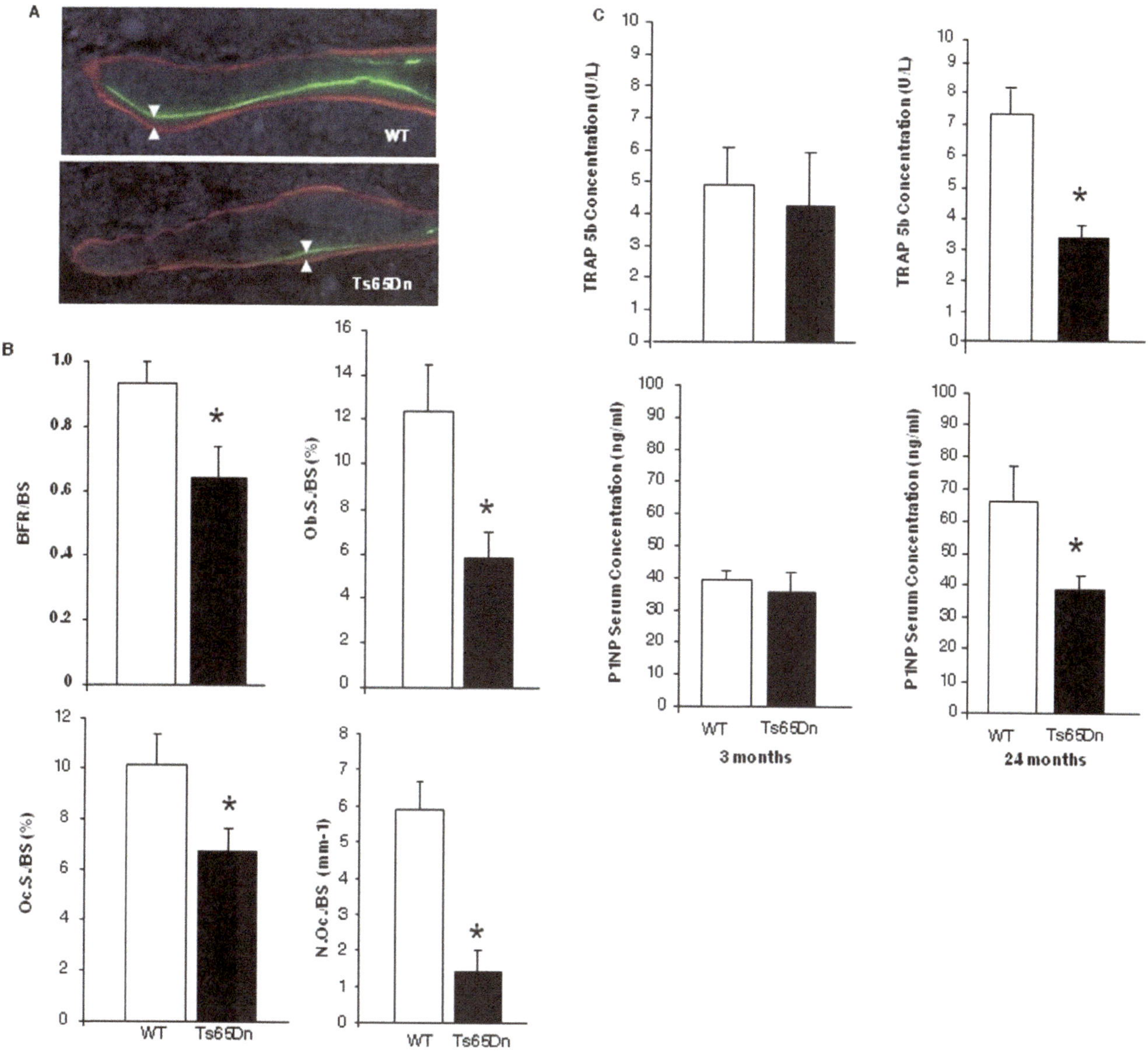

Figure 2. Bone Formation and bone turnover is decreased in Ts65Dn Mice. (**A**). Representative double-fluorochrome-labeled regions of trabecular bone in the proximal tibia of 3 month old WT (top) and Ts65Dn (bottom). *Arrowheads* indicate the distance between the two labels used to calculate the bone formation rate normalized to bone surface (BFR/BS) (um^3/um^2/day). (**B**). Tibial sections (N = 6 per group) were used to quantify BFR/BS, percent osteoblast surface/bone surface (Ob.S./BS), percent osteoclast surface/bone surface (Oc.S./BS) and number of osteoclasts/bone surface (N.Oc./BS.) (**C**). Serum obtained from WT and Ts65Dn mice at 3- and 24-months of age was analyzed for bone resorption, tartrate resistant acid phosphatase 5b (TRAP 5b) and bone formation, procollagen-1 N-terminal peptide (P1NP) markers by ELISA. *, $p<0.05$ vs. respective WT vehicle control.

Tb.N. and Tb.Th. (Figure 4B), as expected for anabolic PTH therapy.

Intermittent PTH treatment caused an approximately equivalent increase in BV/TV in both WT and Ts65Dn mice (Figure 4B). PTH increased bone volume in both metaphyseal trabecular bone (Figure 5B) as well as diaphyseal cortical bone in both WT and Ts65Dn mice (Figure 4C). The magnitude of the PTH-stimulated increase in BMD and cortical thickness in the femur was similar in both WT and Ts65Dn mice. In both groups PTH treatment increased both endocortical and periosteal surfaces, measured by microCT as a decrease in endocortical circumference and a corresponding increase in periosteal circumference (Figure 4C), with no apparent changes in cortical porosity (data not shown).

The observed increase in trabecular bone mass and volume was mediated by a PTH-stimulated increase in mineral apposition rate and bone formation (Figure 5A, B). Osteoblast number/bone perimeter (N.Ob./BPm) was increased significantly in response to PTH treatment in both WT and Ts65Dn animals, indicating an ability of PTH to overcome the suppression in bone formation induced by trisomy 21 (Figure 5C). In contrast, 4 weeks of intermittent PTH treatment did not increase any osteoclast parameter measured, including osteoclast number per bone perimeter (N.Oc./BPm) in either WT or Ts65Dn mice (Figure 5D).

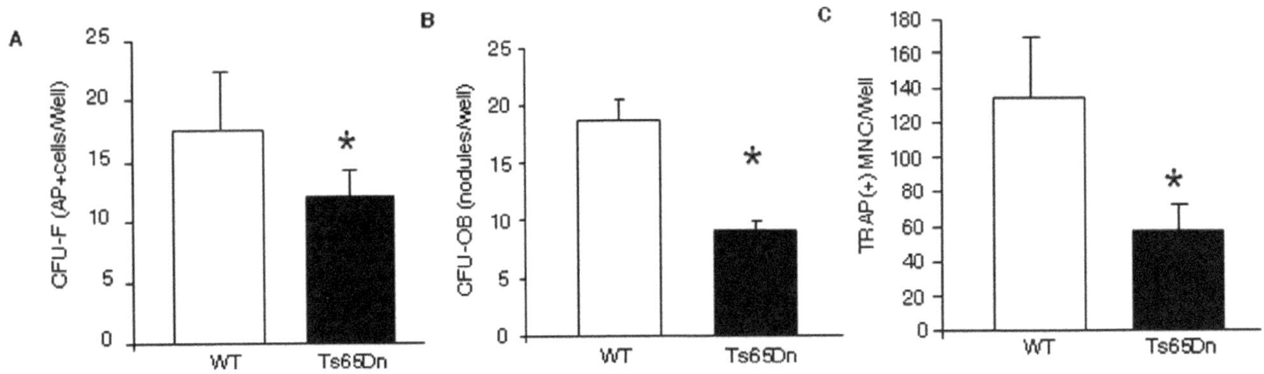

Figure 3. Osteoclast and osteoblast formation is significantly decreased in 3 month old Ts65Dn Mice. (**A**) *Ex vivo* recruitment into the osteoblast lineage was measured at culture day 10 by staining for alkaline phosphatase (AP) and counting the number of AP+ colony forming units (CFU-F) per well. (**B**) *Ex vivo* osteoblast differentiation was assessed at culture day 28 by staining mineralized bone nodules containing differentiated colonies of osteoblasts (CFU-OB) with Alizarin Red and the number of CFU-OB per well enumerated. (**C**) *Ex Vivo* osteoclast differentiation was assessed by staining on day 14 for tartrate resistant acid phosphatase (TRAP) and the number of TRAP+-multinucleated cells per well counted. *, $p<0.05$ vs. WT vehicle control.

Discussion

The present study demonstrated that Ts65Dn DS mice have lower trabecular bone volume and trabecular number and higher trabecular separation in the proximal tibia and distal femur as well as decreased cortical thickness and strength compared with WT littermates. The low bone mass phenotype is consistent with the human DS population that also displays a low BMD due to decreased bone turnover [13]. Histomorphometric analysis of the trabecular bone in Ts65Dn mice revealed a reduction in osteoblast and osteoclast activity and decreased cell numbers on the bone surface, leading to decreased bone turnover markers. These observations result in a significantly lower MAR and BFR in 12 week old Ts65Dn mice, leading to the decreased bone mass and volume observed. Interestingly, histological evaluation also demonstrated the age-related loss of trabecular bone in both WT and Ts65Dn mice, but that the characteristic increase in marrow fat was absent in Ts65Dn. In *ex vivo* bone marrow cultures, the differentiation capacity of osteoblasts and osteoclasts were impaired in Ts65Dn mice, demonstrating the cell intrinsic nature

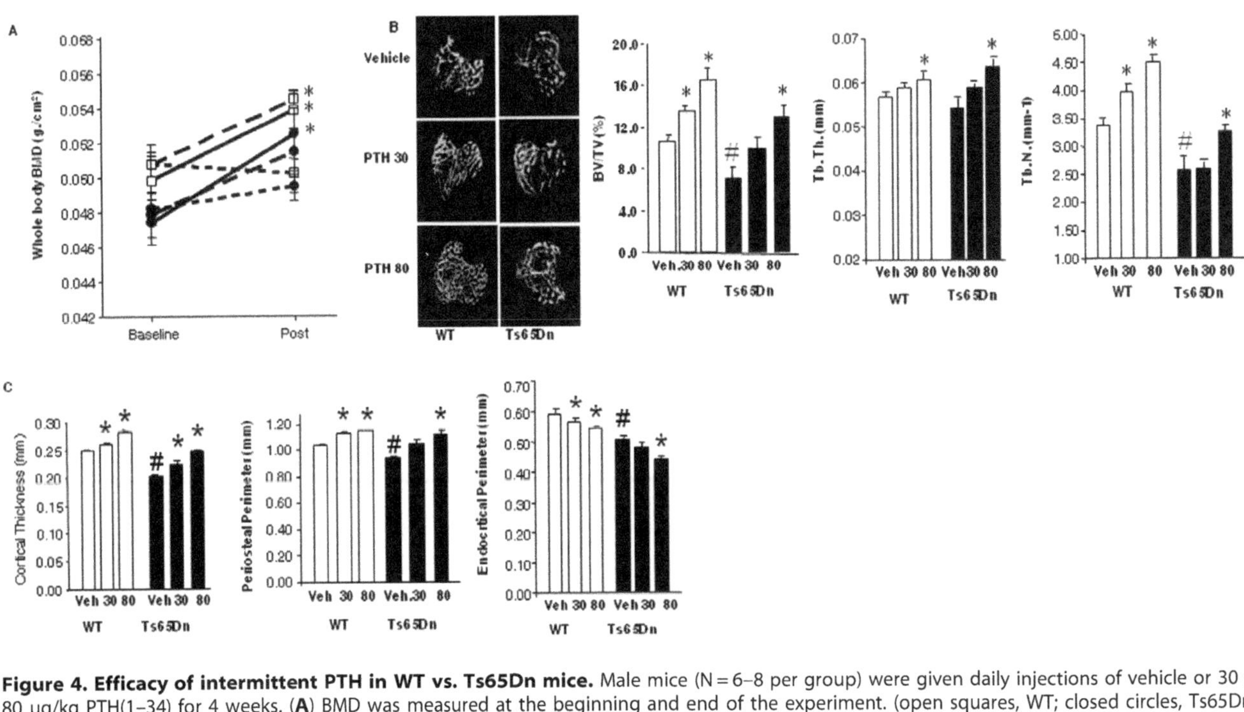

Figure 4. Efficacy of intermittent PTH in WT vs. Ts65Dn mice. Male mice (N = 6–8 per group) were given daily injections of vehicle or 30 or 80 ug/kg PTH(1–34) for 4 weeks. (**A**) BMD was measured at the beginning and end of the experiment. (open squares, WT; closed circles, Ts65Dn). Dotted lines show BMD of vehicle treated animals, dashed lines, 30 ug/kg PTH; solid lines, 80 ug/kg PTH (**B**) % bone volume/tissue volume (BV/TV), trabecular number (Tb.N.) and trabecular thickness (Tb.Th.) were determined in the tibia (open bars WT; solid bars Ts65Dn). Representative superior view of a transverse micro-CT images of the trabecular bone from the proximal tibia of representative animals in each group are shown. (**C**) Micro CT measurements of the effects of PTH treatment on cortical thickness, periosteal perimeter and endocortical perimeter in the distal tibia were performed (open bars WT; solid bars Ts65Dn). *, $p<0.05$ vs. respective vehicle control; #, $p<0.05$ vs. WT vehicle.

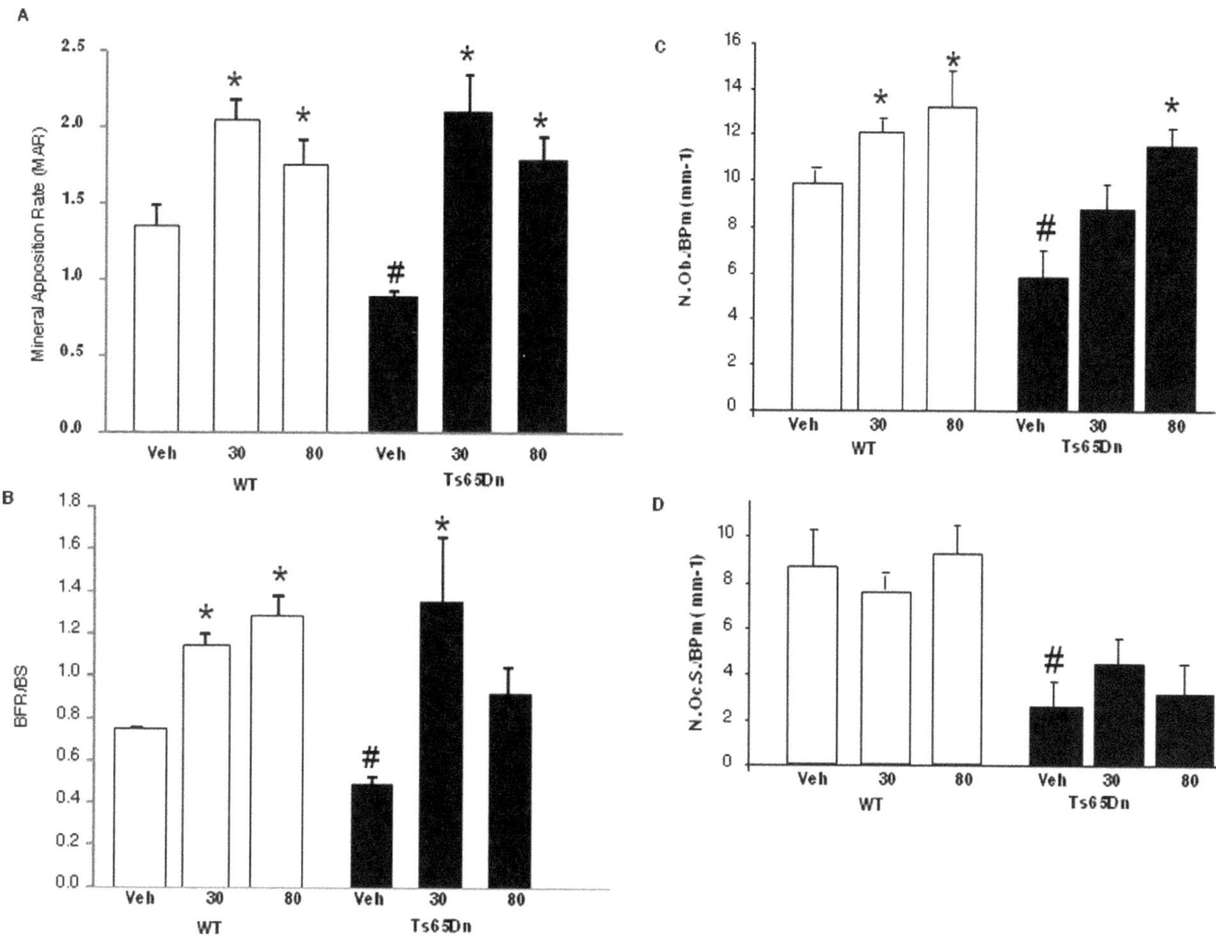

Figure 5. Histomorphometric measurement of bone formation and bone resorption following intermittent PTH in WT and Ts65Dn mice. Male mice (N = 6–8 per group) were given daily injections of vehicle or 30 or 80 ug/kg PTH(1–34) for 4 weeks. (**A**) Mineral apposition rate (MAR) (um^3/um^2/day), (**B**) Bone formation rate/bone surface (BFR/BS) (um^3/um^2/day), (**C**) Number of osteoblasts/bone perimeter (N.Ob./B.Pm), (**D**) Number of osteoclasts/bone perimeter (N.Oc./B.Pm.) were measured in WT and Ts65Dn mice vehicle or PTH treated (30 or 80 ug/kg/day) (open bars, WT; closed bars, Ts65Dn). *, $p<0.05$ vs. respective vehicle control; #, $p<0.05$ vs. WT vehicle.

of the bone phenotype, and confirming both mesenchymal and hematopoetic lineages as targets of trisomy 21. Interestingly, and as reported by others [24], Ts65Dn mice also display significant megakaryocyte hyperplasia, supporting our conclusion of a distorted hematopoietic stem cell compartment in these mice. Thus, the low bone mass of Ts65Dn mice phenocopies the low bone mass observed in DS patients and is the result of low bone turnover; characterized by decreased bone formation and bone resorption. These results are important because they confirm that the Ts65Dn mouse is an accurate model for studying the effects of trisomy on the appendicular skeleton [14] and provide a cellular mechanism for the low bone mass and increased fracture risk of DS patients, that is not related to lifestyle differences, as others have suggested [15,25,26].

Ts65Dn mice at 3-months and 24-months of age have significant decreases in trabecular and cortical bone. The BV/TV and trabecular number are significantly decreased at both ages. With the decreased number of trabeculae, there was a subsequent significant increase in trabecular spacing. Interestingly, trabecular thickness was not significantly affected, suggesting that the fundamental mechanism controlling the development of trabeculae is intact in trisomic Ts65Dn mice, but the rate at which they are generated is decreased. These results extend those of Blazek [14] who analyzed femurs from 6 week and 16 week old Ts65Dn mice and observed an identical decreased bone mass and normal trabecular thickness phenotype and Parsons [27] who analyzed the presphenoid bone, but not the axial or appendicular skeletal elements from a wide age range of Ts65Dn mice. While the differences in cancellous bone in Ts65Dn mice revealed significant osteopenia, analysis of cortical bone demonstrated decreased mechanical integrity. Geometric parameters of the femur were significantly decreased compared to age matched WT control femurs. These results were supported by three-point bending studies that revealed significantly decreased mechanical strength of the femurs of Ts65Dn mice.

Other DS mouse models have been developed and their bone phenotype investigated [7]. These murine DS models (Ts1Rhr and Ms1Rhr) are trisomic and monosomic, respectively for only a small portion of mouse chromosome 16 (MMU16) and contain only 33 trisomic genes that are orthologs to those on human chromosome 21 [7], compared with approximately 100 in Ts65Dn mice. Ts1Rhr mice were similar to normal mice, suggesting that a larger region of trisomy is necessary to recapitulate the DS bone phenotype. Interestingly, 3 week old Ms1Rhr mice like Ts65Dn have a low bone mass phenotype with reduced cortical bone geometry, decreased trabecular bone volume and connectivity and unchanged Tb.N. In contrast to Ts65Dn mice, Tb.Th was decreased in Ms1Rhr mice, which is presumably associated with the different number of trisomic genes in these mice. Unfortunately, the authors did not measure bone turnover markers or perform cellular histomorphometry, so the cellular mechanism responsible for the bone phenotype is unknown [7]. Given the limited number of trisomic genes in Ms1Rhr it is perhaps not surprising that the complete bone phenotype of Ts65Dn or people with DS is not recapitulated, although the overall decrease in bone mass, bone volume and bone strength is maintained.

The low bone mass phenotype of Ts65Dn male mice like people with DS is profound and is the result of decreased bone turnover. The decreased bone turnover is unexpected, given the hypogonadism and infertility associated with the disorder in humans [28] and in Ts65Dn mice [29]. In fact, numerous published studies have yet to completely elucidate the pathophysiology of the infertility in men with Down syndrome [28,30,31,32]. However, it is clear that males with DS are generally infertile and have significant disruption of one or more levels of the hypothalamic-pituitary-gonadal axis resulting in elevated FSH and LH levels and inconsistent testosterone levels that are often in the low-normal range [28]. Whatever the final cause of the hypogonadism and infertility in males with DS, our current understanding of endocrine regulation of bone turnover would suggest increased, not decreased bone turnover in both humans and mice. As such, elucidation of the mechanism driving the low bone mass and low turnover phenotype of Ts65Dn mice warrants continued investigation.

The defect in both osteoblast and osteoclast differentiation in Ts65Dn mice was observed in both *ex vivo* bone marrow cultures and in the histomorphometric analysis of tibias from 3-month old Ts65Dn mice. In *ex vivo* cultures, both osteoblast and osteoclast differentiation was significantly decreased in Ts65Dn compared with control. *In vivo*, osteoblast number per bone surface, osteoclast number per bone surface and bone formation rate were all significantly decreased. These observations suggest an intrinsic defect in both the mesenchymal and the hematopoetic cell lineages. While the defect in megakaryocyotopoiesis in DS has been well studied in humans and is recapitulated in the Ts65Dn mouse [24], this is the first report of a cellular defect in both osteoblastogenesis and osteoclastogenesis in Ts65Dn mice.

Histological evaluation of the bone marrow confirmed the megakaryocyte hyperplasia as has been reported in Ts65Dn mice and in DS patients [2,33], as well as a significant and normal age-related decrease in bone mass in Ts65Dn mice. This is particularly interesting given that DS patients have a life expectancy well into the 5th decade of life and are presenting in increasing numbers with low bone mass and fracture [34]. The effect of trisomy on osteoclast and osteoblast development also inhibited the age-related differentiation of adipocytes in the bone marrow. Our findings are in agreement with a pathologic post-mortem examination of vertebral sections from a 49-year old DS female that reported a complete lack of active osteoclasts and a decreased osteoblast number along the trabeculae [35].

Collectively, these observations provide evidence that the low bone mass observed in humans with DS and Ts65Dn mice is due to a cellular defect in both the hematopoietic and mesenchymal lineages, such that aneuploidy's effects on the available pool of precursor cells decreases their capacity for normal differentiation and function. Thus, fewer cells differentiating into functional osteoblasts and osteoclasts results in the accrual of lower bone mass, which is a mechanism fundamentally distinct from the high bone turnover observed in hypogonadal women and men, where increased numbers and activity of cells leads to low bone mass.

In support of this idea, the Ts65Dn mice demonstrate a lifelong deficit in bone turnover, such that normal peak adult bone mass is never achieved. It is important to note that the serum bone turnover markers of control animals revealed the expected age-dependent increases in both formation and resorption markers, whereas markers in Ts65Dn mice do not increase with age and are consistently lower compared with control throughout the life of the mice. If this temporal difference in bone turnover is recapitulated in humans with DS, it would indicate that low bone turnover is sustained in DS resulting in lower bone accrual and is an area that we are actively investigating. Perhaps most importantly, our studies provide the first data to demonstrate the efficacy of a bone anabolic agent in the treatment of low bone mass in DS and call into question the routine use of bisphosphonates (which decrease bone turnover) in this patient population.

Intermittent PTH therapy increases bone formation by stimulating osteoblast numbers at sites of bone remodeling, where old bone is replaced with new by the concerted efforts of both osteoclasts and osteoblasts [36,37]. In Ts65Dn mice PTH(1–34) treatment significantly increased bone mass and volume at the highest dose tested (80 ug/kg). PTH stimulated both mineral apposition rate and bone formation rate resulting in increased bone mass, consistent with the reported effects of PTH in the treatment of both post menopausal and glucocorticoid-induced osteoporosis [38,39,40]. Interestingly, PTH treatment in both WT and Ts65Dn mice increased bone mass and osteoblastic activity (MAR and BFR) to a similar extent, despite the low BMD and decreased bone turnover status of Ts65Dn mice. The stimulation of bone mass by intermittent PTH treatment demonstrated the efficacy of the intervention in trisomy 21 and supports the idea that PTH or other potential anabolic treatments, such as anti-sclerostin antibody [41,42], may have utility in DS patients with low BMD and low bone turnover.

Thus, these data provide a clearer understanding of the cellular mechanisms leading to the low bone mass in DS, suggest a new direction for treatment and provide a relevant animal model for continued studies of the skeleton in DS. Given the elevated fracture risk and rate in DS patients our data provide the rationale to consider bone anabolic therapies in DS patients with low bone mass.

Methods

Animals and Husbandry

All animal handling and experimentation was performed in accordance with approved University of Arkansas for Medical Sciences (UAMS) institutional guidelines and protocols and approved by the UAMS Institutional Animal Care and Use Committee (IACUC). Ts65Dn male mice and wild type euploid littermate controls were purchased from the Jackson Laboratory (Bar Harbor, ME). Upon arrival they were housed individually with food and water available *ad libitum* and a 12-hr light:dark cycle. Only male mice were evaluated due to the decreased fertility of Ts65Dn male mice and the necessity of Ts65Dn female mice for colony maintenance. Animals were purchased at 6 weeks and aged as required. Some mice were aged and maintained at UAMS for up to 24 months.

For bone phenotyping, animals were sacrificed at 3 months and 24 months and long bones and spines harvested. Some three month old animals were injected with calcein (Sigma, St. Louis, MO) (administered 8 days prior to sacrifice) and alizarin red S (Sigma) or alizarin red complexone (Sigma) (administered 2 days prior to sacrifice), for subsequent determination of dynamic parameters of bone histomorphometry with an inter-label distance of 6 days as described [22]. The BMD of tibia and femur was determined before and after PTH administration with a PIXImus densitometer (GE-Lunar Corp., Madison, WI), as previously described [22]. Synthetic human PTH(1–34) (Creative Peptides, Shirley, NY) was injected daily, i.p., at 30 and 80 ug/kg body weight for 28 days. Weight changes ranged from 2–10% during the course of the experiment in either Ts65Dn or WT control mice and were not significantly different. Vehicle-injected mice of both genotypes served as controls.

Biochemical Markers

In Ts65Dn and WT mice, serum was extracted from blood drawn at sacrifice and serum procollagen-1 N-terminal peptide (P1NP) and tartrate resistant acid phosphatase (TRAP) measured. P1NP was measured using a commercially available enzyme immunoassay (EIA) (Immunodiagnostic Systems) and TRAP using a TRAP-5b solid phase immunofixed enzyme activity assay (Immunodiagnostic Systems) according to the manufacturer's protocol.

Trabecular Bone Assessment by Micro Computed Tomography (CT)

All MicroCT analyses were consistent with current guidelines for the assessment of bone microstructure in rodents using micro-computed tomography [43]. Formalin-fixed tibiae and femora were imaged using a MicroCT 40 (Scanco Medical AG, Bassersdorf, Switzerland) using a 12 μm isotropic voxel size in all dimensions. The region of interest selected for analysis comprised 240 transverse CT slices representing the entire medullary volume extending 1.24 mm distal to the end of the primary spongiosa with a border lying 100 um from the cortex. Three-dimensional reconstructions were created by stacking the regions of interest from each two-dimensional slice and then applying a gray-scale threshold and Gaussian noise filter as described [19] using a consistent and pre-determined threshold with all data acquired at 70 kVp, 114 mA, and 200-ms integration time. Fractional bone volume (bone volume/tissue volume; BV/TV) and architectural properties of trabecular bone (trabecular thickness (Tb.Th., μm), trabecular number (Tb.N., mm-1), and connectivity density (Conn. D, mm-3) were calculated using previously published methods [19].

Cortical Bone Assessment by MicroCT

The MicroCT slices were segmented into bone and marrow regions by applying a visually chosen, fixed threshold for all samples after smoothing the image with a three-dimensional Gaussian low-pass filter ($\sigma = 0.8$, support $= 1.0$) to remove noise, and a fixed threshold (30% of maximal gray scale value). Femoral cortical geometry was assessed in a 1-mm-long region centered at the femoral midshaft. The outer contour of the bone was found automatically using the built-in manufacturer's contouring tool. Total area was calculated by counting all voxels within the contour, bone area by counting all voxels that were segmented as bone, and marrow area was calculated as total area - bone area. This calculation was performed on all 25 slices (1 slice $= \sim 12.5$ μm), using the average for the final calculation. The outer and inner perimeter of the cortical midshaft was determined by a three-dimensional triangulation of the bone surface (BS) of the 25 slices, and cortical thickness and other cortical parameters were determined as described [19].

Histology

After MicroCT analysis, the same tibia and femora, fixed in 10% neutral-buffered formalin, were decalcified in 5% formic acid with agitation until deemed clear by the ammonium oxalate endpoint test [19]. One tibia and one femur were embedded in paraffin, sectioned at 5 um, and stained with hematoxylin and eosin (H&E). The decalcified specimens were then dehydrated through graded ethanol, cleared in methyl salicylate, embedded in paraffin, sectioned (4 μm), and stained with hemotoxylin and eosin (H&E) as described [22].

Bone Histomorphometry

Specimens for plastic embedding and cancellous bone histomorphometry were harvested at sacrifice and the muscle dissected away before fixation in Mallonig's fixative as we have described previously [19,20,22,44,45]. For static histomorphometric analyses, 4–5 um-thick central saggital sections of undecalcified MMA embedded tibiae were stained for TRAP and counterstained with hematoxylin to determine osteoclast numbers and eroded surface, or with Masson's Trichrome for all other measurements, as defined by Parfitt [46] using Osteomeasure software (Osteometrics, Atlanta, GA). Dynamic measurement of bone formation was performed by injecting mice with 30 mg/kg of calcein 8-days before sacrifice and alizarin red S (15 mg/kg) or alizarin red complexone (18 mg/kg) 2-days before sacrifice [39,41]. The proportion of single and double labeled perimeters and the interlabel distance between the fluorophores were measured in the cancellous bone of unstained sections adjacent to those used for static measurements [19,20,22,45]. All cancellous bone measurements were made within the area defined by 700–1500 um distal to the growth plate-metaphyseal junction of the proximal tibia and 150 um away from either endocortical surface. A minimum of eight 20x fields in the proximal tibia were evaluated. Similarly, static cellular measurements of osteoblasts and osteoclasts were obtained as described [19,20,22]. Osteoclasts were enumerated in sections stained for TRAP, with osteoclasts identified as TRAP multinucleated cells, adjacent to bone. Osteoblasts were identified as layers of cuboidal cells aligned along a bone surface. All cellular and dynamic parameters are reported using the terminology recommended by the Histomorphometry Nomenclature Committee of American Society for Bone and Mineral Research [46] and as we have described [19,20].

Whole Femur Mechanical Testing

Mechanical testing was performed to determine bone strength of frozen Ts65Dn intact femora (3 month and 24 month), using standard three-point bending as we have described [19]. The thawed femurs were soaked in saline for 1 hour before testing to ensure hydration and then tested at room temperature using a servohydraulic-testing machine MTS 858 Bionex test systems load frame (MTS, Eden Prairie, MN) with computer control, data logging, and calculations of load to failure using TestWorks version 4.0 (MTS). Femurs were placed anterior side down on two horizontal supports spaced 7 mm apart; the central loading point contacted the posterior surface of the diaphysis at the midpoint of the bone length. The loading point was displaced downward (transverse to the long axis of the bone) at 0.1 mm/second until failure, generating bending in the anteroposterior plane. Load displacement data were recorded at 100 Hz (TestWorks 4.0, MTS), and test curves were analyzed to determine measures of whole-bone strength, primarily peak load and stiffness as we have described [19]. Load-to-failure was reported as the load after a 2% drop from peak load.

Ex vivo Marrow Cultures

Bone marrow cells were harvested from femurs for osteoclastogenic culture as previously described [19,21]. Briefly, cells were flushed from femurs, washed, and cultured in 24-well plates (Becton Dickinson Labware) at a density of 1×10^6 cells per well in α-minimal essential medium (α-MEM), supplemented with 15% fetal calf serum, and 10^{-8} M 1,25-dihydroxyvitamin D3 (1,25(OH)2D3 in quadruplicate wells per treatment. Cells were fed every 3 days with half-volumes of medium, until day 14, when cells were fixed and stained with tartrate resistant acid phosphatase (TRAP) to facilitate determination of the number of TRAP-positive multinucleated (3 or more nuclei) cells formed per well.

For osteoblastogenesis, bone marrow cells were harvested from femurs and seeded in triplicate at 2.5×10^5 cells/cm^2 on six-well tissue culture plates (Becton Dickinson Labware) osteoblast medium (α-MEM +15%FBS containing 10 mM BGP and 50 μM ascorbic acid). The total number of mesenchymal progenitors recruited into the osteoblastic lineage was measured by alkaline phosphatase-positive staining for colony forming unit-fibroblast (CFU-F) at day 10. Replicate cultures were fed every 3 days with half-volumes of medium, until day 28, when cells were fixed and minerals stained with Alizarin Red to facilitate determination of the number of bone nodules representing CFU-osteoblastic (CFU-OB) formed per well [19,21].

Statistical Analyses

All data were analyzed by either Student's t-test or one way ANOVA with post-hoc analyses by Bonferroni post-hoc test as appropriate. Parametric data are presented at mean ± SEM. Differences with P values <0.05 were considered statistically significant and are reported as such. The SigmaStat (SPSS Science) software package was used for all statistical analysis.

Supporting Information

Figure S1 Age-related bone phenotype in Ts65Dn mice. (**A**) Micro CT reconstructions of proximal tibia and femur from 3-month (left column) and 24-month (right column) old WT (top) and Ts65Dn (bottom) mice. Low bone volume and cortical thinning is evident. (**B**). Paraffin-embedded decalcified histological sections of proximal tibia from 3-month (left column) and 24-month (right column) old WT (top) and Ts65Dn (bottom) mice stained with H&E. The expected age-related decrease in trabecular bone is observed in both WT (top) and Ts65Dn (bottom), however, the expected increase in marrow fat is observed in WT (top) but not Ts65Dn (bottom). In contrast, Ts65Dn mice reveal the reported elevation in marrow megakaryocyte number [24] that increases with age (bottom), that is not observed in WT control mice (top). Original magnification 4X

Figure S2 Decreased cortical bone parameters of 24-month old Ts65Dn mice. Determination of femoral midshaft cortical parameters from Micro CT reconstructions of mid shaft femur shows significant decreases compared to WT in (**A**) cortical cross sectional area, (**B**) total cross sectional area, (**C**) periosteal perimeter, (**D**) Peak load (load tolerated at the breaking point adjusted for bone size), (**E**) Stiffness (deformation tolerated before breaking). Open bars WT; solid bars Ts65Dn. *, $p < 0.05$ vs. WT control.

Acknowledgments

We would also like to acknowledge the expert technical assistance of R. Shane Shelton in the PTH treatment experiment.

Author Contributions

Conceived and designed the experiments: KDM LJS GRW DG. Performed the experiments: TWF NSA JVS AWB JWB TS RAS FLS DBL WRH. Analyzed the data: LJS DG NSA TWF. Contributed reagents/materials/analysis tools: KDM DBL. Wrote the paper: LJS DG GAW KDM TWF.

References

1. Down JLH (1866) Observations on an ethnic classification of idiots. Clinical Lecture Reports, London Hospital 3: 259–262.
2. Hawli Y, Nasrallah M, El-Hajj Fuleihan G (2009) Endocrine and musculoskeletal abnormalities in patients with Down syndrome. Nat Rev Endocrinol 5: 327–334.
3. Bittles AH, Glasson EJ (2004) Clinical, social, and ethical implications of changing life expectancy in Down syndrome. Dev Med Child Neurol 46: 282–286.
4. Gonzalez-Aguero A, Vicente-Rodriguez G, Moreno LA, Casajus JA (2011) Bone mass in male and female children and adolescents with Down syndrome. Osteoporos Int 22: 2151–2157.
5. Angelopoulou N, Souftas V, Sakadamis A, Mandroukas K (1999) Bone mineral density in adults with Down's syndrome. Eur Radiol 9: 648–651.
6. Baptista F, Varela A, Sardinha LB (2005) Bone mineral mass in males and females with and without Down syndrome. Osteoporos Int 16: 380–388.
7. Olson LE, Mohan S (2011) Bone density phenotypes in mice aneuploid for the Down syndrome critical region. Am J Med Genet A 155: 2436–2445.
8. Hui SL, Slemenda CW, Johnston CC Jr (1990) The contribution of bone loss to postmenopausal osteoporosis. Osteoporos Int 1: 30–34.
9. Seeman E (1994) Reduced bone density in women with fractures: contribution of low peak bone density and rapid bone loss. Osteoporos Int 4 Suppl 1: 15–25.
10. Kao CH, Chen CC, Wang SJ, Yeh SH (1992) Bone mineral density in children with Down's syndrome detected by dual photon absorptiometry. Nucl Med Commun 13: 773–775.
11. Angelopoulou N, Matziari C, Tsimaras V, Sakadamis A, Souftas V, et al. (2000) Bone mineral density and muscle strength in young men with mental retardation (with and without Down syndrome). Calcif Tissue Int 66: 176–180.
12. Sepulveda D, Allison DB, Gomez JE, Kreibich K, Brown RA, et al. (1995) Low spinal and pelvic bone mineral density among individuals with Down syndrome. Am J Ment Retard 100: 109–114.
13. McKelvey KD, Fowler TW, Akel NS, Kelsay JA, Gaddy D, et al. (2012) Low bone turnover and low bone density in a cohort of adults with Down syndrome Osteoporos Int *In Press*.
14. Blazek JD, Gaddy A, Meyer R, Roper RJ, Li J (2011) Disruption of bone development and homeostasis by trisomy in Ts65Dn Down syndrome mice. Bone 48: 275–280.
15. Antonarakis SE, Lyle R, Dermitzakis ET, Reymond A, Deutsch S (2004) Chromosome 21 and down syndrome: from genomics to pathophysiology. Nat Rev Genet 5: 725–738.
16. Alford KA, Slender A, Vanes L, Li Z, Fisher EM, et al. (2010) Perturbed hematopoiesis in the Tc1 mouse model of Down syndrome. Blood 115: 2928–2937.
17. Reeves RH, Irving NG, Moran TH, Wohn A, Kitt C, et al. (1995) A mouse model for Down syndrome exhibits learning and behaviour deficits. Nat Genet 11: 177–184.
18. Gardiner K, Fortna A, Bechtel L, Davisson MT (2003) Mouse models of Down syndrome: how useful can they be? Comparison of the gene content of human chromosome 21 with orthologous mouse genomic regions. Gene 318: 137–147.
19. Suva LJ, Hartman E, Dilley JD, Russell S, Akel NS, et al. (2008) Platelet dysfunction and a high bone mass phenotype in a murine model of platelet-type von Willebrand disease. Am J Pathol 172: 430–439.
20. Suva LJ, Seedor JG, Endo N, Quartuccio HA, Thompson DD, et al. (1993) Pattern of gene expression following rat tibial marrow ablation. J Bone Miner Res 8: 379–388.
21. Gaddy-Kurten D, Coker JK, Abe E, Jilka RL, Manolagas SC (2002) Inhibin suppresses and activin stimulates osteoblastogenesis and osteoclastogenesis in murine bone marrow cultures. Endocrinology 143: 74–83.
22. Perrien DS, Akel NS, Edwards PK, Carver AA, Bendre MS, et al. (2007) Inhibin A is an endocrine stimulator of bone mass and strength. Endocrinology 148: 1654–1665.

23. Granholm AC, Ford KA, Hyde LA, Bimonte HA, Hunter CL, et al. (2002) Estrogen restores cognition and cholinergic phenotype in an animal model of Down syndrome. Physiol Behav 77: 371–385.
24. Kirsammer G, Jilani S, Liu H, Davis E, Gurbuxani S, et al. (2008) Highly penetrant myeloproliferative disease in the Ts65Dn mouse model of Down syndrome. Blood 111: 767–775.
25. Guijarro M, Valero C, Paule B, Gonzalez-Macias J, Riancho JA (2008) Bone mass in young adults with Down syndrome. J Intellect Disabil Res 52: 182–189.
26. da Silva VZ, de Franca Barros J, de Azevedo M, de Godoy JR, Arena R, et al. (2010) Bone mineral density and respiratory muscle strength in male individuals with mental retardation (with and without Down Syndrome). Res Dev Disabil 31: 1585–1589.
27. Parsons T, Ryan TM, Reeves RH, Richtsmeier JT (2007) Microstructure of trabecular bone in a mouse model for Down syndrome. Anat Rec (Hoboken) 290: 414–421.
28. Stefanidis K, Belitsos P, Fotinos A, Makris N, Loutradis D, et al. (2011) Causes of infertility in men with Down syndrome. Andrologia 43: 353–357.
29. Leffler A, Ludwig M, Schmitt O, Busch LC (1999) Germ cell migration and early development of the gonads in the trisomy 16 mouse–an animal model for Down's syndrome. Ann Anat 181: 247–252.
30. Campbell WA, Lowther J, McKenzie I, Price WH (1982) Serum gonadotrophins in Down's syndrome. J Med Genet 19: 98–99.
31. Sakadamis A, Angelopoulou N, Matziari C, Papameletiou V, Souftas V (2002) Bone mass, gonadal function and biochemical assessment in young men with trisomy 21. Eur J Obstet Gynecol Reprod Biol 100: 208–212.
32. Johannisson R, Gropp A, Winking H, Coerdt W, Rehder H, et al. (1983) Down's syndrome in the male. Reproductive pathology and meiotic studies. Hum Genet 63: 132–138.
33. Roy A, Roberts I, Norton A, Vyas P (2009) Acute megakaryoblastic leukaemia (AMKL) and transient myeloproliferative disorder (TMD) in Down syndrome: a multi-step model of myeloid leukaemogenesis. Br J Haematol 147: 3–12.
34. van Allen MI, Fung J, Jurenka SB (1999) Health care concerns and guidelines for adults with Down syndrome. Am J Med Genet 89: 100–110.
35. Grimwood JS, Kumar A, Bickerstaff DR, Suvarna SK (2000) Histological assessment of vertebral bone in a Down's syndrome adult with osteoporosis. Histopathology 36: 279–280.
36. Lindsay R, Cosman F, Zhou H, Bostrom MP, Shen VW, et al. (2006) A novel tetracycline labeling schedule for longitudinal evaluation of the short-term effects of anabolic therapy with a single iliac crest bone biopsy: early actions of teriparatide. J Bone Miner Res 21: 366–373.
37. Ma YL, Zeng Q, Donley DW, Ste-Marie LG, Gallagher JC, et al. (2006) Teriparatide increases bone formation in modeling and remodeling osteons and enhances IGF-II immunoreactivity in postmenopausal women with osteoporosis. J Bone Miner Res 21: 855–864.
38. Saag KG, Shane E, Boonen S, Marin F, Donley DW, et al. (2007) Teriparatide or alendronate in glucocorticoid-induced osteoporosis. N Engl J Med 357: 2028–2039.
39. Saag KG, Zanchetta JR, Devogelaer JP, Adler RA, Eastell R, et al. (2009) Effects of teriparatide versus alendronate for treating glucocorticoid-induced osteoporosis: thirty-six-month results of a randomized, double-blind, controlled trial. Arthritis Rheum 60: 3346–3355.
40. Neer RM, Arnaud CD, Zanchetta JR, Prince R, Gaich GA, et al. (2001) Effect of parathyroid hormone (1–34) on fractures and bone mineral density in postmenopausal women with osteoporosis. N Engl J Med 344: 1434–1441.
41. Li X, Ominsky MS, Warmington KS, Morony S, Gong J, et al. (2009) Sclerostin antibody treatment increases bone formation, bone mass, and bone strength in a rat model of postmenopausal osteoporosis. J Bone Miner Res 24: 578–588.
42. Ominsky MS, Li C, Li X, Tan HL, Lee E, et al. (2011) Inhibition of sclerostin by monoclonal antibody enhances bone healing and improves bone density and strength of nonfractured bones. J Bone Miner Res 26: 1012–1021.
43. Bouxsein ML, Boyd SK, Christiansen BA, Guldberg RE, Jepsen KJ, et al. (2010) Guidelines for assessment of bone microstructure in rodents using micro-computed tomography. J Bone Miner Res 25: 1468–1486.
44. Mohammad KS, Chen CG, Balooch G, Stebbins E, McKenna CR, et al. (2009) Pharmacologic inhibition of the TGF-beta type I receptor kinase has anabolic and anti-catabolic effects on bone. PLoS One 4: e5275.
45. Rzonca SO, Suva LJ, Gaddy D, Montague DC, Lecka-Czernik B (2004) Bone is a target for the antidiabetic compound rosiglitazone. Endocrinology 145: 401–406.
46. Parfitt AM, Drezner MK, Glorieux FH, Kanis JA, Malluche H, et al. (1987) Bone histomorphometry: standardization of nomenclature, symbols, and units. Report of the ASBMR Histomorphometry Nomenclature Committee. J Bone Miner Res 2: 595–610.

Rapid Diagnosis of Aneuploidy Using Segmental Duplication Quantitative Fluorescent PCR

Xiangdong Kong[1❡], Lin Li[2❡], Lei Sun[3*❡], Kepeng Fu[3], Ju Long[3], Xunjin Weng[3], Xuehe Ye[3], Xinxiong Liu[3], Bo Wang[4], Shanhuo Yan[3], Haiming Ye[3], Zuqian Fan[3]

1 Prenatal Diagnosis Center, the First Affiliated Hospital of Zhengzhou University, Henan, China, **2** Department of Genetic Laboratory, Lin Yi People's Hospital, Shandong, China, **3** Laboratory of Medical Genetics, Qinzhou Maternal and Child Health Care Hospital, Guangxi, China, **4** Genetics Laboratory, Hubei Maternal and Child Health Hospital, Hubei, China

Abstract

The aim of this study was use a simple and rapid procedure, called segmental duplication quantitative fluorescent polymerase chain reaction (SD-QF-PCR), for the prenatal diagnosis of fetal chromosomal aneuploidies. This method is based on the co-amplification of segmental duplications located on two different chromosomes using a single pair of fluorescent primers. The PCR products of different sizes were subsequently analyzed through capillary electrophoresis, and the aneuploidies were determined based on the relative dosage between the two chromosomes. Each primer set, containing five pairs of primers, was designed to simultaneously detect aneuploidies located on chromosomes 21, 18, 13, X and Y in a single reaction. We applied these two primer sets to DNA samples isolated from individuals with trisomy 21 (n = 36); trisomy 18 (n = 6); trisomy 13 (n = 4); 45, X (n = 5); 47, XXX (n = 3); 48, XXYY (n = 2); and unaffected controls (n = 40). We evaluated the performance of this method using the karyotyping results. A correct and unambiguous diagnosis with 100% sensitivity and 100% specificity, was achieved for clinical samples examined. Thus, the present study demonstrates that SD-QF-PCR is a robust, rapid and sensitive method for the diagnosis of common aneuploidies, and these analyses can be performed in less than 4 hours for a single sample, providing a competitive alternative for routine use.

Editor: Osman El-Maarri, University of Bonn, Institut of experimental hematology and transfusion medicine, Germany

Funding: The study was supported by Scientific Research and Technological Development of Guangxi Province (1140003A-48), Then Health Project of Guangxi Province (project no. Z2010032) and Scientific Research and Technological Development of Qinzhou City (20100901 and 20136104). The funders had no role in study design, data collection and analysis, decision to publish, or preparation of the manuscript.

Competing Interests: The authors have declared that no competing interests exist.

* E-mail: sunshijie12345@163.com

❡ These authors contributed equally to this work.

Introduction

Chromosomal aneuploidies cause a number of syndromes attributable to chromosomal aberration, and these abnormalities are typically associated with severe mental retardation, multiple dysmorphic features, growth retardation, etc. The frequency of chromosomal aneuploidy is approximately 1 out of 160 live births in the human population [1]. These diseases cannot be cured, and prenatal diagnosis is important to predict these syndromes. The prenatal diagnosis of chromosome aneuploidies is typically performed using G-band cytogenetic analysis with *in vitro* cultures of nucleated fetal cells retrieved through amniocentesis, chorionic biopsy or fetal blood sampling. This conventional cytogenetic technique detects a wide range of aberrations with high reliability and has become the gold standard for the detection of fetal chromosomal abnormalities since the 1970s [2]. However, conventional cytogenetics is time consuming (up to 2 weeks) and has technical issues, such as culture failure or external contamination. This method is also unable to detect submicroscopic duplications and deletions.

Quantitative methods, measuring the contributions from two different chromosomes, have been used for the rapid detection of trisomy 21 and other chromosome abnormalities. These methods target non-polymorphic sequences rather than polymorphisms, making this method potentially applicable to all human populations [3]. In 1997, homologous gene quantitative polymerase chain reaction (HGQ-PCR) was devised to estimate chromosome numbers for the detection of trisomy 21, showing unique advantages to detection using a single pair of primers [4]. However, a major drawback of this method is that the sequence of the sense primer differs from the PFKL-CH21 gene in exon 8 by one nucleotide, and the antisense primer differs from the PFKM-CH1 gene in exon 9 by one nucleotide. Therefore, the primers could not perfectly bind to the target sequence, making it difficult to maintain the original ratio. Real-time quantitative PCR (RT-PCR) is one of the most robust and versatile tools for the measurement of the copy numbers of nucleic acid sequences. This technology is amenable to automation and high throughput and could potentially reduce turnaround time and avoid issues of contamination [5]. Unfortunately, when dual primer sets and dual Taqman probes are used in a single reaction for amplification, even subtly biased annealing temperatures or DNA quality could produce false negative or ambiguous results [6]. Paralogous sequence quantification and high-resolution melting analyses are alternative techniques based on the use of a single primer to simultaneously amplify sequences from paralogous genes or segmental duplications [7,8]. These tests maintain the original ratio between the target and control chromosomes and can clearly differentiate between samples from patients with common aneuploidies and those from unaffected controls. However, these two tests require several separate PCR reactions for each sample, reducing sample throughput and increasing the probability of handling errors.

Quantitative fluorescence polymerase chain reaction (QF-PCR) is highly accurate and robust, processing 96 samples at one time in an automated system, and the results are available in less than 48 hours [9,10]. However, a major drawback to this technique is that the informative polymorphisms observed in one human population might not be applicable in another [11–13]. Multiplex ligation-dependent probe amplification (MLPA) has been validated for the diagnosis of changes in genomic copy numbers, and this technique has recently been applied for the analysis of chromosomal aneuploidy [14]. However, MLPA requires an overnight step for hybridization to human genomic DNA, making this technique time consuming and difficult to develop [15,16].

To address these drawbacks, we developed two novel segmental duplications for each target chromosome (chromosomes 21, 18, 13, X and Y) to detect aneuploidies. Segmental duplications are two similar sequences with different fragment lengths, located on two different chromosomes. These sequences maintain the original ratio between the two different chromosomes when co-amplified using a single pair of fluorescent primers. The PCR products of different sizes are subsequently analyzed through capillary electrophoresis, and the aneuploidies are determined based on the relative dosage between the two chromosomes in a single reaction. In the present study, we applied this method, called segmental duplication quantitative fluorescent polymerase chain reaction (SD-QF-PCR), to analyze 96 DNA samples. Here, we show that this method is a reliable, simple and high-throughput alternative for the diagnosis of targeted aneuploidies.

Materials and Methods

Ethics Statement

This study was conducted according to the principles expressed in the Declaration of Helsinki. The protocol for this study was approved through the Research Ethics Committee of Qinzhou Maternal and Child Health Hospital. Written informed consent was obtained from each participant for the collection of samples and subsequent analyses.

Samples

A total of 96 samples were collected in this study, of which 36 samples were obtained from patients with trisomy 21 (15 peripheral blood samples; 15 uncultured amniotic fluid samples and 6 cord blood samples); 2 samples were obtained from unbalanced translocation cases, including 46,XX,der(14;21)(q10;q10),+21; 4 cord blood samples were obtained from patients with trisomy 13; 6 samples from patients with trisomy 18 (3 uncultured amniotic fluid samples and 3 cord blood samples); 5 peripheral blood samples were obtained from 45, X patients; 3 peripheral blood samples were obtained from 47, XXX patients; and 2 peripheral blood samples were obtained from 48, XXYY patients. The samples obtained from 40 unaffected individuals (10 peripheral blood samples, 15 uncultured amniotic fluid samples and 15 cord blood samples) were used as unaffected controls. The karyotypes for all samples were previously validated through full karyotyping analysis, and these data were withheld from the technician who performed the SD-QF-PCR assays.

Table 1. Information for primers and amplicons.

Segmental duplications	Amplicon location	Amplicon size (bp)	Primer sequence (5′→3′)
Primer set one 21/11	chr21:38471113-38471259	147	F:GTGCCATTGACACAGGAGGAC
	chr11:66961762-66961889	128	R:FAM-CTTTACCCCCAGCTGTCCC
Primer set two 21/6	chr21:33921446-33921704	259	F:FAM-CAGGACCTGACCCTGGCT
	chr6:156574766-156575012	247	R:CGGGAGACTGCCATTGATGA
Primer set one 18/10	chr18:1362392-1362584	193	F:AGAGGACACACCAAACTAGATCA
	chr10:89514395-89514555	161	R:FAM-AGATGAAATTCGGCCTGTTCA
Primer set two 18/1	chr18:25655313-25655497	185	F:AGAGCTTCAGTTTCTCTGGTCC
	chr1:60749715-60749904	190	R:FAM-TCTAGATCATTGCCCATTGCCC
Primer set one X/Y	chrX:11314897-11315111	215	F:TTGAGGCCAACCATCAGAGC
	chrY:6737876-6738096	221	R:FAM-AGCTACCACCTCATCCTGGG
Primer set two X/Y	chrX:90738412-90738622	211	F:TCTTTTCTACCACTGAAACAGAGT
	chrY:4592828-4593027	200	R:FAM-AGGCGAGTAGCTGTCTATGA
Primer set one 13/11	chr13:90824978-90825215	238	F:AGGAATTCATCTTTCAAGGTCAAAA
	chr11:13751134-13751377	244	R:FAM-TGTTTTGAAGCAGGAGGATTTCT
Primer set two 13/9	chr13:19635510-19635629	120	F:CTTGGGAGAGGCCAAGAAAGA
	chr9:96393435-96393536	102	R:FAM-TGAGGCTGGGTCGAGGG
Primer set one 3/X	chr3:25797801-25798115	315	F:FAM-GGTTTTGCCTAGGTCCAGTG
	chrX:77386140-77386460	321	R:CCTGGTAATACAGCTCAGTGTCA
Primer set two 18/X	chr18:30092561-30092811	251	F:GCACCAGTGAAGATGATGGC
	chrX:79816393-79816660	268	R:FAM-TTGACCTGCCATACGAAGCA

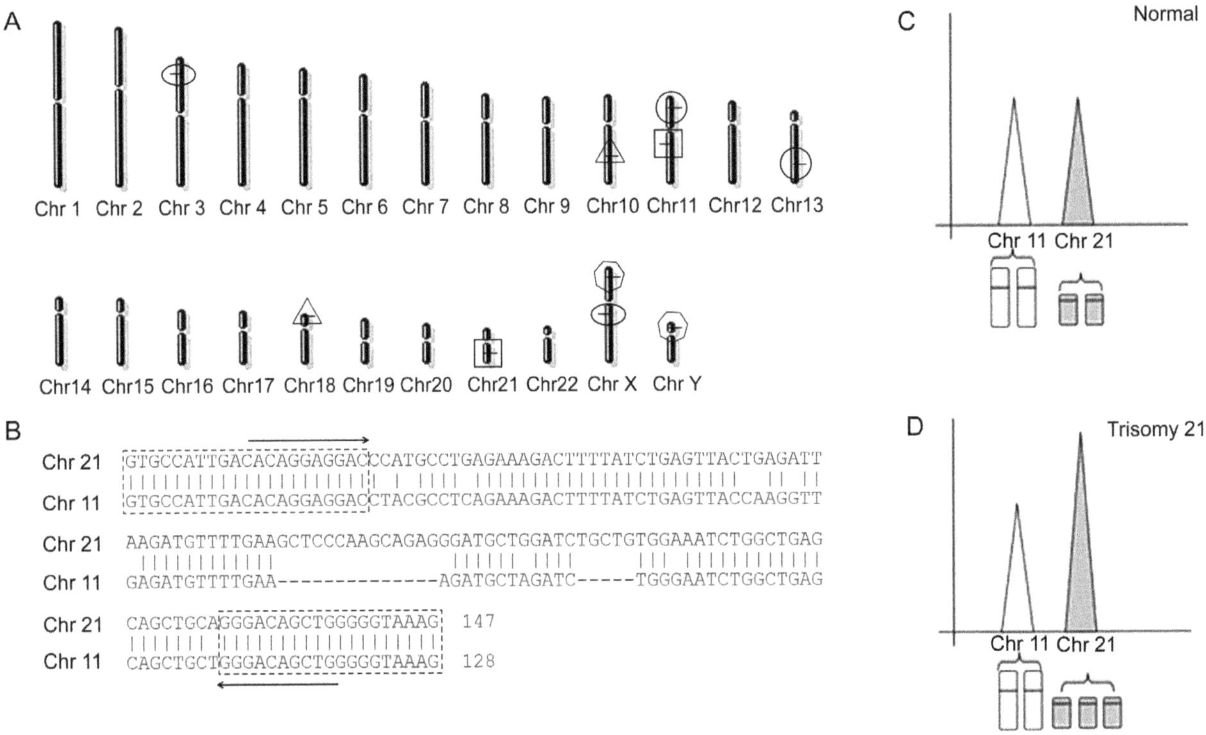

Figure 1. Ideogram of the segmental duplicates. A) The segmental duplications of primer set one located on human chromosomes (Chr). B) A single pair of primers was used to simultaneously amplify a 128-bp sequence on chr 11 and a 147-bp sequence on chr 21 from segmental duplications. C) Normal samples with a 1:1 pattern ratio of chromosome dosages. D) Trisomy 21 samples with a 2:3 pattern ratio of chromosome dosages.

DNA Extraction

DNA was extracted from uncultured amniotic fluid samples and blood samples using the QIAamp DNA Mini Kit (Qiagen) and the QIAamp DNA blood mini kit (Qiagen) according to the manufacturer's instructions. Approximately 5–20 ng of DNA was diluted to 25–50 μL and used in a SD-QF-PCR multiplex-based reaction. The concentration of the extracted genomic DNA was spectrophotometrically determined at an absorbance of 260 nm (Quawell). A total of 96 DNA samples, stored at −80°C, were used in the QF-PCR analysis.

Segmental Duplications and Primers

The segmental duplication sequences were obtained from two public databases: the Segmental Duplication Database (http://humanparalogy.gs.washington.edu/) and NCBI (http://www.ncbi.org/). Two independent primer sets (two segmental duplications per chromosome) were designed to simultaneously detect aneuploidies. The sequences of the PCR primers, available from the NCBI database, are presented in Table 1. One primer was unlabeled, and the other primer was labeled with FAM (6-carboxyfluorescein). All PCR primers and probes were constructed and purified through HPLC at GenScript.

PCR

The PCR amplification was performed using the Gene Amp® PCR System 9700 (Applied Biosystems) in a total reaction volume of 25 μL containing 1×Reaction Master Mix (Tiangen Biotech), 10 ng genomic DNA and 0.5 μmol/L of each forward and reverse primer. The reaction mixture was preheated at 95°C for 3 minutes, followed by 28 cycles of 30 seconds at 95°C, 30 seconds at 60°C, and 30 seconds at 72°C and a final extension step at 72°C for 10 minutes.

Electrophoretic Analysis

Approximately 1 μL of the PCR product was mixed with 24 μL of formamide and 1 μL of the GeneScan 500 Rox size standard (Applied Biosystems). The mixture was denatured at 95°C for 3 minutes and placed on ice to prevent re-annealing until further analysis. The electrophoretic analysis was performed using a POP4 gel (Applied Biosystems) on the ABI 3130×l Genetic Analyzer (Applied Biosystems). The PCR products were separated and visualized using GeneScan Analysis software (Applied Biosystems). GeneMapper® ID Software v3.2 (Applied Biosystems) was used for the data analysis. The relative probe signal ratios were calculated based on the peak area of the segmental duplication (length). The expected value for a euploid sample is 1, and the expected value for a trisomic sample is 1.5, reflecting the additional target chromosome (Figure 1C).

Results and Discussion

Segmental Duplication Selection and Primer Design

Segmental duplications are nearly identical DNA segments widespread throughout the human genome [17,18]. The information for segmental duplications was acquired from the Segmental Duplication Database (http://humanparalogy.gs.washington.edu/). We selected sequences with two hits from the whole genome: one hit must be located on the target chromosome (e.g., primer set one), and the other hit, with different sizes, must be located on a chromosome other than the target chromosome (Figure 1A). In addition, We built a consensus sequence, and

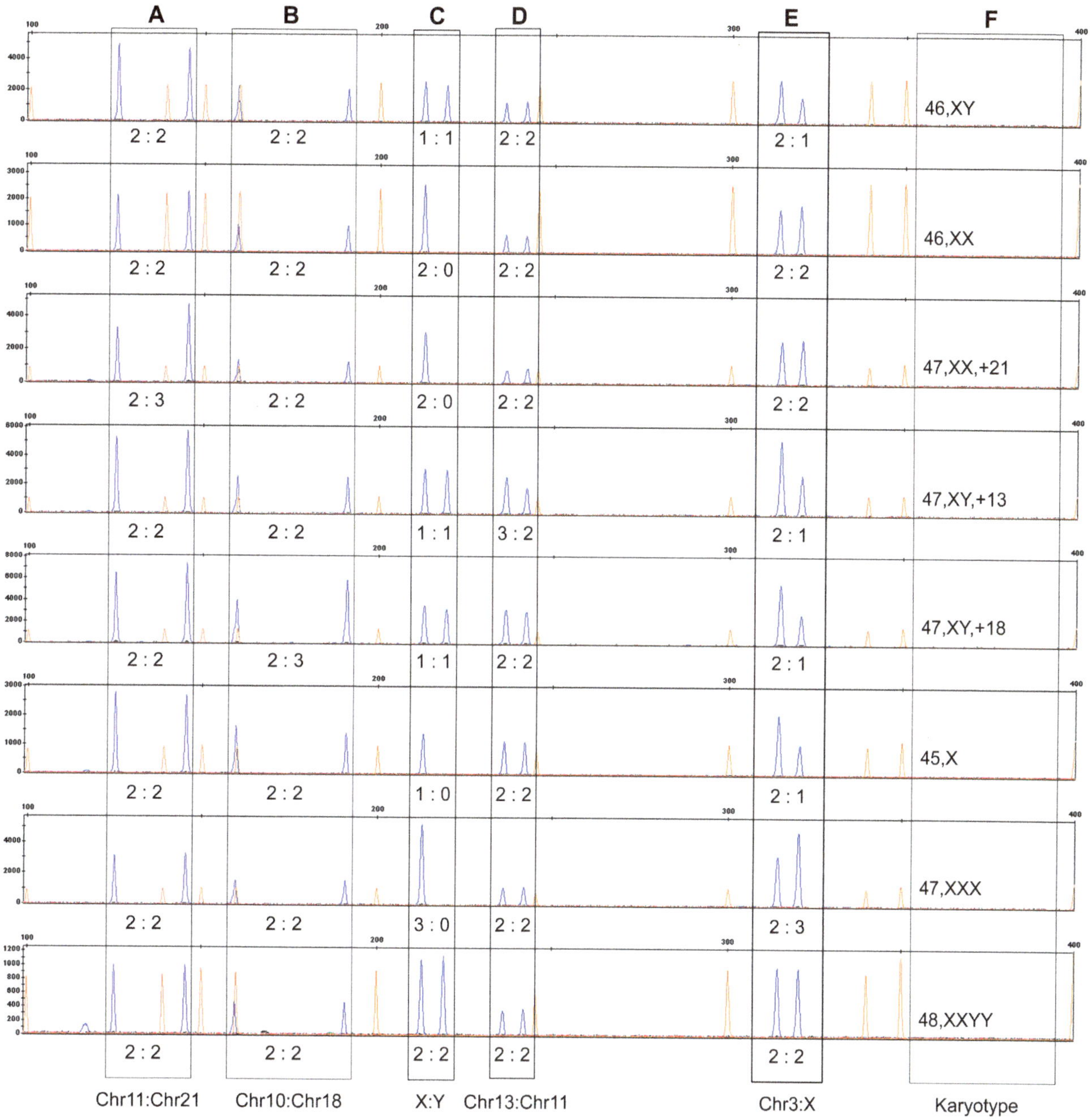

Figure 2. Electrophoretograms of primer set one. The aneuploidies of chromosomes 21, 18 and 13 could be detected using segmental duplications A, B and D, respectively; common sex chromosome aneuploidies could be identified through combinatorial analyses using segmental duplications C and E; F represents the karyotype of each individual.

Table 2. Assay patterns for common sex chromosome abnormalities.

Karyotype	Chr X:Chr Y	Autosome:Chr X
45,X	1:0	2:1
46,XX	2:0	2:2
46,XY	1:1	2:1
48,XXYY	2:2	2:2
47,XXX	3:0	2:3

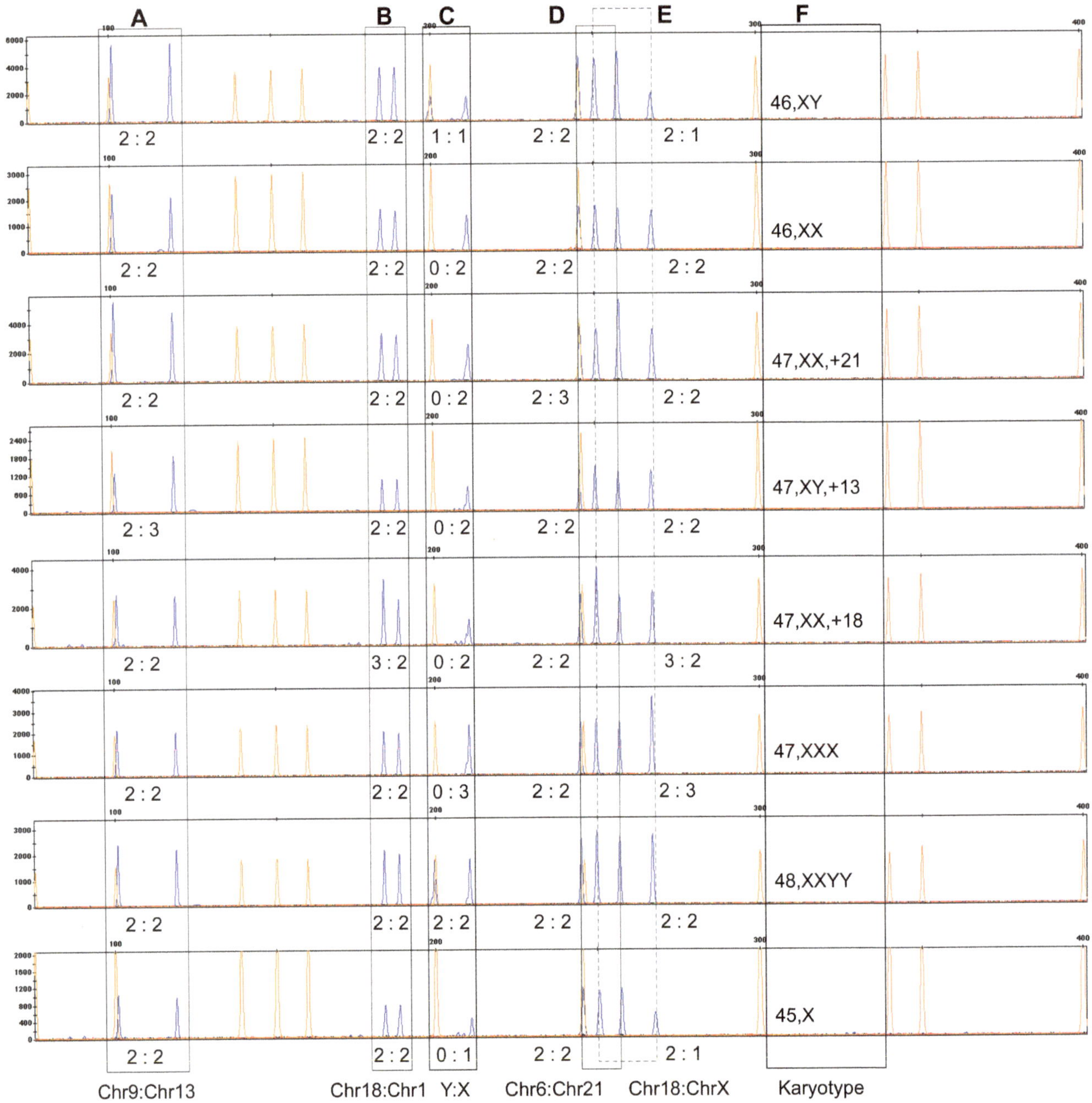

Figure 3. Electropheretograms of primer set two. The aneuploidies of chromosomes 13, 18 and 21 could be detected using segmental duplications A, B and D, respectively; common sex chromosome aneuploidies could be identified through combinatorial analyses using segmental duplications C and E; F represents the karyotype of each individual.

blasted this sequence against the human genome in NCBI (http://www.ncbi.nlm.nih.gov/tools/primer-blast) to obtain a suitable pair of primers, matching both sequences (Figure 1B), which can maintain the original ratio between the target and control chromosomes during amplification (Figure 1C).

We originally designed more than ten pairs of primers for capillary electrophoresis, and these primers were pre-screened under a number of PCR conditions. The following criteria were used to select the primers: (a) no obvious nonspecific primer extension products when the segmental duplications were amplified; (b) segmental duplications were amplified with equal efficiency, with sequence quantifications resulting in a 1:1 ratio; (c) a clear, non-overlapping difference between normal and abnormal samples after electrophoresis; and (d) minimal deviation from the mean. After PCR and capillary electrophoresis, we generated two primer sets (2 primers for each type of aneuploidy) with five pairs of primers each. Each primer met the criteria described above, and both primer sets could simultaneously detect the aneuploidies of chromosomes 21, 18, 13, X and Y in a single reaction (Table 1).

While we did not observe SNPs or CNVs within the target regions of the designed primers, these sequences might appear in some samples due to individual differences. Sequence variants in the primer region could produce false negative or ambiguous

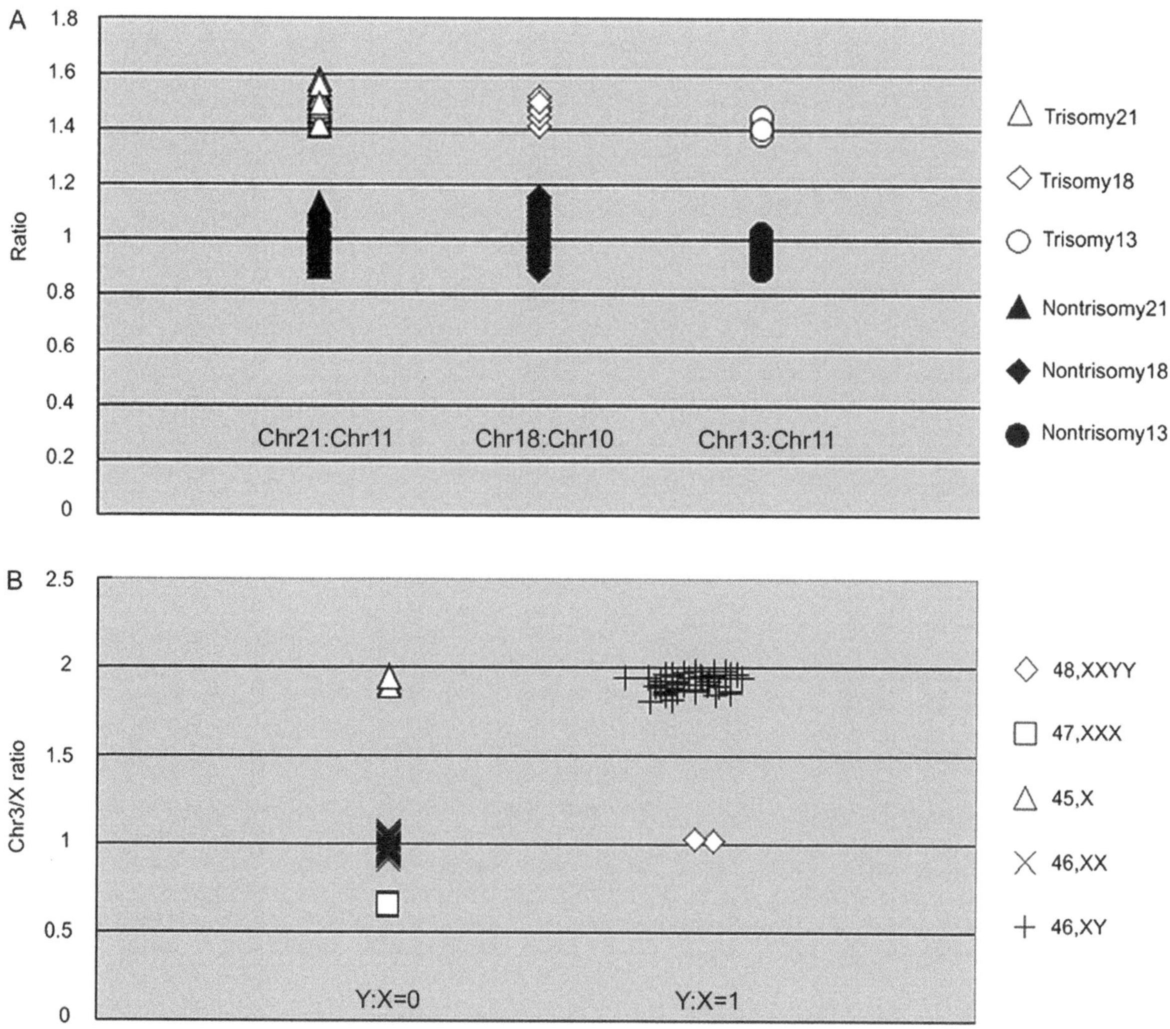

Figure 4. The individual distributions observed in the assays. A) Individual relative ratios of chromosomes 21,18 and 13 in normal and trisomic samples. B) Distribution of the X vs. Y and Chr 3 vs. X ratio; the x-axis represents the X/Y ratio, and the y-axis represents the Chr3/X ratio.

results. To resolve this problem, we analyzed two segmental duplications per chromosome to provide further accuracy in the analysis of a given aneuploidy. To reduce the mutual interference of the primers (which might result in imbalanced amplification and

Table 3. Specificity and sensitivity of the autosomal chromosomes for primer set one.

Primer set	Primer set one		
Segmental duplication	**Chr 21**	**Chr 18**	**Chr 13**
Mean control	1.01	1.03	0.95
SD control	0.06	0.06	0.05
95% CI control	0.96–1.07	0.96–1.09	0.91–0.98
Mean trisomic	1.49	1.47	1.40
SD trisomic	0.05	0.04	0.03
95% CI trisomic	1.44–1.54	1.43–1.51	1.38–1.43
Total samples	96	96	96
Sensitivity	1	1	1
Specificity	1	1	1

a failed experiment), we designed two independent primer sets to simultaneously detect aneuploidies. Thus, this assay design reduces the probability of detecting sequence variants in the two target regions at the same time. Furthermore, in clinical practice, differences between the two assays might reflect structural abnormalities. In such cases, full karyotyping, FISH, or array comparative genomic hybridization should be applied for diagnostic confirmation. The major drawback of this approach, similar to many other PCR-based assays, is that it is possible to miss some cases of structural abnormalities, low-level mosaicism or maternal cell contamination. However, this drawback does not hinder the wide application of this technology.

Detection of the Common Chromosome Aneuploidies

To reduce the probability of a variant in the primer region, we selected two target regions per chromosome and designed two primer sets to simultaneously detect aneuploidies. For primer set one, a series of qualified segmental duplications, located on chromosomes 21 and 11, chromosomes 18 and 10 and chromosomes 13 and 11, were selected to detect the aneuploidies of chromosomes 21, 18 and 13, respectively (Figures 2A, 2B and 2D). To detect abnormalities on the sex chromosomes, we designed two pairs of primers: segmental duplications located on chromosomes X and Y (Figure 2C) were designed to quantify the ratio between the X and Y chromosomes, and segmental duplications located on chromosomes 3 and X were designed to quantify the ratio between chromosomes 3 and X (Figure 2E). In theory, the common abnormalities of sex chromosomes can be identified using these two primers pairs (Table 2).

For primer set two, the segmental duplications located on chromosomes 13 and 9, chromosomes 18 and 1 and chromosomes 21 and 6 were selected to detect the aneuploidies of chromosomes 13, 18 and 21, respectively (Figures 3A, 3B and 3D). Segmental duplications located on chromosomes X and 18 and chromosomes X and Y were designed to detect abnormalities on the sex chromosomes (Figures 3C and 3E).

We examined 96 DNA samples in each of the two assays and obtained a correct and unambiguous diagnosis in all cases. In total, 56 aneuploidies were detected: 36 cases of trisomy 21; 4 cases of trisomy 13; 6 cases of trisomy 18; 5 cases of trisomy 45, X; 3 cases of trisomy 47, XXX; and 2 cases of trisomy 48, XXYY. A total of 40 unaffected DNA controls were also screened in each assay. The diagnostic sensitivity and specificity of all samples was 100%, and the results correlated with their respective karyotypes. We attribute this high reliably to the use of segmental duplications as detection targets. A single pair of primers can perfectly match both loci to co-amplify the segmental duplications located on two different chromosomes, while maintaining almost identical amplification efficiencies between target chromosomes and control chromosomes. Therefore, segmental duplications can be used to reliably detect chromosome abnormalities. For primer set one, the means and standard deviations for the segmental duplications on the autosomal chromosomes are shown in Table 3, and all 96 samples were categorized into different groups according to their mean values (Figure 4).

A total of 36 samples with trisomy 21 were observed, including two unbalanced translocations (46,XX,der(14; 21)(q10;q10),+21) correctly diagnosed as trisomy 21 using SD-QF-PCR. For the determination of trisomy 21, two pairs of segmental duplications (Chr21/Chr11 and Chr21/Chr9) were selected for the identification of additional copies of chromosome 21 (Figure 2A and Figure 3D). The segmental duplications were located on the long arm of chromosome 21 [19]. Thus, these results demonstrate that this approach is not only an acceptable method for detecting an extra target chromosome, but also for detecting the relative dosage of the chromosomes in which the segmental duplications are located, i.e., chromosome deletion or duplication.

Methodology Comparison

Fluorescent in situ hybridization (FISH) is a routine method used for the rapid detection of prenatal aneuploidies in interphase amniocytes. This method avoids the need to culture cells and reduces the time required for diagnosis. However, this technique is relatively labor intensive and requires technical expertise, requirements that prevent the efficient processing of a large number of samples in clinical diagnostic settings [20,21]. These drawbacks have encouraged the development of more rapid and efficient methods for the detection of fetal chromosomal aneuploidies.

QF-PCR and MLPA are the most extensively validated DNA-based techniques described for the rapid detection of fetal chromosomal aneuploidies [9–12]. However, for QF-PCR, based on the amplification of polymorphic microsatellite repeats, the differences in the number of informative polymorphisms might limit the universality of this assay. Segmental duplications are not dependent on multiple informative polymorphism markers, applicable to all human populations. Thus, this method could be considered as an alternative or complement strategy to QF-PCR. MLPA, which requires an overnight step for hybridization, requires approximately 16 hours to detect a single sample. SD-QF-PCR exhibits equal application efficiency and saves more than 12 hours turnaround time, making SD-QF-PCR faster and easier. Compared with conventional karyotype analyses, SD-QF-PCR reduces the turnaround time from 2–4 weeks to less than 4 hours for a single aneuploidy test [2]. Using the current protocol, a single operator can manage at least 96 samples a day and report the results in less than 24 hours, which should meet the needs of most diagnostic laboratories.

Conclusions

In the present study, we designed two novel sets of segmental duplications and described a simple and rapid SD-QF-PCR method as an alternative approach to simultaneously detect the aneuploidies of chromosomes 21, 18, 13, X and Y in a single reaction. This method can process 96 samples at a time in an automated system for each primer set, and the results are available the same day. The retrospective study of 96 DNA samples was entirely consistent with the previous results of conventional cytogenetics. Thus, this procedure represents a competitive alternative diagnostic tool for use in prenatal screening.

Acknowledgments

The authors would like to thank Yangqing Lu at Guangxi University for assistance with the English.

Author Contributions

Conceived and designed the experiments: LS. Performed the experiments: XK LL LS BW XY XL. Analyzed the data: KF JL. Contributed reagents/materials/analysis tools: XW SY HY. Wrote the paper: LS ZF.

References

1. Driscoll DA, Gross S (2009) Clinical practice. Prenatal screening for aneuploidy. N Engl J Med 360: 2556–2562.
2. Caspersson T, Zech L, Johansson C, Modest EJ (1970) Identification of human chromosomes by DNA-binding fluorescent agents. Chromosoma 30: 215–227.
3. Von Eggeling F, Freytag M, Fahsold R, Horsthemke B, Claussen U (1993) Rapid detection of trisomy 21 by quantitative PCR. Hum Genet 91: 567–570.
4. Lee HH, Chang JG, Lin SP, Chao HT, Yang ML, et al. (1997) Rapid detection of trisomy 21 by homologous gene quantitative PCR (HGQ-PCR). Hum Genet 99: 364–367.
5. Zimmermann B, Holzgreve W, Wenzel F, Hahn S (2002) Novel real-time quantitative PCR test for trisomy 21. Clin Chem 48: 362–363.
6. Helmy SM, Ismail S, Bassiouni R, Gaber KR (2009) Sensitivity of DCSR3/GAPDH ratio using quantitative real-time PCR in the rapid prenatal diagnosis for down syndrome. Fetal Diagn Ther 25: 220–223.
7. Deutsch S, Choudhury U, Merla G, Howald C, Sylvan A, et al. (2004) Detection of aneuploidies by paralogous sequence quantification. J Med Genet 41: 908–915.
8. Guo Q, Xiao L, Zhou Y (2012) Rapid diagnosis of aneuploidy by high-resolution melting analysis of segmental duplications. Clin Chem 58: 1019–1025.
9. Mansfield ES (1993) Diagnosis of Down syndrome and other aneuploidies using quantitative polymerase chain reaction and small tandem repeat polymorphisms. Hum Mol Genet 2: 43–50.
10. Mann K, Donaghue C, Fox SP, Docherty Z, Ogilvie CM (2004) Strategies for the rapid prenatal diagnosis of chromosome aneuploidy. Eur J Hum Genet 12: 907–915.
11. Atef SH, Hafez S, Helmy S, Helmy N (2011) QF-PCR as a Rapid Technique for Routine Prenatal Diagnosis of Fetal Aneuploidies. Pediatr Res 70: 412–412.
12. Slater HR, Bruno DL, Ren H, Pertile M, Schouten JP, et al. (2003) Rapid, high throughput prenatal detection of aneuploidy using a novel quantitative method (MLPA). J Med Genet 40: 907–912.
13. Dudarewicz L, Holzgreve W, Jeziorowska A, Jakubowski L, Zimmermann B (2005) Molecular methods for rapid detection of aneuploidy. J Appl Genet 46: 207–215.
14. Schouten JP, McElgunn CJ, Waaijer R, Zwijnenburg D, Diepvens F, et al. (2002) Relative quantification of 40 nucleic acid sequences by multiplex ligation-dependent probe amplification. Nucleic acids res 30: e57.
15. Boormans EM, Birnie E, Oepkes D, Galjaard RJ, Schuring-Blom GH, et al. (2010) Comparison of multiplex ligation-dependent probe amplification and karyotyping in prenatal diagnosis. Obstet Gynecol 115: 297–303.
16. Willis AS, Veyver I, Eng CM (2012) Multiplex ligation-dependent probe amplification (MLPA) and prenatal diagnosis. Prenat Diagn 32: 315–320.
17. She X, Jiang Z, Clark RA, Liu G, Cheng Z, et al. (2004) Shotgun sequence assembly and recent segmental duplications within the human genome. Nature 431: 927–930.
18. Bailey JA, Yavor AM, Massa HF, Trask BJ, Eichler EE (2001) Segmental duplications: organization and impact within the current human genome project assembly. Genome Res 11: 1005–1017.
19. Baldus CD, Liyanarachchi S, Mrózek K, Auer H, Tanner SM, et al. (2004) Acute myeloid leukemia with complex karyotypes and abnormal chromosome 21: Amplification discloses overexpression of APP, ETS2, and ERG genes. PNAS 101: 3915–3920.
20. Caine A, Maltby AE, Parkin CA, Waters JJ, Crolla JA, et al. (2005) Prenatal detection of Down's syndrome by rapid aneuploidy testing for chromosomes 13, 18, and 21 by FISH or PCR without a full karyotype: a cytogenetic risk assessment. Lancet 366: 123–128.
21. Ho SS, Chua C, Gole L, Biswas A, Koay E, et al. (2012) Same-day prenatal diagnosis of common chromosomal aneuploidies using microfluidics-fluorescence in situ hybridization. Prenat Diagn 32: 321–328.

Risk Factors for Hospital Admission with RSV Bronchiolitis in England: A Population-Based Birth Cohort Study

Joanna Murray[1]*, Alex Bottle[1], Mike Sharland[2], Neena Modi[3], Paul Aylin[1], Azeem Majeed[1], Sonia Saxena[1], on behalf of the Medicines for Neonates Investigator Group[¶]

1 Department of Primary Care and Public Health, Imperial College London, London, United Kingdom, **2** Paediatric Infectious Diseases Unit, St. George's Hospital NHS Trust, London, United Kingdom, **3** Section of Neonatal Medicine, Department of Medicine, Imperial College London, London, United Kingdom

Abstract

Objective: To examine the timing and duration of RSV bronchiolitis hospital admission among term and preterm infants in England and to identify risk factors for bronchiolitis admission.

Design: A population-based birth cohort with follow-up to age 1 year, using the Hospital Episode Statistics database.

Setting: 71 hospitals across England.

Participants: We identified 296618 individual birth records from 2007/08 and linked to subsequent hospital admission records during the first year of life.

Results: In our cohort there were 7189 hospital admissions with a diagnosis of bronchiolitis, 24.2 admissions per 1000 infants under 1 year (95%CI 23.7–24.8), of which 15% (1050/7189) were born preterm (47.3 bronchiolitis admissions per 1000 preterm infants (95% CI 44.4–50.2)). The peak age group for bronchiolitis admissions was infants aged 1 month and the median was age 120 days (IQR = 61–209 days). The median length of stay was 1 day (IQR = 0–3). The relative risk (RR) of a bronchiolitis admission was higher among infants with known risk factors for severe RSV infection, including those born preterm (RR = 1.9, 95% CI 1.8–2.0) compared with infants born at term. Other conditions also significantly increased risk of bronchiolitis admission, including Down's syndrome (RR = 2.5, 95% CI 1.7–3.7) and cerebral palsy (RR = 2.4, 95% CI 1.5–4.0).

Conclusions: Most (85%) of the infants who are admitted to hospital with bronchiolitis in England are born at term, with no known predisposing risk factors for severe RSV infection, although risk of admission is higher in known risk groups. The early age of bronchiolitis admissions has important implications for the potential impact and timing of future active and passive immunisations. More research is needed to explain why babies born with Down's syndrome and cerebral palsy are also at higher risk of hospital admission with RSV bronchiolitis.

Editor: Oliver Schildgen, Kliniken der Stadt Köln gGmbH, Germany

Funding: JM was funded through a National Institute for Health Research (NIHR) Programme Grant for Applied Research (RP-PG-0707-10010) held by NM; JM and NM declare financial support from this award for the submitted work. Support for data analysis was received from the Neonatal Data Analysis Unit led by NM. Unrestricted support for the Neonatal Data Analysis Unit from Abbott International and Danone UK is acknowledged. The Dr Foster Unit at Imperial are principally funded via a research grant by Dr Foster Intelligence, an independent healthcare information company and joint venture with the Information Centre of the NHS. The Unit is affiliated with the NIHR Imperial Centre for Patient Safety and Service Quality at Imperial College Healthcare NHS Trust. The Department of Primary Care & Public Health at Imperial College is grateful for support from the NIHR Collaboration for Leadership in Applied Health Research & Care (CLAHRC) for North West London (a partnership between Chelsea and Westminster NHS Foundation Trust and Imperial College London), the NIHR Imperial Biomedical Research Centre (a partnership between Imperial College Healthcare NHS Trust and Imperial College London), and the NIHR Imperial Centre for Patient Safety and Service Quality. SS has an NIHR career development fellowship. This publication presents independent research funded by the National Institute for Health Research (NIHR) under its Programme Grants for Applied Research scheme (RP-PG-0707-10010). The views expressed in this publication are those of the authors and not necessarily those of the NHS, the NIHR or the Department of Health. The funders had no role in the study design, collection, analysis, and interpretation of data, in the writing of the report or in the decision to submit the paper for publication.

Competing Interests: We have the following interests: Unrestricted support for the Neonatal Data Analysis Unit from Abbott International and Danone UK is acknowledged. The Dr Foster Unit at Imperial are principally funded via a research grant by Dr Foster Intelligence, an independent healthcare information company and joint venture with the Information Centre of the NHS. There are no patents, products in development or marketed products to declare.

* E-mail: joanna.murray@imperial.ac.uk

¶ Membership of the Medicines for Neonates Investigator Group is provided in the Acknowledgments.

Introduction

Acute bronchiolitis is the most common lower respiratory tract infection (LRTI) in infants affecting around 10% of children under 1 year [1–5]. It is usually a mild, self-limiting illness but in some infants may be more severe, requiring hospital admission. Bronchiolitis is typically caused by respiratory syncytial virus (RSV) in around 75% of cases [6], with peak incidence during the winter months. Bronchiolitis admission rates in infants under 1 year have previously been estimated from small regional studies to be 30·8 per 1000 in the United Kingdom (UK) [3] and 31·2 per 1000 in the United States (US) [7]. To date, no national studies have reported the disease burden at a population level in the UK.

Children known to be at high risk of developing severe RSV infection include those with chronic lung disease, congenital heart disease, immunodeficiency, low birth weight and those born preterm (approximately 8% of newborns in the UK) [8–11]. Other factors associated with RSV infection include winter births, poverty, malnutrition, tobacco smoke exposure, lack of breast-feeding and multiple gestation [12]. Evidence from the US suggests most children admitted to hospital with RSV infection are healthy, with no risk factors for severe RSV infection [9].

Since there is no effective drug treatment, the mainstay of management for infants with RSV bronchiolitis is supportive care and a small proportion of more severely affected infants are treated in intensive care [1,13–15]. Prophylactic passive immunotherapy with Palivizumab (Synagis®, MedImmune), a monoclonal antibody against RSV infection, is licensed for use in some countries for those most at high risk of RSV infection, but is very expensive (the estimated cost for a single dose of Palivizumab for an infant aged 6 months, weighing 7·5 kg, is £1023·11 [16] so the total cost for 5 doses over the winter season is just over £5000 per patient). The Joint Committee for Vaccination and Immunisation (JCVI) in the UK states Palivizumab use is only cost-effective for a small group of infants at most risk of severe disease [16–18], but there remains a poor evidence base of prognostic factors for hospital admission due to RSV infection [18]. An active immunisation against RSV is currently in phase III trials, also aimed primarily at high-risk groups. However, the difficulty of eliciting immunity in such young infants remains a challenge. The aim of this study was to examine which infants are most at risk of an RSV bronchiolitis admission in England in term, preterm and high-risk infants and to determine the age at and duration of an RSV bronchiolitis admission.

Methods

Data

Hospital Episodes Statistics (HES) is a national administrative database, electronically recording all admissions to NHS hospitals in England since 1989 (www.hesonline.nhs.uk) [19] and has been used extensively for research and measuring quality of healthcare delivery [20,21]. Annual reports from the Office for National Statistics suggest that around 97% of all live births in England occur in NHS hospitals. Coders enter information about clinical diagnoses undertaken using the International Classification of Diseases 10th revision (ICD-10). Maternity data in HES consists of delivery records (for mothers) and birth records (for babies). These contain additional data fields known as the "baby tail", which include information such as birth weight and gestational age [22–24].

Study cohort

We created a birth cohort for all infants born in English NHS hospitals and discharged during a twelve month period (from 1st April 2007 to 31st March 2008). We included only records from live births and excluded infants born in hospitals (85/156) with poor recording (<90% complete) of key indicators (birth weight and gestational age), to enable us to group infants into term and preterm categories [24]. Sensitivity analyses of number of maternity beds, annual number of births, geographic location and infant death rate were conducted to compare hospitals in the study with sites excluded because of poor recording [24]. We linked birth records to subsequent hospital admission records up to a child's first birthday, using a unique personal identifier (HES ID). Linkage to Office of National Statistics (ONS) mortality records allowed us to identify any deaths among the birth cohort during their first year of life, including out-of-hospital deaths.

Outcome and exposure measures

Diagnostic information recorded in individual birth records and any subsequent hospital admission records from the study year was used to group infants into categories of risk factors for severe RSV infection (Appendix S1) using ICD-10 codes or larger subgroups using the Agency for Health Research and Quality's Clinical Classification System (CCS) [25]. Infants were considered preterm if their gestational age at birth was less than 37 weeks (Appendix S1), in accordance with the World Health Organisation (WHO) definition of premature birth [26]. Infants missing gestational age were assumed to be born at full term.

We identified infants admitted as an emergency with a primary diagnosis of acute bronchiolitis using the 'J21' ICD-10 codes ('J210' - acute bronchiolitis due to respiratory syncytial virus, 'J218' - acute bronchiolitis due to other specified organisms and 'J219' - acute bronchiolitis, unspecified). Most bronchiolitis admissions were coded with unspecific aetiology and approximately a third were coded as being due to RSV. We grouped all bronchiolitis codes into a single "RSV bronchiolitis" category as RSV is the commonest cause of bronchiolitis, but specific microbiological diagnoses are poorly coded in HES. We excluded bronchiolitis admissions in children over 1 year because of the uncertain nature of this clinical diagnosis in older infants. We defined infants as being under 1 year of age. We examined age at bronchiolitis admission and calculated the median length of stay (LOS) for bronchiolitis admissions to provide a proxy measure of severity of illness.

Statistical analyses

We calculated the absolute risk of a bronchiolitis admission among infants with and without risk factors for severe RSV infection, including preterm infants and infants with a clinical diagnosis of cystic fibrosis, congenital heart disease, nervous system congenital anomalies, other congenital anomalies, immunodeficiency, cerebral palsy or Down's syndrome (case definitions and codes in Appendix S1). Infants without a particular risk factor condition were considered "healthy". Associated 95% confidence intervals (CI) were calculated using Poisson approximation. We calculated the relative risk (RR) of a bronchiolitis admission, with associated 95% CI for infants in each individual risk group, by comparing with the baseline group of infants without the particular risk factor. Infants may belong to more than 1 of these risk groups, so we controlled for this potential confounding using Poisson regression models to calculate the adjusted RR of bronchiolitis admission for infants in each risk group. To test for significant differences between proportions we used Chi Squared tests and Mann-Whitney tests to compare median values for non-normal data. Data were analysed using the SAS 9·2 software package (SAS Institute, Cary, N.C., USA).

Research Ethics approval

We have permission from the National Information Governance Board (NIGB) under Section 251 of the NHS Act 2006 (formerly Section 60 approval from the Patient Information Advisory Group) to hold confidential data. We have approval to use them for research and measuring quality of delivery of healthcare, from the South East Ethics Research Committee.

Results

The birth cohort included 296618 infants, from 71 NHS hospitals in England. 410 infants in the cohort died during the study year. 51% (151897/296618) of the cohort were boys, 1% (2891) were multiple births and 7·5% (22215) were born preterm before 37 weeks gestation (Table S2, Appendix S2).

Among our birth cohort there were 7189 admissions to hospital with a primary diagnosis of bronchiolitis during their first year of life, 24·2 admissions per 1000 infants (95% CI 23·7 to 24·8). Only 2015 (28·0%) of these were specifically coded as being due to RSV, the remainder were unspecified. In total, 1529 (21·3%) infants admitted with bronchiolitis, had more than one bronchiolitis admission during their first year of life. The modal age of bronchiolitis admission was 1 month (Figure 1) and the median age was 120 days (Inter-quartile range (IQR) = 61 to 209). The median length of hospital stay was 1 day (IQR = 0 to 3 days).

Among infants admitted with bronchiolitis, 15% (1050/7189) were born preterm. Admission rates were higher among infants born preterm (47·3 per 1000 infants (95%CI 44·4–50·2)) compared with those born at term (22·4 per 1000 infants (95%CI 21·8–22·9)) (Table 1). The median length of stay for a bronchiolitis admission among infants born preterm was 1 day (IQR = 0 to 3) and among those born at term it was also 1 day (IQR = 0 to 3). The median age of the bronchiolitis admission among infants born preterm was 136 days (IQR = 71 to 221) compared with 118 days (IQR = 59 to 207) among infants born at term ($p<0·001$).

Among infants admitted with bronchiolitis, 1722 (24·0%) had one or more known risk factors for severe RSV infection. The adjusted RR of a bronchiolitis admission was high among infants with known risk factors for severe RSV disease, including those born preterm (RR 1·9 (95%CI 1·8–2·0)) or with congenital heart conditions (RR 3·4 (95%CI 2·9–3·8)) or chronic lung disease (RR 1·6 (95%CI 1·4–1·8)), compared with healthy infants without the risk factor (Table 1). Other conditions also significantly increased an infant's risk of bronchiolitis admission, including cystic fibrosis (RR = 2·5 (95% CI 1·4 to 4·4)), Down's syndrome (RR 2·5 (95%CI 1·7–3·7)), cerebral palsy (RR 2·4 (95%CI 1·5–4·0)) and other nervous system congenital abnormalities (RR = 1·7 (95% CI 1·3 to 2·4)). A higher proportion of infants born in September (3·9%) or October (3·8%) were admitted with bronchiolitis than among infants born in any other month ($p<0·001$). Bronchiolitis admission rates among infants born in the North East (3·3%) and Yorkshire and the Humber (3·3%) SHAs, were higher ($p<0·001$) compared with in infants born in London (1·6%) (Figure 2).

Discussion

Main findings

Most (85%) of the infants who are admitted to hospital with bronchiolitis in England are born at term, with no known predisposing risk factors for severe RSV infection, although risk of admission is higher in known risk groups. Babies born with Down's syndrome, cerebral palsy and cystic fibrosis are also at higher risk of hospital admission with RSV bronchiolitis. The early age of bronchiolitis admissions has important implications for the potential impact and timing of future active and passive immunisations.

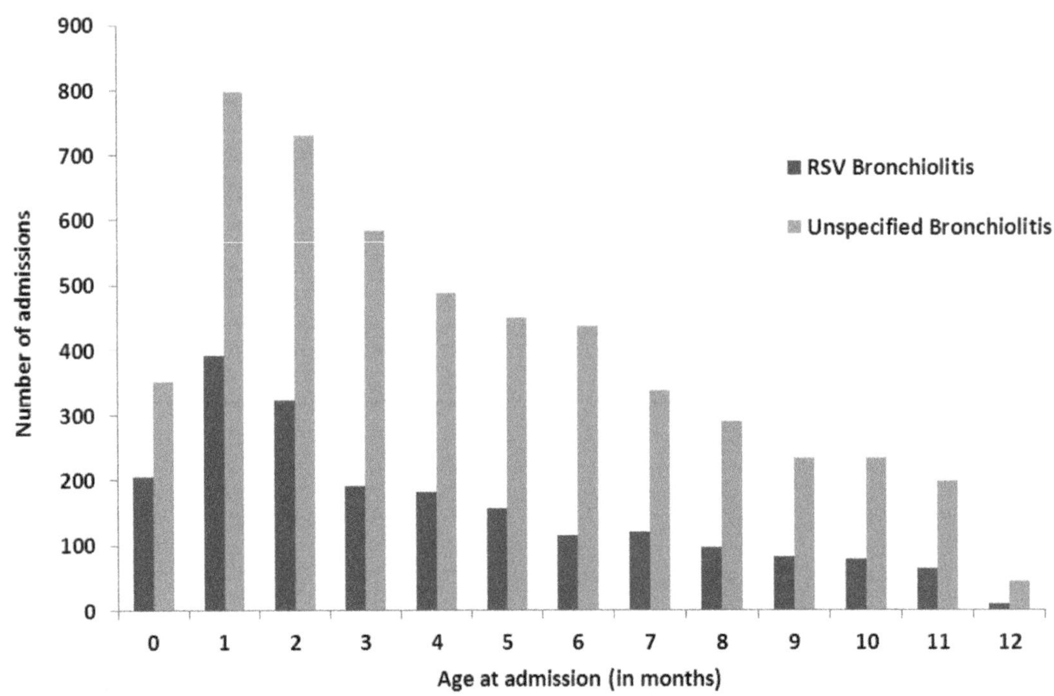

Figure 1. Age of bronchiolitis admission in months, for admissions coded as RSV or unspecified bronchiolitis.

Table 1. Rates and relative risk of a bronchiolitis hospital admission among infants in different risk groups.

Risk Group†	Number of bronchiolitis admissions (% of infants in risk group)	Total number of infants in risk group (% of whole birth cohort)	Median length of stay in days (IQR)	Rate of bronchiolitis admission per 1000 infants under 1 year (95% CIs)	RR† (95% CIs)	Adjusted RR (95%CI)
Born at term	6139 (2·2)	274403 (92·5)	1 (0 to 3)	22·4 (21·8 to 22·9)	–	–
Premature birth	1050 (4·7)	22215 (7·5)	1 (0 to 3)	47·3 (44·4 to 50·2)	2·11 (1·98 to 2·26)	1.89 (1·77 to 2·02)
Cystic fibrosis	11 (6·4)	171 (0·1)	2 (0 to 14)	64·3 (32·1 to 115·1)	2·66 (1·33 to 4·76)	2·45 (1·36 to 4·43)
Congenital heart Disease	272 (12·1)	2239 (0·8)	2 (0 to 5)	121·5 (107·5 to 136·8)	5·17 (4·56 to 5·84)	3·35 (2·92 to 3·84)
Chronic lung disease	282 (5·6)	5016 (1·7)	2 (0 to 4)	56·2 (49·9 to 63·2)	2·37 (2·10 to 2·67)	1·61 (1·42 to 1·82)
Immunodeficiency	7 (11·7)	60 (0·0)	8 (1 to 58)	116·7 (46·9 to 240·4)	4·82 (1·94 to 9·93)	1·69 (0·80 to 3·58)
Nervous system congenital anomalies	42 (8·6)	489 (0·2)	2 (1 to 4)	85·9 (61·9 to 116·1)	3·56 (2·56 to 4·82)	1·73 (1·26 to 2·36)
Down's syndrome	28 (15·4)	182 (0·1)	3 (0 to 9)	153·9 (102·2 to 222·4)	6·37 (4·23 to 9·21)	2·53 (1·72 to 3·72)
Cerebral Palsy	16 (10·7)	149 (0·1)	3 (1 to 5)	107·4 (61·4 to 174·4)	4·44 (2·54 to 7·21)	2·43 (1·48 to 3·99)

†Relative risk compared with infants without risk factor of interest.

Strengths and weaknesses

This is among the first studies reporting the population burden of bronchiolitis across NHS hospitals in England. The main strength of our cohort is that use of HES birth records provides a large, nationally representative sample of births across England during this time, when compared with ONS live births data [27]. We assumed infants with unknown gestational age and birth weight were not born preterm, as infants in this unknown group had similarly short length of stay at birth to infants born at term. Despite incomplete recording of gestational age in some birth records, 7·5% of our cohort were born at <37 weeks gestation which is consistent with ONS data reporting that around 7·7% of live births annually are delivered preterm [28]. This suggests under-reporting of gestational age in HES birth records appears to be mostly among term babies. Similarly, rates of congenital heart disease, chronic lung disease and other risk factors for severe RSV disease compare well with published UK population data [3,29,30].

However, there are a number of important limitations to our study. Our case definition for bronchiolitis and co-morbidity is dependent on the accuracy of clinical coding and recording in diagnosis fields in HES records, although improvements in the quality of HES coding have been demonstrated in recent years [31]. We combined RSV and unspecified bronchiolitis, presenting data on *all* bronchiolitis admissions. Only 28% of the bronchiolitis admissions were coded as being due to RSV, the remainder having

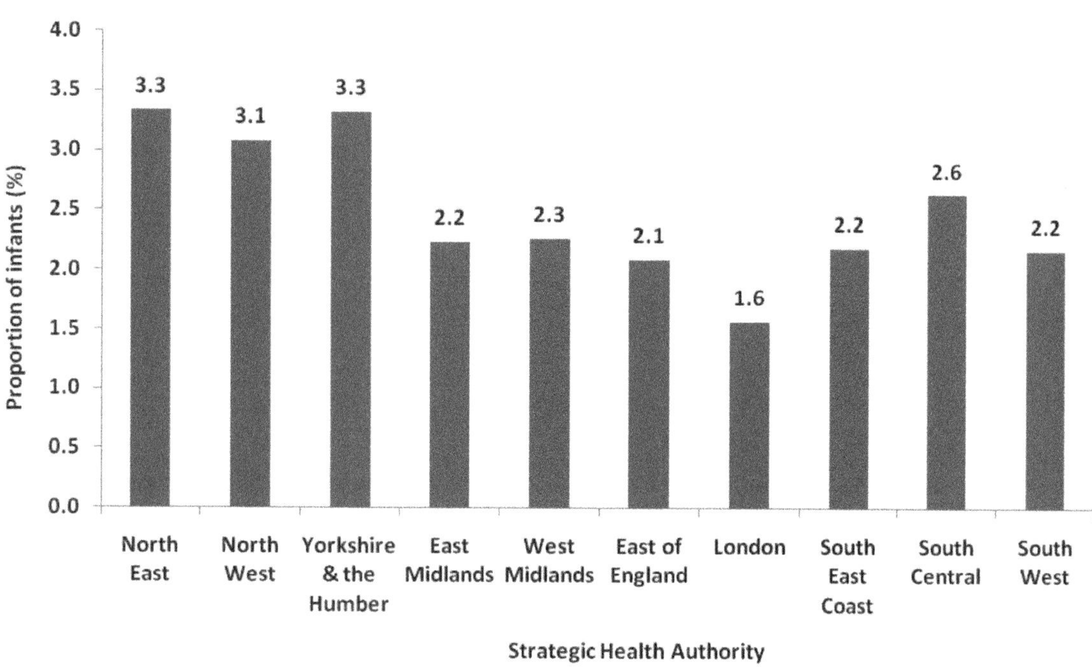

Figure 2. Proportion of bronchiolitis hospital admissions among birth cohort, by Strategic Health Authority (SHA) of admission.

unspecific bronchiolitis codes. No linked microbiological data to confirm the presence of RSV was available. A previous study in the UK has estimated that around 75% of unspecified bronchiolitis admissions were RSV related [32]. Globally it is estimated that only between 4% and 28% of children admitted with LRTI are tested for RSV [4].

A limitation of the cohort study design is attrition, as it was not possible to identify bronchiolitis admissions occurring outside NHS hospitals in England, or to identify individuals who migrated elsewhere, though we estimate this number should be low with only one year of follow-up. Using linked ONS mortality data it was possible to identify the small number of individuals in the cohort who died during the study period. The number of infant deaths directly attributable to RSV infection is reported to be very low [33]. There is potentially some inherent selection bias in our study, through the inclusion of only hospitals with good completeness of recording of birth record fields, but sensitivity analyses showed few differences between included and excluded sites in terms of supply factors (such as number of maternity beds and number of deliveries). No data were available to identify any individuals who had received Palivizumab prophylaxis against RSV infection. There are very strict criteria for Palivizumab use in the UK due to its significant cost, which means that very few babies in the cohort are likely to have received it.

Findings in relation to other studies

We found no comparable national studies to compare our estimates of bronchiolitis hospital admission rates in the UK but one previous study from Shropshire reported a bronchiolitis hospital admission rate of 30·8 per 1000 infants in this region of England [3], compared with our estimate of 24·2 admissions per 1000 infants. Our estimate may be slightly lower because we applied a narrow case definition including only infants admitted with a primary diagnosis of bronchiolitis (ICD-10 'J21'codes). This is likely to underestimate the total burden of RSV illness in infancy, as we have excluded pneumonias due to RSV and non-specific, symptomatic clinical codes from our bronchiolitis case definition, though some of these admissions may in reality have been related to RSV infection. A study from the United States has reported a bronchiolitis admission rate of 31·2 per 1000 infants under 1 year [7], but a more recent study in Texas reported higher bronchiolitis admission rates of 5·5% among children under 2 years [34]. These higher incidence estimates are likely to be due to the wider inclusion of children aged 12 to 24 months in their study, coupled with variation in the clinical definition of bronchiolitis used in the US compared with that used in UK [13].

21% of infants admitted with bronchiolitis, had more than one bronchiolitis admission during their first year of life. Previous infection with RSV only confers partial immunity, so it is possible for individuals to be re-infected with the same or different RSV strains over the course of one season. Re-admissions for bronchiolitis among older infants may in reality be incorrectly diagnosed episodes of post-bronchiolitic wheezing. The modal age of bronchiolitis admission was 1 month and the median was 4 months, confirming findings reported elsewhere which show increased risk of RSV admission with younger age [13,35–37]. It is unclear why RSV may be affecting babies at a younger age than has previously been reported. It could be associated with changes to the virus itself or maternal immunological priming, but further investigation into what may be driving this trend is needed. The median age of bronchiolitis admission was 4 months which is consistent with other studies where RSV hospital admissions are typically reported during the first 3 to 6 months of life [8,38]. However, there is some debate regarding the most common age of RSV admissions [37]. A population-based cohort in Denmark found the median age of admission for RSV infections was 6 months [39]. Similarly, a recent prognostic birth cohort study reported that the median age at time of RSV LRTI was 6 months [40]. Unplanned short stay hospital admissions in this age group have been increasing [20]. In 2006 the unplanned admission rate among children less than 1 year in England was 181 per 1000 child years [20]. Our findings suggest that approximately 1 in 6 of these unplanned admissions was for bronchiolitis.

We found the majority of infants admitted with bronchiolitis were not in high-risk groups, with only 24% (1722/7189) having one or more recognised risk factors for severe RSV infection. In a smaller US study, 34% of RSV-infected patients (189/564) had at least one high-risk condition for RSV infection [9]. Preterm infants accounted for only 15% of bronchiolitis admissions in our study. Infants with chronic lung disease or congenital heart disease each accounted for around 4% of bronchiolitis admissions. This is consistent with findings reported elsewhere, suggesting that the majority of infants with severe RSV infection do not have any underlying risk factors [9]. Low rates of bronchiolitis admissions in some high-risk groups may also be driven by Palivizumab use, however no national prescribing data for Palivizumab is available for us to estimate the number of admissions its use may have prevented. The median age of bronchiolitis admission was only 18 days later in preterm infants (136 days) compared with those born at term (118 days), so onset of RSV disease appears to occur at a similar corrected age. Median LOS for bronchiolitis admissions was calculated as a proxy marker of severity of illness and was found to be similarly short (1 day) among both term and preterm born infants.

Geographical variation in bronchiolitis admission rates may be a proxy for other risk factors for hospital admission with severe RSV infection, such as maternal smoking or deprivation. We think this finding is most likely driven by variation in clinical practice, with different thresholds for admission in different regions as there are no national evidence based guidelines giving criteria for admission. Indeed, widespread variation in hospital management of bronchiolitis has previously been reported [13].

Implications and future research

Our study has highlighted that the burden of RSV bronchiolitis hospital admissions among infants in England predominantly affects those born at term, without any risk factors for severe RSV infection and the age at admission appears to be significantly lower now than previously reported. Since the majority of infants hospitalised with bronchiolitis are below 6 months of age, this will limit the impact of any future vaccine which is unlikely to be capable of eliciting immunity in such young infants. This has important implications for future vaccination strategies, suggesting that the cost benefit of both active and passive vaccines needs detailed evaluation. We found that the median length of stay for bronchiolitis admissions was only 1 day. Improved management of symptoms in the community, through both primary care and A & E services may reduce the need for admission still further. Further studies examining the clinical burden of bronchiolitis in the community are needed and could confirm the clinical and health service burden to be greater still [13,16,18]. Improved management of RSV is achievable through the use of improved, evidence-based guidelines [1]. The regional variation in bronchiolitis admission rates we have presented suggests admission criteria vary widely and there is a need for clearer guidance about which infants to admit to hospital in the UK.

Our findings suggest that in addition to the recognised risk factors for RSV bronchiolitis hospital admission, namely congenital heart disease, chronic lung disease and preterm birth, several other clinical conditions may also increase risk. The factors we have identified are cerebral palsy, cystic fibrosis and Down's syndrome. We suggest further investigation is warranted, into whether infants with these conditions would also benefit from Palivizumab immunoprophylaxis.

Conclusion

Bronchiolitis is an important cause of hospital admissions among infants in the UK. Several clinical subgroups are at increased risk of hospital admission, but the majority of bronchiolitis cases in England are among infants born at term, with no known risk factors for severe RSV infection. The early age of bronchiolitis admissions has important implications for the potential impact of future active and passive immunisations. More research is needed to explain why babies born with Down's syndrome and cerebral palsy are also at higher risk of hospital admission with RSV bronchiolitis.

What's known on this subject

Well known predisposing risk factors for RSV bronchiolitis include preterm birth, chronic lung disease, congenital heart disease and immune deficiency. Passive immunotherapy is indicated for those at highest risk of severe infection.

What this study adds

Most infants admitted to hospital with bronchiolitis are born at term and have no risk factors for severe RSV infection. There is a peak in bronchiolitis admissions at the age of 1 month.

Research Ethics approval

We have permission from the NIGB under Section 251 of the NHS Act 2006 (formerly Section 60 approval from the Patient Information Advisory Group) to hold confidential data. We have approval to use them for research and measuring quality of delivery of healthcare, from the South East Ethics Research Committee.

Supporting Information

Appendix S1 Identifying at-risk groups (ICD-10 code lists).

Appendix S2 Table S1: Characteristics of birth cohort and infants hospitalised with bronchiolitis.

Acknowledgments

Members of the Medicines for Neonates Investigator Group:

Neena Modi[3], Peter Brocklehurst[4], Jane Abbott[5], Kate Costeloe[6], Elizabeth Draper[7], Azeem Majeed[1], Jacquie Kemp[8], Deborah Ashby[9], Alys Young[10], Stavros Petrou[11].

1 Department of Primary Care and Public Health, Imperial College London, London, United Kingdom;

2 Paediatric Infectious Diseases Unit, St. George's Hospital NHS Trust, London, United Kingdom;

3 Section of Neonatal Medicine, Department of Medicine, Imperial College London, London, United Kingdom;

4 Director of the Institute for Women's Health, University College London;

5 BLISS charity;

6 Barts and the London School of Medicine and Dentistry, Queen Mary University of London;

7 University of Leicester, Department of Health Sciences;

8 London Specialised Commissioning Group;

9 Imperial Clinical Trials Unit, School of Public Health, Imperial College London;

10 Manchester Academic Health Sciences Centre, University of Manchester;

11 Division of Health Sciences, Warwick Medical School, University of Warwick

Author Contributions

Contributed reagents/materials/analysis tools: JM AB MS NM PA AM SS. Wrote the paper: JM AB MS NM PA AM SS. Conceived and designed the study: JM AB MS SS. Acquisition of data: AB PA. Performed all analyses: JM. Supervised the analyses: AB. Acquisition of funding: AB NM PA AM SS. Revised and approved the manuscript: JM AB MS NM PA AM SS.

References

1. Barben J, Kuehni CE, Trachsel D, Hammer J (2008) Management of acute bronchiolitis: can evidence based guidelines alter clinical practice? Thorax 63:1103–1109.
2. Bush A, Thomson AH (2007) Acute bronchiolitis. BMJ 335(7628):1037–1041.
3. Deshpande SA, Northern V (2003) The clinical and health economic burden of respiratory syncytial virus disease among children under 2 years of age in a defined geographical area. Arch Dis Child 88(12):1065–1069.
4. Nair H, Nokes DJ, Gessner BD, Dherani M, Madhi SA, et al. (2010) Global burden of acute lower respiratory infections due to respiratory syncytial virus in young children: a systematic review and meta-analysis. The Lancet 375(9725):1545–1555.
5. Koehoorn M, Karr CJ, Demers PA, Lencar C, Tamburic L, et al. (2008) Descriptive Epidemiological Features of Bronchiolitis in a Population-Based Cohort. Pediatrics 122(6):1196–1203.
6. Papadopoulos NG, Moustaki M, Tsolia M, Bossios A, Astra E, et al. (2002) Association of Rhinovirus Infection with Increased Disease Severity in Acute Bronchiolitis. Am J Respir Crit Care Med 165(9):1285–1289.
7. Shay DK, Holman RC, Newman RD, Liu LL, Stout JW, et al. (1999) Bronchiolitis-associated hospitalizations among US children, 1980-1996. JAMA 282(15):1440–1446.
8. Smyth RL, Openshaw PJ (2006) Bronchiolitis. Lancet 368(9532):312–322.
9. Hall CB, Weinberg GA, Iwane MK, Blumkin AK, Edwards KM, et al. (2009) The Burden of Respiratory Syncytial Virus Infection in Young Children. The New England Journal of Medicine 360(6):588–598.
10. Hall CB (2010) Respiratory syncytial virus in young children. The Lancet 375(9725):1500–1502.
11. Office for National Statistics. News Release on preterm births. 24-5-2007. http://www.statistics.gov.uk/pdfdir/preterm0507.pdf Accessed June 2012.
12. Law BJ, Carbonell-Estrany X, Simoes EA (2002) An update on respiratory syncytial virus epidemiology: a developed country perspective. Respir Med 96 Suppl B: S1–S7.
13. Scottish Intercollegiate Guidelines Network (SIGN). Bronchiolitis in children - A national clinical guideline. 2006. http://www.sign.ac.uk/pdf/sign91.pdf Accessed June 2012. Report No 91, SIGN.
14. Spurling GK, Fonseka K, Doust J, Del MC (2007) Antibiotics for bronchiolitis in children. Cochrane Database Syst Rev (1):CD005189.
15. Patel H, Platt R, Lozano JM, Wang EE (2004) Glucocorticoids for acute viral bronchiolitis in infants and young children. Cochrane Database Syst Rev (3):CD004878.
16. Wang D, Bayliss S, Meads C (2011) Palivizumab for immunoprophylaxis of respiratory syncitial virus (RSV) bronchiolitis in high-risk infants and young children: a systematic review and additional economic modelling of subgroup analyses. Health Technol Assess 15(5):1–124.
17. Joint Committee on Vaccination and Immunisation - Respiratory Syncitial Virus (RSV) Subgroup. Minutes of the RSV subgroup on 8th June 2010. 8-6-2010.
18. Wang D, Cummins C, Bayliss S, Sandercock J, Burls A (2008). Immunoprophylaxis against respiratory syncytial virus (RSV) with palivizumab in children: a systematic review and economic evaluation. Health Technol Assess 12(36):iii, ix–86.
19. Aylin P, Williams S, Bottle A, Jarman B (2004). Counting hospital activity: spells or episodes? BMJ 329(7476):1207.
20. Saxena S, Bottle A, Gilbert R, Sharland M (2009). Increasing short-stay unplanned hospital admissions among children in England; time trends analysis '97–'06. PLoS One 4(10):e7484.
21. Bottle A, Aylin P (2009). Application of AHRQ patient safety indicators to English hospital data. Qual Saf Health Care 18(4):303–308.

22. The NHS Information Centre for Health and Social Care HESonline Hospital Episode Statistic. NHS Maternity Statistics. 2010. http://www.hesonline.nhs.uk/Ease/servlet/ContentServer?siteID = 1937&categoryID = 1475 Accessed June 2012.
23. The NHS Information Centre for Health and Social Care. HES Online Data Dictionary: Inpatients. 2009. http://www.hesonline.nhs.uk/Ease/servlet/ContentServer?siteID = 1937&categoryID = 571 Accessed June 2012.
24. Murray J, Saxena S, Modi N, Majeed A, Aylin P, et al. (2013) Quality of routine hospital birth records and the feasibility of their use for creating birth cohorts. J Public Health (Oxf) 35(2):298–307
25. Agency for Healthcare Research and Quality (AHRQ). Clinical Classifications Software for ICD-10 Data. 2003. http://www.ahrq.gov/data/hcup/icd10usrgd.htm Accessed June 2012.
26. Beck S, Wojdyla D, Say L, Betran AP, Merialdi M, et al. (2010) The worldwide incidence of preterm birth: a systematic review of maternal mortality and morbidity. Bull World Health Organ 88(1):31–38.
27. Office for National Statistics. Birth statistics: Births and patterns of family building England and Wales (FM1). 15-12-2008. http://www.statistics.gov.uk/downloads/theme_population/FM1_36/FM1-No36.pdf Accessed June 2012.
28. Office for National Statistics. News Release: 1 in 13 live births in England and Wales are born preterm. 24-5-2007. Accessed June 2012.
29. Wren C, Richmond S, Donaldson L (2000) Temporal variability in birth prevalence of cardiovascular malformations. Heart 83(4):414–419.
30. Manktelow BN, Draper ES, Annamalai S, Field D (2001) Factors affecting the incidence of chronic lung disease of prematurity in 1987, 1992, and 1997. Archives of Disease in Childhood - Fetal and Neonatal Edition 85(1):F33–F35.
31. Audit Commission. An Evaluation of Three Years of the PbR Data Assurance Framework. 2011. http://www.audit-commission.gov.uk/sitecollectiondocuments/downloads/20110120AnEvaluationOfThreeYearsOfThePbRDataAssuranceFramework.pdf Accessed June 2012. 1-10-2011.
32. Muller-Pebody B, Edmunds WJ, Zambon MC, Gay NJ, Crowcroft NS (2002) Contribution of RSV to bronchiolitis and pneumonia-associated hospitalizations in English children, April 1995–March 1998. Epidemiol Infect 129(1):99–106.
33. Ladhani S, Pebody RG, Ramsay ME, Lamagni TL, Johnson AP, et al. (2010) Continuing impact of infectious diseases on childhood deaths in England and Wales, 2003–2005. Pediatr Infect Dis J 29(4):310–313.
34. Garcia CG, Bhore R, Soriano-Fallas A, Trost M, Chason R, et al. (2010) Risk factors in children hospitalized with RSV bronchiolitis versus non-RSV bronchiolitis. Pediatrics 126(6):e1453–e1460.
35. Figueras-Aloy J, Carbonell-Estrany X, Quero J, IRIS Study Group (2004) Case-Control Study of the Risk Factors Linked to Respiratory Syncytial Virus Infection Requiring Hospitalization in Premature Infants Born at a Gestational Age of 33–35 Weeks in Spain. The Pediatric Infectious Disease Journal 23(9).
36. Carbonell-Estrany XAVI, Quero JOS, The IRIS Study Group (2001) Hospitalization rates for respiratory syncytial virus infection in premature infants born during two consecutive seasons. The Pediatric Infectious Disease Journal 20(9).
37. Bont L, Houben ML (2011) Commentary: why are young healthy term infants protected against respiratory syncytial virus bronchiolitis? Pediatr Infect Dis J 30(9):785–786.
38. Tregoning JS, Schwarze J (2010) Respiratory viral infections in infants: causes, clinical symptoms, virology, and immunology. Clin Microbiol Rev 23(1):74–98.
39. Stensballe LG, Hjuler T, Andersen A, Kaltoft M, Ravn H, et al. (2008) Hospitalization for respiratory syncytial virus infection and invasive pneumococcal disease in Danish children aged <2 years: a population-based cohort study. Clin Infect Dis 46(8):1165–1171.
40. Houben ML, Bont L, Wilbrink B, Belderbos ME, Kimpen JL, et al. (2011) Clinical prediction rule for RSV bronchiolitis in healthy newborns: prognostic birth cohort study. Pediatrics 127(1):35–41.

21

DNA-Methylation Profiling of Fetal Tissues Reveals Marked Epigenetic Differences between Chorionic and Amniotic Samples

Christel Eckmann-Scholz[1], Susanne Bens[2], Julia Kolarova[2], Sina Schneppenheim[2], Almuth Caliebe[2], Simone Heidemann[2], Constantin von Kaisenberg[1,3], Monika Kautza[4], Walter Jonat[1], Reiner Siebert[2], Ole Ammerpohl[2]*

1 Department of Gynecology & Obstetrics, Christian-Albrechts-University Kiel & University Hospital Schleswig-Holstein, Kiel, Germany, **2** Institute of Human Genetics, Christian-Albrechts-University Kiel & University Hospital Schleswig-Holstein, Kiel, Germany, **3** Department of Obstetrics, Gynecology and Reproductive Medicine, Hannover Medical School, Hannover, Germany, **4** Praxis of Human Genetics, Kiel, Germany

Abstract

Epigenetic mechanisms including DNA methylation are supposed to play a key role in fetal development. Here we have investigated fetal DNA-methylation levels of 27,578 CpG loci in 47 chorionic villi (CVS) and 16 amniotic cell (AC) samples. Methylation levels differed significantly between karyotypically normal AC and CVS for 2,014 genes. AC showed more extreme DNA-methylation levels of these genes than CVS and the differentially methylated genes are significantly enriched for processes characteristic for the different cell types sampled. Furthermore, we identified 404 genes differentially methylated in CVS with trisomy 21. These genes were significantly enriched for high CG dinucleotid (CpG) content and developmental processes associated with Down syndrome. Our study points to major tissue-specific differences of fetal DNA-methylation and gives rise to the hypothesis that part of the Down syndrome phenotype is epigenetically programmed in the first trimester of pregnancy.

Editor: Wolfgang Wagner, RWTH Aachen University Medical School, Germany

Funding: This study was made possible by intramural funding of the Medical Faculty of the Christian-Albrechts-University Kiel to the involved institutions. The funders had no role in study design, data collection and analysis, decision to publish, or preparation of the manuscript.

Competing Interests: The authors have declared that no competing interests exist.

* E-mail: oammerpohl@medgen.uni-kiel.de

Introduction

The epigenetic composition of the fetus has gained much attention in the recent past. In particular, the patterns of DNA methylation and their changes during normal and pathologic fetal development are subject of studies in various fields of research. These include reproduction failure, effects of assisted reproduction, disturbances of the maternal-fetal interface, disorders of development, syndromes caused by errors in imprinting, fetal programming of behavior or disease or the impact of maternal factors on fetal development [1–4].

Compared to its sequence the methylation of DNA shows a much higher plasticity both intra- and interindividually. DNA methylation patterns differ between tissues and epigenetic modifications are supposed to be major determinants of the cell type-specific gene expression program and, thus, to imprint the cellular protein expression, function and destiny [5,6]. Consequently, DNA methylation patterns can be influenced by internal and external factors allowing cellular differentiation and response to exogenic stimuli. The latter is directly linked to the interindividual differences in DNA methylation which have been shown to increase with ageing by twin studies [7–9]. Considering this epigenetic plasticity it is intriguing to speculate that differences in DNA methylation patterns could explain (part of the) phenotypic differences observed between individuals carrying the same genetic change. E.g., despite carrying a third chromosome 21 only 40–60% of individuals with Down syndrome are affected by congenital heart defects, mostly an atrial (ventricular) septal defect [10–12].

This figure - besides through the effect of modifier genes - could well be explained by a secondary epigenetic mark influencing cardiac development established or erased directly or indirectly through the effect of a gene on chromosome 21.

DNA methylation patterns can also be of relevance for diagnostics. In this regard, a series of locus-specific and genome-wide DNA methylation profiling studies has been performed in the recent past in order to detect methylation patterns differentiating fetuses with chromosomal aberrations from those with normal karyotypes. This led to the development of novel approaches for noninvasive prenatal diagnosis of e.g. trisomy 21 by analysis of fetal-specific DNA methylation in maternal blood [13].

It is remarkable, that description of fetal trisomic and non-trisomic fetal DNA methylation patterns, respectively, has so far been almost exclusively based on the analysis of a limited number of placental DNA both from first and third trimester pregnancies [14–18]. Nevertheless, it is well known from prenatal chromosomal testing that placental tissue e.g. derived from chorionic villi sampling (CVS) is a peculiar fetal tissue to study because of the mixture of ectodermal and mesodermal cells, recurrent mosaicism and the contamination of fetal tissue by maternal cells. In contrast to those placental cells which are more distantly related to the fetus, cells obtained by amniocentesis (AC) which are epithelial cells derived from the epiblast of the inner cell mass are supposed to reflect closely the true composition of the fetus [19].

In order to characterize and compare DNA methylation patterns between amniotic and chorionic tissue samples we performed an array-based methylation profiling study in an extensive series of 63 fetal tissues derived from routine prenatal AC and CVS sampling. Through analysis of CVS samples from fetuses with trisomy 21 we unravel potential novel markers for non-invasive prenatal testing. Finally, by describing the molecular features shared by the genes differentially methylated between the different tissues as well as the CVS samples with and without trisomy 21 we provide initial insights into the biological processes underlying epigenetic patterns in normal fetal differentiation and development as well as potentially in the manifestation of the typical phenotype of Down syndrome.

Materials and Methods

Study Population

The study was performed on 63 samples from 61 different women left over from routine prenatal cytogenetic testing. This included 47 chorionic villi samples (CVS) and 16 samples derived from amniocentesis (AC). CVS and AC sampling was performed with written informed consent of the patients according to standard methods. The main indications for invasive prenatal testing were advanced maternal age as well as abnormal ultrasound findings such as elevated nuchal translucency (NT) or abnormal first trimester screening. Clinical details on the pregnancies as well as pregnancy outcome are summarized in Table S1. For control purposes peripheral blood samples from normal female and male individuals were included. The study was approved by the Ethics Committee of the Medical Faculty of the Christian-Albrechts-University Kiel (IRB No: D447/09, D402/09).

DNA Extraction

DNA was extracted from native CVS tissue left over after setting up direct preparations and long-term cultures for cytogenetic analyses as well as from long-term cultured AC cells. Samples were cryopreserved until DNA extraction. DNA extraction was performed centrally by a single person to widely exclude batch effects applying the High Pure PCR Template Preparation Kit (Roche Diagnostics, Mannheim, Germany).

DNA Methylation Analysis

DNA methylation analysis using the HumanMethylation27k BeadChip (Illumina Inc., San Diego, CA, USA) was performed using a custom service provided by AROS Applied Biotechnology AS (Aarhus, DK). The HumanMethylation27 BeadChip was developed to assay 27,578 CpG sites selected from more than 14,000 genes in parallel [20]. Two samples were analyzed in duplicates using different batches of the HumanMethylation27 BeadChip. Array data are available in a MIAMI compliant format from GeneOmnibus (GSE35327).

Processing of Data and Bioinformatic Analyses

Raw hybridisation signals were processed using GenomeStudio software (ver. 2011.1; Illumina Inc.) applying the default settings. Further analyses were performed using the R-package [21] and RStudio (ver. 0.94.102) using raw data obtained from the GenomeStudio analysis. Color balance adjustment and data normalization (*simple scaling normalization*) were done using the lumi package for R [22–24]. CpG loci with detection p-values<0.001 in at least one of the samples analyzed were excluded from further analyses. Finally, 22234 CpG loci in 63 samples entered analysis. Data obtained from samples analyzed in duplicates were averaged. Subsequent principal component (PCA) and hierarchical cluster analyses were performed using Qlucore's Omics Explorer 2.1 (Version 2.1(25); Qlucore, Lund, Sweden). Genes were considered being differentially methylated between two data sets if the false discovery rate (FDR) was below $q<0.01$ (t-test). The R-package was used to perform Pearson's product-moment correlation.

Bioinformatic Characterisation of Groups of Differentially Methylated Genes

To analyze whether promoter regions of differentially methylated genes showed different CpG compositions, we used a previously described classification into promoters with high (HCP), intermediate (ICP) and low (LCP) CpG content [25,26]. Proportions of PRC2 target genes and promoter classes in the groups of genes differentially methylated and all genes present on the HumanMethylation27 Bead Chip were compared using the chi-square test (two-sided; GraphPad Prism, ver. 4.02). A genome-wide mapping of PRC2 genes in embryonic stem cells is available as supplemental material in the study by Lee et al. [27]. Imprinted genes were identified from publicly available databases (http://igc.otago.ac.nz/home.html26 and http://www.geneimprint.com/site/genes-by-species27) and a previously published review [28]. Gene ontology analysis has been performed using GOrilla [29] with a list of genes present on the BeadChip acting as background list.

Bisulfite Pyrosequencing of KIAA0575, ECEL1, SOX11 and STG4

Bisulfite conversion of genomic DNA was performed using the EpiTect Bisulfite Conversion Kit (Qiagen, Hilden, Germany) according to the manufacture's protocol. Bisulfite Pyrosequencing was performed according to previously published protocols [30]. Primer sequences and precise PCR conditions are available from the authors on request. DNA-methylation of *KIAA0575*, *ECEL1*, *SOX11* and *STG4* has been analyzed in this study.

GeneScan analysis of the *AMELX/AMELY* locus. To determine the content of fetal tissue in CVS samples obtained from male fetuses we performed a PCR based GeneScan analysis on the *AMEL* gene locus using primers yielding different sized PCR fragments from the X-chromosomal (*AMELX*, Xp22.2) and Y-chromosomal (*AMELY*, Yp11.2) copy of the gene. PCR fragments were analyzed using an ABI 3100 (Applied Biosystems, Carlsbad, CA). DNAs from peripheral blood of normal males (n = 6), normal females (n = 5) as well as mixtures of normal male and female DNA (ratio: 1:1, n = 5) acted as control. The ratios of the peak area of X- and Y-chromosomal specific peaks were calculated. Using the controls as standard values in a regression analysis, the content of fetal tissue in CVS samples has been determined in CVS samples from male fetuses.

Results

Applying the "Infinium HumanMethylation27 BeadChip" we investigated 27,578 CpG sites selected from more than 14,000 genes in a series of 63 fetal tissues left over from routine prenatal genetic testing. In particular, we investigated 47 chorionic villi samples (CVS) and 16 samples derived from amniocentesis (AC). Besides samples from fetuses with normal male or female karyotype these included six cases with trisomy 18 (5 CVS, 1 AC) and three cases with trisomy 21 (all CVS). One CVS sample was derived from a fetus with a gonosomal chromosome pattern typical for Turner Syndrome. Two samples (1 AC, 1 CVS with trisomy 21) were obtained from pregnancies induced by intracytoplasmatic sperm injection (ICSI). None of the chromosomal aberrations was mosaic. Clinical details are summarized in Table S1.

The reproducibility and validity of the applied array platform for determination of DNA-methylation levels has been extensively demonstrated by us in previous studies using different types of samples and comparison to alternative techniques like methylation specific PCR, bisulfite pyrosequencing or bisulfite sequencing [31–33]. In addition, we here investigated the reproducibility by analyzing two pairs of CVS samples in duplicate (CV21 and 19; CV26 and 10; Table S1) using two different batches of the array. This comparison yielded Pearson correlation coefficients of 0.96 and 0.97, respectively, indicating good reproducibility also in the fetal samples under study (Figure S1). Moreover, to test the validity of the DNA methylation values derived from the array we here examined the status of 6 CpG loci in 3 randomly selected AC und 7 CVS samples by bisulfite pyrosequencing (Figure S2).

Having established the technical validity of the array we aimed in a first step at comparing the DNA-methylation between the amniotic cells and the chorionic samples with a regular karyotype. To this end, we excluded all samples with a chromosomal aberration. Moreover, we excluded the samples of pregnancies derived after ICSI in order to avoid putative effects of in vitro fertilization on the epigenetic pattern. Already an unsupervised principal component analysis (PCA) of the complete data set from the remaining 50 samples clearly separated AC from CVS samples (Figure 1a). This indicates that the methylation patterns of the samples investigated are much stronger associated with the origin of the fetal tissue than other factors like sex of the fetus despite the X-chromosome undergoing DNA-methylation in females is being included in the analysis. A supervised comparison identified 2418 CpG loci corresponding to 2014 individual genes to be significantly ($FDR < 1 \times 10^{-15}$, t-test) differentially methylated between AC and CVS (Figures 1b and 1c). Like in the unsupervised analysis the samples clustered independently from the sex of the fetus (Figure 1c). We conclude that there are major differences in the DNA-methylation patterns between the fetal tissues obtained by routine invasive prenatal testing.

Interestingly, inspection of the heatmap (Figure 1c) suggested that the methylation values of the genes differentially methylated between amniotic and chorionic samples are more extreme in AC than those in CVS. To further investigate this observation, we plotted the means of the normalized methylation values in AC and CVS of all differentially methylated 2418 CpG loci. As shown in Figure 2, these loci were preferentially (2054 of 2418 CpG loci) intermediately methylated in CVS but either lowly or highly DNA-methylated in AC samples. In contrast, genes not differentially methylated between CVS and AC showed a similar DNA methylation distribution pattern in both sample types (Figure S3). We conclude that the genes differentially methylated between AC and CVS are predominately characterized by more extreme DNA-methylation levels in the former and more intermediate levels in the latter samples.

The more intermediate methylation levels of the genes differentially methylated between amniotic and chorionic samples could be due to the fact that tissue sampled by CVS is a mixture of various embryonic and also maternal cell compartments. In contrast, cells derived from AC usually lack maternal contamination if the sample is not contaminated by blood. The potential differences in the contribution of maternal cells between AC and CVS prompted us to investigate the correlation of the DNA-methylation patterns with fetal sex. Unsupervised analysis of the 50 samples already suggested that fetal sex was less visible in the methylation pattern of CVS than in AC. To corroborate this observation we focused on the X-chromosomal genes as many (but not all) of those are being methylated in 50% of the X-chromosomes of females due to X-inactivation not present in normal males. In an unsupervised approach both AC and CVS samples separated according to fetal sex based on the methylation levels of the X-chromosomal genes. Nevertheless, three CVS samples from male fetuses clustered separately from the other CVS samples of male fetuses (Figure 3, arrow). These three samples showed a mixture of male and female X-chromosomal methylation patterns likely due to maternal cells contaminating the CVS sample. We conclude that varying maternal contribution affects the DNA methylation pattern of CVS samples. This is further supported by a GeneScan analysis of the *AMELX/AMELY* locus in CVS samples derived from male fetuses revealing a detectable maternal contamination of between 0% and 29% (median 17%).

Next we wondered whether the 2014 genes differentially methylated between amniotic and chorionic samples share certain biological features. Several studies demonstrated that genes with promoters either containing a high CpG content (HCP) or a low CpG content (LCP) show different DNA methylation properties [31–33]. The 628 genes found hypermethylated in CVS compared to AC were significantly enriched for polycomb repressor complex 2 (PRC2) target genes in embryonic stem cells ($p < 0.0001$; $OR = 3.88$, $RR = 3.51$) and imprinted genes ($p < 0.0001$, $OR = 2.69$, $RR = 2.50$), while LCP genes were depleted ($p = 0.0213$, $OR = 0.77$, $RR = 0.78$). In contrast, the 1406 genes hypermethylated in AC in comparison to CVS were significantly enriched for genes with LCPs ($p < 0.0001$, $OR = 4.39$, $RR = 3.62$) but depleted for HCP genes ($p < 0.0001$, $RR = 0.29$, $OR = 0.26$) and PRC2 target genes in embryonic stem cells ($p < 0.0001$, $RR = 0.35$, $OR = 0.33$).

We further investigated whether genes differentially methylated between AC and CVS were enriched for certain biological functions by performing a gene ontology analysis. This approach revealed that the 2014 genes differentially methylated between AC and CVS were significantly enriched for genes involved in various regulatory and developmental processes including e.g. regulation of adenylate cyclase activity which might point e.g. to hormonal or neuronal signaling (Table S2). In addition, the physiologic properties of the cell compartments analyzed are reflected by significant enrichment of the differentially methylated genes for processes "(cellular) response to nitric oxide" (5.3–6.3fold; containing predominately genes encoding surfactant proteins), "keratinization" (2.8fold) or "female pregnancy" (2.4fold). A detailed list of loci aberrantly methylated in CVS samples with trisomy 21 and trisomy 18 along with the corresponding DNA methylation values of the respective loci in normal peripheral blood is available from the supplement (Table S4). Applying a threshold of $delta.beta > 0.2$ we identified 89 loci with differential methylation between CVS with trisomy 21 and both normal CVS as well as peripheral blood samples from normal females. All of these loci were hypermethylated in trisomy 21 samples.

One single locus (CACNA1H, cg25760229) was differentially methylated between CVS with trisomy 18 and both normal CVS and peripheral blood samples from normal females (hypermethylated in trisomy 18 samples).

Finally, we wondered whether maternal factors could be associated with methylation differences in CVS and AC samples with normal karyotype. Due to the tissue differences shown above we treated both sample sources differently. By PCA we failed to detect any significant effect of maternal age, BMI or smoking

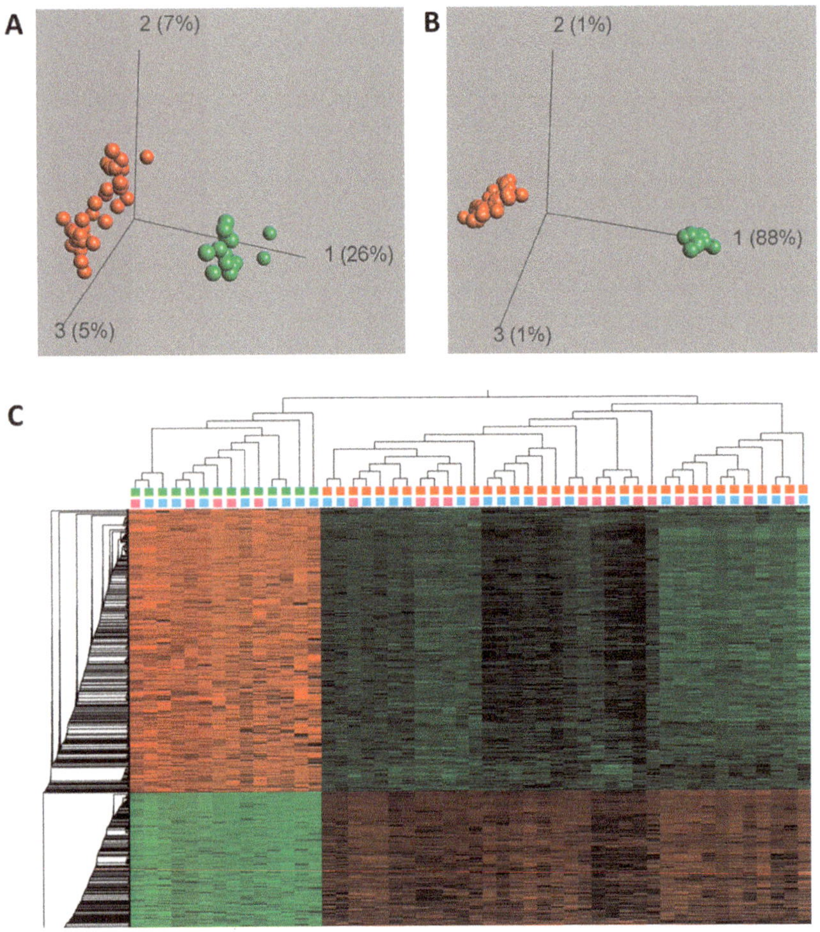

Figure 1. DNA methylation differs between AC and CVS samples. (A) Principal component analysis (PCA) of 22,234 CpG loci which passed quality tests and entered the analysis. Unsupervised analysis separated AC (green spheres) from CVS samples (red spheres). (B) Differential methylation analysis to separate AC from CVS samples (t-test, FDR$<1\times10^{-15}$). (C) Hierarchic cluster analysis of the 2418 CpG loci shown in (B). The upper panel on top of the heatmap indicates the sample type (green: AC, red:CVS) while the second panel indicates the fetuses' sex (pink: female, cyan: male). Green color in the heatmap indicates low DNA-methylation, black intermediate and red high DNA-methylation values. Samples with known chromosomal aberrations and samples from ICSI were excluded. AC and CVS differ significantly in their DNA methylation pattern.

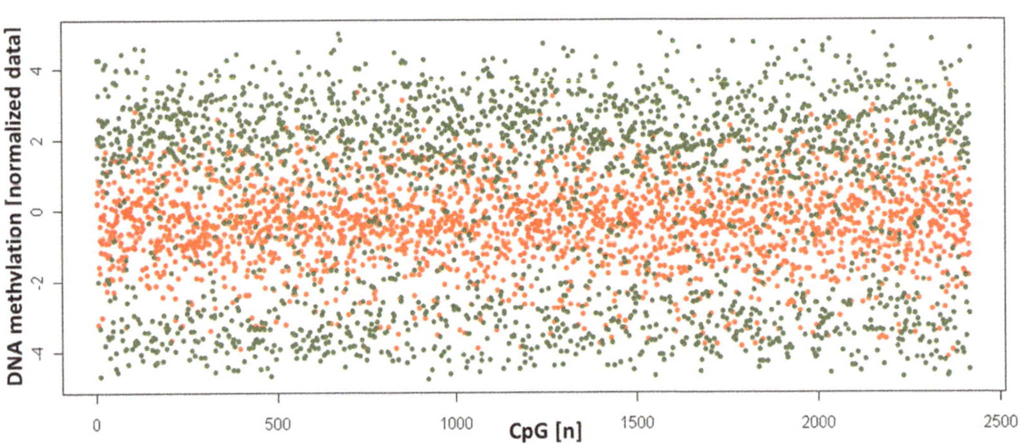

Figure 2. CpG loci differentially methylated between AC and CVS samples preferentially show an intermediate methylation level in CVS. Scatter plot of the means of DNA methylation values of all 2418 CpG loci differentially methylated between samples obtained by amniocentesis (AC, green circle) and chorionic villi biopsy (CVS, red circle) samples (FDR$<1\times10^{-15}$). For all loci the means have been calculated in AC and CVS separately and subsequently plotted. Most CpG loci are characterized by either a high or a low DNA methylation value in AC but an intermediate DNA methylation value in CVS.

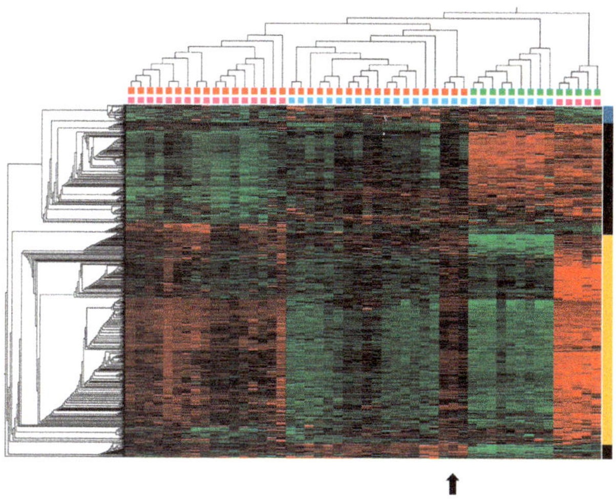

Figure 3. Hierarchic cluster analysis of DNA methylation values of 767 X-chromosomal CpG loci present on the array. The upper panel on top of the heatmap indicates the sample type (green: AC, red: CVS) while the second panel indicates the fetuses' sex (pink: female, cyan: male). Samples with known chromosomal aberrations and samples from ICSI were excluded. Three CVS samples from male fetuses show a DNA methylation pattern similar to female samples (arrow). A blue bar at the right site indicates genes methylated specifically in male fetuses, an orange bar genes methylated in female samples and a black bar genes with tissue- specific DNA methylation.

status on the methylation pattern in AC and CVS, respectively (data not shown). Probably, the number of samples under investigation was too low to get a conclusive significant result.

Having determined the methylation patterns in AC and CVS samples with normal karyotypes we aimed in the second part of the analyses at investigating whether fetal trisomies were associated with an altered DNA-methylation pattern. We limited the bioinformatic analyses to the CVS samples as the number of fetuses with a trisomy in the AC population was too low. In the three CVS samples with a fetal trisomy 21 (including one conceived by ICSI) a total of 464 loci (Figure 4; $q<0.01$) corresponding to 404 genes were differentially methylated as compared to CVS samples with a normal karyotype. Remarkably, the vast majority (387/404) of the genes was hypermethylated in the trisomic samples and only 17 hypomethylated. The 387 hypermethylated genes in trisomy 21 were significantly enriched for genes with HCP content ($p=0.0244$, $OR=1.27$, $RR=1.28$), known PRC2 target genes in embryonic stem cells ($p<0.0001$, $OR=4.37$, $RR=4.07$) and (known or suggested) imprinted genes ($p<0.0001$, $OR=3.23$, $RR=3.03$), while genes with LCP were significantly depleted ($p=0.0002$, $OR=0.55$, $RR=0.56$). In contrast the 17 hypomethylated genes were significantly enriched only for genes with HCP content ($p=0.0146$, $OR=5.93$, $RR=5.92$). Gene ontology analysis of all 404 aberrantly methylated genes in cases with trisomy 21 showed a significant enrichment of several processes in development, embryogenesis and signaling which could be associated with the typical phenotype of Down syndrome, including "neuron fate determination" (15.2fold), "meso/metanephros development" (9.4fold, 5.9fold), "heart morphogenesis" (5.5fold), "eating/feeding behavior" (11.9fold, 6.2fold) or "embryonic digestive tract morphogenesis" (9.5fold) (Table S3).

In contrast to the samples with trisomy 21, an analysis comparing the five CVS samples with trisomy 18 to the normal controls identified only 15 significantly differentially methylated loci, corresponding to 14 genes (Figures 4c and 4d). No significant enrichment of any properties of the genes was detected.

Finally, we wondered whether the single sample of AC with trisomy 18, the CVS sample with a gonosomal chromosome pattern typical for Turner Syndrome and the AC samples derived from a pregnancy after ICSI showed peculiar patterns of methylation. Obviously, bioinformatic analysis of single samples is meaningless. Nevertheless, displaying the methylation pattern of the X-chromosomal genes in the Turner sample as compared to the mean values of the normal male and female CVS samples showed lack of both, the typical female X-inactivation pattern and of the male methylation pattern (Figure S4). Finally, displaying the two ICSI samples as compared to the normal AC and CVS samples with regard to the genes differentially methylated between both tissues showed a remarkable loss of methylation in the ICSI derived AC sample (Figure S5). This might point to changes in the DNA methylation detectable in AC samples derived from ICSI patients but warrants further investigation.

Discussion

In the present study we performed array-based methylation profiling on an extensive series of fetal samples with normal and aberrant karyotypes obtained by routine prenatal CVS and AC sampling. Obviously, relying on left-over samples from routine prenatal testing implements a certain selection bias as with few exceptions only fetuses at risk for chromosomal aberrations and/or with abnormal ultrasound findings or maternal serum screenings will be sampled due to ethical considerations. Thus, the present series was enriched for pregnancies with normal karyotype but abnormal ultrasound ($n=12$), aberrant first trimester screen ($n=23$) or advanced maternal age ($n=41$) (multiple answers were permitted). Moreover, samples with known chromosomal aberrations were included on purpose. Thus, the analyses provided here reflect the findings of an "at-risk" cohort rather than of the normal distribution of pregnancies.

Moreover, it needs to be taken into account that whereas native (cryopreserved) CVS samples were investigated without prior culturing the AC cells had to be cultured to obtain sufficient amounts of DNA for the analyses. In this regard it needs to be considered that amplification of unmodified DNA prepared from uncultured AC cells would not have been suitable for the methylation arrays applied as by the amplification process the DNA methylation marks get lost. In turn, amplification of bisulfite treated DNA might have introduced experimental biases due to selective amplification of methylated or unmethylated DNA. The minute DNA amounts left over after routine diagnostics from uncultured amniotic cells might also be the reason why hitherto genome-wide methylation profiling studies focused on CVS or placental samples. Obviously, culturing cells harbors the risk of changing the DNA methylation pattern. Nevertheless, based on our own and others reports on lymphoblastoid cell lines as compared to normal lymphocytes we think that the culture-induced methylation changes are minor as compared to the tissue-specific differences which were in the focus of the present study [31]. To further evaluate this assumption we determined the predicted cumulative population doublings, predicted passages and the predicted time in culture using the tool available at http://www.molcell.rwth-aachen.de/dms. Based on the DNA methylation values of seven CpG loci present on the HumanMethylation27k Bead Chip Koch et al. developed an algorithm to investigate these parameters from in vitro cultured cells [34]. As calculated by this tool, the cumulative population doublings

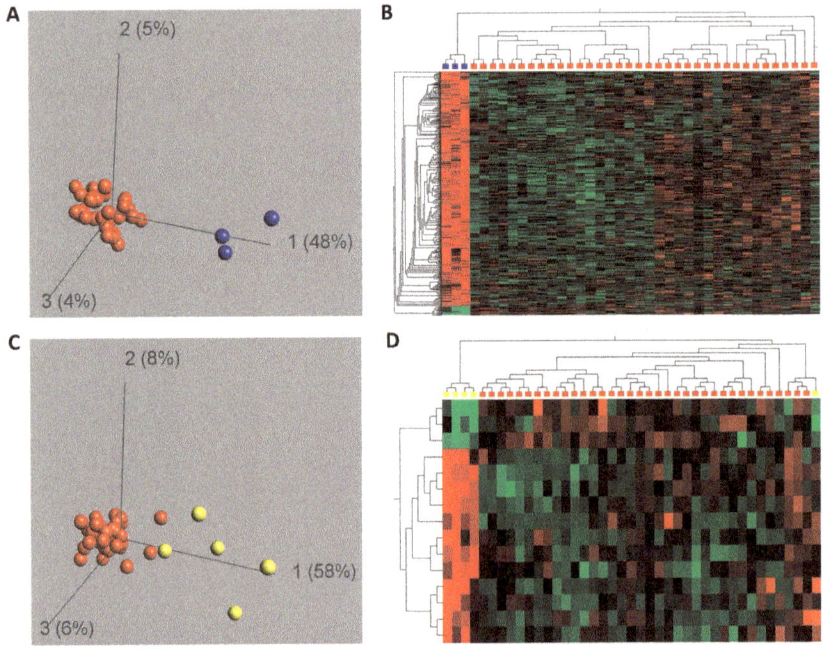

Figure 4. DNA methylation patterns in CVS samples with chromosomal imbalances. PCA (A) and Hierarchic cluster analysis (B) of DNA methylation values of 464 CpG loci differentially methylated between chorionic villi biopsy samples without chromosomal imbalances (red spheres or red squares, respectively) and samples with trisomy 21 (47,XY+21; blue spheres or blue squares, respectively) (FDR<0.01). While in cases with trisomy 21 numerous epigenetic alterations could be identified, in cases with trisomy 18 (47,XX+21/47,XY+21, yellow spheres or yellow squares) only 15 differentially methylated loci have been found (C and D). Green color in the heatmap indicates low DNA-methylation, black intermediate and red high DNA-methylation values.

ranged from 1 to 26 (median = 9), the predicted passages from −2 to 12 (median = 2) and the predicted time in culture from 18 to 64 (median = 7.5) in AC samples. All these values were lower than those calculated from uncultured CVS cells supporting our assumption that the methylome of the in vitro cultured AC samples might not be heavily altered in culture.

Even taking into account potential sampling and culturing artifacts the differences in the methylation patterns between CVS and AC samples with normal karyotype were striking. Investigating nearly 800 selected genes using the Illumina GoldenGate DNA Methylation Cancer Panel I array, Yuen et al. [35] recently identified 195 sites (23%) to be differentially methylated between various fetal studies. Here 2418 CpG loci corresponding to 2014 individual genes, i.e. almost 11% of all CpGs on the array, showed a differential methylation between the two tissues studied. This strong difference is most likely attributed to the fact that CVS samples derive from chorionic ectoderm (trophoblast) and extra-embryonic mesoderm and blood whereas cells sampled by AC are all of embryonic ectodermal origin including epithelial cells from the embryonic surfaces and from the amnion [19]. Indeed, the gene ontology analyses support this view showing on the one hand enrichment of genes involved in more fetal ectodermal or epithelial functions like keratinization or response to nitric oxide (mediated by surfactant proteins) and on the other hand more trophoblastic and extra-embryonic functions including many pregnancy associated hormones and proteins (see Table S2).

A striking feature of loci differentially methylated between CVS and AC were the preferentially intermediate methylation levels of these loci in CVS in contrast to the extreme DNA-methylation levels in AC samples (Figure 2). DNA methylation in normal tissues shows for the majority of genes a bimodal distribution, i.e. full methylation or no methylation [20,31]. This pattern was indeed observed in both AC and CVS samples. The enrichment of intermediate methylation levels in the genes differentially methylated between AC and CVS is inherent to this set of genes. A technical bias seems unlikely as the validity of the array has been proven previously and in the present set of samples by independent techniques. Also a bioinformatic bias seems unlikely due to the fact that intermediate methylation levels in CVS were present in 85% of the differentially methylated genes and in AC only in 15% of those genes. Moreover, the DNA methylation pattern of these CpG loci in AC was similar to the pattern found in peripheral blood of adults (data not shown). Finally, the genes hypermethylated in AC were significantly enriched for genes with LCPs (but depleted for HCP and PRC2 target genes in embryonic stem cells) suggesting a role in somatic tissue-specificity. Overall, these observations are in remarkable agreement with a recent report by Novakovic et al. [36] who showed that there is a progressive increase in average methylation in human placentas from first to third trimester. Using also the Infinium HumanMethylation27 BeadChip these authors have demonstrated that this progress particularly affects genes with an intermediate (beta value >0.6) methylation level and non-CpG island (i.e. LCP) genes. AC samples are usually obtained 2–10 weeks later in pregnancy than CVS samples. Therefore the intermediate methylation levels characteristic of CVS samples might reflect the different origin of the cells in such a sample. A different explanation is that in earlier weeks of pregnancy there is a higher epigenetic instability, comparable to the increased propensity for chromosomal mosaicism in the early placenta. The latter might be supported by the fact, that placental tissue also genetically is frequently mosaic [37].

Another feature which explains intra-sample heterogeneity might be contamination with maternal cells. By analysis of X-chromosomal methylation patterns we show (here) that such contamination might be variable and can even affect detection of the fetal sex via methylation-based X-inactivation patterns. In contrast to the CVS samples cultured cells derived from AC usually lack maternal contamination.

We failed to identify any association of maternal factors like maternal age, BMI or smoking status on the methylation pattern in AC and CVS likely due to the small size of the cohort for such analyses. In line with this, targeted analysis of the *F2RL3* locus recently shown to be differentially methylated in peripheral blood with regard to the smoking status [38] showed no different methylation levels in samples depending on the maternal smoking status.

Analyses of the association of karyotypic aberrations with DNA methylation levels had to be restricted to CVS samples due to the low number of AC samples with such changes. The intra-sample variability of CVS samples described above might be the cause that we only detected 15 loci, corresponding to 14 genes (Figures 4c and 4d) significantly differentially methylated between CVS samples with and without trisomy 18. In contrast, we identified a total of 464 loci (Figure 4; $q<0.01$) corresponding to 404 genes which were differentially methylated in samples with trisomy 21 as compared to CVS samples with a normal karyotype. It needs to be emphasized that the array applied in this study aims at a genome-wide coverage whereas several previous studies comparing DNA methylation between trisomic and normal CVS/placental samples focused on CpGs on the affected chromosomes, i.e. 18 or 21 [14,23,39]. A recent postnatal study investigated peripheral blood samples and isolated T-cells of individuals with Down syndrome as compared to controls on the same array platform like the one applied by us identified 108 genes (118 probes) and 140 CpGs (134 genes) to be differentially methylated in Down syndrome [40]. Nevertheless differences in the methylation profiles between individuals with and without trisomy 21 have been shown to be tissue specific [35].

Remarkably, in trisomy 21 fetuses studied herein more than 95% (387/404) of the differentially methylated genes were hypermethylated as compared to normal CVS samples. Only 3/387 hypermethylated (*COL6A2, H2BFS, RUNX1*) and 1/17 hypomethylated (*MCM3AP*) genes are located on chromosome 21. Thus, the trisomy 21 is associated with a genome-wide perturbance of DNA methylation not restricted to chromosome 21 that predominately leads to hypermethylation. This is in line with the pattern of differentially methylated genes observed by Kerkel et al. [40] on postnatal blood samples of individuals with trisomy 21. None of the nine genes identified by Kerkel et al. being aberrantly methylated in peripheral blood samples of patients with trisomy 21 have been identified by us. However, the focus of the study by Kerkel et al. and this study differs in the stage of development and the tissues analyzed. In our study, only 112 of the 404 genes belong to the 2014 genes showing tissue-specific differential methylation between CVS and AC suggesting that the deviation from the physiologic pattern in CVS might also be representative for other tissues. Remarkably, both differentially hypo- and hypermethylated genes in trisomy 21 were enriched for HCP content. Moreover, the 387 hypermethylated genes in trisomy 21 were significantly enriched for known PRC2 target genes in embryonic stem cells while genes with LCP were significantly depleted. This might suggest that many of those genes differentially methylated in trisomy 21 are indeed relevant for prenatal development. In line with this, the aberrantly methylated genes in cases with trisomy 21 show a remarkable enrichment of genes involved in processes of neuronal, heart, kidney, gut or facial bone (e.g. palate) development. Considering the phenotype of Down syndrome which frequently includes developmental disorders of the named organs it is intriguing to speculate that trisomy 21 exerts its pleiotropic effects via deregulation of an epigenetic modifier. Such a modifier might be localized in the Down syndrome critical region in chromosome 21 or could be deregulated indirectly e.g. through a transcript located on chromosome 21. Indeed, such a hypothesis could explain to a considerable extend the intra-individual variation in the Down syndrome phenotype as the levels of DNA methylation and its distribution in different tissues might vary and thus could explain differences in expressivity.

In summary, our extensive array-based survey of fetal sample obtained by routine prenatal invasive testing points to major tissue-specific differences of fetal DNA-methylation and gives rise to the hypothesis that part of the Down syndrome phenotype is epigenetically programmed in the first trimester of pregnancy.

Supporting Information

Figure S1 Reproducibility of the BeadArray based DNA methylation analyses as measured by Pearson coefficients. Two CVS samples have been hybridized separately in independent experiments using different batches of arrays.

Figure S2 Verification of results obtained from BeadArray analysis by bisulfite pyrosequencing (BPS). 6 CpG loci have been analyzed both by BPS (A, upper table, values represent % methylation) and by BeadChip technology (A, lower table; average beta values are shown) in the same samples. The color code indicates methylation value (green: low, black: intermediate, red: high DNA methylation). (B) Scatter plots of results obtained in (A). Pearson's product-moment correlation $r^2 = 0.69$

Figure S3 The majority of CpG loci present on the array are comparably methylated in CVS and AC samples. Histograms showing the frequency of the DNA methylation values in CVS (A) and AC (B). Scatter plot comparing DNA methylation values of CVS and AC samples (C). Histograms and scatter plots show DNA methylation values of CpG loci not differentially methylated between AC and CVS ($FDR>1\times10^{-15}$, t-test). Pearson's product-moment correlation $r^2 = 0.94$.

Figure S4 Hierarchic cluster analysis of DNA methylation values of 767 X-chromosomal CpG loci present on the array. The upper panel on top of the heatmap indicates the sample type (green: AC, red: CVS) while the second panel indicates the fetuses' sex (pink: female, cyan: male). The third panel indicates normal karyotype (yellow) versus Turner syndrome (black). Three CVS samples from male fetuses show a DNA methylation pattern similar to female samples (arrow). A blue bar at the right site indicates genes methylated specifically in male fetuses, an orange bar genes methylated in female samples and a black bar genes with tissue- specific DNA methylation.

Figure S5 The AC sample derived from a pregnancy after ICSI showed a peculiar pattern of methylation. PCA (A) and hierarchic cluster analysis of DNA methylation values of 2418 CpG loci differentially methylated between AC (green sphere (A) or green square (B)) and CVS (red sphere (A) or red square (B)) (t-test, $FDR<1\times10^{-15}$). One AC sample from ICSI is indicated by a blue sphere (A) or a blue square (B), respectively.

Table S1 Clinical characteristics of the samples included in the study.

Table S2 Gene ontology terms (GO) significantly enriched in the group of genes differentially methylated between CVS and AC samples as compared to the entirety of loci present on the array (p<0.001, GOrilla tool: GOprocess).

Table S3 Gene ontology terms (GO) significantly enriched in the group of genes differentially methylated between CVS samples without chromosomal imbalances and samples with known trisomy 21 as compared to the entirety of loci present on the array (p<0.001, GOrilla tool: GOprocess).

Table S4 DNA methylation values (avg.beta and normalized data) of loci differentially aberrantly methylated in trisomy 21 (sheet 1) and trisomy 18 (sheet 2). Data from CVS (trisomy and CVS) as well as from peripheral blood samples from normal female and male donors are included.

Acknowledgments

The authors thank the technical staff of the prenatal cytogenetic, molecular genetic and epigenetic laboratories of Institute of Human Genetics for expert assistance.

Author Contributions

Conceived and designed the experiments: OA RS. Performed the experiments: CES SB JK CvK SS MK. Analyzed the data: OA. Contributed reagents/materials/analysis tools: CES WJ RS SH AC. Wrote the paper: RS OA.

References

1. Chowdhury S, Erickson SW, MacLeod SL, Cleves MA, Hu P, et al. (2011) Maternal genome-wide DNA methylation patterns and congenital heart defects. PloS one 6: e16506.
2. Banister CE, Koestler DC, Maccani MA, Padbury JF, Houseman EA, et al. (2011) Infant growth restriction is associated with distinct patterns of DNA methylation in human placentas. Epigenetics 6: 920–7.
3. Lambertini L, Lee TL, Chan WY, Lee MJ, Diplas A, et al. (2011) Differential methylation of imprinted genes in growth-restricted placentas. Reprod Sci 18: 1111–7.
4. Rexhaj E, Bloch J, Jayet PY, Rimoldi SF, Dessen P, et al. (2011) Fetal programming of pulmonary vascular dysfunction in mice: role of epigenetic mechanisms. Am J Physiol Heart Circ Physiol 301: H247–52.
5. Christophersen NS, Helin K (2011) Epigenetic control of embryonic stem cell fate. J Exp Med 207: 2287–95.
6. Hirabayashi Y, Gotoh Y. (2011) Epigenetic control of neural precursor cell fate during development. Nat Rev Neurosci 11: 377–88.
7. Poulsen P, Esteller M, Vaag A, Fraga MF, (2007) The epigenetic basis of twin discordance in age-related diseases. Pediatr Res 61: 38R–42R.
8. Bocklandt S, Lin W, Sehl ME, Sanchez FJ, Sinsheimer JS, et al. (2011) Epigenetic predictor of age. PloS one 6: e14821.
9. Martin GM (2005) Epigenetic drift in aging identical twins. Proc Natl Acad Sci U S A 102: 10413–4.
10. Ali S (2011) Echocardiographic diagnosis of atrioventricular septal defect without primum atrial septal defect: a relatively "common" congenital heart defect in Down's syndrome. Anadolu Kardiyol Derg 11: 183–5.
11. Joziasse IC, Smith KA, Chocron S, van Dinther M, Guryev V, et al. (2011) ALK2 mutation in a patient with Down's syndrome and a congenital heart defect. Eur J Hum Genet 19: 389–93.
12. Howard CM, Davies GE, Farrer MJ, Cullen LM, Coleman MM, et al. (1993) Meiotic crossing-over in nondisjoined chromosomes of children with trisomy 21 and a congenital heart defect. Am J Hum Genet 53: 462–71.
13. Papageorgiou EA, Karagrigoriou A, Tsaliki E, Velissariou V, Carter NP, et al. (2011) Fetal-specific DNA methylation ratio permits noninvasive prenatal diagnosis of trisomy 21. Nat med 17: 510–3.
14. Chim SS, Jin S, Lee TY, Lun FM, Lee WS, et al. (2008) Systematic search for placental DNA-methylation markers on chromosome 21: toward a maternal plasma-based epigenetic test for fetal trisomy 21. Clin Chem 54: 500–11.
15. Tsui DW, Lam YM, Lee WS, Leung TY, Lau TK, et al. (2010) Systematic identification of placental epigenetic signatures for the noninvasive prenatal detection of Edwards syndrome. PloS one 5: e15069.
16. Tong YK, Ding C, Chiu RW, Gerovassili A, Chim SS, et al. (2006) Noninvasive prenatal detection of fetal trisomy 18 by epigenetic allelic ratio analysis in maternal plasma: Theoretical and empirical considerations. Clin Chem 52: 2194–202.
17. Papageorgiou EA, Fiegler H, Rakyan V, Beck S, Hulten M, et al. (2009) Sites of differential DNA methylation between placenta and peripheral blood: molecular markers for noninvasive prenatal diagnosis of aneuploidies. Am J Pathol 174: 1609–18.
18. Chu T, Burke B, Bunce K, Surti U, Allen Hogge W, et al. (2009) A microarray-based approach for the identification of epigenetic biomarkers for the noninvasive diagnosis of fetal disease. Prenat Diagn 29: 1020–30.
19. Gardner RJM, Sutherland GR (2004) Chromosome abnormalities and genetic counseling. Oxford University Press New York. 577 p.
20. Bibikova M, Lin Z, Zhou L, Chudin E, Garcia EW, et al. (2006) High-throughput DNA methylation profiling using universal bead arrays. Genome Res 6: 383–93.
21. R Development Core Team (2011) R: A language and environment for statistical computing. R Foundation for Statistical Computing, Vienna, Austria. ISBN 3-900051-07-0, URL http://www.R-project.org/.
22. Du P, Kibbe WA, Lin SM (2008) lumi: a pipeline for processing Illumina microarray. Bioinformatics 24: 1547–8.
23. Du P, Zhang X, Huang CC, Jafari N, Kibbe WA, et al. (2010) Comparison of Beta-value and M-value methods for quantifying methylation levels by microarray analysis. BMC Bioinformatics 11: 587.
24. Lin SM, Du P, Huber W, Kibbe WA (2008) Model-based variance-stabilizing transformation for Illumina microarray data. Nucleic Acids Research 36: e11.
25. Weber M, Hellmann I, Stadler MB, Ramos L, Paabo S, et al. (2007) Distribution, silencing potential and evolutionary impact of promoter DNA methylation in the human genome. Nature Genet 39: 457–66.
26. Martin-Subero JI, Ammerpohl O, Bibikova M, Wickham-Garcia E, Agirre X, et al. (2009) A comprehensive microarray-based DNA methylation study of 367 hematological neoplasms. PloS one 4: e6986.
27. Lee TI, Jenner RG, Boyer LA, Guenther MG, Levine SS, et al. (2006) Control of developmental regulators by Polycomb in human embryonic stem cells. Cell 125: 301–13.
28. Murphy SK, Jirtle RL (2003) Imprinting evolution and the price of silence. Bioessays 25: 577–88.
29. Eden E, Navon R, Steinfeld I, Lipson D, Yakhini Z (2009) GOrilla: a tool for discovery and visualization of enriched GO terms in ranked gene lists. BMC Bioinformatics 10: 48.
30. Tost J, Gut IG (2007) DNA methylation analysis by pyrosequencing. Nat Protoc 2: 2265–75.
31. Martin-Subero JI, Kreuz M, Bibikova M, Bentink S, Ammerpohl O, et al. (2009) New insights into the biology and origin of mature aggressive B-cell lymphomas by combined epigenomic, genomic, and transcriptional profiling. Blood 113: 2488–97.
32. Ammerpohl O, Haake A, Pellissery S, Giefing M, Richter J, et al. (2012) Array-based DNA methylation analysis in classical Hodgkin lymphoma reveals new insights into the mechanisms underlying silencing of B cell-specific genes. Leukemia 26: 185–8.
33. Ammerpohl O, Pratschke J, Schafmayer C, Haake A, Faber W, et al. (2012) Distinct DNA methylation patterns in cirrhotic liver and hepatocellular carcinoma. Int J Cancer 130: 1319–28.
34. Koch CM, Joussen S, Schellenberg A, Lin Q, Zenke M, et al. (2012) Monitoring of cellular senescence by DNA-methylation at specific CpG sites. Aging Cell 11: 366–9.
35. Yuen RK, Neumann SM, Fok AK, Penaherrera MS, McFadden DE, et al. (2011) Extensive epigenetic reprogramming in human somatic tissues between fetus and adult. Epigenetics Chromatin 4: 7.
36. Novakovic B, Yuen RK, Gordon L, Penaherrera MS, Sharkey A, et al. (2011) Evidence for widespread changes in promoter methylation profile in human placenta in response to increasing gestational age and environmental/stochastic factors. BMC Genomics 12: 529.
37. Churakov G, Kriegs JO, Baertsch R, Zemann A, Brosius J, et al. (2009) Mosaic retroposon insertion patterns in placental mammals. Genome Res 19: 868–75.
38. Breitling LP, Yang R, Korn B, Burwinkel B, Brenner H (2011) Tobacco-smoking-related differential DNA methylation: 27K discovery and replication. Am J Hum Genet 88: 450–7.
39. Tong YK, Jin S, Chiu RW, Ding C, Chan KC, Leung TY, et al. (2010) Noninvasive prenatal detection of trisomy 21 by an epigenetic-genetic chromosome-dosage approach. Clin Chem 56: 90–8.
40. Kerkel K, Schupf N, Hatta K, Pang D, Salas M, et al. (2010) Altered DNA methylation in leukocytes with trisomy 21. PLoS Genet 6: e1001212.

Whole-Genome Array CGH Evaluation for Replacing Prenatal Karyotyping in Hong Kong

Anita S. Y. Kan[1,2]*, Elizabeth T. Lau[1,2], W. F. Tang[1], Sario S. Y. Chan[2], Simon C. K. Ding[2], Kelvin Y. K. Chan[1,2], C. P. Lee[1,2], Pui Wah Hui[1,2], Brian H. Y. Chung[2,3], K. Y. Leung[4], Teresa Ma[4], Wing C. Leung[5], Mary H. Y. Tang[1,2]

1 Department of Obstetrics and Gynaecology, Li Ka Shing Faculty of Medicine, The University of Hong Kong, Hong Kong Special Administrative Region, China, **2** Department of Obstetrics and Gynaecology, Queen Mary Hospital, Hong Kong Special Administrative Region, China, **3** Department of Paediatrics and Adolescent Medicine, Queen Mary Hospital, Li Ka Shing Faculty of Medicine, The University of Hong Kong, Hong Kong Special Administrative Region, China, **4** Department of Obstetrics and Gynaecology, Queen Elizabeth Hospital, Hong Kong Special Administrative Region, China, **5** Department of Obstetrics and Gynaecology, Kwong Wah Hospital, Hong Kong Special Administrative Region, China

Abstract

Objective: To evaluate the effectiveness of whole-genome array comparative genomic hybridization (aCGH) in prenatal diagnosis in Hong Kong.

Methods: Array CGH was performed on 220 samples recruited prospectively as the first-tier test study. In addition 150 prenatal samples with abnormal fetal ultrasound findings found to have normal karyotypes were analyzed as a 'further-test' study using NimbleGen CGX-135K oligonucleotide arrays.

Results: Array CGH findings were concordant with conventional cytogenetic results with the exception of one case of triploidy. It was found in the first-tier test study that aCGH detected 20% (44/220) clinically significant copy number variants (CNV), of which 21 were common aneuploidies and 23 had other chromosomal imbalances. There were 3.2% (7/220) samples with CNVs detected by aCGH but not by conventional cytogenetics. In the 'further-test' study, the additional diagnostic yield of detecting chromosome imbalance was 6% (9/150). The overall detection for CNVs of unclear clinical significance was 2.7% (10/370) with 0.9% found to be de novo. Eleven loci of common CNVs were found in the local population.

Conclusion: Whole-genome aCGH offered a higher resolution diagnostic capacity than conventional karyotyping for prenatal diagnosis either as a first-tier test or as a 'further-test' for pregnancies with fetal ultrasound anomalies. We propose replacing conventional cytogenetics with aCGH for all pregnancies undergoing invasive diagnostic procedures after excluding common aneuploidies and triploidies by quantitative fluorescent PCR. Conventional cytogenetics can be reserved for visualization of clinically significant CNVs.

Editor: Harriet Wikman, University Medical Center Hamburg-Eppendorf, Germany

Funding: The authors would like to acknowledge the Hospital Authority of Hong Kong and also S. K. Yee Medical Research Fund for their support. The funders had no role in study design, data collection and analysis, decision to publish, or preparation of the manuscript.

Competing Interests: The authors have declared that no competing interests exist.

* E-mail: kansya@hku.hk

Introduction

Conventional cytogenetics has been the gold standard for detecting chromosomal abnormalities in prenatal diagnosis. It enables the examination of genome-wide numerical and structural abnormalities at microscopic level, and can achieve a resolution of 5–10 Mb [1]. However, the method is labour intensive, with a turn-around time of 14 to 21 days. Various molecular cytogenetic techniques, such as Quantitative Fluorescent Polymerase Chain Reaction (QF-PCR) [2,3] and Fluorescent In Situ Hybridization (FISH) technology, could complement the detection of chromosomal abnormalities and offer faster turn-around times. However, these methods are targeted to detect specific chromosomal abnormalities and are dependent on the chromosomal probe used. In contrast, whole-genome array comparative hybridization (aCGH) not only provides high resolution detection of genomic alterations, but also allows refinement of breakpoints on chromosome rearrangements.

Chromosomal microarray to assess DNA copy number variations has been suggested as the first-tier clinical diagnostic test in the postnatal setting for individuals with developmental disabilities or congenital anomalies because of an increased diagnostic yield of 12 to 15% compared to conventional karyotyping [4,5]. The clinical utility of aCGH in the prenatal setting has been demonstrated in systematic reviews [6–8], a large scale prospective randomized controlled trial [9] and also in recent research [10]. The major challenge for the large-scale implementation of these techniques appears to lie in interpretation of the results [11]. Thus genetic counseling and ethical issues [12,13] are significant in offering whole-genome aCGH in prenatal diagnosis. Essentially, there is a need for consensus in determining which patient groups should be offered in routine prenatal practice, and international guidance on interpretation and reporting of copy number variations for prenatal population [11]. This evaluation study demonstrates the advantages and disadvantages of aCGH and argues that whole-genome oligonucleotide aCGH is able to replace conventional cytogenetics in prenatal diagnosis in the local population of Hong Kong.

In this study, the use of aCGH for prenatal diagnosis is evaluated in two models: (1) as a first-tier test and, (2) as a 'further-test' analyzing prenatal samples of patients with abnormal fetal ultrasound findings and normal karyotypes. Results from aCGH are compared with those from conventional cytogenetics in order to determine the concordance of results and the additional diagnostic yield of aCGH over karyotyping.

Methods

Patients and samples

Approval was granted by the Institutional Review Board, University of Hong Kong/Hospital Authority, Hong Kong for the study to be conducted within 3 hospitals: Tsan Yuk Hospital, Queen Elizabeth Hospital, and Kwong Wah Hospital. Written informed consent was obtained from participants, who were recruited between January 2011 and November 2012. Informed consent and counseling on the benefits and limitations of the test, test methodology, reporting time, and possible test results (clinically significant, unclear clinical significance, benign) and outcomes of the investigation were explained to the participants by medical staff. Parental blood samples were obtained at the time of consent in case information on inheritance of CNV is necessary for further interpretation of prenatal results. Prenatal samples of 370 patients (Figure 1) with indications for chromosome studies were tested using whole-genome aCGH analysis at the Prenatal Diagnostic Laboratory, Tsan Yuk Hospital. Of those 370 prenatal samples, 220 patients had been prospectively recruited for the first-tier test study prior to the invasive procedure. In addition, 150 subjects with abnormal fetal ultrasound findings were retrospectively recruited into the 'further-test' study once conventional cytogenetic results had shown a normal karyotype on invasive testing. A total of 193 parental blood samples were used to categorize unclear CNVs identified in the corresponding prenatal samples in the evaluation study. In addition to the evaluation study, abnormal findings of 12 prenatal samples tested by conventional cytogenetics and requiring characterization were assessed using aCGH.

Conventional cytogenetics was performed by Giemsa banded (G-banded) karyotyping as a clinical service on all prenatal samples at Prenatal Diagnostic Laboratory, Tsan Yuk Hospital. As per protocol, optimally, 3–5 mg of dissected chorionic villi or 30 ml amniotic fluid was obtained to set up for karyotype, QF-PCR and aCGH. Cultured cells in flasks were used when either a) there were not enough cells in the primary sample, or b) in retrospective samples for the 'further-test' study, or c) in retrospective samples required for characterization studies. Eleven placental tissue samples and 2 skin biopsy samples obtained from pregnancies which were terminated after abnormal fetal ultrasound findings were processed for aCGH analysis.

Indications for recruitment to the study

Prenatal patients with clinical indications for further diagnoses were recruited to the research study. The reasons included abnormal findings on fetal ultrasound; positive Down syndrome screening; or maternal anxiety concerning advanced maternal age, family history of genetic disorder or previous child with anomalies. Some patients met more than one of the indications for study. In categorizing the indications as shown in Figure 1, ultrasound abnormality preceded positive Down syndrome screening and in turn over maternal anxiety.

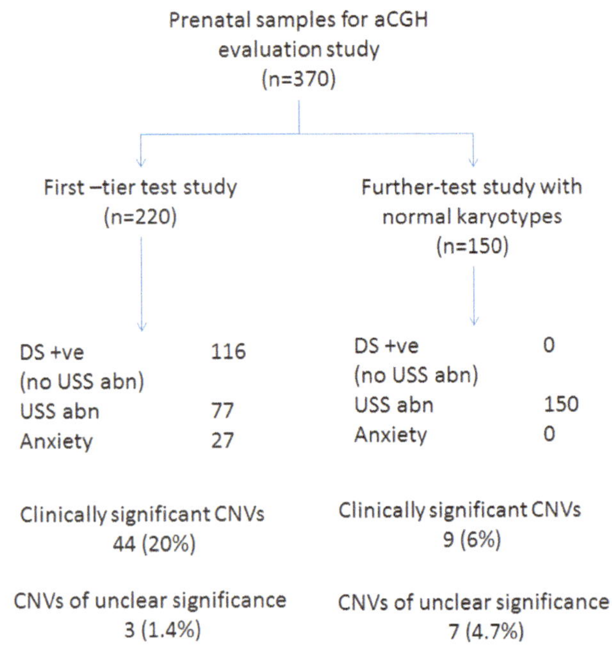

Figure 1. A schematic diagram showing the indications for recruitment to the study and CNVs detected in the evaluation study. The samples were subjected to first-tier test and 'further-test', with the clinical indications of testing and findings stated. aCGH, array CGH; CNVs, copy number variants; n, number of samples; DS +ve, Down syndrome screening positive; USS abn, ultrasound abnormality; Anxiety: maternal anxiety. Details on the clinically significant CNVs and CNVs of uncertain clinical significance are listed in Tables 1, 2, 3, 4, 5, 6.

Methods of DNA extraction

Cells were pelleted from 5 ml amniotic fluid by centrifugation at 400×g for 10 min. DNA was extracted by Gentra Puregene Tissue Kit (QIAGEN, USA) following manufacturer's instruction. Uncultured chorionic villi, tissue or cultured cells were pelleted by centrifugation at 3000×g for 5 min, lysed in 300 µl of lysis buffer (100 mM Tris, pH 8.5, 5 mM EDTA, 0.2% SDS, 200 mM NaCl) with Proteinase K at final concentration of 2 mg/ml. The lysate was incubated at 55°C overnight, added with 7 µl of RNase A solution (Qiagen, USA) and incubated at 37°C for 60 to 120 min. DNA was precipitated by the addition of 2.5 volume of cold 100% ethanol, spooled, washed twice with 1 ml of 70% ethanol and air dried. The DNA pellet was dissolved in Tris EDTA (TE) buffer (10 mM Tris, 0.1 mM EDTA, pH 7.5). For the blood samples, 3 ml of EDTA blood were diluted to 9 ml with 1X PBS. The diluted blood was overlaid onto 6 ml of Ficoll-Paque Plus (GE Healthcare Life Sciences) and centrifuged at 600×g for 30 min. The mononuclear cells at the interphase were transferred to a fresh tube and washed twice with 15 ml of 1X PBS. Cells were pelleted by centrifugation at 400×g for 10 min. The cells were lysed in 1 ml of lysis buffer (100 mM Tris, pH 8.5, 5 mM EDTA, 0.2% SDS, 200 mM NaCl) and DNA was precipitated and processed as above. Where DNA extraction was deemed urgent, for example in advanced gestations, a commercial kit (QIAmp DNA blood kit, Qiagen, USA) was used. The concentration of DNA samples was measured by NanoDropND-1000 spectrophotometer (NanoDrop Technologies, USA) and the quality of DNA samples was analyzed by agarose gel electrophoresis to exclude degradation or RNA contamination.

Array CGH analysis and interpretation

All samples were tested by NimbleGen CGX-135K arrays which were designed by Signature Genomics (Perkin Elmer, USA) following manufacturer's instructions. The coverage of the array has an average resolution of 140 kb across the genome and 40 kb or less in regions of clinical relevance. It evaluates over 245 known genetic syndromes and over 980 gene regions of functional significance in human development. The data were analyzed by Genoglyphix software (Signature Genomics, Spokane, USA). The gender of the prenatal samples was examined using QF-PCR [14] to determine the gender-matched reference DNA used in aCGH. The control DNA was from pooled gender-matched DNA from Promega (Madison, Wisconsin, USA).

Copy number variants (CNVs) detected by aCGH were systematically evaluated for clinical significance by comparison with information in the Signature Genomics' proprietary Genoglyphix Chromosome Aberration Database (Signature Genomics, Spokane, WA, USA), the internal laboratory database at Tsan Yuk Hospital, and the publicly available databases [Database of Genomic Variant (DGV), International Standards for Cytogenomic Arrays Consortium Database (ISCA), Children Hospital of Philadelphia database (CHOP), Database of Chromosomal Imbalance and Phenotype in Humans using Ensembl Resources (DECIPHER)]. Categorization of CNVs was based on available information concerning the fetal phenotypes and by comparison of phenotypes with known genes in the region of copy gain or loss. This was ascertained from searching Online Mendelian Inheritance in Man (OMIM), PubMed, RefSeq and the University of California Santa Cruz (UCSC) genome browser. A CNV was considered to be: (1) benign if it was reported in healthy subjects in the databases searched; if there are no genes involved; or if involved genes were unrelated to the phenotype and have no apparent clinical relevance; (2) clinically significant if it corresponded to a region known to be of clinical relevance or had a gene of clinical relevance; (3) of unclear clinical significance if there is insufficient evidence to categorize as clinically significant or benign at the time of reporting. When CNVs of unclear clinical significance were detected in a prenatal sample, parental blood samples were processed to provide additional information for interpretation.

Confirmation of CNVs

Clinically significant copy number gains and losses not detectable by karyotyping were confirmed by Fluorescent In Situ Hybridization (FISH) studies whenever possible. Microdeletion and telomeric FISH probes were obtained from Abbott Diagnostics (USA) and FISH probes from bacterial artificial chromosome clones from The Centre for Applied Genomics at the Hospital for Sick Children (Toronto, Canada). Homozygous alpha thalassemia deletion was confirmed by standard laboratory protocol [15].

Microarray data are available in the ArrayExpress database (www.ebi.ac.uk/arrayexpress) under accession number E-MTAB-2156.

Results

Clinically significant CNVs identified by aCGH in the prenatal samples from both the first-tier test study and from the 'further-test' study are shown in Figure 1. The initial turn-around time for aCGH was 8–10 days, while conventional cytogenetics took 14–21 days (data not shown).

First-tier test study

Two hundred and twenty prenatal samples were examined using whole-genome aCGH methodology together with routine culture for G-banded karyotyping with or without QF-PCR rapid aneuploidy testing. One hundred and sixteen samples (52.7%) were positive for Down syndrome screening with no apparent fetal ultrasound anomalies at the time of testing; whilst 77 prenatal samples (35.0%) had fetal ultrasound anomalies detected prior to invasive prenatal diagnosis. Forty of these fetal malformations concerned a single organ system and 37 had abnormalities involving more than one organ system. In 27 prenatal samples (12.3%), maternal anxiety was the clinical indication for invasive testing and inclusion into the study (Figure 1).

Clinically significant CNVs were detected in 44 (20%) out of 220 samples (Table 1). Common aneuploidies were detected in 21 prenatal samples (9.5%) with six cases of trisomy 21; seven cases of trisomy 18; four cases of trisomy 13; and four cases of monosomy X. Twenty three prenatal samples (10.5%) had other chromosomal imbalances, as summarized in Table 2, 3, 4. There were 7 (3.2%) prenatal samples with CNVs detected by aCGH which had been undetected by karyotyping (Table 2, Case no. 1–7). In 9 (4.1%) samples, aCGH revealed additional information over G-banded karyotyping (Table 3, Case no. 8–16). These included 4 complex chromosomal rearrangements (Table 3, Case no. 8–11) involving 2 or more chromosome segments not attributed to unbalanced translocations, one additional marker chromosome (Table 3, Case no. 12), 2 additional ring structures (Table 3, Case no. 13 and 14), one mosaic ring chromosome 18 (Table 3, Case no. 15) and one unbalanced translocation which aCGH helped to define a small deletion in the derivative chromosome (Table 3, Case no. 16). In 7 samples (3.2%), aberrations were detected both by aCGH and karyotyping. These included 4 unbalanced translocations (Table 4, Case no. 17–20), trisomies involving chromosome 7 or 16 (Table 4, Case no. 21, 22) and one case with terminal deletion of chromosome 13 was identified (Table 4, Case no. 23). The result of the first-tier study showed an additional diagnostic yield of 3.2% (7/220) for aCGH over conventional G-banded karyotyping. One triploidy was not detected by aCGH.

The clinically significant results were analyzed and categorized according to the clinical indications for the investigations. There were six cases of patients who had screened positive for Down syndrome without fetal ultrasound anomalies being evident (Table 1). Three cases had common aneuploidies (one each of trisomy 13, 18, 21) and the remaining three had other chromosomal imbalances including ring structures and trisomy 7 (Table 3, Case no. 14, 15, and Table 4 Case no. 21). In 77 prospective samples with fetal ultrasound anomalies detected (Table 1), 38 (49.4%) showed clinically significant chromosomal imbalances. Of these, 18 were common aneuploidies (three trisomy 13, six trisomy 18, five trisomy 21 and four monosomy X). In addition, 20 had other chromosomal imbalances (Table 2, Case no. 1–7, Table 3, Case no. 8–13, 16, Table 4, Case no. 17–20, 22 and 23). Eleven out of the 20 cases had fetal ultrasound anomalies in more than one organ system (including the neck and body fluid, central nervous system, cardiovascular, craniofacial, gastrointestinal, genitourinary, musculoskeletal, thoracic, or other

Table 1. Clinically significant CNVs detected in the first-tier test study.

		Clinically significant CNV*		
Indication	**Samples**	**Common aneuploidies (%)**	**Other abnormalities (%)**	**Total (%)**
DS positive (no USS abn)	116	3 (2.6)	3 (2.6)	6 (5.2)
USS abn	77	18 (23.4)	20 (26.0)	38 (49.4)
Anxiety	27	0	0	0
Total	220	21 (9.5)	23 (10.5)	44 (20.0)

DS: Down syndrome screening; USS abn: ultrasound abnormality;
*percentage of clinical significant CNV found in the indication category.

anomalies including intrauterine growth restriction). Where invasive testing was indicated for maternal anxiety, no chromosomal imbalance was detected in the 27 samples studied.

Further-test study after normal karyotyping

In 150 patients with normal karyotyping and abnormal fetal ultrasound findings, nine clinically significant CNVs were identified using aCGH. All of the patients had fetal ultrasound detected anomalies in more than one organ system (Table 5). These included one 1p32 microdeletion resulting in *NFIA* haploinsufficiency [16]; one 22q11.2 microdeletion, one deletion in chromosome 14 resulting in paternal uniparental disomy 14-like phenotype; one 8p23.1 microdeletion; one unbalanced translocation detected after an apparent normal karyotype and four samples with microdeletion in 16p13.3 resulting in Hemoglobin Bart's disease. With the exception of the unbalanced translocation which was undetected on chorionic villus karyotyping, but identified by aCGH of the amniotic fluid and cytogenetic study, the remaining CNVs detected were <5 Mb in size and submicroscopic, beyond the detection resolution of conventional karyotyping. The additional diagnostic yield of aCGH over conventional cytogenetics was found to be 6%.

CNV of unclear clinical significance

The detection rate for CNVs of unclear significance identified during the evaluation study using the 135 K whole-genome array was 2.7% (10/370), with 1.4% (3/220) detected for the first-tier test and 4.7% (7/150) for 'further-test' (Table 6). Six of these 10 samples had CNVs associated with microdeletions or microduplications with incomplete penetrance and variable expressivity (Table 6, Case no. 1, 2, 4–7). Eight samples involved genes or loci which may be associated with neurodevelopmental problems (Table 6, Case no. 1–8). Two samples involved genes associated with structural abnormalities of organ systems that may or may not have relevance to the phenotype (Table 6, Case no. 7, 8). One de novo microdeletion of 1q21.1 with susceptibility for thrombocytopenia-absent radius (TAR) was classified as a CNV of unclear significance having determined that the fetal radii were present on the follow-up ultrasound scan (Table 6, Case no. 7). Where CNVs of unclear clinical significance were identified, the incidence of de novo CNVs was found to be 0.9% of the total in the study (3/370).

Characterization by aCGH on samples with abnormal karyotypes

During the study period, in addition to the 370 samples for the evaluation study, twelve prenatal samples were identified with abnormal karyotypes during conventional cytogenetics. These were further examined by aCGH. Breakpoints were established for two samples with unbalanced translocations and three samples with interstitial deletions. One sample used aCGH to confirm suspected deletion of chromosome 16 pter which had been undetermined by G-banding. This sample was found to have a balanced translocation between chromosome 2 and chromosome 10 which was inherited from the father. It was reassuring that no submicroscopic changes were evident. Three samples showed complex rearrangements, one involved a marker chromosome derived from chromosome X, one involved a marker chromosome derived from chromosome 15 which had the same array findings as Case no. 8 in Table 3. One complex chromosomal rearrangement involved translocation of a 1.76 Mb segment from chromosome 19 to a duplicated segment of chromosome 2. These three complex rearrangements would not have been accurately detected by conventional karyotyping.

Common benign CNVs

A total of 563 samples (370 prenatal and 193 parental) were performed using aCGH for the first-tier test, 'further-test' studies and for abnormal chromosomal characterization. These studies established common benign CNVs at eleven loci in patients of Hong Kong (Table 7). The most common locus with chromosomal gain or loss found in Hong Kong was at 8p11.23, and was detected at a frequency of up to 78% (Table 7, no. 5) reflecting the homogeneity of the local population. The proportion of parental samples required to be performed was 144 out of 193 (74.6%) in the first half period of evaluation and 49 out of 193 (25.4%) in the second half. The knowledge of common benign CNVs in the local population reduced the need for parental sample testing and could minimize cost if aCGH use in prenatal diagnosis is launched as clinical service.

Increased nuchal translucency (NT)

Among all 382 prenatal samples, 27 of them had NT of 3.5 mm or above. In seven of these 27 prenatal samples Down syndrome screening results were not available. The remainders were screened positive for Down syndrome. There were three findings of trisomy 21, in addition to three samples with clinically significant CNVs detectable by karyotyping. There were three samples with CNVs of unclear clinical significance (Table 6, Case no. 3, 4, 6), one of which had structural abnormality on fetal ultrasound scan. Therefore aCGH did not yield increased detection of clinically significant CNVs compared to karyotyping in this specific number of samples with increased nuchal translucency.

Discussion

This evaluation study demonstrated the effectiveness of the whole-genome oligonucleotide aCGH in prenatal diagnosis for the

Table 2. Clinically significant CNVs other than common aneuploidies detected in the first-tier test study which were not detected by karyotyping.

Case No.	Gest (w)	Sample type	Indication for study	Initial Karyotype	Array results	CNV size and type/syndrome or locus	Outcome	Phenotype and other information
1	18+6	AF	USS: ventriculomegaly, partial agenesis of corpus callosum	46,XY	arr 1q43q44(236,811,017–247,174,728)×1 dn	10.36 Mb loss/1q44 microdeletion syndrome	TOP at 22 w	Postmortem: agenesis of corpus callosum. Updated karyotype: 46,XY,del(1)(q43)
2	22	Placental Tissue	USS: hypoplastic tibiae and fibulae	46,XX	arr 19p13.3q13.43(213,080–63,703,259)×2~3 dn	mos +19	TOP at 21 w	Clinical diagnosis: brachyphalangy, polydactyly and tibial aplasia/hypoplasia syndrome. Updated karyotype: mos 47,XX,+19 [6]/46,XX [94]
3	16+4	Cultured AF	DS +ve, USS: early onset IUGR, fetal heart in right thorax, NT 4.6 mm in first trimester	46,XX	arr 2p25.3q11.2(26,551–100,807,481)×2~3 dn	mos 100.78 Mb gain/mos +2p	TOP	Postmortem: fetal heart in right thorax, diaphragmatic hernia, left lung hypoplasia, ASD, 1A1V.Updated karyotype: mos 47,XX,+del(2)(q11.2) [3]/46,XX [27]
4	17+5	AF	Alpha thalassaemia couple, USS: increased cardio-thoracic ratio	46,X,inv(X)(p21q22.1)	arr Xq22.1(99,482,878-99,663,419)×3 dn, 16p13.3(162,893-169,832)×0	217 kb gain at Xp21.1, 180 kb gain at Xq22.1/Unclear epilepsy & Intellectual disability restricted to female, 6.94 kb 2-copy loss at 16p13.3/Hb Bart's disease	TOP at 18 w	Hb Bart's disease
5	24	AF	USS: holoprosencephaly, proboscis, hypotelorism	46,XY	arr 8q23.3q24.12(113,718,332-122,076,557) ×1 dn	8.36 Mb loss in 8q23.3-8q24.12/Langer-Giedion/Trichorhinophalangeal	TOP at 23w	No information
6	20+2	AF	USS: Bilateral hand deformity, missing middle finger, compatible with ectrodactyly	46,XX	arr 17p13.3(1,059,027-1,218,853)×4 mat,17p13.3(2,260,944-2,366,399)×4 mat	Two copy gain 159.83 kb gain in 17p13.3	TOP at 23 w	Postmortem: bilateral ectrodactyly
7	13+4	CV	USS: enlarged fetal bladder 1.03×1.08×0.8 cm. Dilated renal pelvis	46,XY	arr 16q24.1(83,708,997-85,428,578)×1 dn	1.72 Mb loss	TOP at 19+3 w	Postmortem: bilateral low set ears, urethral atresia, bilateral hydroureters and renal dysplasia, malrotation of gastrointestinal tract, rectal atresia

AF: amniotic fluid; ASD: atrial septal defect; CV: chorionic villi; DCDA: dichorionic diamniotic; DS: Down syndrome screening; FB: fetal blood; Gest: Gestation; IUGR: intrauterine growth restriction; PPROM: preterm premature rupture of membranes; TOP: termination of pregnancy; USS: ultrasound scan findings; w: weeks; +ve: positive.

Table 3. Clinically significant CNVs other than common aneuploidies detected in the first-tier test study with additional information provided by aCGH over karyotyping.

Case No.	Gest (w)	Sample type	Indication for study	Initial Karyotype	Array results	CNV size and type/ syndrome or locus	Outcome	Phenotype and other information
8	32	Cultured AF	USS: fetal hydrops, pleural effusion, lung hypoplasia, ascites, bilateral hydrocele, polyhydramnios	46,XY,15q+dn	arr 15q11.2q13.2(20,372,901-28,138,979)×4 dn,15q13.2q13.3(28,927,707-30,226,405) ×3 dn	7.77 Mb 2-copy gain/ 15q11-q13 Microduplication region 1.3 Mb gain/15q13.3 Microdeletion region	Stillborn at 32+2w	Postmortem: hydrops fetalis with severe interstitial edema and hypoplastic lungs
9	17	CV	Maternal age, USS: DCDA twins - one IUGR, the other reduced because of acrania	46,XX,16p-	arr 16p13.3p13.2(2,912,285-7,697,824)×1 dn, 16p13.2(7,702,318-8,933,435)×1~2 dn, 16p13.13(11,323,756-12,017,936)×2~3 dn	4.79 Mb loss/16p13.3 Microdeletion-Severe Rubinstein-Taybi syndrome, 1.23 Mb mosaic loss, 694.18 kb mosaic gain	TOP at 19w	Postmortem: hypertelorism with prominent slanting of upper and lower inner epicanthic folds, wide mouth and roundish receding chin, pre-axial polydactyly of right hand, 11 pairs of ribs, ventricular septal defect, right renal and right ovarian agenesis, single umbilical artery
10	35+4	Cultured AF	DS -ve, USS: strawberry head, absent vermis, short long bones, abnormal heart	47,XY,+mar dn	arr 9p24.3p23(199,254-24,838,669)×4, 9p21.3p21.1(24,871,570-38,751,949)×3	24.6 Mb 2-copy gain, 13.87 Mb gain/+9p	TOP	Baby abnormal
11	22+4	Placental Tissue	USS: truncus arteriosus, dilated cerebral ventricles, hydronephrosis, absent nasal bone	46,XX,der(8)(qter-> q21.3::p23->qter)dn	arr 8p23.3p23.1(192,262-10,096,394)×1 dn, 8p23.1(10,620,658-11,895,875)×4 dn, 8q21.3q24.3(91,500,429-146,264,292)×3 dn	9.9 Mb loss/8p23.1 microdeletion(CDH2) syndrome, 1.28 Mb 2-copy gain/8p23.1 microduplication syndrome, 54.76 Mb gain	TOP at 22+4w	Postmortem: hypertelorism, flattened nasal bridge, down slanting palpebral fissure, micrognathia, high arched palate, midline alveolar cleft, truncus arteriosus type I with ventricular septal defect, atretic left pulmonary trunk origin, mild thymic hypoplasia, hydrocephalus with dilated lateral ventricles and fourth venticle and dilated renal pelves
12	10+3	Cultured CV	Maternal age, USS: mild ventriculomegaly 11-12 mm, micrognathia	47,XX,+mar	arr 9p24.3q22.31(199,254-94,915,798)×3	94.72 Mb gain	TOP	Updated karyotype: 47,XX,+ del(9)(q22)
13	35	Fetal blood	IUGR	46,XX [27]/47,XX,+mar dn [79]	arr 18q11.1q21.32(16,796,771-54,412,918)×3	37.62 Mb gain	TOP	Updated karyotype: mos 46,XX/47,XX,+r(18)
14	16+6	Cultured AF	DS +ve, CVS: mos 47,XX,+mar [8]/46,XX [22]	mos 47,XX,+mar dn [20]/46,XX [20]	arr 1p13.1p12(116,138,882-120,311,704)×2~3 dn	4.17 Mb gain	TOP	Abortus: facial asymmetry with hypoplasia of the left face and jaw, club feet; Updated karyotype: mos 47,XX,+r(1)dn [20]/46,XX [20]

Table 3. Cont.

Case No.	Gest (w)	Sample type	Indication for study	Initial Karyotype	Array results	CNV size and type/ syndrome or locus	Outcome	Phenotype and other information
15	20+3	Cultured AF	DS +ve, CVS: mosaicism with 3 cell lines: 45,XY,-18 (36.67%), 46,XY,r(18)(p11.3q23)(63.33%), 47,XY,r(18)×2(3.33%)	mos 45,XY,-18 [9]/46,XY,r(18)(p11.3q23) [27]	arr 18p11.32p11.21(131,491-14,107,537)×1, 18q11.1q23(16,796,771-74,503,562)×1~2, 18q23 (74,508,960-76,114,684)×1	13.98 Mb loss in 18p11.32p11.21, mos 57.71 Mb loss at 18q11.1q23, 1.61 Mb loss at 18q23	TOP at 20w	Postmortem: low set ears
16	23	AF	USS: thickened myocardium with thin rim of pericardial effusion	46,XY,18q+	arr 2p25.3p23.2(26,551-27,758,445)×3, 18q23(75,373,273-76,114,684)×1	27.73 Mb gain at 2p, 741.41 kb loss at 18q	TOP at 23w	Postmortem: patent ductus arteriosus. Updated karyotype: 46,XY,der(18)t(2;18)(p23;q23)pat

AF: amniotic fluid; ASD: atrial septal defect; CV: chorionic villi; DCDA: dichorionic diamniotic; DS: Down syndrome screening; FB: fetal blood; Gest: Gestation; IUGR: intrauterine growth restriction; PPROM: preterm premature rupture of membranes; TOP: termination of pregnancy; USS: ultrasound scan findings; w: weeks; +ve: positive.

analysis of chromosome imbalance at high resolution. During the first-tier test, a detection rate of 20% was determined amongst patients with clinical indications for testing. Clinically significant imbalances were found to be common aneuploidies (9.5%), whilst 10.5% involved other chromosomal abnormalities (Table 1). Rapid aneuploidy testing such as QF-PCR is able to exclude common aneuploidies prior to testing using aCGH. This would make aCGH more cost effective. Scott *et al.* also proposed the use of combined QF-PCR and aCGH as first-line prenatal diagnostic testing [17]. Our detection rate of 10.5% clinically significant CNVs other than common aneuploidy was double that of Scott *et al.* (2013). It is considered that this may be related to different patient characteristics, different indications for prenatal testing, in addition to using whole-genome rather than targeted array. CNVs only detectable by aCGH were also higher in our evaluation study (3.2% in this study versus 1.2% pathogenic CNVs) [17].

Array CGH helped to precisely delineate breakpoints, characterize marker chromosomes and detect mosaicism within a shorter time frame compared to G-banded cytogenetics. There were five samples with chromosome mosaicism in the study. Mosaic trisomy 19 and mosaic trisomy 7 (Table 2, Case no. 2 and Table 4 Case no. 21) were results confined to placental mosaicism where studies on skin fibroblast and in the amniotic fluid sample respectively indicated normal karyotypes. Of interest was a mosaic ring chromosome 18 finding with aCGH of one copy number gain for the chromosome 18 segment (Table 3, Case no. 13), not matching the mosaic ratio, but the FISH study found a small number of double rings in the cell population which explained the array result.

Four complex chromosomal rearrangements were determined in the first-tier test study, and three complex rearrangements were identified from prenatal samples with abnormal karyotypes requiring characterization. This highlighted the advantage of higher resolution aCGH in chromosome analysis. There were two samples with identical complex rearrangement comprising 2-copy gain at the Prader Willi/Angelman syndrome region (15q11.2–q13.2) and one copy gain at the 15q13.3 Microdeletion region (15q13.2–q13.3, Figure 2). Karyotyping of the first sample (Figure 2 Sample A; Table 3, Case no. 8) showed 15q+ while the chromosomal gain in the second sample (Figure 2 Sample B) performed using aCGH for characterization was in a marker chromosome. Although aCGH showed the same chromosomal imbalances, the phenotypes of the 2 samples were very different. In the latter sample choroid plexus cyst was the only anomaly. Since other CNVs detected in Case no. 8 (Table 3) were benign and apparently common in the local population, the severe phenotype may have been caused by small mutation in another chromosomal region or an interruption of the region 15q11.2–q13.2 by a complex rearrangement. The 15q proximal region is known for its instability due to the presence of repeating DNA elements [18,19] which may give rise to the triplication from centromere to breakpoint (BP) 4 plus duplication from BP4 to BP5 in these samples. Further investigation into the association of phenotypes and the manifestation of the copy number gain and imprinting [20] can be made on similar samples with rearrangements in the region. The finding also demonstrated the advances of complementary use of both aCGH and karyotyping in analyzing samples with multiple significant CNVs.

There were 4 cases of Hemoglobin Bart's disease with clinically significant aCGH findings in the 'further-test' study. While routine prenatal screening for thalassaemia by mean corpuscular volume (MCV) is offered in our locality, one case presented late in the third trimester (Table 5, Case no. 9) and was a result of non-paternity. This

Table 4. Clinically significant CNVs other than common aneuploidies detected in the first-tier test study with abnormalities detected by both aCGH and karyotyping.

Case No.	Gest (w)	Sample type	Indication for study	Initial Karyotype	Array results	CNV size and type/ syndrome or locus	Outcome	Phenotype and other information
17	23+3	Cultured AF	USS: diaphragmatic hernia, hyperextended right knee	46,XX,der(15)t(4;15)(p15.2;q26.1)pat	arr 4p16.3p15.1(33,860-28,155,263)×3 dn, 15q26.1q26.3(87,502,509-100,208,480)×1 dn	28.12 Mb gain at 4p, 12.71 Mb loss at 15q/Congenital diaphragmatic hernia	TOP at 23w	Postmortem: low set ears, receded chin, clenched fists, right knee dislocation, rocker-bottom feet, left diaphragmatic hernia, lung hypoplasia
18	11+2	CV	USS: cystic hygroma	46,XX,der(7)t(7;11)(q35;p12)pat	arr 7q35q36.3(146,772,782-158,816,094)×1, 11p15.5p12 (195,983-42,558,628)×3	12.04 Mb loss at 7q, 42.36 Mb gain at 11p	Miscarriage at 16w	Abortus: cleft lip
19	13+1	CV	USS: cardiomegaly, club feet at 13w. No obvious fetal abnormalities seen at 16w. Previous child with 46,XX,t(5;9)(p15.2;p21)mat	46,XY,der(5)t(5;9)(p15.2;p21)mat	arr 5p15.33p15.2(108,467-13,978,254)×1, 9p24.3p21.1 (199,254-29,362,821)×3	13.87 Mb loss in 5p, 29.16 Mb gain in 9p	TOP at 16w	Postmortem: no anatomical abnormality
20	21+6	AF	USS: bilateral complete cleft lip and bilateral cleft palate	46,XX,4p-	arr 4p16.3p16.1(33,860-8,772,114)×1,8p23.3p23.1 (192,262-6,907,722)×3	8.74 Mb loss in 4p/Wolf Hirschhorn syndrome, 6.72 Mb gain in 8p	TOP	Postmortem: bilateral cleft lip and palate. Updated karyotype: 46,XY,der(4)t(4;8)(p16;p23)dn
21	12+6	CV	Maternal age, DS +ve	47,XX,+7	arr 7p22.3q36.3(136,363-158,816,094)×2~3	mos +7 (60%)	Cervical incompetence; spontaneous miscarriage at 21w	Postmortem: single umbilical artery
22	14+2	Placental tissue	DS +ve, USS: mild cardiomegaly, pericardial effusion, increased placental thickness	mos 47,XX,+16 [8]/46,XX [14]	arr 12q22q23.1(93,607,866-95,066,901)×3 Trisomy 16	+16	PPROM at 14w and TOP performed	No information
23	22+5	AF	USS: abnormal brain with echoic shadow 3.9 cm, ? absent corpus callosum, holoprosencephaly	46,XY,13q-	arr 13q32.1q34(96,486,944-114,109,838)×1	17.62 Mb loss in 13q32.1-13q34	TOP at 23w	Postmortem: holoprosencephaly, ASD. Updated karyotype: 46,XY,del(13)(q32)dn

AF: amniotic fluid; ASD: atrial septal defect; CV: chorionic villi; DCDA: dichorionic diamniotic; DS: Down syndrome screening; FB: fetal blood; Gest: Gestation; IUGR: intrauterine growth restriction; PPROM: preterm premature rupture of membranes; TOP: termination of pregnancy; USS: ultrasound scan findings; w: weeks; +ve: positive.

Table 5. Overview of the clinical aspects of the fetuses with clinically significant CNVs detected in the further-test study with normal karyotype.

Case No.	Gest (w)	Sample type	DS +ve	Ultrasound abnormalities	Karyotype	Array results	CNV size and type	Locus/syndrome	Outcome	Phenotype and other information
1	23+4	AF	Y	Absent corpus callosum, prominent posterior horn of lateral ventricle. MRI fetal brain: Absent cerebellar vermis, complete absence of corpus callosum	46,XX	arr 1p32.1p31.3(60,638,478-64,100,969)×1 dn	3.46 Mb loss	*NFIA* haplo-insufficiency	TOP at 23+4w	Postmortem: absence of cerebellar vermis and corpus callosum
2	21	AF	N	Left axis deviation, TOF with VSD, over-riding aorta, small PA	46,XY	arr 22q11.21(17,299,469-19,790,658)×1	2.49 Mb loss	22q11.2 microdeletion	TOP at 22w	Postmortem: TOF
3	33	AF	N	Polyhydramnios, short limbs, small stomach bubble	46,XY	arr 14q32.2q32.31(99,890,594-101,081,825)×1 mat	1.19 Mb loss	UPD(14)pat-like phenotype	Live birth at 34w, 2.41 kg	Newborn with pharyngolaryngomalacia and obstructive sleep apnoea syndrome
4	12+2	CV	Y	Cystic hygroma, subcutaneous oedema, exomphalos	46,XY	arr 8p23.1(8,146,273-11,895,875)×1	3.75 Mb loss	8p23.1 Microdeletion	Live birth at 39w, 2.96 kg	Secundum ASD.
5	12+	CV	N	Skin oedema and NT 6 mm	46,XY	arr 10p15.3p13(128,680-15,889,188)×3,13q33.1q34 (102,510,400-114,109,838)×1	15.76 Mb gain in 10p; 11.60 Mb loss in 13q	Unbalanced translocation (10;13)	TOP at 23w	USS at 21w: bilateral pleural effusion and ascites, amniocentesis performed for aCGH. Missed karyotype in CV, detected after aCGH in AF. Postmortem: hydrops fetalis (bilateral pleural effusion and ascites), polydactyly of right hand. Updated karyotype: 46,XY,der(13)t(10;13)(p13;q33)pat
6	13	CV	N	Fetal cardiomegaly, placentomegaly	46,XX	arr 16p13.3(162,893-169,832)×0	6.94 kb 2-copy loss	Hb Bart's disease	TOP at 14w	No information
7	16+2	AF	N	Placenta thickened, increased CT ratio, abnormal hands+feet	46,XX	arr 16p13.3(162,893-169,832)×0	6.94 kb 2-copy loss	Hb Bart's disease	TOP at 17w	Abnormal hands & feet, cardiac hypertrophy
8	13+1	CV	N	Placentomegaly, cardiomegaly	46,XX	arr 16p13.3(162,893-169,832)×0	6.94 kb 2-copy loss	Hb Bart's disease	TOP at 14w	Cardiomegaly
9	32	FB	N	USS: fetal hydrops with ascites & cardiomegaly, dilated RA, left to right shunt, MCA PSV normal	46,XX	arr 16p13.3(162,893-169,832)×0	6.94 kb 2-copy loss	Hb Bart's disease	Emergency Caesarean section at 32+1w, 1.48 kg, NND	Postmortem: ASD and pulmonary hypoplasia, placental hydrops

AF: amniotic fluid; ASD: atrial septal defect; CT: cardio-thoracic; CV: chorionic villi; DORV: double outlet right ventricle; DS: Down syndrome screening; FB: fetal blood; FU: follow up; Gest: Gestation; Hb: haemoglobin; N: not DS +ve or not mentioned; NND: neonatal death; PA: pulmonary artery; PS: pulmonary stenosis; TOF: Tetralogy of Fallot; TOP: termination of pregnancy; USS: ultrasound: VSD: ventricular septal defect; w: weeks; Y:yes; +ve: positive.

Table 6. Overview of the clinical aspects of the fetuses with CNVs of unclear clinical significance.

Category	Case No.	Gest (w)	Sample type	DS +ve	Ultrasound abnormalities	Karyo-type	Array results	CNV size and type	OMIM Genes/ Locus	Outcome	Phenotype and other information
First-tier test	1	19+2	AF	Y	DS+ve risk 1:105	46,XX	arr 1q21.1(144,998,070-146,193,043)×1 mat	1.19 Mb loss	1q21.1 microdeletion	Live birth at 37+6w, 3.14 kg	No abnormality at birth. FU paediatricians for failure to thrive. Growth parameters below 3rd centile.
	2	20	AF	N	USS: early onset IUGR	46,XX	arr 16p11.2(29,564,890-30,100,123)×1 dn	535.23 kb loss	16p11.2 microdeletion	TOP at 24w	No information
	3	13+5	CV	Y	DS +ve 1st tri, risk 1:190, USS: increased NT 4.1 mm	46,XY	arr 3p26.3(76,277-3,092,911)×1 pat,9p24.3(485,809-551,031)×1 pat	3.02 Mb loss at 3p, 65.22 kb loss at 9p	*CHL1, CNTN6, CNTN4, IL5RA, KANK1*	Live birth at 39+5w, 3.92 kg	No abnormality at birth. Last update of baby normal.
Further test	4	12+3	Cultured CV	Y	USS: 12wk scan showed cystic hygroma, NT 5.6 mm, 18wk scan showed TOF	46,XY	arr 16p12.1(21,857,845-22,336,067)×1 dn	478.22 kb loss	16p12.1 microdeletion	TOP at 20w	Postmortem: TOF
	5	22+1	Cultured AF	N	USS: increased cisterna magnum 1.03 cm	46,XY	arr 16p13.11p12.3(15,419,888-18,054,322)×3 mat	2.63 Mb gain	16p13.11 microduplication	Live birth at 38+6w, 3.32 kg	No abnormality at birth.
	6	17+2	Cultured AF	N	USS: Increase NT 5.2 mm in 1st trimester. Previous child with bilateral SVC, dysmorphism, global developmental delay	46,XY	arr 15q11.2(20,372,901-20,636,841)×1 pat	263.94 kb loss	15q11.2 microdeletion	Live birth at 40+6w, 2.84 kg	Noted bilateral preauricular sinuses at birth. FU paediatricians for 15q11.2 microdeletion from paternal origin (tested at another unit). Last update of baby normal.
	7	22+5	Cultured AF	N	USS: TOF, small thymus	46,XX	arr 1q21.1(144,100,334-144,458,066)×1 dn	357.73 kb loss	1q21.1 microdeletion with susceptibility for thrombocytopenia-absent radius (TAR)	Live birth at 38w, 2.22 kg.	Last FU at 9 months: 6 kg. TOF with surgical correction done; left indirect inguinal hernia with herniotomy done; clefting of soft palate; poor feeding with recurrent projectile vomiting; failure to thrive with short stature; insucking of chest since birth
	8	21+6	Cultured AF	N	USS: TGA	46,XX	arr 2q13(111,114,738-112,817,963)×1 mat	1.7 Mb loss	*BUB1, BCL2L11, ANAPC1, MERTK, FBLN7*	TOP at 23+6w	Postmortem: TGA
	9	19	Cultured AF	N	USS: large omphalocoele with liver herniation, TOF	46,XY	arr 2q21.1(130,769,854-131,199,432)×3 pat	429.6 kb gain	*CCDC115, IMP4, PTPN18, CFC1*	TOP at 23+2w	Postmortem: omphalocoele, TOF, single umbilical artery
	10	22	Cultured AF	N	USS: bilateral club feet. Right hand held in fixed flexion position with overlapping finger	46,XX	arr 2p21(45,025,361-45,129,076)×3 pat,15q13.3q14(30,846,564-31,432,930)×3 mat	98.46 kb gain, 586.4 kb gain	*SIX3, SIX2, FMN1, RYR3*	TOP at 23+4w	Postmortem: low set ears, multiple joint contractures, compatible with arthrogryposis multiplex congenita

AF: amniotic fluid; CM: cisterna magna; CV: chorionic villi; DS: Down syndrome screening; FU: follow up; Gest: Gestation; IUGR: intrauterine growth restriction; N: not DS +ve or not mentioned; NT: nuchal translucency; SVC: superior vena cava; TGA: transposition of great arteries; TOF: Tetralogy of Fallot; TOP: termination of pregnancy; USS: ultrasound; Y: yes; +ve: positive.

Table 7. Common benign CNVs found in Hong Kong.

No.	Region size (Kb)	Cytoband Location	Genome coordinates	Event	Genes	Frequency of gain/ loss (%)
1	194	1q31.1	chr1:187592011–187776739	Loss	0	9
2	37	1q44	chr1:246644054–246914515	Gain/Loss	1	29/13
3	122	6p25.3	chr6:210793–321392	Gain/Loss	1	7/18
4	171	7p22.3	chr7:136,363–325,833	Gain	0	14
5	97–125	8p11.23	chr8:39310297–39531197	Gain/Loss	1–2	51/27
6	68–504	14q11.2	chr14:21388121–22089869	Gain/Loss	0–2	23/12
7	3–180	16p12.1	chr16:22534936–22689740	Gain/Loss	0	1/11
8	320	17q21.31	chr17:41507230–42147712	Gain/Loss	1	2/55
9	83	19p12	chr19:20408868–20518856	Loss	0	20
10	123	Xp22.33	chrX:3761569–3863478	Gain/Loss	1	9/34
11	105–109	Xq28	chrX:153064828–153168166	Gain/Loss	3	23/9

Kb: Kilobase.

highlighted one potential use of the test to diagnose Hemoglobin Bart's disease in circumstances of non-paternity [21].

Uncertain CNVs tend to be a concern for clinicians in counseling. Adequate pre and post-test information and counseling by trained counselors, and a team approach involving obstetricians, clinical geneticists and laboratory scientists in CNV interpretation is beneficial and is adopted in our setting. In this evaluation study, both CNVs of clinical significance and CNVs of unclear significance were reported to referring doctors. In the 10 cases with CNVs of unclear clinical significance, 5 of the pregnancies, all with major ultrasound abnormalities, were terminated (Table 6). Maternal cell contamination was not determined during the evaluation study. However the impact of contamination on the interpretation of prenatal microarray has been reported [22]. Taking this into account, our laboratory has adopted the policy to routinely exclude

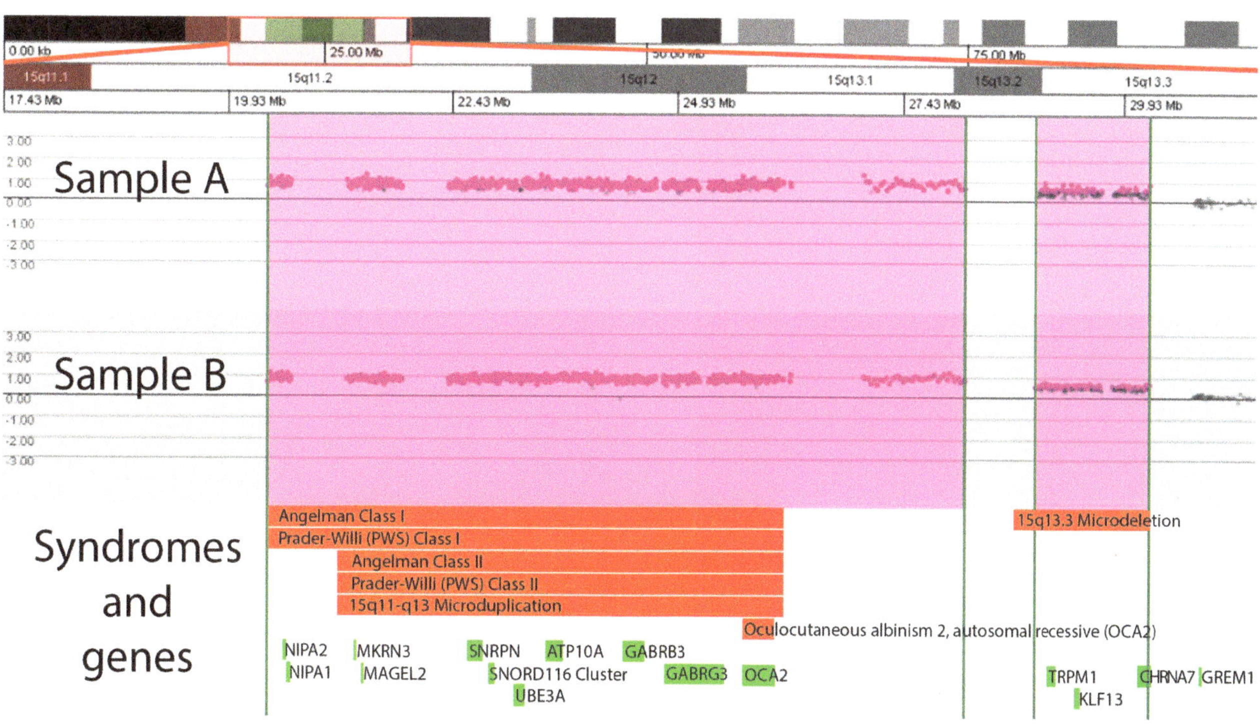

Figure 2. Identical complex chromosomal rearrangements in chromosome 15 found in 2 prenatal samples with different karyotypes and phenotypes. Sample A karyotype is 46,XY,15q+ dn (Table 3, Case no. 8); Sample B karyotype is 47,XX,+mar from characterization study. Each dot on the X-axis represents one oligonucleotide probe on the respective chromosome position. Two-copy gain is detected at 15q11.2q13.2 with minimum gain of 7.77 Mb. Single copy gain is detected at 15q13.2q13.3 with minimum gain of 1.3 Mb. No probe is located in the segment between the 2 regions of copy gains, therefore the exact number of copy gained is unknown in the segment. The genetic syndromes (red boxes) and genes (green boxes) in the region denoted by Signature Genomics Genoglyphix software are shown in the lower panel.

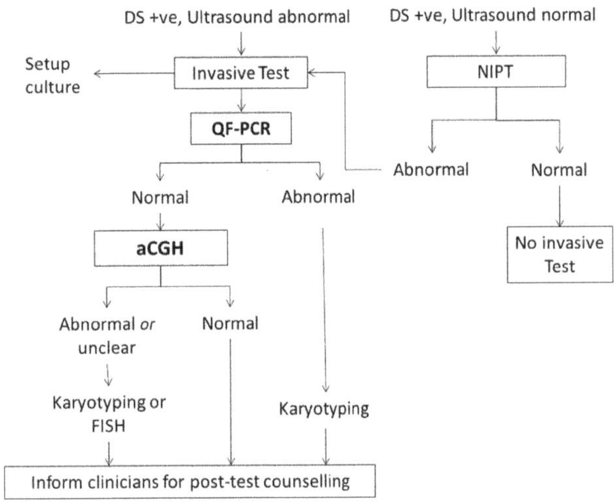

Figure 3. Proposed workflow for replacing karyotyping with aCGH in prenatal testing in Hong Kong. Pregnancies with Down syndrome screening positive without ultrasound abnormalities can be subjected to non-invasive prenatal testing; while pregnancies with Down syndrome screening positive in the presence of ultrasound abnormalities can be subjected to invasive test by QF-PCR to exclude common aneuploidy and maternal contamination, followed by aCGH as shown. aCGH, array CGH; DS+ve, Down syndrome screening positive; FISH, fluorescent in-situ hybridization; NIPT, non-invasive prenatal testing; QF-PCR, quantitative fluorescent-polymerase chain reaction for common aneuploidy detection.

maternal cell contamination by examining STR markers of 13, 18 and 21 in fetal and maternal samples.

Various authorities already approved the offering of aCGH as an adjunct diagnostic tool in prenatal cases with fetal ultrasound abnormalities [23–24]. The additional diagnostic yield of 6% in our further-test study is consistent with 5.2 to 10% increased detection by aCGH in fetuses with ultrasound abnormalities and normal karyotype reported in the literature [6,7]. Data from a review study showed the overall detection rate of about 1% for significant submicroscopic aberrations in low risk pregnancies [10]. This consequently caused microarrays to be identified as a first-line diagnostic test in women choosing the test irrespective of clinical indication [9,10,25]. This is in line with the latest recommendations from the American College of Obstetricians and Gynecologists and the Society of Maternal-Fetal Medicine [26]. Based on these findings and reports in the literature [6–10,25] on the potential of aCGH to detect chromosomal abnormalities beyond G-banded karyotyping, it is proposed that whole-genome aCGH would be suitable to replace conventional cytogenetics in prenatal diagnosis in Hong Kong (Figure 3). In a prenatal diagnostic setting, women screened positive for fetal Down syndrome may be offered an option of having noninvasive prenatal testing for fetal trisomy assessment by maternal plasma DNA if there is no ultrasound abnormality. In cases where ultrasound examination shows fetal abnormalities which require additional information from aCGH, an invasive diagnostic test could be performed. Rapid aneuploidy testing of the sample with QF-PCR would exclude common aneuploidies, triploidy and maternal contamination before aCGH analysis. This rapid test would identify triploidy which cannot be identified by aCGH. Cultures would be set up for cytogenetic study and karyotyping for all clinically significant CNVs (20.0%, Table 1) detected by aCGH if the CNV is large (>10 Mb). In cases where the CNV is small (<10 Mb), metaphase and interphase FISH could be performed. Conventional cytogenetics performed for abnormal QF-PCR findings (9.5% of samples, Table 1) would be needed to assess whether there is a parental balanced translocation carrier state in order to determine recurrence risk. This approach would reduce conventional cytogenetic testing by around 80% of the cases in Hong Kong. The disadvantages would include the potential for non-detection of balanced translocation or an inversion carrier status, low level mosaicism or small heterochromatic marker chromosomes of the fetus. Whilst non-detection of balanced translocation or inversion carrier status would be unlikely to affect the health of the fetus, low level mosaicism detection is a limitation of all prenatal investigation techniques. Further cost-benefit analysis and review of the staffing requirements of a cytogenetic laboratory may help to define the value of using microarrays for our prenatal diagnostic service provision.

NimbleGen has, however, phased out production of oligonucleotide 135 K arrays in favor of transitioning to Agilent oligonucleotide 8×60 K array, which has a lower backbone resolution. It is therefore anticipated that fewer CNVs of unclear significance will be detected for prenatal samples, with a shorter hybridization and faster turn-around time expected. Further studies will be required to confirm these effects.

Conclusions

This evaluation study showed that the whole-genome 135 K aCGH platform increased the diagnostic yield of 3.2% using aCGH over conventional cytogenetics in the first-tier test study, and by 6.0% in the 'further-test' study for the Hong Kong population. It also offered a higher resolution karyotyping for prenatal diagnosis in both study models and results are comparable to recent published studies. It is proposed that aCGH should replace karyotyping for use in prenatal testing where invasive procedures are required, after excluding common aneuploidies and triploidies by quantitative fluorescent PCR. Conventional cytogenetics can be reserved for visualization of clinically significant CNVs.

Acknowledgments

We thank all participating patients and medical staff from the hospitals and private clinics for recruiting to the study. Appreciation goes to all colleagues from the Prenatal Diagnostic Laboratory for supporting the study.

Author Contributions

Conceived and designed the experiments: ASYK ETL WFT MHYT. Performed the experiments: ETL WFT SSYC SCKD KYKC. Analyzed the data: ASYK ETL WFT SSYC SCKD KYKC. Contributed reagents/materials/analysis tools: ASYK CPL PWH BHYC KYL TM WCL MHYT. Wrote the paper: ASYK ETL WFT SSYC SCKD KYKC CPL PWH BHYC KYL TM WCL MHYT.

References

1. Kirchhoff M, Rose H, Lundsteen C (2001) High resolution comparative genomic hybridisation in clinical cytogenetics. J Med Genet 38: 740–744.
2. Mann K, Ogilvie CM (2012) QF-PCR: application, overview and review of the literature. Prenat Diagn 32: 309–314. doi: 10.1002/pd.2945.
3. Hills A, Donaghue C, Waters J, Waters K, Sullivan C, et al. (2010) QF-PCR as a stand-alone test for prenatal samples: the first 2 years' experience in the London region. Prenat Diagn 30: 509–517. doi: 10.1002/pd.2503.
4. Miller DT, Adam MP, Aradhya S, Biesecker LG, Brothman AR, et al. (2010) Consensus statement: Chromosomal microarray is a first-tier clinical diagnostic

test for individuals with developmental disabilities or congenital anomalies. Am J Hum Genet 86: 749–764. doi: 10.1016/j.ajhg.2010.04.006.
5. Manning M, Hudgins L (2010) Array-based technology and recommendations for utilization in medical genetics practice for detection of chromosomal abnormalities. Genet Med 12: 742–745. doi: 10.1097/GIM.0b013e3181f8baad.
6. Hillman SC, Pretlove S, Coomarasamy A, McMullan DJ, Davison EV, et al. (2011) Additional information from array comparative genomic hybridization technology over conventional karyotyping in prenatal diagnosis: a systematic review and meta-analysis. Ultrasound Obstet Gynecol 37: 6–14. doi: 10.1002/uog.7754.
7. Hillman SC, McMullan DJ, Hall G, Togneri FS, James N, et al. (2013) Use of prenatal chromosomal microarray: prospective cohort study and systematic review and meta-analysis. Ultrasound Obstet Gynecol 41: 610–620. doi: 10.1002/uog.12464.
8. de Wit MC, Srebniak MI, Govaerts LC, Van Opstal D, Galjaard RJ, et al. (2013) The additional value of prenatal genomic array testing in fetuses with (isolated) structural ultrasound abnormalities and a normal karyotype: a systematic review of the literature. Ultrasound Obstet Gynecol doi: 10.1002/uog.12575.
9. Wapner RJ, Martin CL, Levy B, Ballif BC, Eng CM, et al. (2012) Chromosomal microarray versus karyotyping for prenatal diagnosis. N Engl J Med 367: 2175–2184. doi: 10.1056/NEJMoa1203382.
10. Callaway JL, Shaffer LG, Chitty LS, Rosenfeld JA, Crolla JA (2013) The clinical utility of microarray technologies applied to prenatal cytogenetics in the presence of a normal conventional karyotype: a review of the literature. Prenat Diagn 33: 1119–1123. doi: 10.1002/pd.4209.
11. Vetro A, Bouman K, Hastings R, McMullan DJ, Vermeesch JR, et al. (2012) The introduction of arrays in prenatal diagnosis: A special challenge. Hum Mutat 33: 923–929. doi: 10.1002/humu.22050.
12. Wapner RJ, Driscoll DA, Simpson JL (2012) Integration of microarray technology into prenatal diagnosis: counselling issues generated during the NICHD clinical trial. Prenat Diagn 32: 396–400. doi: 10.1002/pd.3863.
13. McGillivray G, Rosenfeld JA, McKinlay Gardner RJ, Gillam LH (2012) Genetic counselling and ethical issues with chromosome microarray analysis in prenatal testing. Prenat Diagn 32: 389–395. doi: 10.1002/pd.3849.
14. Lau ET, Tang L, Wong C, Yung Hang L, Ghosh A, et al. (2009) Assessing discrepant findings between QF-PCR on uncultured prenatal samples and karyotyping on long-term culture. Prenat Diagn 29: 151–155. doi: 10.1002/pd.2194.
15. Chong SS, Boehm CD, Higgs DR, Cutting GR (2000) Single-tube multiplex-PCR screen for common deletional determinants of alpha-thalasseamia. Blood 95: 360–362.
16. Shek NWM, Tan TY, Ding CK, Chung BHY, Lau ETK, et al. (2013) Prenatal diagnosis of agenesis of the corpus callosum and cerebellar vermian hypoplasia associated with a microdeletion on chromosome 1p32. Case Rep in Perinat Med 2: 39–45. doi: 10.1515/crpm-2012-0032.
17. Scott F, Murphy K, Carey L, Greville W, Mansfield N, et al. (2013) Prenatal diagnosis using combined quantitative fluorescent polymerase chain reaction and array comparative genomic hybridization analysis as a first-line test: results from over 1000 consecutive cases. Ultrasound Obstet Gynecol 41: 500–507. doi: 10.1002/uog.12429.
18. Battaglia A. (2008) The inv dup (15) or idic (15) syndrome (Tetrasomy 15q). Orphanet J Rare Dis 3: 30. doi: 10.1186/1750-1172-3-30.
19. Mignon-Ravix C, Depetris D, Luciani JJ, Cuoco C, Krajewska-Walasek M, et al. (2007) Recurrent rearrangements in the proximal 15q11-q14 region: a new breakpoint cluster specific to unbalanced translocations. Eur J Hum Genet 15: 432–440.
20. Hogart A, Leung KN, Wang NJ, Wu DJ, Driscoll J, et al. (2009) Chromosome 15q11–13 duplication syndrome brain reveals epigenetic alterations in gene expression not predicted from copy number. J Med Genet 46: 86–93. doi: 10.1136/jmg.2008.061580.
21. Kou KO, Lee H, Lau B, Wong WS, Kan A, et al. (2013) Two unusual cases of haemoglobin Bart's hydrops fetalis due to uniparental disomy or non-paternity. Fetal Diagn Ther doi:10.1159/00354808.
22. Lamb AN, Rosenfeld JA, Coppinger J, Dodge ET, Dabell MP, et al. (2012) Defining the impact of maternal cell contamination on the interpretation of prenatal microarray analysis. Genet Med 14(11): 914–21. doi: 10.1038/gim.2012.77.
23. Duncan A, Langlois S (2011) Use of array genomic hybridization technology in prenatal diagnosis in Canada. J Obstet Gynaecol Can 33: 1256–1259.
24. Novelli A, Grati FR, Ballarati L, Bernardini L, Bizzoco D, et al. (2011) Microarray application in prenatal diagnosis: a position statement from the cytogenetics working group of the Italian Society of Human Genetics (SIGU), November 2011. Ultrasound Obstet Gynecol 39: 384–388. doi: 10.1002/uog.11092.
25. Fiorentino F, Napoletano S, Caiazo F, Sessa M, Bono S, et al. (2013) Chromosomal microarray analysis as a first-line test in pregnancies with a priori low risk for the detection of submicroscopic chromosomal abnormalities. Eur J Hum Genet 21: 725–730. doi: 10.1038/ejhg.2012.253.
26. American College of Obstetricians and Gynecologists (2013) Committee opinion no. 581: the use of chromosomal microarray analysis in prenatal diagnosis. Obstet Gynecol 122: 1374–1377. doi: 10.10971/01.AOG.0000438962.16108.d1.

Extensive Natural Variation for Cellular Hydrogen Peroxide Release Is Genetically Controlled

Homa Attar[1]*, Karen Bedard[2¤a], Eugenia Migliavacca[1,3], Maryline Gagnebin[1], Yann Dupré[1], Patrick Descombes[4¤e], Christelle Borel[1¤b], Samuel Deutsch[1¤c], Holger Prokisch[5], Thomas Meitinger[5], Divya Mehta[5¤d], Erich Wichmann[5,6,7], Jean Maurice Delabar[8], Emmanouil T. Dermitzakis[1], Karl-Heinz Krause[2], Stylianos E. Antonarakis[1]*

1 Department of Genetic Medicine and Development, University of Geneva Medical School, Geneva, Switzerland, **2** Department of Pathology and Immunology, University of Geneva Medical School and University Hospitals, Geneva, Switzerland, **3** Swiss Institute of Bioinformatics, University of Lausanne, Dorigny, Switzerland, **4** Genomics Platform, NCCR Frontiers in Genetics, University of Geneva Medical School, Geneva, Switzerland, **5** Institute of Epidemiology I, Helmholtz Zentrum München, German Research Center for Environmental Health, Neuherberg, Germany, **6** Institute of Medical Informatics, Biometry and Epidemiology, Chair of Epidemiology, Ludwig-Maximilians-Universität, Munich, Germany, **7** Klinikum Grosshadern, Munich, Germany, **8** Functional and Adaptive Biology, Université Paris Diderot-Paris7 and CNRS, Paris, France

Abstract

Natural variation in DNA sequence contributes to individual differences in quantitative traits. While multiple studies have shown genetic control over gene expression variation, few additional cellular traits have been investigated. Here, we investigated the natural variation of NADPH oxidase-dependent hydrogen peroxide (H_2O_2 release), which is the joint effect of reactive oxygen species (ROS) production, superoxide metabolism and degradation, and is related to a number of human disorders. We assessed the normal variation of H_2O_2 release in lymphoblastoid cell lines (LCL) in a family-based 3-generation cohort (CEPH-HapMap), and in 3 population-based cohorts (KORA, GenCord, HapMap). Substantial individual variation was observed, 45% of which were associated with heritability in the CEPH-HapMap cohort. We identified 2 genome-wide significant loci of Hsa12 and Hsa15 in genome-wide linkage analysis. Next, we performed genome-wide association study (GWAS) for the combined KORA-GenCord cohorts (n = 279) using enhanced marker resolution by imputation (>1.4 million SNPs). We found 5 significant associations ($p<5.00\times10-8$) and 54 suggestive associations ($p<1.00\times10-5$), one of which confirmed the linked region on Hsa15. To replicate our findings, we performed GWAS using 58 HapMap individuals and ~2.1 million SNPs. We identified 40 genome-wide significant and 302 suggestive SNPs, and confirmed genome signals on Hsa1, Hsa12, and Hsa15. Genetic loci within 900 kb from the known candidate gene p67phox on Hsa1 were identified in GWAS in both cohorts. We did not find replication of SNPs across all cohorts, but replication within the same genomic region. Finally, a highly significant decrease in H_2O_2 release was observed in Down Syndrome (DS) individuals ($p<2.88\times10-12$). Taken together, our results show strong evidence of genetic control of H_2O_2 in LCL of healthy and DS cohorts and suggest that cellular phenotypes, which themselves are also complex, may be used as proxies for dissection of complex disorders.

Editor: Sunil K. Ahuja, South Texas Veterans Health Care System and University Health Science Center San Antonio, United States of America

Funding: The work was supported by grants from the Swiss National Science Foundation, the National Center for Competence in Research (NCCR) "Frontiers in Genetics," and the European Union FP6 "AnEUploidy" integrated project. The funders had no role in study design, data collection and analysis, decision to publish, or preparation of the manuscript.

Competing Interests: The authors have declared that no competing interests exist.

* E-mail: Stylianos.Antonarakis@unige.ch (SA); homa.attar@gmail.com (HA)

¤a Current address: Department of Pathology, Dalhousie University, Halifax, Canada
¤b Current address: Department of Genetics and Genomic Sciences, Mount Sinai School of Medicine, New York, New York, United States of America
¤c Current address: DOE Joint Genome Institute, Walnut Creek, California, United States of America
¤d Current address: Molecular Genetics of Depression, Max-Planck-Institut für Psychiatrie, München, Germany
¤e Current address: Functional Genomics Core, Nestle Institute of Health Sciences, Lausanne, Switzerland

Introduction

Recent genome-wide association studies (GWAS) using clinical phenotypes have identified a large number of DNA polymorphisms that convey an increased risk for common diseases. Identified genetic loci, however, explain only a small fraction of the overall observed phenotypic variability even when assessing very large sample sizes [1–8] owing to biological complexity [9] and low penetrance of common genomic variants [10]. Small-scale studies (<100 individuals) indicate that gene expression is genetically controlled [11–13] emphasizing the direct link between phenotypic and genotypic variation. Despite these findings, how individual genes affect disease mechanisms remains poorly understood. Working with end-members of the phenotypic spectra (gene expression or clinical phenotypes) may not be sufficient to understand disease mechanisms. To remedy some of these shortcomings, we propose to explore the genetic control of cellular phenotypes (endophenotypes) as a trait of intermediate complexity. Our study will explore hydrogen peroxide (H_2O_2) release which is associated with multiple diseases as a proxy for a complex phenotype.

Hydrogen peroxide (H_2O_2) release is a quantitative cellular phenotype with known implications in multiple diseases [14]. H_2O_2 release, as measured at the extra-cellular level, includes reactive oxygen species (ROS) generation, and superoxide metabolism and degradation, all fundamental components of innate immunity. Causative associations between the phagocyte NADPH-dependent oxidase NOX complex and multiple diseases are known [14–17]. Both, low and high levels of ROS are detrimental and confer susceptibility to distinct diseases. Among these, low levels of ROS production have been shown to be associated with X-linked chronic granulomatous disease (CGD), autosomal recessive CGD, autoimmunity, and arthritis [18–23]. High ROS levels have been attributed to cardiovascular disease, hypertension, and neurodegenerative disorders [24–32]. The first evidence for genetic factors involved in ROS level regulation comes from a family-based study assessing heredity of ROS levels in essential hypertension [24]. This study found that 20–35% of the observed variation could be attributed to genetic factors. Down Syndrome (DS) individuals also show a ROS alteration suggesting that genetic loci on Homo sapiens (Hsa) chromosome 21, or loci on other chromosomes interacting with Hsa21, may be key players in ROS regulation. Despite efforts to characterize both the genetic and the molecular basis of altered ROS production in DS, insight into disease mechanisms are still lacking [33,34]. Some of the phenotypes of DS might be related to unbalanced redox-states. However, the role, impact, and consequences of low or high ROS levels in various cell types of this chromosomal abnormality remain obscure [35–39].

The major source of ROS production in lymphoblastoid cells is NOX2-dependent. NOX2-deficient lymphocytes from chronic granulomatous disease (CGD) patients produce very low levels of ROS. Expressed co-factors of NOX2 and NOX homologues in lymphoblastoid cell lines include $p22^{phox}$, $p47^{phox}$, $p67^{phox}$, $p40^{phox}$, RAC1, and RAC2. Intracellular superoxide produced by this enzyme can not diffuse through cell membranes. However, superoxide is readily converted both spontaneously and enzymatically, to hydrogen peroxide (H_2O_2), which is membrane permeable. Superoxide dismutase (SOD), catalase, and peroxidases are associated with ROS metabolism and degradation. In this study, we measure ROS production and H_2O_2 release by detecting H_2O_2 release at the extra-cellular level.

The aim of this study is to evaluate the use of a cellular quantitative phenotype as a proxy to complex phenotypes by taking H_2O_2 release in EBV transformed lymphoblastoid cell lines (LCL) as an example. We aim at identifying human genetic factors underlying the variability of H_2O_2 release, and thus the susceptibility to infectious diseases, through a whole genome linkage and association analysis in the general healthy population. Furthermore, we evaluated levels and differences of H_2O_2 release in LCL derived from Down Syndrome individuals, and identify regulatory loci which may provide insights into the biological pathways of H_2O_2 variation.

Results

Phenotypic distribution of H_2O_2 release in four population-based cohorts

We observed extensive natural variation of NADPH oxidase-dependent H_2O_2 release in LCL of four population-based cohorts: KORA, GenCord, HapMap, and DS (**Figure 1**). KORA is a cohort of newly established LCL derived from unrelated healthy adults, GenCord is a cohort of newly established LCL derived from unrelated newborns, and HapMap is part of a three-generational sample cohort, from which unrelated LCL from healthy adults were used for genome wide association (GWA) analysis. A cohort of newly established LCL derived from unrelated Down Syndrome individuals were used to quantify the difference of these individuals to healthy cohorts. All cohorts are of Caucasian origin. A description of each cohort's demographic, phenotypic, and genotypic characteristics is shown in **Table 1**. We observed a mean and standard deviation for H_2O_2 release (arbitrary units) of 0.51 in the KORA cohort (± 0.64, $N = 199$), 0.47 (± 0.38, $N = 80$) in GenCord, 1.22 (± 1.15, $N = 58$) in HapMap, and 0.23 (± 0.31, $N = 75$) in DS individuals (**Figure 1, Table 1, File S1**). To quantify the degree to which this observed variation was individual-specific and reproducible, we assessed phenotypes in 21 LCL of unrelated HapMap individuals in two independent experiments. We found a 28-fold inter-individual difference, and high reproducibility (ratio of coefficient of variance >28, $p<1.00\times10^{-4}$, **File S2A**, Pearson correlation coefficient $= 0.89$, $p<1.00\times10^{-4}$, **File S2B**). The phenotypic distribution of H_2O_2 release in the DS cohort differed from all other healthy cohorts, with a significantly different distribution compared to the HapMap (Wilcoxon rank sum test, $p<2.88\times10^{-12}$), the GenCord ($p<3.11\times10^{-9}$), and the KORA cohort ($p<5.35\times10^{-9}$, **Figure 1**).

We next aimed at identifying the genetic contribution to this natural variation in H_2O_2 release. Linkage analysis was used as a first step to assess the genetic basis of H_2O_2 release in the family-based HapMap-CEPH cohort, and genome-wide association analysis was conducted to refine and replicate results in the KORA, GenCord, and HapMap cohorts.

Hydrogen peroxide release heritability and linkage analysis

We measured H_2O_2 variation in human LCL from 10 CEPH-HapMap three-generation families ($N = 113$). We observed extensive variation in H_2O_2 release that ranged from 0.001 to 6.035 (arbitrary units). To estimate what fraction of this natural phenotypic variation could be attributed to genetic components, we performed a variance-component linkage analysis [40] and found genome-wide estimated sample heritability (h^2) of 45%. This finding suggests that 45% of all H_2O_2 release variation can be attributed to genetic factors in the cell lines used herein. In a linkage analysis of LCL of these same individuals, we identified two significant and two suggestive LOD scores on chromosomes Hsa1, Hsa12, Hsa15 and Hsa19 (**Figure 2**) with the use of 2723 SNP markers. Nominal genome-wide significance level was assessed by performing 1000 simulations in which we shuffled the phenotypes but kept the genotypes, allele frequency, and family structure constant. A LOD score of 4.48 was obtained for the nominal genome-wide significance threshold. The significant linkage signals were on Hsa12 with LOD score of 4.64 ($p<1.00\times10^{-6}$ for marker TSC0795922 at position 10,950 kb) and on Hsa15 with LOD score 4.81 ($p<1.00\times10^{-6}$ for marker TSC0181040 at position 37,068 kb). However, marker density in this linkage analysis was not sufficient to assign candidate genes. Furthermore, the linked region on Hsa12 is very gene-rich. The identified locus on Hsa15 is located 115 kb upstream of the transcription start site of MEIS2. The suggestive hit on Hsa1 had a LOD score of 4.17 ($p<1.00\times10^{-5}$, TSC0343078 at position 4,389 kb), the second suggestive linkage signal was identified on Hsa19 with a LOD score of 3.26 ($p<5.00\times10^{-5}$, TSC1058872 at position 54,754 kb).

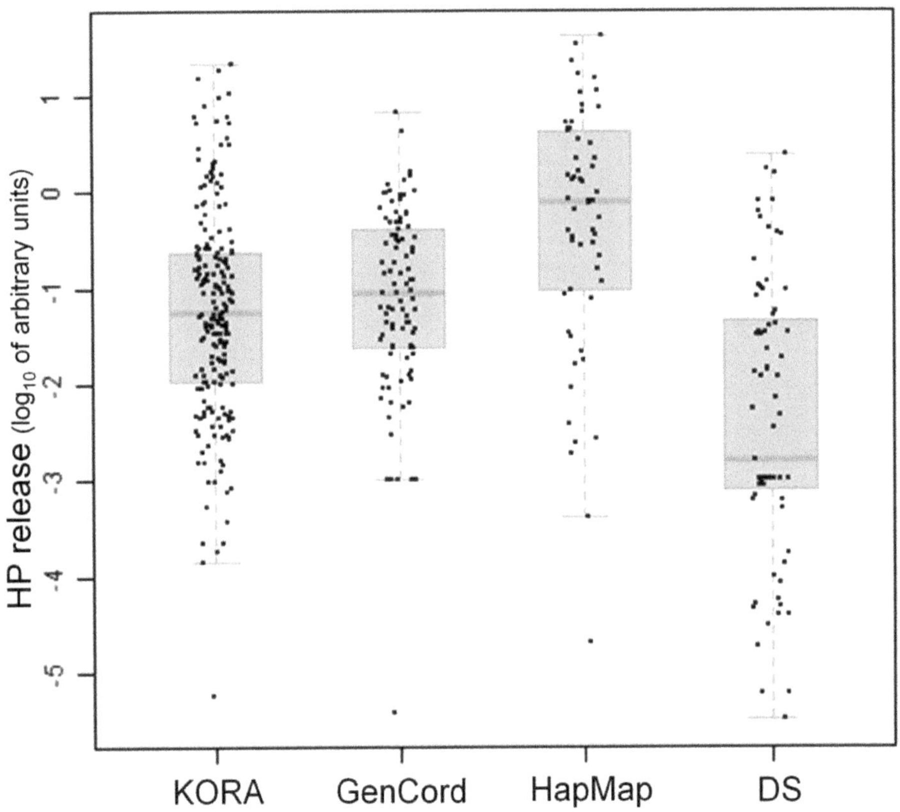

Figure 1. Distribution of H_2O_2 release in sample cohorts KORA, GenCord, HapMap and Down Syndrome. Box plots (in light grey) for the sample cohorts KORA, GenCord, HapMap and Down Syndrome (DS) show the distribution of H_2O_2 variation across cohorts. Each black dot corresponds to an individuals' mean of 4 measures of H_2O_2 release. The median is shown as a dark grey line, the low and upper end of the box plots (in light grey) indicate the first and third quartile of the distribution. The whiskers indicate the lower and upper end of the distribution The distribution of H_2O_2 in the Down Syndrome cohort shows a significant decrease as compared to HapMap (Wilcoxon rank sum test, $p<2.88\times10^{-12}$).

Genome-wide association analysis for KORA-GenCord

We used the KORA and GenCord cohorts as an initial combined cohort for GWA analysis and we used HapMap (N = 58) as a replication cohort (see discussion). As all three cohorts were genotyped on different platforms, we obtained a common and larger set of SNPs by imputation using the HapMap Phase II genotypes as a reference (see methods, **File S3**). After applying quality filters for imputed SNPs (R>0.9), a total set of 1.4 out of 2.1 million SNPs was included for GWAS. We performed principal component analysis to detect outliers for each cohort separately, and excluded one sample from the GenCord cohort. Next, we assessed whether the use of multiple cohorts and imputation of SNPs did not lead to population substructure, or clustering of called versus imputed SNPs by performing both principal component analysis and multidimensional scaling for the combined three cohorts. For the PCA analysis, a random selection of 500 K SNPs, and a centered approach was used. No evident substructure was detected by visual inspection among the three cohorts (**File S4**), and by analysis of proportions of variance of components 1 to 18. The cumulative proportion of variance of the first 10 components explained only 0.039 of the observed variation (data not shown), and increased slowly with increasing components.

We found 5 significant associations ($p<5\times10^{-8}$) and 54 suggestive associations with p-values of less than 1.00×10^{-5} (**Figure 3, Figure 4**) with the use of a linear genetic association model and median centered phenotypic distribution (see discussion for the choice of the design and the genetic model). These associated loci are located in 21 genetic clusters when defining a cluster as 1 mega-base of size (**Table 2** shows the top 15 clusters). Nominal unadjusted p-values from the WALD test statistics are reported. The strongest association hit was found on Hsa14 with a cluster of 7 SNPs on position 86,942 kb (top signal rs17741027, $p = 1.23\times10^{-9}$), followed by Hsa10 with 4 SNPs at position 52,264 kb (rs16909866, $p = 1.66\times10^{-8}$). Among these top associations ($p<1.00\times10^{-5}$), we could not find association on Hsa12 and Hsa15 within the genetic regions linked in the CEU-CEPH family-based cohort, but we found an overlap with a known candidate gene, p67^{phox} (also called NOXA2 or NCF2) on Hsa1. Three SNPs are located 913 kb downstream of the candidate gene p67phox on Hsa1 (position 181,791 kb), with the strongest signal for SNP rs1535133 ($p = 5.97\times10^{-7}$, position 182,704 kb (**Figure 4**). To replicate these findings, and to investigate whether the previously linked regions were population-specific, we subsequently analyzed the population-based HapMap cohort in a GWAS.

Genome-wide association analysis for HapMap

We used 60 unrelated LCL of Caucasian origin from the CEPH-Hapmap cohort as a replication cohort. We determined the H_2O_2 release in 58 samples and performed a GWAS using a total of 2,124,999 SNPs with minor allele frequency of more than 5% [41,42]. We detected highly significant association signals in this analysis (**Figure 3, Figure 5**). Overall, 40 SNPs reached

Table 1. Demographic characteristics for all four population-based cohorts.

	GENCORD	KORA	CEPH-HapMap	Down Syndrome
Cohort characteristics				
Origin cohort	University of Geneva, Laboratory of Prof. Antonarakis SE, Geneva, Switzerland	German Research Center for Environmental Health, Neuherberg, Germany	Coriell Cell Repositories, Camden, USA	AnEUploidy collection, Paris, France; Galliera Genetic Bank of Genoa, Italy; Emory University School of Medicine, Atlanta, USA and CSS-Mendel Institute in Rome, Italy
Origin population	Caucasian	Caucasian	Caucasian	Caucasian
Sample size	99	200	58	75
Individual's age (category)	1 day	40–60 years	>60 years	<40
Immune status	immature	mature	mature	mixed
Recently established cell line	yes	yes	no	yes
Gender (% female)	49%	56%	52%	-
Phenotypic characteristics (H_2O_2 release)				
Mean	0.47	0.51	1.22	0.22
Standard deviation	±0.38	±0.64	±1.15	±0.31
Range	0.004–2.28	0.005–3.73	0.009–4.97	0.004–1.45
Genotypic characteristics				
Plateform	Illumina 550 K	Affymetrix 6.0 500 K	multiple plateforms	no genotypes
Number called SNPs	480,455	413,877	2.1 million	-
Number called and imputed SNPs	1.4 million	1.4 million	2.1 million	-

Demographic, phenotypic and genotypic characteristics for each cohort are indicated.

genome-wide significance of $p<5.00\times10^{-8}$, and 302 suggestive SNPs of less than $p<1.00\times10^{-5}$ that correspond to 90 clusters (**Table 3** shows the top 15 clusters). The most significant loci with p-values of less than 1.00×10^{-12} were rs12022620 on Hsa1 (intronic SNP within *SIPA1L2*) and rs12528870 on Hsa6 (intergenic SNP, **Figure 5**). The function of *SIPA1L2* (signal-induced proliferation-associated 1 like) is not well characterized yet. Among the other strong statistical signals, we identified association signals within the genomic regions of the linked regions. We found a cluster on Hsa12 ($p<1.4\times10^{-10}$) with 12 SNPs at position 4,690 kb close to *KCNA6* and *GALNT8*, and on Hsa21 (rs12483177, $p<1.8\times10^{-8}$) with 11 SNPs at position at 43,587 kb close to *SIK1* and *HSF2BP* (**Figure 5**). *KCNA6* (voltage-gated potassium channel) mediates the voltage-dependent potassium ion permeability of excitable membranes (UniProtKB for KCNA6_HUMAN). The role of *GALNT8* (polypeptide N-acetylgalactosaminyltransferase 8) is not described in the literature. *SIK1* (salt-inducible kinase 1) has a transient role during the earliest stages of myocardial cell differentiation and/or primitive chamber formation [43] and may also be important for the earliest stages of skeletal muscle growth and/or differentiation and in G2/M cell cycle regulation [44]. In computational studies investigating Hidden Markov Chain predictions and fold recognition algorithms for kinases on HSA21, *SIK1* and three other kinases were identified to be members of a novel mitogen-activated kinase pathway (MAPK) [45].

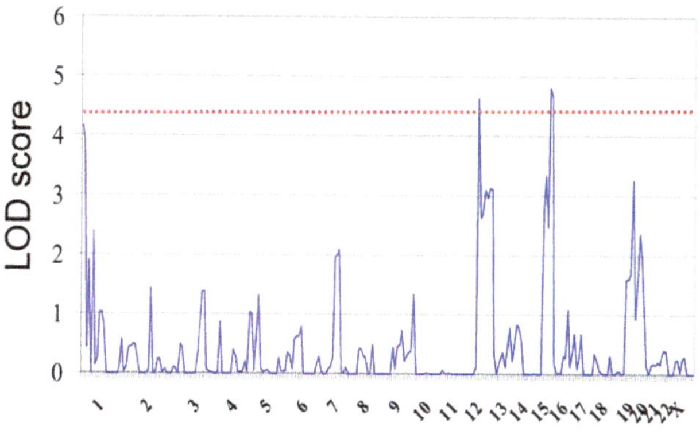

Figure 2. Two significant and two suggestive LOD scores on Hsa12, Hsa15, Hsa1, and Hsa19. LOD scores of genome-wide linkage analyses using the CEPH-HapMap family-cohort of three generations are plotted for all autosomal chromosomes (in blue). The blue line shows the maximal LOD score within a window size of 10 kb. The red dotted line indicates the significance level identified through 1'000 simulations.

Comparisons across all linkage, association studies and known candidate genes

We identified replication between the top linkage findings for four loci in the HapMap samples on Hsa1 (rs2500247 at position 3,172 kb, $p=4.65\times10^{-6}$), Hsa12 (rs10492058, 4,756 kb, $p=1.45\times10^{-10}$), and on two loci on Hsa15 (rs2075814, 22,717 kb, $p=4.2\times10^{-7}$; rs16947598, 43,816 kb, $p=1.70\times10^{-7}$). Of the known candidate genes expressed in LCL, $p67^{phox}$ (Hsa1, pos = 183,525 kb) overlapped with two top association signals in the KORA-GenCord GWAS and in the HapMap GWAS (KORA-GenCord, rs10489726, 913 kb downstream, $p=5.97\times10^{-7}$; and HapMap, rs528846, 932 kb upstream, $p=8.63\times10^{-6}$). We did not detect strong association findings in KORA-GenCord samples that overlapped with the

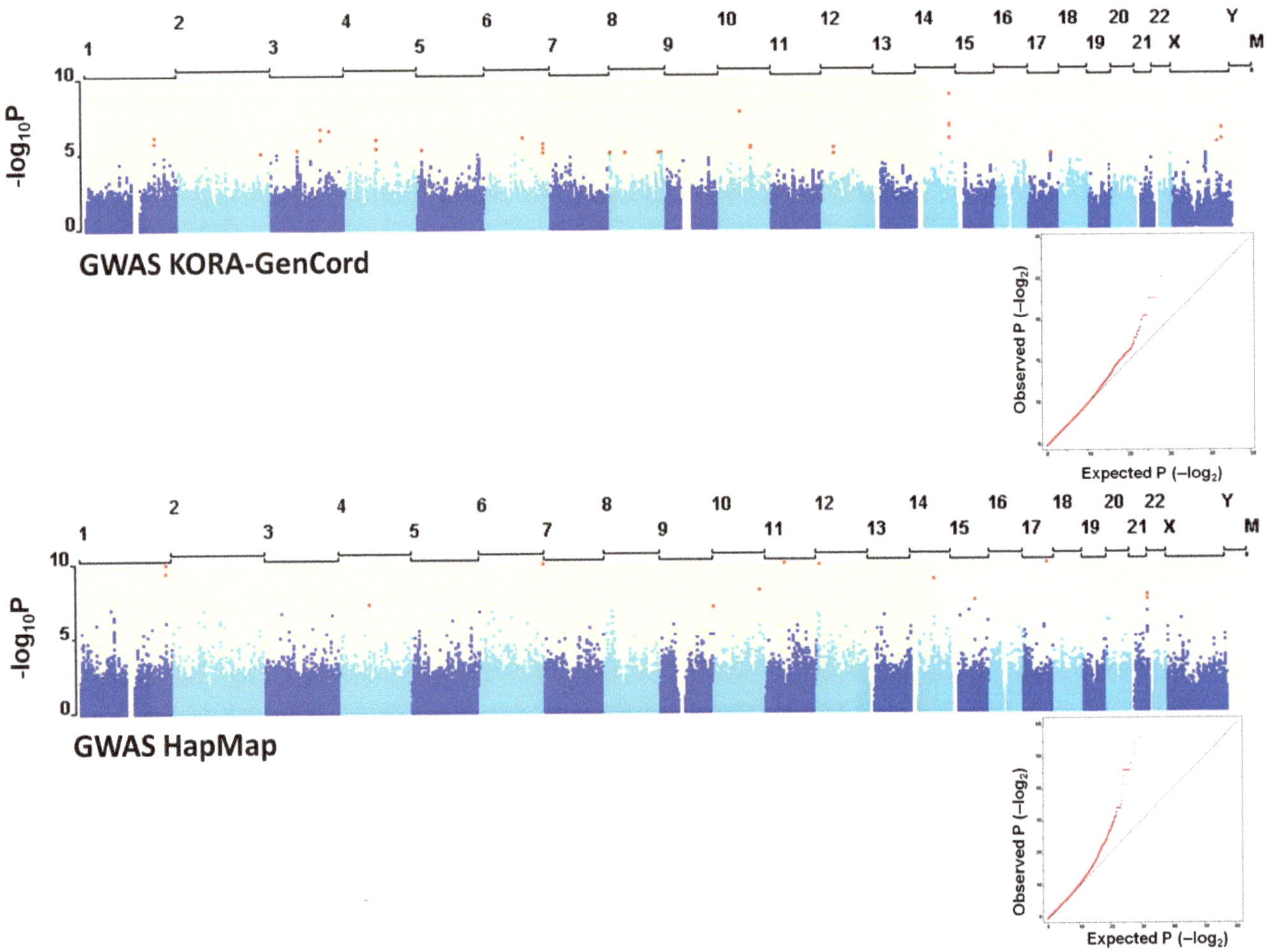

Figure 3. Genome-wide association results for natural variation of H_2O_2 release in KORA-GenCord and HapMap cohorts. Manhattan dot plots show results for genome-wide association analysis for the KORA-GenCord and the HapMap sample cohorts. The blue dots represent the association finding of one single SNP with natural variation in H_2O_2 release. Light and dark blue colors distinguish subsequent chromosomes. We did not analyze genetic markers for mitochondrial SNPs in this study. We show results of a genetic additive model indicating the unadjusted nominal $-\log_{10}$ of p-values. Quantile plots show the observed versus the expected distribution of GWAS for both analyses.

linkage findings. Neither did we find the same replicated SNPs nor genetic regions among the two GWA studies within a distance of 1 Mb. **Table 4** indicates replicated loci among linkage and GWA.

Given the lack of replication of the top SNPs across the two GWA studies, we next asked whether we could detect enrichment of lower p-values of these top SNPs of the KORA-GenCord in the GWA HapMap. We observed an enrichment for p-values of $p<0.2$ in HapMap GWAS (data not shown). A similar pattern was observed when comparing top HapMap signals with p-values of all KORA-GenCord. This pattern suggests enrichment for repeated associated loci across GWAS, but this enrichment is not significant.

Covariate analysis

To assess the impact of potential co-variates (immune status, time of cell line establishment, individuals' age, and gender) on H_2O_2 distribution, we combined all samples after median centered normalization, and estimated the relative contribution of each of the co-variates in an univariate linear regression model with a cluster effect on the population. We found that none of the covariates had a significant effect on the trait distribution. We found the following relative order of correlation: Time of establishment of cell lines (B-coefficient = 0.142, p = 0.231), status of immune system ((B-coefficient = 0.139, p = 0.127), individuals' age (B-coefficient = 0.109, p = 0.072), and gender (B-coefficient = 0.052, p = 0.499). To estimate whether a statistical model with adjustment for all co-variate was different than a model for the main variate only, we performed a randomized set of 100'000 SNPs using a multivariate linear regression model with adjustment for all co-variates and a cluster effect on the population. We compared the results of this model with an univariate model with no adjustment for co-variates. We found no significant differences between the two models for the 100'000 randomly selected SNPs. This analysis suggested that covariates did not represent a confounding factor.

Discussion

The most essential outcome of this study is the finding of extensive natural phenotypic variation in healthy individuals for H_2O_2 release, and evidence for a genetic basis to the observed variation in LCL of the cohorts used herein. This finding is in line with several studies reporting large natural phenotypic variation, such as for gene expression level variation, many of which were

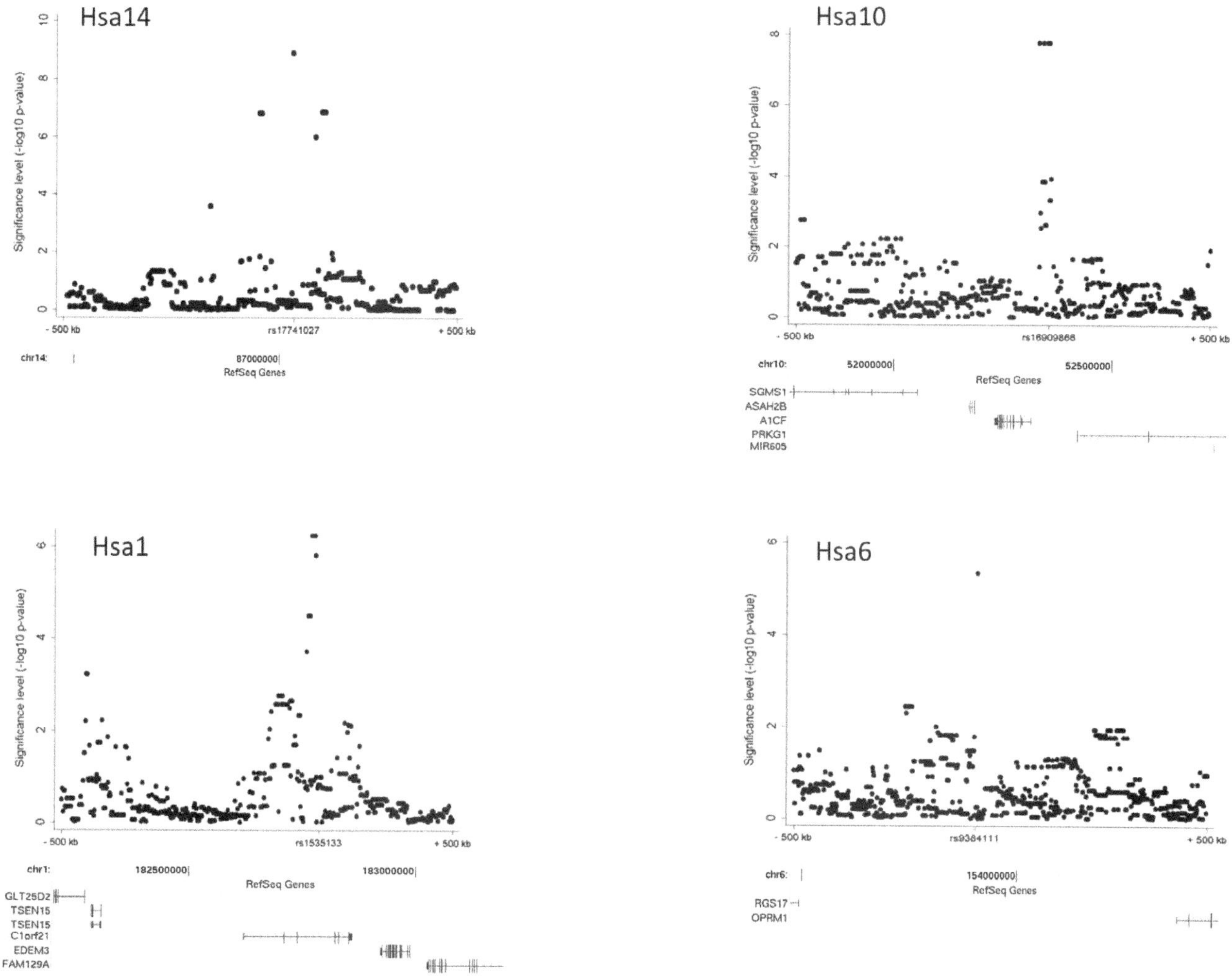

Figure 4. Examples of significant association findings in KORA-GenCord GWA. The significance level ($-\log_{10}$ P) of the top two association findings and two examples of top hits overlapping with either linkage, top GWA in HapMap, overlap with known candidate genes, or top findings on Hsa21 are shown within a genetic region of 1 Mb (±500 kb around the significantly associated SNP). The chromosome, SNP ID, location and genic context (RefSeq genes, using UCSC genome browser) are indicated for each depicted SNP.

repeatedly shown to be shaped by genetic polymorphisms [46–50]. It may be conceivable that many traits maintain natural variation for response to selection pressure [51]. The measurements of the phenotypic spectra of H_2O_2 release in more than 500 individuals in 4 healthy cohorts and in a DS cohort confirm previously reported differences in H_2O_2 release of primary neutrophils of healthy individuals and individuals with chronic granulomatous disease [52], and on altered redox-states in DS individuals.

In the study of the Kuhns DB, et al., 10–20 fold differences in primary neutrophils from peripheral blood of healthy individuals were detected in comparison to individuals with chronic granulomatous disease. Also, large inter-individual differences were detected, and correlated to genotypes. This correlation was reported to be a strong predictor for overall survival of CGD patients. Our genetic study of natural variation in H2O2 release revealed 45% of heritability, and we detected genomic regions on Hsa1, Hsa12 and Hsa15 as significant and replicated regions in more than one cohort. Results from GWAS in HapMap samples indicated an associated genetic locus close to the gene *SIK1* on Hsa21. *SIK1* is encoding a kinase known for its involvement in cardiomyogenesis by regulating cardiomyoblast cell cycle [43,44], but it could also exert additional unknown functions. Further experiments are necessary to replicate and to assess the functional consequences of this association in DS and in healthy individuals. In our study, we did not find significant association signals on Hsa21 or any other markers close to *SIK1* in the combined KORA-GenCord GWA.

H_2O_2 release, an endophenotype more closely related to sequence variation (as opposed to a clinical phenotype) may be a complex trait in itself. The detection of multiple genome-wide significant loci suggests a polygenic trait. The strongest linkage results indicate loci on Hsa1, Hsa12, Hsa15 and Hsa19, two of which (Hsa1 and Hsa15) were also significantly associated in either the KORA-GenCord or HapMap GWAS, or both. However, we did not detect the same associated SNPs in the three cohorts, but replication within the same genomic regions. This may indicate either a lack of power to detect genetic loci due to the relatively small sample size, or reflect the complex genetic architecture of H_2O_2 with multiple loci contributing small proportions to the observed phenotypic variation. Our study design focused on the detection of common alleles with a genetic effect of more than 5% given an allele frequency of 0.15, and with our study design, we

Table 2. Results from GWAS for the KORA-GenCord cohort.

SNP ID	Chr	Pos (bp)	type	Closest gene (within 1 MB)	Unadjusted p-value	Number SNPs/cluster
rs17741027	14	86941588	INTERGENIC	GALC	1.23×10−9	7
rs16909866	10	52263776	INTRONIC	ACF_HUMAN	1.66×10−8	4
rs1400014	3	132414349	INTRONIC	NEK11	2.27×10−7	2
rs3859991	X	130050216	INTRONIC	RHGXX_HUMAN	2.64×10−7	3
rs6801020	3	153876452	INTERGENIC	P2RY1	2.68×10−7	1
rs1535133	1	182704057	INTRONIC	C1orf21	5.97×10−7	3
rs9372321	6	97600416	INTRONIC	KLHL32	8.6×10−7	1
rs11728249	4	83760349	INTERGENIC	C4orf11	1.7×10−6	2
rs5909759	X	116093601	INTERGENIC	U6	2.13×10−6	3
rs9479282	6	152642425	INTRONIC	SYNE1;C6orf98	2.23×10−6	7
rs10887721	10	82035334	INTRONIC	MAT1A	3.17×10−6	2
rs4930939	12	30893752	INTERGENIC	CAPRIN2	4.58×10−6	3
rs9384111	6	153924030	INTERGENIC	U6	4.59×10−6	1
rs4701883	5	10816656	UPSTREAM	DAP	5.43×10−6	1
rs17006293	3	69777596	INTERGENIC	MITF	5.88×10−6	3

We show the results of the top 15 out of the 21 clusters of significantly associated genetic loci ($p<5.00\times10^{-8}$) and with suggestive associations ($p<1.00\times10^{-5}$) from genome-wide association analyses. We associated natural variation in H_2O_2 release measured in the KORA-GenCord cohort (n = 279 individuals) with more than 1.4 million markers (called and imputed SNPs). SNP ID, chromosome and position are indicated. Also, the type of SNP, the closest gene (within 1 MB), unadjusted p-value and the number of SNPs per cluster are indicated. SNP annotations were done by using the software WGAViewer (build 36, Ensembl core database *homo sapiens core 46 36h*, Ensembl variation database *homo sapiens variation 46 36h*, and Ensembl gene ontology database *ensemble go 46*).

have 80% of power to detect such a quantitative trait locus while using 300 individuals [53].

Our study design considered the use of a combined GWA of 279 individuals to increase sample size, and to replicate findings in a follow-up cohort of 58 HapMap individuals. Even though all cohorts used herein are of Caucasian origin, and population substructure did not appear to be a confounding factor, differences among these cohorts may have reduced the power to detect the same loci across cohorts. Co-variate analysis showed that the effect of the SNP on association was significant in shaping the H_2O_2 trait, and suggests that despite differences in the origin of cohorts, cell line establishment and age of the cell lines the underlying genetics is the predominant factor. Further evidence for a strong genetic effect, rather than differences in cellular phenotypes in different cohorts, comes from a study by Dimas, et al. [13] showing that 83% of detected eQTLs in HapMap were replicated in GenCord samples. This finding was crucial to our study design and validates the use of the GenCord cohort as a comparable cohort to the HapMap cohort. We cannot exclude that H_2O_2 release may underlie different cellular covariates than gene expression levels, leading to population-specific differences that we could not fully correct for. We investigated multiple genetic models for assessing the best method for normalization of the phenotypic distribution. We expected all cohorts to show similar distributions of H_2O_2 release, as all individuals were of European ancestry, and we measured all phenotypes under standardized and highly controlled conditions. No substantial differences among cohorts could be attributed to population substructure or to known covariates. The non-normal distribution of phenotypes may probably be due to the relative small sample size, as departure from normal distribution was largest for HapMap (N = 58) and smallest for KORA (N = 199). As shown in Figure 1, the distribution of H_2O_2 release is enriched for extreme phenotypes with individuals with either very high or very low phenotypes. To assess the impact of the phenotypic distribution on our results, and to exclude false positive signals due to departure from model assumptions, we have considered three different methods of normalization across cohorts. Also, we compared results from parametric and non-parametric association models. We conducted log transformation, median centered and inverse variance normalization, and median centered normalization only. Log transformation did not lead to a normal distribution. When using median and inverse variance normalization we lost all association signals, leading to the hypothesis that the genetic signal may be associated with the high and low end distribution of the phenotypes. Therefore, we chose to use the median centered approach, while keeping the internal variation of each population untouched. The median centered approach does not fully support the assumption for normal distribution. To assess whether results differed due to model assumptions, we compared these results with a non-parametric regression model using the Spearman rank correlation. We found the same top association signals with both models, with the only difference of slightly lower p-values (mostly at one order of magnitude for the top signals), showing that results did not depend on model assumptions.

LCL represent a relevant physiological cell type for ROS production [14], and LCL express mainly NOX2-dependent ROS [54–56]. A study by Kobayashi, et al. [57] compared fresh neutrophils, fresh B-lymphocytes, and EBV transformed B-lymphocytes from the same individuals to compare the relative expression of NOX2. They reported that B-lymphocytes have 1.1% of the NOX2 and 2.6% of the p22 that a neutrophil has, and that this is further decreased when the cells are EBV transformed. They showed that regardless of the amount of NOX2 the neutrophil expressed, the relative expression level in a B-cell of the same individual was correlated. This study would not have been feasible without the use of immortalized cell lines for both large families and population-based collections with more than 2 million

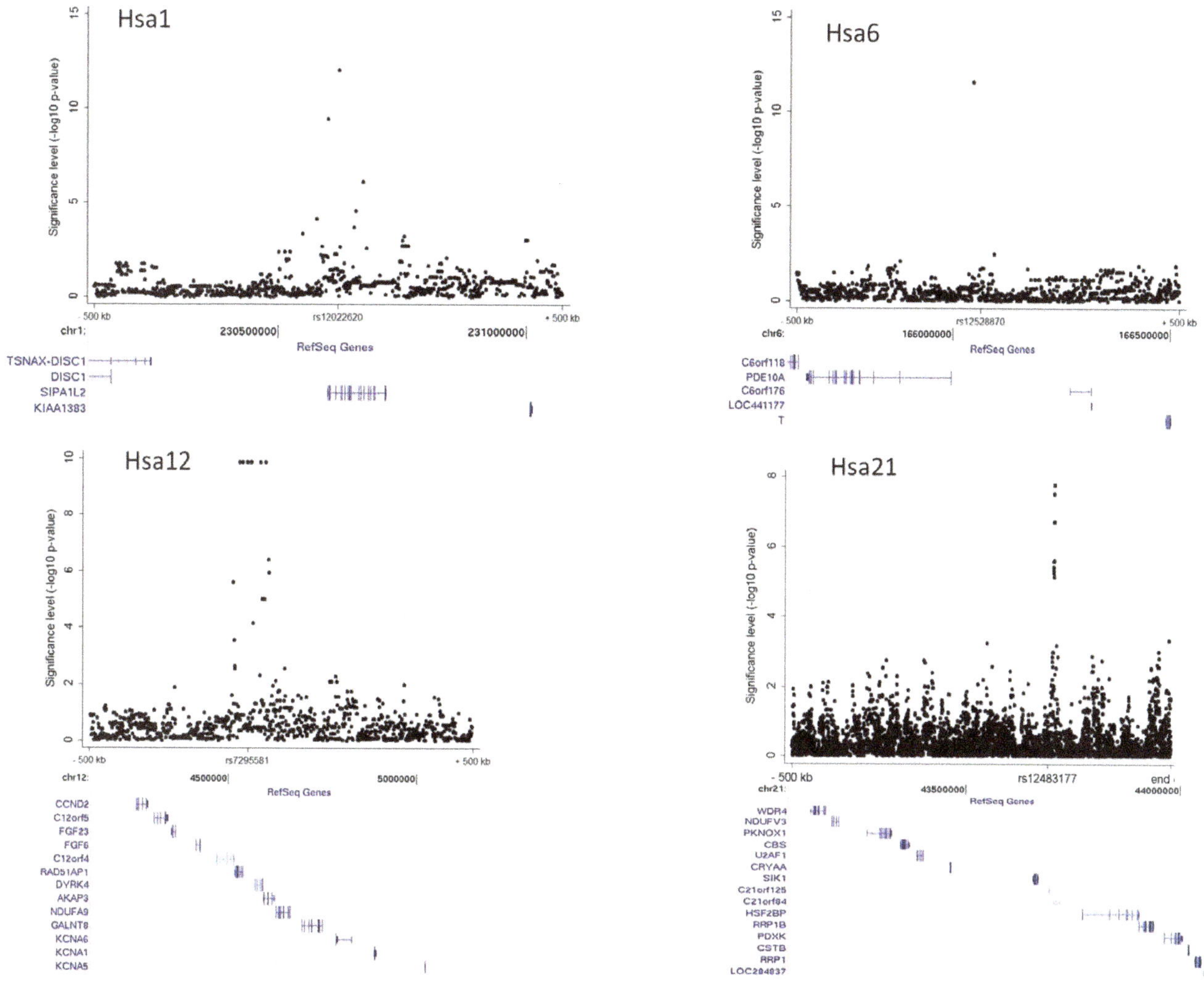

Figure 5. Examples of significant association findings in HapMap GWA. The significance level ($-\log_{10}$ P) of the top two association findings and two examples of top hits overlapping with either linkage, top GWA in KORA-GenCord, overlap with known candidate genes, or top findings on Hsa21 are shown within a genetic region of 1 Mb (($\pm$500 kb around the significantly associated SNP). The chromosome, SNP ID, location and genic context (RefSeq genes, using UCSC genome browser) are indicated for each depicted SNP.

genetic markers. As for all genome-wide studies using cell lines, it is a first step into identifying the genetic basis and requires validation in further cohorts, functional analysis, and ultimately verification in primary cells from healthy and diseased individuals. Potential confounding factors due to EBV-transformation remain a subject of debate and need to be considered. Also, we measured H_2O_2 levels after PMA stimulation, and genetic variation involved in the *protein kinase C*, through which PMA acts directly, cannot be fully excluded. However, heritability would not have been detected if EBV transformation or PMA stimulation would affect pathways in a random way. Finally, H_2O_2 release is an endophenotype with multiple levels of metabolism. Our assay relied on extracellular measures of hydrogen peroxide release which is the joint result of ROS production, metabolism, and degradation. Each step of these mechanisms may involve few or many genes, and thus contribute to the complexity of the phenotype.

We did not find genome-wide significant associations for loci of the NADPH-dependent NOX2 and other NOX related genes. We identified a locus 1 Mb from p67phox (or NCF2) as the closest hit for NOX2 members expressed in LCL (p22^{phox}, p40^{phox}, p47^{phox}, p67^{phox}, and homologues RAC1 and RAC2). These results suggest that variation in other genetic loci have stronger impact on natural variation of H_2O_2 as compared to the known genes identified in studies of Mendelian disorders. Previous case-control studies investigating the molecular basis of either H_2O_2 or ROS applied candidate gene approaches with contradictory results. Some studies identified mutations or polymorphisms associated with ROS generation within the NADPH-dependent NOX2 gene or its cofactors, while others found no association [31]. Recently, it has been suggested that haplotype rather than single SNP analysis may capture more of the relevant biological effects of phenotypic traits. Indeed, in the case of NOX2 dependent ROS generation, Bedard and coworkers [16] report an association between p22^{phox} (also called *CYBA*) haplotypes, rather than single polymorphisms. The associated haplotype was shown to act, at least in part, through an effect on protein expression levels. While this approach shed some light on the contradictory results reported so far on the involvement of NADPH-dependent NOX components in ROS generation, the large observed natural variation could not solely be attributed to the NADPH-dependent NOX2 and its cofactors, leading to the hypothesis that other loci are involved in regulatory mechanisms.

Table 3. Results from GWAS for the HapMap cohort.

SNP ID	Chr	Pos (bp)	type	Closest gene (within 1 MB)	Unadjusted p-value	Number SNPs/cluster
rs12022620	1	230616732	INTRONIC	SIPA1L2	$1.00\times10-12$	3
rs12528870	6	166117266	INTERGENIC	U6	$3.00\times10-12$	1
rs12602262	17	62290605	INTERGENIC	CACNG5	$1.20\times10-11$	1
rs11039359	11	47704385	INTRONIC	FNBP4	$4.80\times10-11$	1
rs7295581	12	4690362	INTERGENIC	GALNT8	$1.45\times10-10$	12
rs17833323	14	58415000	INTERGENIC	DACT1	$1.32\times10-9$	32
rs10749212	10	118166653	INTERGENIC	PNLIPRP3	$7.27\times10-9$	7
rs12483177	21	43586879	INTERGENIC	Q6ZN03_HUMAN	$1.75\times10-8$	13
rs6494367	15	61002704	INTERGENIC	TLN2	$3.6\times10-8$	1
rs17001416	4	77250823	INTRONIC	ART3	$4.84\times10-8$	20
rs2297721	9	138776337	INTRONIC	NP_976222.1	$8.64\times10-8$	3
rs17005290	2	81322921	INTERGENIC	5S_rRNA	$1.45\times10-7$	3
rs466886	6	33348677	INTRONIC	RPS18	$1.67\times10-7$	1
rs16947598	15	43815915	INTERGENIC	SQRDL	$1.70\times10-7$	1
rs333036	8	19026645	INTERGENIC	PSD3	$1.76\times10-7$	11

Results show the top 15 out of the 90 clusters of significantly associated genetic loci ($p<5.00\times10^{-8}$) and with suggestive associations ($p<1.00\times10^{-5}$) from genome-wide association analyses. We associated natural variation in H_2O_2 release measured in the HapMap cohort (n = 58 individuals) with more than 2.2 million markers. SNP ID, chromosome and position are indicated. Also, the type of SNP, the closest gene (within 1 MB), the unadjusted p-value and the number of SNP per cluster are indicated. SNP annotations were done by using the software WGAViewer (build 36, Ensembl core database *homo sapiens core 46 36h*, Ensembl variation database *homo sapiens variation 46 36h*, and Ensembl gene ontology database *ensemble go 46*).

Taken together, our results indicate that there is a substantially large contribution of genetic factors at the basis of H_2O_2 release among healthy individuals in the cohorts used in this study. Our results suggest that this trait, even though an endophenotype, is complex and that multiple genes or regulatory elements are probably acting in concert to shape its expression. The herein identified association findings, together with the closeby genes may be enriched for biologically significant genes, and/or genetic loci

Table 4. Overlap between top hits from linkage and GWAS.

Results for linkage and overlap with GWAS	Hsa1	Hsa12	Hsa15	Hsa19
Linkage results (LOD>3)	**TSC0774051 - TSC0393286**	**TSC0795922 - TSC0431222**	**TSC0453546 - TSC1202583**	**TSC1058872 -TSC0057999**
	1,864 kb–7'905 kb	10,841–13'493 kb	21,775–21'897 kb	59,446–59,469 kb
	LOD = 4.17	LOD = 4.64	LOD = 3.34	LOD = 3.26
		TSC0796032-TSC0014204	**TSC0181040-TSC0940969**	
		54,428–54,474 kb	34,855–37,771 kb	
		LOD = 3.09	LOD = 4.81	
		TSC0209972-TSC0621539	**TSC0577078**	
		96,905–99,714 kb	43,404 kb	
		LOD = 3.12	LOD = 4.4	
KORA-GenCord (top associations) overlap with linkage	-	-	-	-
HapMap (top associations) overlap with linkage	**rs2500247**	**rs10492058**	**rs2075814**	-
	3,172 kb	4,756 kb	22,717 kb	
	$p = 4.65\times10^{-6}$	$p = 1.45\times10^{-10}$	$p = 4.2\times10^{-7}$	
			rs16947598	
			43,816 kb	
			$p = 1.70\times10^{-7}$	

This table indicates replicated genetic regions identified through GWA in KORA-GenCord and in HapMap. Top hits for GWAS are shown when the loci overlap within 5 Mb of distance from top linkage hits. The chromosome, the genetic marker, the position and the LOD score or the p-value is shown.

relevant to pathogen defense and signaling, and pathway analysis may constitute the next step into the understanding of the regulation of H_2O_2 release. More generally, the elucidation of the genetic control of some heritable cellular traits may also be a complex problem that requires combined approaches and extensive sample sizes.

Materials and Methods

Sample collections and genotyping

CEPH_HapMap sample collection: We acquired EBV-transformed lymphoblastoid cell lines (beta-LCL) of 10 families (1333, 1334, 1340, 1341, 1345, 1346, 1347, 1362, 1408, 13292) and of 60 unrelated individuals of Caucasian origin from the Coriell Cell Repositories (Coriell Cell Services, Coriell Institute for Medical Research, Camden, NJ, USA; http://ccr.coriell.org). These are considered as healthy individuals and form part of the Caucasians of European Ancestry (CEPH) and the Haplotype Map (HapMap) Project [41,42]. Genotypes of the 10 families were downloaded from the CEPH database [50]. A total of 2723 single nucleotide polymorphisms (SNPs) were used for subsequent linkage analyses. For the 60 unrelated individuals, we used 2'124'999 million SNPs from publicly available databases, and from HapMart, NCBI_Build36 (http://snp.cshl.org/linkage_maps; www.hapmap.org; [41,42].

KORA sample collection: KORA S4 (Cooperative Health Research in the Augsburg Region) is a sample collection of a population-based project conducted from 1999–2001 for which beta-LCL of healthy adults from the Augsburg region in Germany were established [58]. Two hundred LCL from this collection were used; these samples were genotyped with the Affymetrix 500 K oligonucleotide array containing a total of 500,568 SNPs (Affymetrix 6.0 chips). Genotypes were determined using the software BRLMM version 1.4.0 with standard settings proposed by the manufacturer. A total of 413,877 SNPs passed quality control filters and were used for further analysis.

GenCord sample collection: The GenCord (Geneva Cord sample collection, University of Geneva, Medical School, Geneva, Switzerland) sample collection is a population-based collection of LCL derived from umbilical cords of 200 healthy newborns of Western European origin. The sample collection was approved by the institutional ethics committee, and all mothers provided their informed consent prior to sample collection [13]. There are no phenotypic data on these newborns. DNA samples were extracted from cord tissue LCL with the Puregene cell kit (Gentra-Qiagen, Venlo, The Netherlands). Genotyping was performed with the illumina 550 K SNP (Illumina, San Diego, CA) array following the instructions of the manufacturers. From a total of 555,352 SNPs, 480,455 SNPs passed quality filters and were used for subsequent analysis.

Filter settings for genotype quality required accuracy of sample call rates of more than 98% were (estimated based on 5 duplicated genotyping of samples). Any SNP with a call rate of less than 99% call rate was excluded, as well as all SNPs called less than in 1% of all samples. Separation of homozygote and heterozygote SNPs was verified and corrected if needed (cluster separation >0.3 was required). The range of excess of heterozygosity was verified and SNPs not falling into the range of -0.1 to -1, and 0.1 to 1 were excluded. MAF was set to $>5\%$; to exclude samples with cryptic relatedness, IBD was set to >0.125; and deviation of Hardy Weinberg equilibrium was defined as <0.05. We verified the specified gender, and visualized a random set of 100 SNPs for quality checking.

Down syndrome sample collection: 33 Down syndrome (DS) LCL samples were acquired from the Galliera Genetic Bank of Genoa, Emory University School of Medicine in Atlanta, and CSS-Mendel Institute in Rome [59] and 42 LCL from the AnEUploidy collection in Paris, France. Full trisomy was assessed by karyotyping. We excluded potential clustering effects of H_2O_2 release due to the multiple origins of these samples, no substructure was detected.

Cell culture: The LCL of all three populations were cultured in RPMI 1640 with Glutamax I medium (Invitrogen) supplemented with 10% fetal calf serum and 1% mix of penicillin, fungizone, and streptomycin (Invitrogen). All cell lines were grown and maintained for at least 2 weeks at a constant density of 200–400,000 cells/ml. Cells were washed once with PBS (Invitrogen) to reduce accumulation of cell debris 4–5 days prior to measuring ROS production.

AmplexRed ROS measurements: Cell lines were assessed for H_2O_2 release using AmplexRed (Invitrogen), a quantitative enzymatic assay that detects H_2O_2 in the culture media. Ninety minutes prior to AmplexRed measurements, cell lines were centrifuged at 1000 rpm for 10 min and transferred to 2,5 ml Hanks' balanced salt solution (HBSS) media (containing 5% of glucose) and kept on ice. 0.5 ml of each cell line was used for measuring cell number by Fluorescent Activated Cell Sorting (FACS). Beads were added at a known concentration to obtain absolute values of cell number. Cells were diluted to a final concentration of 500,000 cells/ml.

AmplexRed measurements were performed according to manufacturers' instructions with minor modifications. In brief, 50,000 cells were plated in 0.2 ml volume of HBSS containing 25 mM AmplexRed and 0.005 U/ml horseradish peroxidase. NADPH oxidase activity was stimulated with 0.1 mM phorbol 12-myristate 13-acetate (PMA). In 1 of 5 replicates per individual cell line, 10 mM diphenyleneiodonium (DPI), an NADPH oxidase inhibitor [60], was added prior to stimulation. Fluorescence was recorded every minute for a minimum of 30 min with excitation and emission wavelengths of 550 nm and 600 nm, respectively in a BMG Fluostar microplate reader at 37°C.

Experimental design and normalization of H_2O_2: Each well-plate was set up with 12 individual cell lines. Each cell line was measured in 4 replicates in addition to one replicate that was inhibited with DPI. From the 4 replicates per sample, one was removed based on an outlier detection procedure, and the average of the remaining 3 replicates was used as the phenotypic read-out. We defined the phenotypic read-out as the maximal slope over 5 time points within 30 min of measurements. The standard curve of H_2O_2 was used to transform relative H_2O_2 measures to absolute values for each individual plate, thus allowing for comparison among different plates. Experiments for which regression of the standard curve of H_2O_2 did not reach R^2 of 0.99 were excluded. For normalization across plates, the same 2 individuals (GM0755 and GM07341) were measured on every plate and served as a reference for normalization. As a negative control cell line, an LCL of a patient with chronic granulomatous disease (CGD) was tested to ensure specificity of the assay for NOX2-dependent H_2O_2 detection.

Statistical analysis

Linkage analysis and heritability estimate: Heritability analysis was performed with MERLIN software [40]. We assessed 113 individuals and their corresponding ROS production from 10 CEPH-HapMap families. Genetic markers for 2723 SNPs from the CEPH database (http://snp.cshl.org/linkage_maps); [61] were used. Mendelian inconsistencies and unlikely genotypes were removed using PEDCHECK and PEDWIPE software [62,40].

For genome-wide linkage analysis, the same phenotypes and genotypes were used for multipoint variance component analysis [40]. Empirical significance of the linkage results were obtained from 1000 simulations by randomly redistributing the phenotypes and recalculating the maximal linkage signal genome-wide. We extracted the lowest p-value from each simulation to obtain a null distribution. Observed and expected p-values were compared to assess the nominal genome-wide significance threshold. All simulations were performed using R on a cluster of 32 HP/Intel Itanium 2 based servers at the Vital-IT Center, Lausanne, Switzerland (http://www.vital-it.ch). Mapping positions of these markers correspond to NCBI36/hg18.

Normalization of phenotypes across populations: We applied a median centered transformation for the phenotypes before combining the data from KORA and GenCord populations. HapMap samples were used as a replication cohort and were analyzed separately; and also analyzed with a median centered transformation.

Association studies: Imputation of SNPs across all 3 populations. We imputed SNPs from unphased alleles for 337 individuals by using the BEAGLE 3.0.4 software [63]. The HapMap sample collection with 2.2 million SNPs was used as the reference to impute SNPs for the KORA and GenCord collections. All SNPs were mapped to the same strand as the reference and A/T, C/G SNPs were discarded, resulting in 456,122, and 311,949 SNPs for KORA and GenCord, respectively. We set a threshold for the inclusion of an imputed SNP at allelic $R^2>0.9$ to ensure high quality imputation. Of all 2.2 million imputed SNPs, 1.4 million were retained for further analyses.

Principal component analysis: Principal component analysis was first performed for samples of each cohort, and we excluded one sample from the GenCord population after visual inspection of the first 10 components. Principal component analysis of a random set of 500,000 SNPs was then used to test for population substructure among all three cohorts. Visual inspection of the first to the 8th component did not reveal evidence for substantial population substructures.

Genome-wide association studies: We performed linear regression analyses and an additive genetic model to perform association between H_2O_2 levels and each SNP using PLINK software [64]. SNPs were coded 0, 1, or 2 for homozygous rare, heterozygous, and homozygous common alleles, respectively. For this additive model, we fitted a linear regression of the form

$$Y_i = b_0 + b_1 X_i + \varepsilon_i$$

We report the nominal *p*-value of the test of no association, i.e., $b_l = 0$ where Yi are the H_2O_2 release for each sample i, Xi are the genotypes coded as 0,1,2 and ε_i are assumed to be independent normally distributed random errors with mean 0 and constant variance. Mapping positions of GWA markers for KORA/GenCord and for HapMap correspond to NCBI36/hg18.

Covariate analysis: We combined all samples from HapMap, KORA and GenCord after median transformation of the H_2O_2 release phenotype (N = 337), The following covariates were assigned to each individual: The status of the immune system of the individual ("mature" for HapMap and KORA, "immature" for GenCord); gender; the time of cell lines establishment prior to use in this study ("old" for HapMap, "new" for KORA and GenCord); the age of the individual (">60 years" for HapMap, "40–60 years" for KORA, "1 day" GenCord). A clustering effect was set for each of the three populations. We conducted a general linear mixed effect regression model with a clustering effect for the population and adjustment for immune status, gender, cell line age, and individual age. We performed univariate mixed effect linear regression with a cluster effect on populations for each co-variate. We then used a multivariate mixed effect linear regression with adjustment for all co-variates and a cluster effect on populations for a randomized set of 100'000 SNPs. This model was compared to a univariate mixed effect linear regression using the SNP only.

Supporting Information

File S1 Sample collection identifiers and phenotypes. All individuals used in this study are indicated with their identifier and their phenotype. H2O2 release indicates normalized hydrogen peroxide release levels, units are arbitrary.

File S2 Extensive inter-individual variation and high reproducibility for H_2O_2 phenotypes. (**A**) H_2O_2 release for 21 CEPH-HapMap unrelated individuals, each of which was measured in 4 replicates is shown. Each bar corresponds to the normalized H_2O_2 release of an individual, and standard deviations of three replicates per individual are indicated in red. The coefficient of variance is >28 with a p-value of $p<1.00\times10^{-4}$, indicating that there is 28 times more variation among individuals than among replicates. (**B**) H_2O_2 release for the same 21 individuals was measured several weeks later, to estimate the reproducibility of the phenotype. Comparison for individuals of both experimental sets indicates a coefficient of correlation of more than 0.89 (Pearson correlation test, $p<1.00\times10^{-4}$).

File S3 Overlap of SNPs among the three sample cohorts and genotyping platforms. This schematic figure displays the number of individuals genotyped for each cohort, and the number of SNPs genotyped per population. The overlap between the circles shows the numbers and percentages of overlapping SNPs among populations and genotyping platforms.

File S4 Principal component analysis indicates no apparent substructure. A random set of 500,000 SNPs of 337 individuals from three cohorts was analyzed using centered principal component analysis (PCA). Here we show PC1 versus PC2. No evident substructure is apparent among cohorts.

Acknowledgments

We thank Lena Serrander and Laetitia Fioraso-Cartier for assistance with establishing the H_2O_2 assay, and Josiane Wyniger for technical assistance in genotyping. We thank Bernd Kranz for providing cell lines for KORA, and Clementine Ripoll for technical assistance in cell line processing for the Down Syndrome cohort. Denis Cohen assisted in data managing, and Rosemary Sudan helped editing the manuscript.

Author Contributions

Advised on study design and analysis: SEA KHK ETD. Conceived and designed the experiments: HA SEA KB KHK. Performed the experiments: HA KB. Analyzed the data: HA EM KB. Contributed reagents/materials/analysis tools: SEA KHK EW HP TM JMD MG YD PD CB SD DM. Wrote the paper: HA SEA.

References

1. Hindorff LA, Sethupathy P, Junkins HA, Ramos EM, Mehta JP, et al. (2009) Potential etiologic and functional implications of genome-wide association loci for human diseases and traits. Proc Natl Acad Sci U S A. Jun 9;106(23):9362–7.
2. Risch NJ and Merikangas K (1996) The future of genetic studies of complex human diseases. Science. 273, pp. 1516–1517.
3. Risch NJ (2000) Searching for genetic determinants in the new millenium. Nature. 405, pp. 847–856.
4. McCarthy MI, Abecasis GR, Cardon LR, Goldstein DB, Little J, et al. (2008) Genome-wide association studies for complex traits: consensus, uncertainty and challenges. Nat Rev Genet. May;9(5):356–69.
5. McCarthy MI, Hirschhorn JN (2008) Genome-wide association studies: potential next steps on a genetic journey. Hum Mol Genet. Oct 15;17(R2):R156–65.
6. Altshuler D, Daly MJ, Lander ES (2008) Genetic mapping in human disease. Science. Nov 7;322(5903):881–8.
7. Visscher PM, Hill WG, Wray NR (2008) Heritability in the genomics era–concepts and misconceptions. Nat Rev Genet. Apr;9(4):255–66.
8. Manolio TA, Collins FS, Cox NJ, Goldstein DB, Hindorff LA, et al. (2009) Finding the missing heritability of complex diseases. Nature. Oct 8;461(7265):747–53.
9. Carlson CS, Eberle MA, Kruglyak L, Nickerson DA (2004) Mapping complex disease loci in whole-genome association studies. Nature. May 27;429(6990):446–52.
10. Antonarakis SE, Chakravarti A, Cohen JC, Hardy J (2010) Mendelian disorders and multifactorial traits: the big divide or one for all? Nat Rev Genet. May;11(5):380–4.
11. Stranger BE, Forrest MS, Clark AG, Minichiello MJ, Deutsch S, et al. (2005) Genome-wide associations of gene expression variation in humans. PLoS Genet. Dec;1(6).
12. Dermitzakis ET, Clark AG (2009) Genetics. Life after GWA studies. Science. Oct 9;326(5950):239–40.
13. Dimas AS, Deutsch S, Stranger BE, Montgomery SB, Borel C, et al. (2009) Common regulatory variation impacts gene expression in a cell type-dependent manner. Science. Sep 4;325(5945):1246–50.
14. Bedard K, Krause KH (2007) The NOX family of ROS-generating NADPH oxidases. Physiol Reviews. 87: 245–313, 2007.
15. Holland SM (2010) Chronic granulomatous disease. Clin Rev Allergy Immunol. Feb;38(1):3–10.
16. Bedard K, Attar H, Bonnefont J, Jaquet V, Borel C, et al. (2009) Three common polymorphisms in the CYBA gene form a haplotype associated with decreased ROS generation. Hum Mutat. Jul;30(7):1123–33.
17. Piirila H, Valiaho J, Vihinen M (2006) Immunodeficiency mutation databases (IDbases). Hum Mutat. 27:1200–8.
18. Dinauer MC, Curnutte JT, Rosen H, Orkin SH (1989) A missense mutation in the neutrophil cytochrome b heavy chain in cytochrome-positive X-linked chronic granulomatous disease. J Clin Invest. Dec;84(6):2012–6.
19. Dinauer MC, Pierce EA, Erickson RW, Muhlebach TJ, Messner, et al. (1991) Point mutation in the cytoplasmic domain of the neutrophil p22-phox cytochrome b subunit is associated with a nonfunctional NADPH oxidase and chronic granulomatous disease. Proc Natl Acad Sci U S A. Dec 15;88(24):11231–5.
20. Noack D, Rae J, Cross AR, Muñoz J, Salmen S, et al. (1999) Autosomal recessive chronic granulomatous disease caused by novel mutations in NCF-2, the gene encoding the p67-phox component of phagocyte NADPH oxidase. Hum Genet. Nov;105(5):460–7.
21. Olofsson P, Holmberg J, Tordsson J, Lu S, Akerström B, et al. (2003) Positional identification of Ncf1 as a gene that regulates arthritis severity in rats. Nat Genet. Jan;33(1):25–32.
22. Hultqvist M, Bäcklund J, Bauer K, Gelderman KA, Holmdahl R (2007) Lack of reactive oxygen species breaks T cell tolerance to collagen type II and allows development of arthritis in mice. J Immunol. Aug 1;179(3):1431–7.
23. Hultqvist M, Olofsson P, Holmberg J, Bäckström BT, Tordsson J, et al. (2004) Enhanced autoimmunity, arthritis, and encephalomyelitis in mice with a reduced oxidative burst due to a mutation in the Ncf1 gene. Proc Natl Acad Sci U S A. Aug 24;101(34):12646–51.
24. Lacy F, Kailasam MT, O'Connor DT, Schmid-Schonbein GW, Parmer RJ (2000) Plasma hydrogen peroxide production in human essential hypertension: role of heredity, gender, and ethnicity. Hypertension. 36:878–84.
25. Dominiczak AF, Brain N, Charchar F, McBride M, Hanlon N, et al. (2004) Genetics of hypertension: lessons learnt from mendelian and polygenic syndromes. Clin Exp Hypertens. Oct–Nov;26(7–8):611–20.
26. Mein CA, Caulfield MJ, Dobson RJ, Munroe PB (2004) Genetics of essential hypertension. Hum Mol Genet. Apr 1;13 Spec No 1:R169–75.
27. Del Campo M, Antonell A, Magano LF, Muñoz FJ, Flores R, et al. (2006) Hemizygosity at the NCF1 gene in patients with Williams-Beuren syndrome decreases their risk of hypertension. Am J Hum Genet. Apr;78(4):533–42.
28. Moreno MU, San José G, Fortuño A, Beloqui O, Díez J, et al. (2006) The C242T CYBA polymorphism of NADPH oxidase is associated with essential hypertension. J Hypertens. Jul;24(7):1299–306.
29. Deng AY (2007) Genetic basis of polygenic hypertension. Hum Mol Genet. Oct 15;16 Spec No. 2:R195–202.
30. Krause KH (2007) Aging: a revisited theory based on free radicals generated by NOX family NADPH oxidases. Exp Gerontol. 42:256–62.
31. San Jose G, Fortuno A, Beloqui O, Diez J, Zalba G (2008) NADPH oxidase CYBA polymorphisms, oxidative stress and cardiovascular diseases. Clin Sci (Lond). 114:173–82.
32. Arca M, Conti B, Montali A, Pignatelli P, Campagna F, et al. (2008) C242T polymorphism of NADPH oxidase p22phox and recurrence of cardiovascular events in coronary artery disease. Arterioscler Thromb Vasc Biol. 28:752–7.
33. Antonarakis SE, Lyle R, Dermitzakis ET, Reymond A, Deutsch S (2004) Chromosome 21 and down syndrome: from genomics to pathophysiology. Nat Rev Genet. Oct;5(10):725–38.
34. Antonarakis SE, Epstein CJ (2006) The challenge of Down syndrome. Trends Mol Med. Oct;12(10):473–9).
35. Kedziora J, Bartosz G (1988) Down's syndrome: a pathology involving the lack of balance of reactive oxygen species. Free Radic Biol Med. 4(5):317–30.
36. Elroy-Stein O, Groner Y (1988) Impaired neurotransmitter uptake in PC12 cells overexpressing human Cu/Zn-superoxide dismutase. Implication for gene dosage effects in Down syndrome. Cell. 52 pp. 259–267.
37. Busciglio J, Pelsman A, Wong C, Pigino G, Yuan M, et al. (2002) Altered metabolism of the amyloid-precursor protein is associated with mitochondrial dysfunction in Down's syndrome. Neuron. 33(5):677–88.
38. Busciglio J, Yankner BA (1995) Apoptosis and increased generation of reactive oxygen species in Down's syndrome neurons in vitro. Nature. Dec 21–28;378(6559):776–9.
39. Helguera P, Pelsman A, Pigino G, Wolvetang E, Head E (2005) ets-2 promotes the activation of a mitochondrial death pathway in Down's syndrome neurons. J Neurosci. 25(9):2295–303.
40. Abecasis GR, Cherny SS, Cookson WO, Cardon LR (2002) Merlin–rapid analysis of dense genetic maps using sparse gene flow trees. Nat Genet. Jan;30(1):97–101.
41. The International HapMap Consortium (2005) A Haplotype Map of the Human Genome. Nature. Oct 27;437(7063):1299–320.
42. International HapMap Consortium, Frazer KA, Ballinger DG, Cox DR, Hinds DA, et al. (2007) A second generation human haplotype map of over 3.1 million SNPs. Nature. Oct 18;449(7164):851–61.
43. Romito A, Lonardo E, Roma G, Minchiotti G, Ballabio A, et al. (2010) Lack of sik1 in mouse embryonic stem cells impairs cardiomyogenesis by down-regulating the cyclin-dependent kinase inhibitor p57kip2. PLoS One. Feb 3;5(2):e9029.
44. Stephenson A, Huang GY, Nguyen NT, Reuter S, McBride JL, et al. (2004) snf1lk encodes a protein kinase that may function in cell cycle regulation. Genomics. Jun;83(6):1105–15.
45. Pellegrini-Calace M, Tramontano A (2006) Identification of a novel putative mitogen-activated kinase cascade on human chromosome 21 by computational approaches. Bioinformatics. Apr 1;22(7):775–8.
46. Cheung VG, Conlin LK, Weber TM, Arcaro M, Jen KY, et al. (2003) Natural variation in human gene expression assessed in lymphoblastoid cells. Nat Genet. Mar;33(3):422–5.
47. Schadt EE, Monks SA, Drake TA, Lusis AJ, Che N, et al. (2003) Genetics of gene expression surveyed in maize, mouse and man. Nature. 422:297–302.
48. Monks SA, Leonardson A, Zhu H, Cundiff P, Pietrusiak P, et al. (2004) Genetic Inheritance of Gene Expression in Human Cell Lines. Am J Hum Genet. 75 (6):1094–105.
49. Morley M, Molony CM, Weber TM, Devlin JL, Ewens KG, et al. (2004) Genetic analysis of genome-wide variation in human gene expression. Nature. 12;430(7001):743–7.
50. Spielman RS, Bastone LA, Burdick JT, Morley M, Ewens WJ, et al. (2007) Common genetic variants account for differences in gene expression among ethnic groups. Nat Genet. 39(2):226–31.
51. Stearns SC, Byars SG, Govindaraju DR, Ewbank D (2010) Measuring selection in contemporary human populations. Nat Rev Genet. 2010 Sep;11(9):611–22.
52. Kuhns DB, Alvord WG, Heller T, Feld JJ, Pike KM, et al. (2010) Residual NADPH oxidase and survival in chronic granulomatous disease. N Engl J Med. Dec 30;363(27):2600–10.
53. Purcell S, Cherny SS, Sham PC (2003) Genetic Power Calculator: design of linkage and association genetic mapping studies of complex traits. Bioinformatics. Jan;19(1):149–50.
54. Piccoli C, Ria R, Scrima R, Cela O, D'Aprile A, et al. (2005) Characterization of mitochondrial and extra-mitochondrial oxygen consuming reactions in human hematopoietic stem cells. Novel evidence of the occurrence of NAD(P)H oxidase activity. J Biol Chem. 280: 26467–26476.
55. Gruhne B, Sompallae R, Marescotti D, Kamranvar SA, Gastaldello S, et al. (2009) The Epstein-Barr virus nuclear antigen-1 promotes genomic instability via induction of reactive oxygen species. Proc Natl Acad Sci U S A. Feb 17;106(7):2313–8.
56. Winterbourn CC (2008) Reconciling the chemistry and biology of reactive oxygen species. Nat Chem Biol. May;4(5):278–86.
57. Kobayashi S, Imajoh-Ohmi S, Kuribayashi F, Nunoi H, Nakamura M, et al. (1995). Characterization of the superoxide-generating system in human peripheral lymphocytes and lymphoid cell lines. J Biochem. 1995 Apr;117(4):758–65.

58. Wichmann HE, Gieger C, Illig T (2005) KORA-gene–resource for population genetics, controls and a broad spectrum of disease phenotypes. Gesundheitswesen. 67(Suppl 1):S26–30.
59. Prandini P, Deutsch S, Lyle R, Gagnebin M, Delucinge Vivier C, et al. (2007) Natural gene-expression variation in Down syndrome modulates the outcome of gene-dosage imbalance. Am J Hum Genet. Aug;81(2):252–63.
60. Hancock JT, Jones OT (1987) The inhibition by diphenyleneiodonium and its analogues of superoxide generation by macrophages. Biochem J. Feb 15;242(1):103–7.
61. Matise TC, Sachidanandam R, Clark AG, Kruglyak L, Wijsman E, et al. (2003) A 3.9-centimorgan-resolution human single-nucleotide polymorphism linkage map and screening set. Am J Hum Genet. Aug;73(2):271–84.
62. O'Connell JR, Weeks DE (1998) PedCheck: a program for identification of genotype incompatibilities in linkage analysis. Am J Hum Genet. Jul;63(1):259–66.
63. Browning BL, Browning SR (2011) A fast, powerful method for detecting identity by descent. Am J Hum Genet. Feb 11;88(2):173–82.
64. Purcell S, Neale B, Todd-Brown K, Thomas L, Ferreira MA, et al. (2007) PLINK: a tool set for whole-genome association and population-based linkage analyses. Am J Hum Genet. Sep;81(3):559–75.

24

Noninvasive Prenatal Diagnosis of Fetal Trisomy 21 by Allelic Ratio Analysis Using Targeted Massively Parallel Sequencing of Maternal Plasma DNA

Gary J. W. Liao[1,2], K. C. Allen Chan[1,2], Peiyong Jiang[1,2], Hao Sun[1,2], Tak Y. Leung[3], Rossa W. K. Chiu[1,2], Y. M. Dennis Lo[1,2]*

1 Centre for Research into Circulating Fetal Nucleic Acids, Li Ka Shing Institute of Health Sciences, The Chinese University of Hong Kong, Shatin, New Territories, Hong Kong, China, **2** Department of Chemical Pathology, The Chinese University of Hong Kong, Shatin, New Territories, Hong Kong, China, **3** Department of Obstetrics and Gynaecology, The Chinese University of Hong Kong, Shatin, New Territories, Hong Kong, China

Abstract

Background: Plasma DNA obtained from a pregnant woman contains a mixture of maternal and fetal DNA. The fetal DNA proportion in maternal plasma is relatively consistent as determined using polymorphic genetic markers across different chromosomes in euploid pregnancies. For aneuploid pregnancies, the observed fetal DNA proportion measured using polymorphic genetic markers for the aneuploid chromosome would be perturbed. In this study, we investigated the feasibility of analyzing single nucleotide polymorphisms using targeted massively parallel sequencing to detect such perturbations in mothers carrying trisomy 21 fetuses.

Methodology/Principal Findings: DNA was extracted from plasma samples collected from fourteen pregnant women carrying singleton fetuses. Hybridization-based targeted sequencing was used to enrich 2 906 single nucleotide polymorphism loci on chr7, chr13, chr18 and chr21. Plasma DNA libraries with and without target enrichment were analyzed by massively parallel sequencing. Genomic DNA samples of both the mother and fetus for each case were genotyped by single nucleotide polymorphism microarray analysis. For the targeted regions, the mean sequencing depth of the enriched samples was 225-fold higher than that of the non-enriched samples. From the targeted sequencing data, the ratio between fetus-specific and shared alleles increased by approximately 2-fold on chr21 in the paternally-derived trisomy 21 case. In comparison, the ratio is decreased by approximately 11% on chr21 in the maternally-derived trisomy 21 cases but with much overlap with the ratio of the euploid cases. Computer simulation revealed the relationship between the fetal DNA proportion, the number of informative alleles and the depth of sequencing.

Conclusions/Significance: Targeted massively parallel sequencing of single nucleotide polymorphism loci in maternal plasma DNA is a potential approach for trisomy 21 detection. However, the method appears to be less robust than approaches using non-polymorphism-based counting of sequence tags in plasma.

Editor: Cees Oudejans, VU University Medical Center, Netherlands

Funding: The study was supported by the University Grants Committee of the Government of the Hong Kong Special Administration Region, China, under the Areas of Excellence Scheme (AoE/M-04/06) and an additional sponsored research agreement with Sequenom. YMDL was supported by an Endowed Chair from the Li Ka Shing Foundation. The funders had no role in study design, data collection and analysis, decision to publish, or preparation of the manuscript.

Competing Interests: The authors have read the journal's policy and have the following conflicts: KCAC, RWKC and YMDL have filed patent applications on the detection of fetal nucleic acids in maternal plasma for noninvasive prenatal diagnosis. Part of this patent portfolio has been licensed to Sequenom. YMDL is a consultant to and holds equities in Sequenom.

* E-mail: loym@cuhk.edu.hk

Introduction

Prenatal screening and diagnosis of fetal aneuploidies, such as trisomy 21 (T21), is an established part of modern obstetrics care. Conventional prenatal screening is built on parameters such as maternal age, sonographic and biochemical markers [1]. Since these parameters are mainly based on phenotypic features, which are essentially epiphenomena associated with the core molecular pathology, their diagnostic performance is usually suboptimal. Pregnancies stratified as high risk by the above screening approaches require further investigation of fetal genetic materials obtained via invasive procedures, such as chorionic villus sampling (CVS) and amniocentesis. These latter procedures carry small, but definite, risk of miscarriage [2]. The demonstration of fetal DNA in maternal plasma in 1997 has opened up possibilities for noninvasive prenatal diagnosis (NIPD) [3].

Maternal plasma DNA contains a mixture of fragmented maternal and fetal genomic DNA [4]. The large background of maternal DNA represents a challenge for the interrogation of fetal chromosomal status. Early studies for NIPD of T21 were polymorphism-based, requiring the measurements of allelic ratios and comparing them with the expected normal values [5–7]. These early methods were based on fetal-specific molecular signatures such as DNA methylation markers [5] and RNA markers [6], or required one to attempt to increase the fractional fetal DNA concentration to a sufficiently high level such as using formaldehyde treatment of maternal plasma [7]. However, for the last approach, there are controversies on the effectiveness of formaldehyde treatment because this method could not be replicated consistently by different groups [8–10]. Therefore, the clinical applicability of such a method remains unclear.

An alternative approach for NIPD of T21 is to measure the proportion of chromosome 21 (chr21)-derived DNA molecules in a maternal plasma sample. If a mother is carrying a T21 fetus, the additional copy of chr21 from the fetus would contribute an additional amount of chr21 DNA molecules to the maternal plasma sample, leading to an increased proportion of chr21 sequences [11]. The advent of massively parallel sequencing (MPS) enhances the precision of DNA quantification to an unprecedented level, and has enabled the detection of aberrant quantities of fetal DNA derived from an aneuploid chromosome using a tag-counting approach [11–14]. Therefore, it is an opportune time to reinvestigate the feasibility of the allelic ratio approach for the NIPD of T21 by using MPS. Since single nucleotide polymorphisms (SNPs) only account for approximately 1.6% of the human genome according to the dbSNP Build 135 for human (http://www.ncbi.nlm.nih.gov/projects/SNP/), conventional non-targeted MPS would only include SNP alleles in a small proportion of sequence reads. In our previous publication, by using a hybridization-based targeted MPS platform, we demonstrated the enrichment of DNA molecules within the targeted regions, as well as the preservation of the allelic ratios of the targeted SNPs in maternal plasma after target enrichment [15]. Therefore, in this study, we investigated the feasibility of the allelic ratio approach by using targeted MPS to preferentially sequence selected SNP loci in maternal plasma DNA for fetal T21 detection.

Materials and Methods

Ethics statement

Approvals were obtained from the institutional review board of the Joint Chinese University of Hong Kong - New Territories East Cluster Clinical Research Ethics Committee. All participants gave informed written consent.

Subjects and sample collection

We recruited fourteen pregnant women with singleton fetuses (gestational age ranging from 12 weeks to 13 weeks and 5 days) from the Department of Obstetrics and Gynaecology, Prince of Wales Hospital, Hong Kong. Maternal peripheral blood samples were collected prior to CVS. Following CVS, fetal genomic DNA samples were obtained from the chorionic villi. The aneuploidy or euploidy status were confirmed by full karyotyping. Among the fourteen cases, seven were T21 fetuses and the rest were euploid.

DNA extraction

Maternal peripheral blood samples (5–10 mL) were centrifuged at 1 600 g for 10 min at 4°C. The plasma portion (2–5 mL) was recentrifuged at 16 000 g for 10 min at 4°C. We removed any residual plasma from the blood cell portion by recentrifugation at 2 500 g for 5 min [16]. Plasma DNA was extracted with the DSP DNA Blood Mini Kit (Qiagen), as described previously [11]. Fetal and maternal genomic DNA was extracted from chorionic villi and peripheral blood cells, respectively, with the QIAamp DNA Blood Mini Kit (Qiagen) according to the manufacturer's protocol. The extracted plasma DNA was quantified by real-time PCR using an ABI 7300 Sequence Detector (Applied Biosystems). A β-globin real-time PCR assay was performed as described previously [4]. A conversion factor of 6.6 pg of DNA per cell was used to calculate the amount of the extracted plasma DNA.

Targeted MPS of plasma DNA libraries

As the plasma DNA molecules were already fragmented in nature, no additional fragmentation step was required. 10–30 ng plasma DNA for each case was used for DNA library construction by the Genomic DNA Sample Preparation Kit (Illumina) as previously described [15], except for the replacement of the adaptors and primers with the oligonucleotides from the Multiplexing Sample Preparation Oligonucleotide Kit (Illumina) and the SureSelect Target Enrichment System Kit (Agilent) according to the manufacturer's instructions. In order to obtain high fold sequencing coverage for SNPs, the SureSelect Target Enrichment System (Agilent) was applied for capturing SNPs in the targeted regions. As a proof-of-principle study, approximately 5% of the probes were designed to target a total of 2 906 SNP loci on chr7 (313 SNPs), chr13 (564 SNPs), chr18 (592 SNPs) and chr21 (1 437 SNPs), while the remaining probes were designed for another project. The above 2 906 SNPs represented a subset of the SNPs in the Genome-Wide Human SNP Array 6.0 (Affymetrix) (Table S2). 500 ng of each constructed plasma DNA library was incubated with the probes for 24 h at 65°C. After hybridization, the captured DNA molecules were eluted and amplified by a 12-cycle PCR according to manufacturer's instructions. Libraries with and without target enrichment were indexed for multiplex sequencing on a Genome Analyzer IIx (Illumina) in 50-bp×2 paired-end format. An additional 7 cycles of sequencing were performed to decode the index sequence. All sequenced reads were aligned to the unmasked human reference genome (Hg18) (http://genome.ucsc.edu) with the aid of SOAPaligner/soap2 (http://soap.genomics.org.cn). Two mismatches were allowed during alignment. The range of fragment sizes of paired-end reads was defined as 50–600 bp. Duplicated paired-end reads (e.g., reads with identical sequences and start–end coordinates) were considered clones of the same original plasma DNA template. All but one of the duplicated reads were filtered, leaving only 1 copy for subsequent bioinformatics analysis as previously described [15]. The allele counting in plasma DNA was based on the SNP loci contained in the microarray. Since we already knew the position for each SNP locus, we directly counted the alleles in plasma DNA according to the maternal and fetal genotyping information which served as the gold standard. For example, if maternal genotype was AA and fetal genotype was AB for one SNP, we counted the copy number of A and B alleles for this SNP locus in plasma DNA for subsequent analysis.

F-S ratio calculation

We define a SNP as informative if it is homozygous in the mother (e.g., genotype AA) and heterozygous in the fetus (e.g., genotype AB). In this scenario, the B allele is the fetus-specific allele and the A allele is the allele shared by the mother and fetus. Informative SNPs were identified according to maternal and fetal genotyping information. The fetus-specific allelic counts and shared allelic counts for the informative SNPs were obtained from the plasma DNA sequencing data, and were used to calculate the ratio between the fetus-specific alleles and the shared alleles (expressed as F-S ratio) for chr21 (expressed as FSR_{21}) and the reference chromosomes (expressed as FSR_{Ref}). In this study, reference chromosomes included all autosomes except chr21 in the non-targeted sequencing data analysis, and included chr7, chr13 and chr18 in the targeted sequencing data analysis. If a mother is carrying a euploid fetus, the ratio between FSR_{21} and FSR_{Ref} (expressed as FSR^{21}_{Ref}) should be equal to 1 (Figure 1). If a mother is carrying a T21 fetus with an additional chr21 from the father (referred in this manuscript as paternally-derived T21), the fetal genotype on chr21 would become ABB. The additional copy of the fetus-specific allele would increase the FSR^{21}_{Ref} to 2 (Figure 1). If the extra copy of chr21 is from the mother (referred in this manuscript as maternally-derived T21), the fetal genotype on chr21 would become AAB. The additional copy of the shared allele would reduce the FSR^{21}_{Ref} to less than 1 (Figure 1).

Microarray genotyping

Maternal and fetal genomic DNA samples were genotyped with the Genome-Wide Human SNP Array 6.0 (Affymetrix). The parental origin of the additional copy of chr21 in seven T21 fetuses was determined using microarray analysis of the chorionic villus samples in which the allelic signal intensities for SNPs on chr21 were analyzed. If the fetus has paternally-derived T21, the signal intensity of the fetus-specific allele (B allele) should be 2-fold higher than the shared allele (A allele), because the fetal genotype would become ABB on chr21, and vice versa. Using this approach, one fetus was identified as a paternally-derived T21, while six were maternally-derived T21.

Computer simulation

Computer simulation was employed to investigate the accuracy of the F-S ratio analysis for T21 detection. The statistical model is based on the assumption that the numbers of fetus-specific and shared allelic counts should follow a binomial distribution, according to the fractional fetal DNA concentration in both the paternally- and maternally-derived T21 models. For example, assuming the fractional fetal DNA concentration in the reference chromosomes (chrRef) is f, the probability of detecting the fetus-specific allele for an informative SNP would be f/2 on chrRef irrespective of the aneuploidy status of the fetus. On the other hand, the probability of detecting the fetus-specific allele on chr21 would be f/2 if the mother is carrying a euploid fetus, 2f/(2+f) if the mother is carrying a paternally-derived T21 fetus, and f/(2+f) if the mother is carrying a maternally-derived T21 fetus (Figure 1). For illustration purposes, we assumed equal amounts of informative allelic counts (the summation of fetus-specific and shared allelic counts) were obtained from chr21 and chrRef. Based on the above assumptions, 1 000 euploid and 1 000 T21 cases were simulated each time for different fractional fetal DNA concentrations to investigate the detection accuracy in both the paternally- and maternally-derived T21 models.

Results

Efficiency of target enrichment

We defined sequencing depth as the mean number of times each base had been sequenced in a particular region. On average, 3.1 million and 2.9 million paired-end reads in non-enriched and enriched samples, respectively, were mapped uniquely to the reference human genome (Hg18). After filtration of the duplicated paired-end reads, we calculated the sequencing depth of the targeted region by dividing the total number of sequenced bases within the targeted region by the length of the targeted region. The mean sequencing depth was 0.12 time for the non-enriched samples and 27 times for the enriched samples, indicating a mean enrichment of 225-fold (Table S1). This finding was consistent with our previous publication [15].

Estimation of fractional fetal DNA concentrations

We calculated the fractional fetal DNA concentrations (also referred to as the fetal DNA proportion) in the non-enriched samples by using the informative SNPs from all autosomes except for chr21, according to the equation: fractional fetal DNA concentration = fetus-specific allelic counts ×2/(fetus-specific allelic counts + shared allelic counts) ×100%. The median fractional fetal DNA concentration for the fourteen cases analyzed in this study was 15.5% (range: 9.1%–19.7%).

F-S ratio calculation using non-targeted sequencing data

Based on maternal and fetal genotyping information, informative SNPs were identified on chr21 (range amongst the samples: 1 044 to 1 775 SNPs), and chrRef which included all autosomes except chr21 (range amongst the samples: 99 581 to 106 950 SNPs). Within the above informative SNPs, fetus-specific allelic counts (expressed as FC) and shared allelic counts (expressed as SC) were determined for chr21 (FC_{21} = 2 to 19, SC_{21} = 87 to 213) and chrRef (FC_{Ref} = 390 to 1 622, SC_{Ref} = 6 880 to 18 892). We then calculated the FSR_{21}, FSR_{Ref} and FSR^{21}_{Ref} (Table S1). As shown in Figure 2A, the paternally-derived T21 case

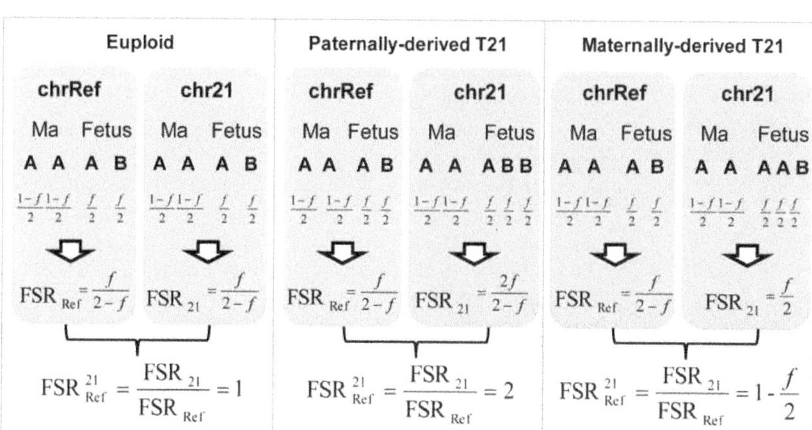

Figure 1. Schematic of T21 detection by F-S ratio calculation. Assuming the fractional fetal DNA concentration in chrRef is f, the F-S ratio would be f/(2-f) on chrRef irrespective of the aneuploidy status of the fetus. On the other hand, the F-S ratio on chr21 would be f/(2-f) if the mother is carrying a euploid fetus, 2f/(2-f) if the mother is carrying a paternally-derived T21 fetus, and f/2 if the mother is carrying a maternally-derived T21 fetus. Therefore, the FSR^{21}_{Ref} would be 1 if the mother is carrying a euploid fetus, would become 2 if the mother is carrying a paternally-derived T21 fetus, and would become (1-f/2) if the mother is carrying a maternally-derived T21 fetus.

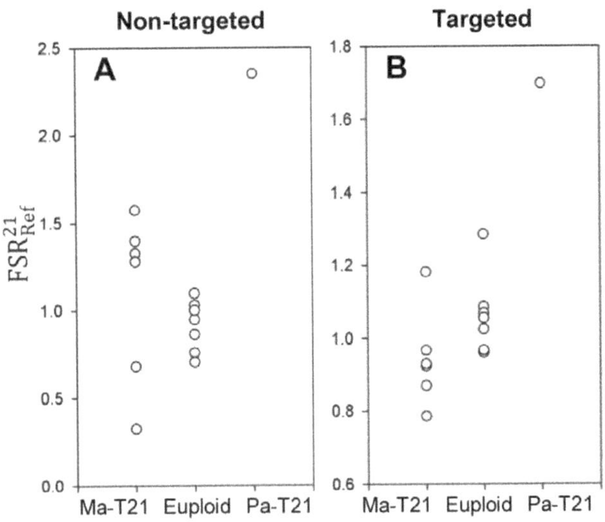

Figure 2. T21 detection by F-S ratio in non-targeted and targeted sequencing data. FSR^{21}_{Ref} values were calculated to differentiate the paternally- and maternally-derived T21 from the euploid fetuses in non-targeted (A) and targeted (B) sequencing data. (Ma-T21: maternally-derived T21. Pa-T21: paternally-derived T21.).

($FSR^{21}_{Ref} = 2.35$) could be differentiated from the euploid group (FSR^{21}_{Ref} mean 0.91, median 0.96, range: 0.70 to 1.10). On the other hand, the maternally-derived T21 cases (FSR^{21}_{Ref} mean 1.10, median 1.30, range: 0.33 to 1.57) overlapped with the euploid cases (Mann-Whitney rank sum test, $p = 0.366$).

F-S ratio calculation using targeted sequencing data

Among the 1 437 targeted SNP loci on chr21 and 1 469 SNP loci on chrRef (including chr7, chr13 and chr18), informative SNPs (chr21 = 151 to 273 SNPs, chrRef = 145 to 182 SNPs) were identified for each case. The number of sequenced reads with the fetus-specific and shared alleles were determined for chr21 ($FC_{21} = 197$ to 761, $SC_{21} = 3$ 610 to 7 740) and chrRef ($FC_{Ref} = 154$ to 473, $SC_{Ref} = 2$ 786 to 5 557) (Table S1). As shown in Figure 2B, the paternally-derived T21 case ($FSR^{21}_{Ref} = 1.68$) could be differentiated from the euploid group (FSR^{21}_{Ref} mean 1.06, median 1.06, range: 0.95 to 1.29). Although the maternally-derived T21 group appeared to have lower FSR^{21}_{Ref} values (FSR^{21}_{Ref} mean 0.94, median 0.93, range: 0.78 to 1.17) (Mann-Whitney rank sum test, $p = 0.051$), there was still significant overlapping with the euploid group.

Computer simulation

We used computer simulation to determine the parameters that would further improve the accuracy of the allelic ratio approach for T21 detection. First, we fixed the fractional fetal DNA concentration at 15% and gradually increased the numbers of informative allelic counts on chr21 and chrRef to investigate the detection accuracy for fetal T21. Additional informative allelic counts would improve the detection accuracy in both the paternally- and maternally-derived T21 models. In order to obtain accurate detection (sensitivity >99%, specificity >99%), more informative allelic counts were required for the maternally-derived T21 detection (informative allelic counts = 130 000) than the paternally-derived T21 detection (informative allelic counts = 1 100) (Figure 3A). If the fractional fetal DNA concentration was reduced to 5%, the corresponding informative allelic counts would need to be increased to 3 600 000 for detecting maternally-derived T21 and 3 500 for detecting paternally-derived T21 (Figure 3B). When the fractional fetal DNA concentration in maternal plasma was gradually decreased from 40% to 1%, the minimal number of informative allelic counts would need to be increased in both the paternally- and maternally-derived T21 scenarios, in order to maintain a high detection rate (sensitivity >99%, specificity >99%). The required increase was higher for the maternally-derived T21 scenario than that for the paternally-derived one (Figure 4). The sensitivity and specificity chosen for this analysis were chosen to mirror the recently reported performance of the non-polymorphic tag counting approach [12–14].

Discussion

In this study, we investigated if the analysis of chromosome-specific allelic ratio would be useful for the NIPD of fetal chromosomal aneuploidy. The paternally-derived T21 case was successfully detected in both non-targeted and targeted sequencing data. For the maternally-derived T21 cases, this approach became less effective. Although the mean FSR^{21}_{Ref} values was lower in the maternally-derived T21 cases, there was significant overlapping in the FSR^{21}_{Ref} values between the euploid and the maternally-derived T21 cases. The difference in performances between paternally- and maternally-derived T21 detection was mainly due to the magnitude of the change in FSR^{21}_{Ref}, which was increased by 2-fold for paternally-derived T21 and decreased by f/2-fold for maternally-derived T21 (Figure 1). Since fetal DNA represents a minor population in maternal plasma, the lower fractional concentration of fetal DNA would diminish the degree of FSR^{21}_{Ref} change in maternally-derived T21. For example, assuming the fractional fetal DNA concentration is 5%, the FSR^{21}_{Ref} of maternally-derived T21 would become 0.975, which is very close to that of a euploid case ($FSR^{21}_{Ref} = 1$).

Since maternally-derived T21 accounts for the majority of T21 cases in clinical practice, it is necessary to investigate how one could improve its detection accuracy using the allelic ratio method [1,17]. One approach is to increase the fractional concentration of fetal DNA, which would enlarge the magnitude of FSR^{21}_{Ref} change in maternally-derived T21. Although an early study attempted to enrich the fetal DNA proportion by formaldehyde treatment of maternal plasma [7], this method is not ready for use because it has not been consistently reproduced by different groups [8–10]. Alternatively, the accuracy of detecting maternally-derived T21 can be improved by increasing the number of informative allelic counts. According to our simulation analysis, additional informative allelic counts would, to some extent, compensate for the loss of detection accuracy caused by the decrease in fractional fetal DNA concentration (Figure 4). Two approaches can be used to increase the number of informative allelic counts, namely, recruiting more informative SNPs and sequencing each locus deeper.

The number of informative SNPs is determined by two factors: the total number of SNPs on the chromosome of interest for detection and the frequency of informative SNPs. The latter is the percentage of detectable informative SNPs amongst a group of analyzed SNPs. As a proof-of-principle study, we directly used the fetal genotype information, as determined by microarray-based analysis of chorionic villus DNA, to maximize the frequency of informative SNPs. Amongst the fourteen cases recruited for this study, the mean proportions of SNPs that were informative were 11.9% (range: 11.3% to 12.1%) in all autosomes and 12.9% (range: 11.0% to 15.0%) in targeted SNP loci. However, the fetal genomic material would not be available beforehand for actual NIPD. Therefore, informative SNPs would need to be deduced

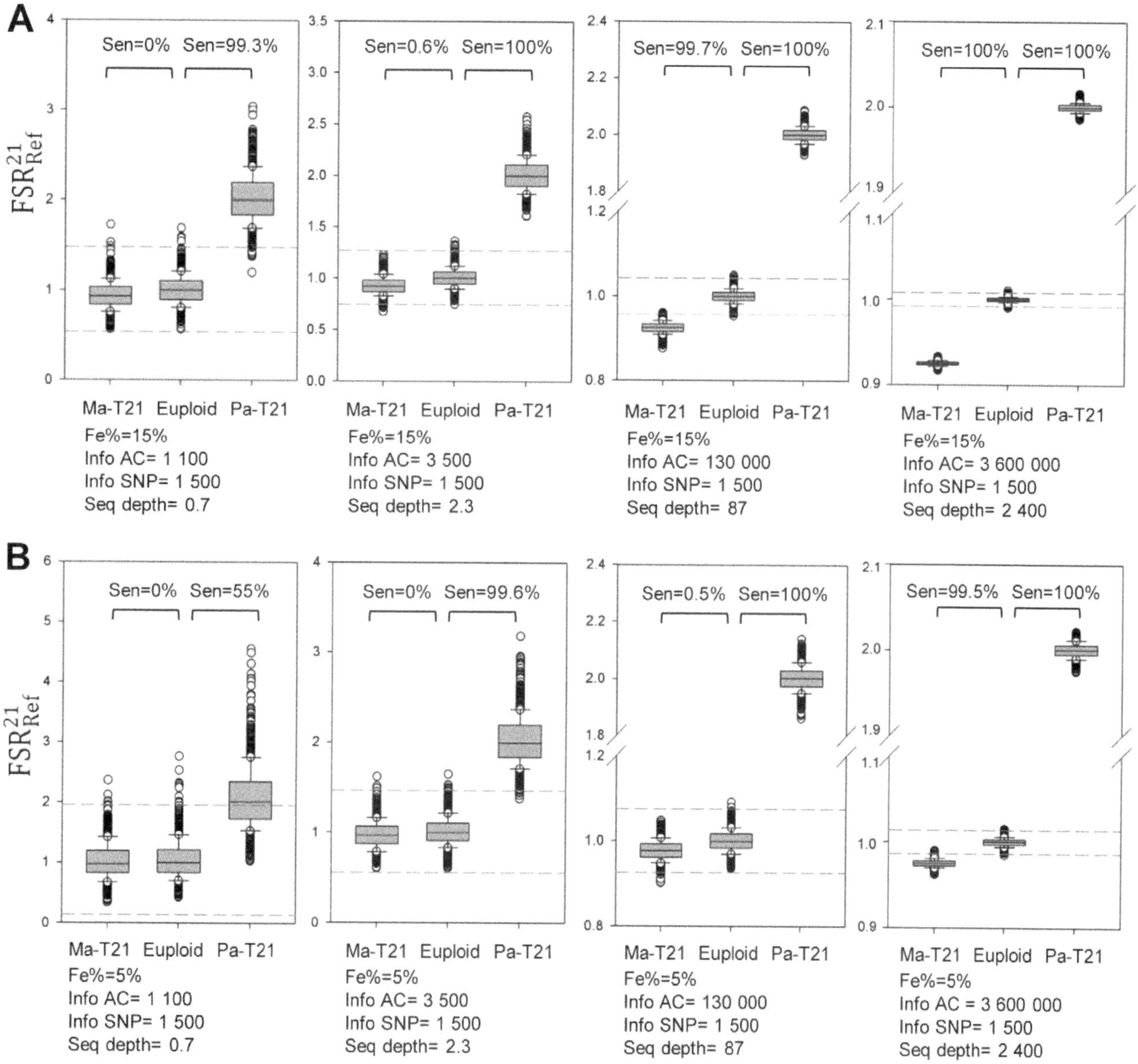

Figure 3. Computer simulation for T21 detection for fractional fetal DNA concentrations of 5% and 15%. In order to obtain a specificity of greater than 99%, the cutoffs for T21 differentiation were chosen at 3 standard deviations above and below the mean F-S ratio of the euploid group. The sensitivity for paternally- and maternally-derived T21 detection was investigated on different numbers of informative allelic counts on chr21 and chrRef, respectively, for a fractional fetal DNA concentration of 15% (A). Similar analysis was performed for a fractional fetal DNA concentration of 5% (B). (Ma-T21: maternally-derived T21. Pa-T21: paternally-derived T21. Sen = sensitivity. Fe% = fractional fetal DNA concentration. Info AC = informative allelic counts on each of chr21 and chrRef. Info SNP = informative SNPs on each of chr21 and chrRef. Seq depth = sequencing depth. Info AC = Info SNP × Seq depth).

indirectly, for example, by selecting SNPs in which the parents are both homozygous but with different alleles (e.g., mother is AA and father is BB). In this scenario, the frequency of informative SNPs would decrease, because such an approach would exclude any SNPs in which the father is heterozygous.

In terms of targeted analysis of SNPs, we demonstrated in this study the feasibility of the hybridization-based enrichment system. In this proof-of-principle study, we only employed a relatively small number of probes to capture 2 906 SNP loci on the target chromosomes. However, it is possible to increase the number of analyzed SNP loci. For example, if we design probes to cover all chr21 SNP loci (12 930 SNPs) on the Genome-Wide Human SNP Array 6.0 (Affymetrix), we could increase the number of informative SNPs on chr21 to approximately 1 500 SNPs for each case in the current dataset. If we obtain the same number of informative SNPs on chrRef and sequence the plasma DNA to a depth of 87 times, we would harvest approximately 130 000 informative allelic counts (1 500×87) on chr21 and chrRef, respectively. Such numbers would allow the relatively robust classification of maternally-inherited T21 from the euploid cases, assuming a fractional fetal DNA concentration of 15% or above (Figure 3A). Given that in this study the mean frequency of informative SNPs is approximately 12% and approximately 50% reads could be mapped back to the targeted regions (with the

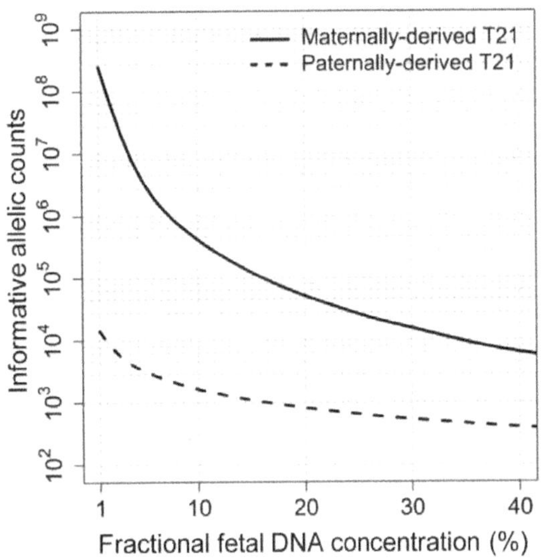

Figure 4. Computer simulation to investigate the minimal number of informative allelic counts for T21 detection. The solid curve represents the minimal number of informative allelic counts required on each of chr21 and chrRef (Y axis), in order to achieve a reliable detection in maternally-derived T21 (sensitivity >99%, specificity >99%) according to a given fractional fetal DNA concentration (X axis). The dash curve represents the paternally-derived T21 model.

remaining reads being off-target), the total number of reads required to obtain 130 000 informative allelic counts would be approximately 4.3 million (130 000 reads ×2/(12% ×50%)), which was comparable to that of the tag counting approach [12–14]. However, if the fractional fetal DNA concentration is reduced to 5%, the number of reads would need to be increased to approximately 120 million (Figure 3B), which was more than that needed for the non-polymorphic tag counting approach [12–14]. 5% and 15% were analyzed here because 5% is close to the lower limit for the non-polymorphism-based tag counting approach at the depth of sequencing used in a number of recent studies, and 15% is the approximate mean fractional fetal DNA concentration in the published clinical trials based on the tag counting approach [12–14].

In order to obtain a sufficient number of allelic counts, an alternative approach is to sequence more deeply each locus with a relatively small number of informative SNPs. According to our previous publication, we demonstrated that each milliliter of plasma contained approximately 1 000 genome-equivalents of DNA, which would give rise to 2 000 allelic counts for each locus [4]. If we could count all of the alleles for each locus in 5 mL plasma, we would obtain 10 000 allelic counts for each locus. In this scenario, 26 informative SNPs (13 SNPs on chr21, 13 SNPs on chrRef) could provide sufficient informative allelic counts for maternally-derived T21 detection in a sample containing 15% fetal DNA, representing 130 000 informative allelic counts (10 000×13) on chr21 and chrRef, respectively. The number of informative SNPs would need to be increased to 720 (360 SNPs on chr21, 360 SNPs on chrRef) for a sample containing a fractional fetal DNA concentration of 5%. Due to the high read depth required by this strategy (i.e. 10 000 counts per informative allele), PCR-based approaches for target enrichment might be alternative methods for this type of application [18,19].

The targeted massively parallel sequencing of SNP loci in plasma DNA is thus a feasible method for the NIPD of fetal aneuploidies. However, when compared with published work based on tag counting of nonpolymoprhic loci for T21 detection [12–14], this approach appears to be less effective and robust because it requires the parental genotyping information and needs more sequencing reads if the fractional fetal DNA concentration is low as illustrated in this proof-of-principle study. In addition, the costs and time required for target enrichment would need to be taken into account. Nevertheless, this study has also outlined the strategies that one could use to further improve this approach.

Supporting Information

Table S1 Sequencing data and allelic information for plasma DNA libraries with and without target enrichment.

Table S2 Information of SNPs used for targeted sequencing.

Author Contributions

Conceived and designed the experiments: GJWL KCAC RWKC YMDL. Performed the experiments: GJWL. Analyzed the data: GJWL KCAC PJ HS. Contributed reagents/materials/analysis tools: TYL. Wrote the paper: GJWL KCAC YMDL.

References

1. Driscoll DA, Gross S (2009) Prenatal screening for aneuploidy. N Engl J Med 360: 2556–2562.
2. Mujezinovic F, Alfirevic Z (2007) Procedure-related complications of amniocentesis and chorionic villous sampling: a systematic review. Obstet Gynecol 110: 687–694.
3. Lo YMD, Corbetta N, Chamberlain PF, Rai V, Sargent IL, et al. (1997) Presence of fetal DNA in maternal plasma and serum. Lancet 350: 485–487.
4. Lo YMD, Tein MSC, Lau TK, Haines CJ, Leung TN, et al. (1998) Quantitative analysis of fetal DNA in maternal plasma and serum: implications for noninvasive prenatal diagnosis. Am J Hum Genet 62: 768–775.
5. Tong YK, Ding CM, Chiu RWK, Gerovassili A, Chim SSC, et al. (2006) Noninvasive prenatal detection of fetal trisomy 18 by epigenetic allelic ratio analysis in maternal plasma: theoretical and empirical considerations. Clin Chem 52: 2194–2202.
6. Lo YMD, Tsui NBY, Chiu RWK, Lau TK, Leung TN, et al. (2007) Plasma placental RNA allelic ratio permits noninvasive prenatal chromosomal aneuploidy detection. Nat Med 13: 218–223.
7. Dhallan R, Guo X, Emche S, Damewood M, Bayliss P, et al. (2007) A non-invasive test for prenatal diagnosis based on fetal DNA present in maternal blood: a preliminary study. Lancet 369: 474–481.
8. Benachi A, Yamgnane A, Olivi M, Dumez Y, Gautier E, et al. (2005) Impact of formaldehyde on the in vitro proportion of fetal DNA in maternal plasma and serum. Clin Chem 51: 242–244.
9. Chinnapapagari SKR, Holzgreve W, Lapaire O, Zimmermann B, Hahn S (2005) Treatment of maternal blood samples with formaldehyde does not alter the proportion of circulatory fetal nucleic acids (DNA and mRNA) in maternal plasma. Clin Chem 51: 652–655.
10. Chung GTY, Chiu RWK, Chan KCA, Lau TK, Leung TN, et al. (2005) Lack of dramatic enrichment of fetal DNA in maternal plasma by formaldehyde treatment. Clin Chem 51: 655–658.
11. Chiu RWK, Chan KCA, Gao YA, Lau VYM, Zheng WL, et al. (2008) Noninvasive prenatal diagnosis of fetal chromosomal aneuploidy by massively parallel genomic sequencing of DNA in maternal plasma. Proc Natl Acad Sci U S A 105: 20458–20463.
12. Chiu RWK, Akolekar R, Zheng YWL, Leung TY, Sun H, et al. (2011) Non-invasive prenatal assessment of trisomy 21 by multiplexed maternal plasma DNA sequencing: large scale validity study. BMJ 342: 9.
13. Palomaki GE, Kloza EM, Lambert-Messerlian GM, Haddow JE, Neveux LM, et al. (2011) DNA sequencing of maternal plasma to detect Down syndrome: an international clinical validation study. Genet Med 13: 913–920.

14. Bianchi DW, Platt LD, Goldberg JD, Abuhamad AZ, Sehnert AJ, et al. (2012) Genome-wide fetal aneuploidy detection by maternal plasma DNA sequencing. Obstet Gynecol. In press doi: 10.1097/AOG.0b013e31824fb482.
15. Liao GJW, Lun FMF, Zheng YWL, Chan KCA, Leung TY, et al. (2011) Targeted massively parallel sequencing of maternal plasma DNA permits efficient and unbiased detection of fetal alleles. Clin Chem 57: 92–101.
16. Chiu RWK, Poon LLM, Lau TK, Leung TN, Wong EMC, et al. (2001) Effects of blood-processing protocols on fetal and total DNA quantification in maternal plasma. Clin Chem 47: 1607–1613.
17. Antonarakis SE (1991) Parental origin of the extra chromosome in trisomy 21 as indicated by analysis of DNA polymorphisms. N Engl J Med 324: 872–876.
18. Mamanova L, Coffey AJ, Scott CE, Kozarewa I, Turner EH, et al. (2010) Target-enrichment strategies for next-generation sequencing. Nat Methods 7: 111–118.
19. Tewhey R, Warner JB, Nakano M, Libby B, Medkova M, et al. (2009) Microdroplet-based PCR enrichment for large-scale targeted sequencing. Nat Biotechnol 27: 1025–1031.

25

Prevention of Neural Tube Defects: A Cross-Sectional Study of the Uptake of Folic Acid Supplementation in Nearly Half a Million Women

Jonathan P. Bestwick, Wayne J. Huttly, Joan K. Morris, Nicholas J. Wald*

Wolfson Institute of Preventive Medicine, Barts and the London School of Medicine and Dentistry, Queen Mary University of London, London, United Kingdom

Abstract

Background: Taking folic acid supplements before pregnancy to reduce the risk of a neural tube defect (NTD) is especially important in countries without universal folic acid fortification. The extent of folic acid supplementation among women who had antenatal screening for Down's syndrome and NTDs at the Wolfson Institute of Preventive Medicine, London between 1999 and 2012 was assessed.

Methods and Findings: 466,860 women screened provided details on folic acid supplementation. The proportion of women who took folic acid supplements before pregnancy was determined according to year and characteristics of the women. The proportion of women taking folic acid supplements before pregnancy declined from 35% (95% CI 34%–35%) in 1999–2001 to 31% (30%–31%) in 2011–2012. 6% (5%–6%) of women aged under 20 took folic acid supplements before pregnancy compared with 40% of women aged between 35 and 39. Non-Caucasian women were less likely to take folic acid supplements before pregnancy than Caucasian women; Afro-Caribbean 17% (16%–17%), Oriental 25% (24%–25%) and South Asian 20% (20%–21%) compared with 35% (35%–35%) for Caucasian women. 51% (48%–55%) of women who previously had an NTD pregnancy took folic acid supplements before the current pregnancy.

Conclusions: The policy of folic acid supplementation is failing and has led to health inequalities. This study demonstrates the need to fortify flour and other cereal grain with folic acid in all countries of the world.

Editor: Cheryl S. Rosenfeld, University of Missouri, United States of America

Funding: These authors have no support or funding to report.

Competing Interests: The authors have declared that no competing interests exist.

* E-mail: n.j.wald@qmul.ac.uk

Introduction

In 1991 the results of the Medical Research Council Vitamin Study were published. This randomised controlled trial showed that taking folic acid before conception reduced the risk of a neural tube defect (NTD) pregnancy by an estimated 72% [1]. A high enough daily intake of folate to provide such a reduction in risk cannot easily be obtained by dietary changes so supplementation is necessary, particularly in countries where folic acid fortification has not been implemented. Mandatory fortification has been introduced in over 70 countries including the US, Canada and Australia [2], but despite evidence that such fortification is effective [3–5], over 120 countries have not introduced mandatory folic acid fortification, including all countries in the European Union, so women of child bearing age need to take folic acid supplements before pregnancy to reduce their risk of an NTD pregnancy. In 1998, 6 years after the UK Department of Health recommendation on the intake of folic acid before pregnancy [6] the proportion of women from one hospital screened at the Wolfson Institute of Preventive Medicine, London who took folic acid supplements before pregnancy was reported to be 42% (523/1238) [7]. We here assess the extent of folic acid supplementation using data from almost half a million women screened at the Wolfson Institute between 1999 and 2012.

Methods

Ethics Statement

The results in the paper arose out of an audit of our screening service for which no explicit consent was sought but women screened were informed that data arising from the screening programme might be used to make improvements to the services provided. All the data were anonymous and no enquiries or procedures were performed other than those that formed part of the routine service so ethical approval was not required.

In 1998 the antenatal Down's syndrome and NTD screening service at the Wolfson Institute of Preventive Medicine, London introduced a question on screening request forms asking whether women had (i) started taking folic acid supplements before pregnancy, (ii) started once pregnancy was confirmed or (iii) not taken folic acid supplements. Between January 1999 and December 2012 520,570 pregnant women were routinely screened at the Wolfson Institute for Down's syndrome using the late first trimester (11–13 weeks' gestation) Combined test (61%; median gestational age 12 weeks, 5 days) or the early second trimester (15–

20 weeks' gestation) Quadruple test (39%; median gestational age 16 weeks, 3 days). Women screened with the Quadruple test were also screened for NTDs using maternal serum alphafetoprotein, collected as part of the Quadruple test, and a further 867 women were screened for NTDs only. A total of 466,860 (90%; lower proportion in earlier years as the new request forms were being introduced) provided data on folic acid supplement status. The proportion of women who started taking folic acid supplements before pregnancy was determined for each calendar year. Data on the following specified factors that are routinely collected as part of the screening service were used to determine the independent effects of each: previous NTD pregnancy (yes/no), previous Down's syndrome pregnancy (yes/no), ethnicity (Caucasian, Afro-Caribbean, South Asian [Indian, Pakistani, Bangladeshi or Sri-Lankan], Oriental [Chinese, Japanese or South East Asian] or Other), insulin dependent diabetes mellitus (yes/no), in-vitro fertilisation (IVF, yes/no), smoker (yes/no), maternal weight (five 10 kg categories) and maternal age (seven 5-year categories), region of residence (categorised as strategic health authorities and the Isle of Man), and time of screening (first or second trimester). The relative use of taking folic acid supplements before pregnancy versus not taking folic acid supplements before pregnancy was calculated according to these factors and categories. Adjusted relative use estimates were calculated using multivariate Poisson regression with robust variances [8]. The average marginal effects were calculated to estimate the adjusted percentages of women taking folic acid before pregnancy i.e. the percentages independent of the specified factors. All analyses were performed in Stata version 12 (StatCorp, College Station, Texas).

Results

Figure 1 shows the strategic health authorities of England, and the Isle of Man where women provided blood samples for screening. Fifty-eight percent of women were from London, 27% from the South East, 11% from the North West, with the remainder from the East of England, Isle of Man and the South West.

All factors were statistically significantly associated with taking folic acid supplements before pregnancy (all $p<0.001$) and each factor, adjusting for all other factors, remained statistically significant (all $p<0.001$; see Table S1). Figure 2 shows that between 1999–2001 and 2002–2004 the observed proportion of women taking folic acid supplements before pregnancy reduced from 35% (95% CI 34%–35%) to 31% (30%–31%) and in the following ten years the proportion remained stable. The adjusted percentage taking folic acid supplements before pregnancy reduced in each period from 40% (39%–41%) in 1999–2001 to 28% (28%–28%) in 2011–2012.

Figure 3 shows that younger women were less likely to take folic acid supplements before pregnancy than older women; 6% (5%–6%) of women aged under 20 and 40% of women aged between 35 and 39. The adjusted percentage of women taking folic acid supplements before pregnancy peaked at 38% (38%–38%) in women aged 35–39 and was 31% (29%–33%) in women aged 45 or older.

Figure 4a shows that non-Caucasian women were less likely to take folic acid supplements before pregnancy than Caucasian women; 35% (35%–35%) of Caucasian women took folic acid supplements before pregnancy compared with 17% (16%–17%) of Afro-Caribbean women, 20% (20%–21%) of South Asian women, 25% (24%–25%) of Oriental women and 23% (22%–23%) of women of other ethnic groups. Adjusted percentage estimates were similar to the unadjusted values.

Figure 4b shows that 51% (48%–55%) of women with a previous NTD affected pregnancy took folic acid supplements before their current pregnancy compared with 30% (30%–30%) of women without a previous NTD affected pregnancy (adjusted figures similar).

Table S1 shows results for other factors and gives unadjusted and adjusted relative use of folic acid supplements before pregnancy, from which adjusted percentages were derived. These results show that (i) women who had undergone IVF were most likely to take folic acid supplements prior to pregnancy, but despite being under close medical supervision 20% of them were not doing so, (ii) women who had previously had a pregnancy affected with Down's syndrome were more likely to take folic acid supplements before pregnancy than those who had not, but the proportion was still only about half, (iii) insulin dependent diabetic women were more likely to take folic acid supplements before pregnancy than non-insulin dependent diabetic women, (iv) smokers were less likely to take folic acid supplements before pregnancy than non-smokers and (v) women who were screened in the second trimester were less likely to take folic acid supplements than women screened in the first trimester, possibly because a greater proportion of women who had second trimester screening had unplanned pregnancies that were confirmed later in gestation.

Discussion

This study has four main findings. Firstly, relatively few women are taking folic acid supplements before pregnancy, with the proportion declining over the study period, from 35% in 1991–2001 to about 30% in 2011–2012. However, as women are having children at older ages and more women are having IVF, and these women were more likely to take folic acid supplements before pregnancy, the extent of the year-specific downwards trend is concealed. Perhaps more relevant is the observation that the adjusted percentage of women taking folic acid supplements before pregnancy declined from 40% in 1999–2001 to 28% in 2011–2012. Secondly non-Caucasian women were about half as likely as Caucasian women to take folic acid supplements before pregnancy. This probably reflects socio-economic status, demonstrating an example of health inequalities. Thirdly, whilst women who had previously had an NTD pregnancy were more likely to take folic acid supplements before pregnancy than women who had not, only about half of them did. Further, 16 women had had two previous NTD pregnancies; only five of them took folic acid supplements before pregnancy. Fourthly, younger women were far less likely to take folic acid supplements before pregnancy; women younger than 20 were five times less likely to take folic acid supplements before pregnancy than women aged 30 or over. This may be partly due to more unplanned pregnancies and less knowledge of the benefits of folic acid supplementation in younger women. After adjustment the percentage of women aged 45 or older taking folic acid supplements prior to pregnancy was 31%, lower than the percentage of women aged 40–44 (36%) despite the unadjusted percentages being the same (40%). The main contributor to the lower adjusted percentage for women aged 45 or older compared with women aged 40–44 is the proportion of women who had undergone IVF treatment (who were most likely to take folic acid before pregnancy) in the 45 or older age group; 34% compared with 7% of women aged 40–44.

During the study period the proportion of women who started taking folic acid supplements after pregnancy had been confirmed increased from 45% to 62% (see Table S1). However, to prevent NTDs folic acid supplements need to be taken before pregnancy; there is little to no benefit of taking folic acid supplements after

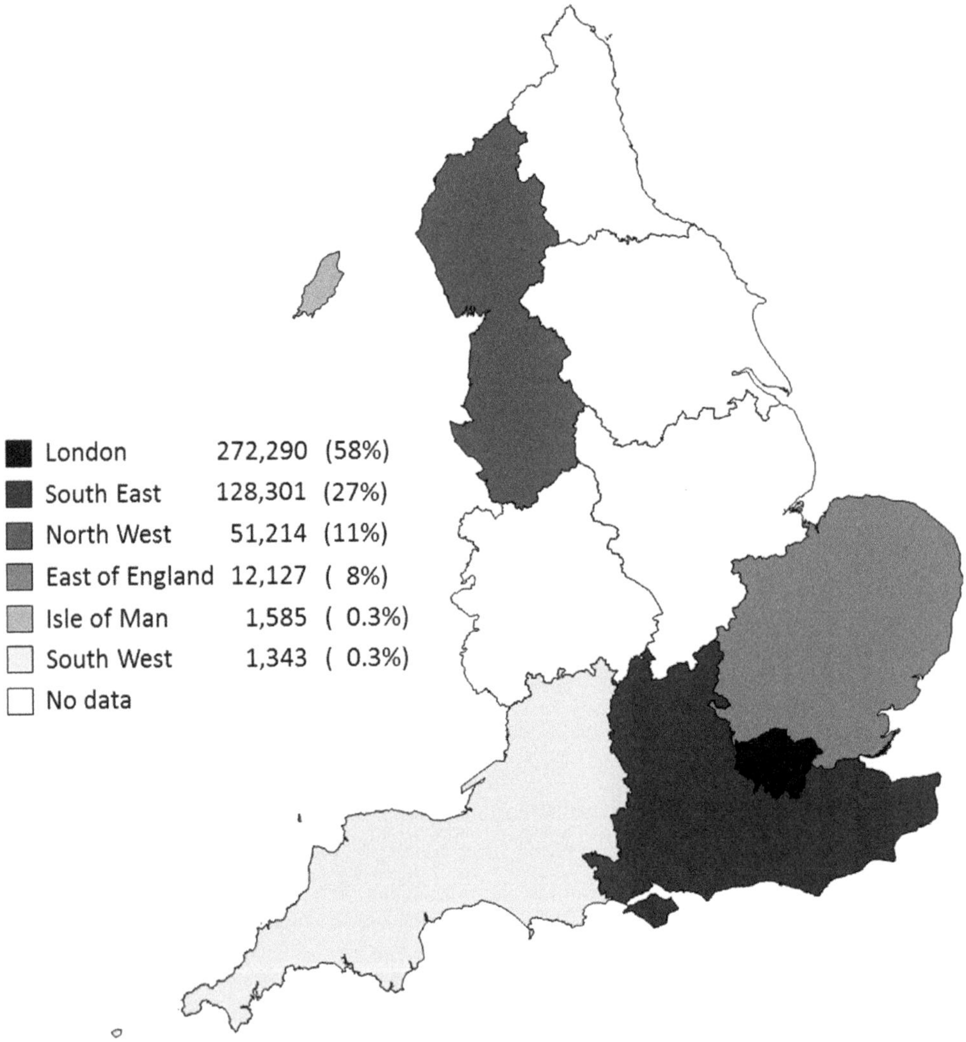

Figure 1. Number of women who provided folic acid supplement status according to strategic health authority and the Isle of Man.

pregnancy has been confirmed as the neural tube (and any defect) will have formed by around 8 weeks of pregnancy.

A strength of this study is the large sample size; almost half a million pregnancies resulting in very narrow confidence intervals of our estimates and even small differences are highly statistically significant. The results show that the policy of folic acid supplementation has failed. The policy exacerbates health inequalities among ethnic minorities and younger women. Our study is based on women from England and the Isle of Man, but the results are similar to other countries; a review of 34 studies conducted in 8 countries between 1992 and 2001 showed that nowhere was the proportion of women taking folic acid supplements before pregnancy greater than 50% and that overall it was about 25% [9]. Our results show that over the past decade the proportion has decreased in England. A weakness of this study is that it is limited to women that had antenatal screening for Down's syndrome and neural tube defects. Uptake of screening in England and Wales was 53% in 2007, increasing to 74% in 2011 [10].

The global number of spina bifida and anencephaly births has been estimated at 300,000 to 400,000 per year [11]. In the 20 years since the publication of the MRC Vitamin Study 1,800,000 cases could have been prevented on the basis that fortification alone would prevent one-third of cases. Among women that took folic acid supplements this would be even higher. In contrast, an estimated worldwide total of 10,000 people were disabled from thalidomide [12] and this led to transformation of the drug regulatory system. It is a public health tragedy that in spite of the fortification initiative in many countries most have not introduced mandatory folic acid fortification [2].

It is widely judged that folic acid fortification and supplementation is safe. Concerns over the possible increased risk of cancer being associated with folic acid fortification are not justified [13,14] and a large meta-analysis of placebo-controlled randomised trials of folic acid (median daily dose 2.0 mg over an average 5 years of follow-up) showed no increase in cancer incidence in those taking folic acid [15]. Moreover there is evidence that the generally recommended daily dose of folic acid supplementation is too low at 0.4 mg; about 80% of all NTDs could be prevented if it were 5 mg instead of about 50% with 0.4 mg [16]. Therefore fortification would offer additional protection against NTDs for women taking the current recommended daily dose.

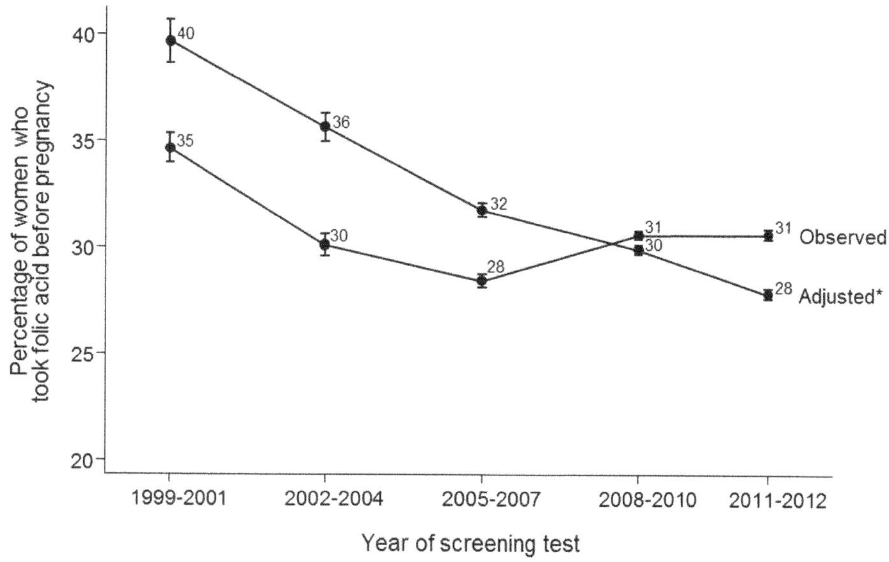

Number of women: 17,862 30,854 87,120 180,054 150,970

*Adjusted for maternal age, maternal weight, ethnicity, previous NTD pregnancy, previous Down's syndrome pregnancy, IVF, diabetes, smoking, Down's syndrome screening test and region of England.

Figure 2. Observed and adjusted* percentage of women taking folic acid supplements before pregnancy according to year.

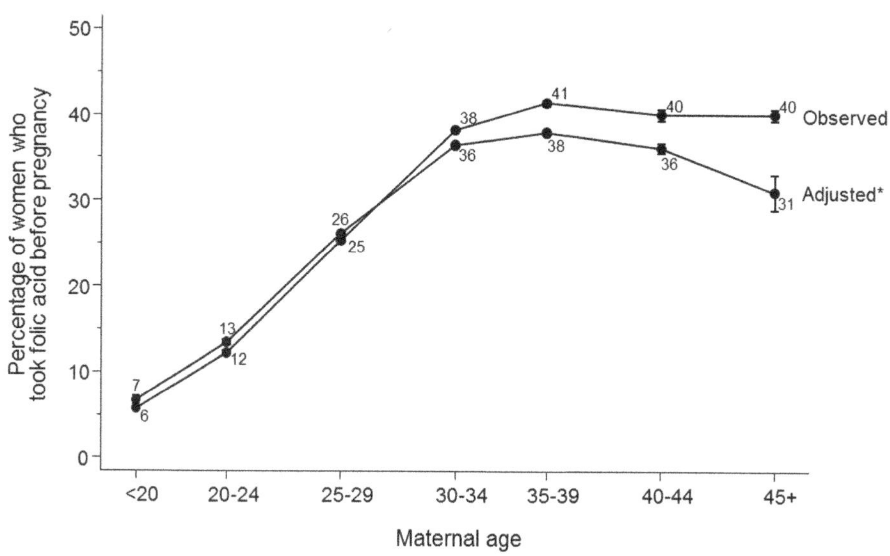

Number of women: 18,111 69,354 122,785 149,428 86,949 19,177 1,055

*Adjusted for year screened, maternal weight, ethnicity, previous NTD pregnancy, previous Down's syndrome pregnancy, IVF, diabetes, smoking, Down's syndrome screening test and region of England.

Figure 3. Observed and adjusted* percentage of women taking folic acid supplements before pregnancy according to maternal age.

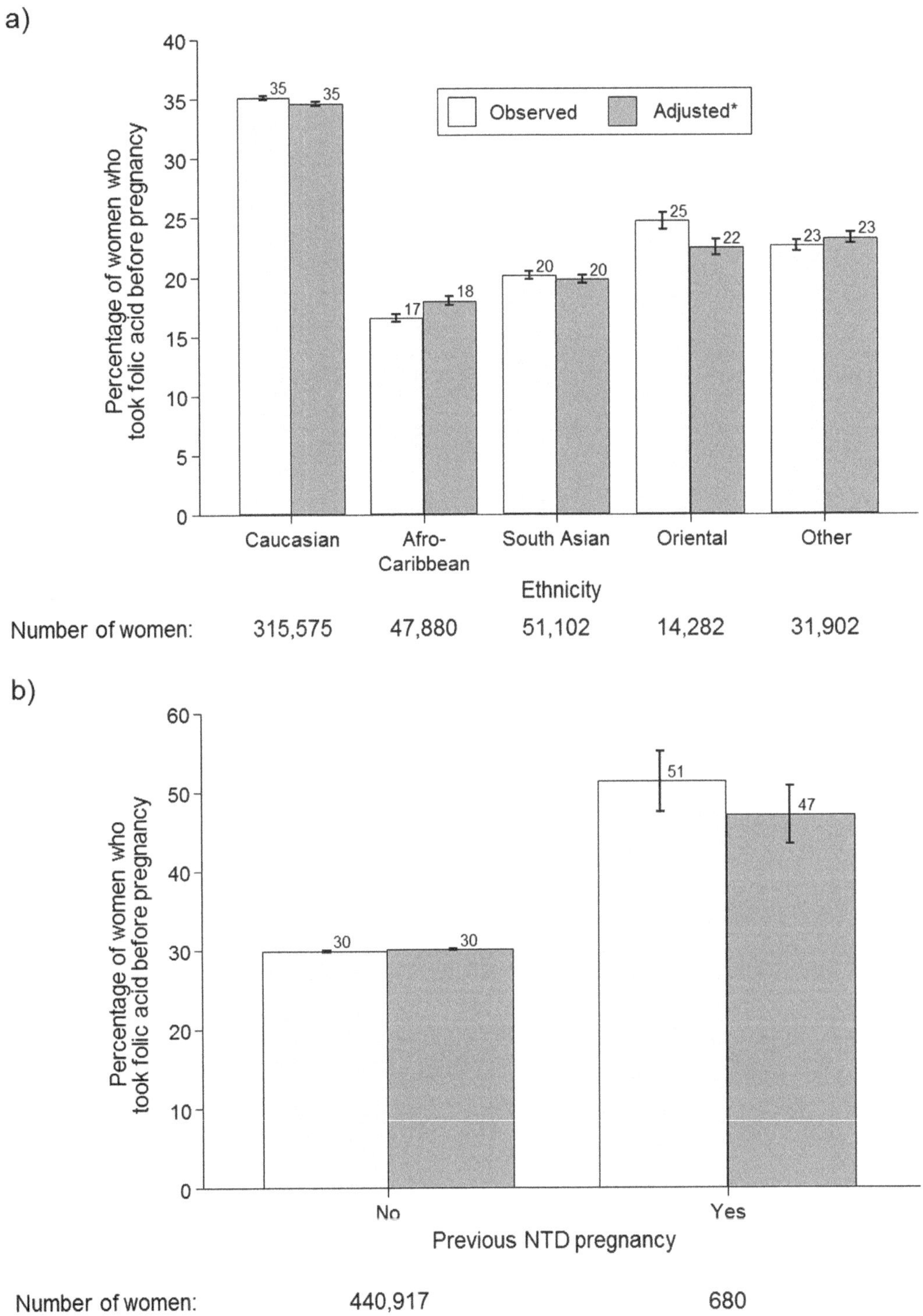

* Adjusted for year screened, maternal age, maternal weight, previous Down's syndrome pregnancy, IVF, diabetes, smoking, Down's syndrome screening test and region of England; (a) also adjusted for previous NTD pregnancy, (b) also adjusted for ethnicity

Figure 4. Observed and adjusted* percentage of women taking folic acid supplements before pregnancy according to ethnicity (a) and previous neural tube defect (NTD) pregnancy (b).

The prevention of neural tube defects is a global problem. Our results show that public health policy cannot rely on pre-pregnancy folic acid supplementation alone. Improved education in communities with particularly low rates of pre-pregnancy folic acid supplementation may increase the rates but for all women to benefit countries that have not introduced folic acid fortification should do so to avert a preventable serious birth defect responsible for still births, severe physical disability and needless therapeutic abortions.

Supporting Information

Table S1 Percentage of women taking folic acid before pregnancy, once pregnancy confirmed or not at all with unadjusted and adjusted relative use compared with reference categories.

Author Contributions

Conceived and designed the experiments: JB NW. Performed the experiments: JB NW. Analyzed the data: JB JM NW. Wrote the paper: JB NW. Collated and managed the data: WH.

References

1. MRC Vitamin Study Research Group (1991) Prevention of neural tube defects: results of the Medical Research Council Vitamin Study. Lancet 338: 131–137.
2. Flour Fortification Inititative. Global Progress. Available: http://www.ffinetwork.org/global_progress/. Accessed 9 October 2013.
3. Honein MA, Paulozzi LJ, Matthes TJ, Erickson JD, Wong LY (2001) Impact of folic acid fortification of the US food supply on the occurrence of neural tube defects. JAMA 285: 2981–6.
4. Lopez-Camelo JS, Orioli IM, da Graca Dutra M, Nazer-Herrera J, Rivera N, et al. (2005) Reduction of birth prevalence rate of neural tube defects after folic acid fortification in Chile. Am J Med Genet A 135: 120–5.
5. De Wals P, Tairou F, Van Allen MI, Uh SH, Lowry RB, et al. (2007) Reduction in neural-tube defects after folic acid fortification in Canada. New Engl J Med 357: 135–42.
6. Expert Advisory Group (1992) Folic acid and the prevention of neural tube defects. London: Department of Health.
7. Huttly WJ, Wald NJ, Walters JC (1999) Folic acid supplementation before pregnancy remains inadequate. BMJ 319: 1499.1.
8. Zou G (2004) A modified poisson regression approach to prospective studies with binary data. Am J Epidemiol 159: 702–6.
9. Ray JG, Singh G, Burrows RF (2004) Evidence for suboptimal use of periconceptional folic acid supplements globally. BJOG 111: 399–408.
10. NHS (2012) NHS Fetal Anomaly Screening Programme Annual report 2011–2012. Available: fetalanomaly.screening.nhs.uk/getdata.php?id = 11702. Accessed 28 January 2014.
11. Oakley GP Jr (1998) Folic-acid-preventable spina bifida and anencephaly. Bull World Health Organ (suppl 2): 116–7.
12. Therapontos C, Erskine L, Gardner ER, Figg WD, Vargesson N (2009) Thalidomide induces limb defects by preventing angiogenic outgrowth during early limb formation. Proc Natl Acad Sci 106: 8573–8.
13. Bayston R, Russell A, Wald NJ, Hoffbrand AV (2007) Folic acid fortification and cancer risk. Lancet 370: 2004.
14. Bayston R, Russell A, Wald NJ, Hoffbrand AV (2007) Folic acid fortification and cancer risk. Lancet 371: 1335–6.
15. Vollset SE, Clarke R, Lewington S, Ebbing M, Halsey J, et al (2013) Effects of folic acid supplementation on overall and site-specific cancer incidence during the randomised trials: meta-analyses of data on 50000 individuals. Lancet 381: 1029–36.
16. Wald NJ, Law MR, Morris JK, Wald DS (2001) Quantifying the effect of folic acid. Lancet 358: 2069–73.

Permissions

All chapters in this book were first published in PLOS ONE, by The Public Library of Science; hereby published with permission under the Creative Commons Attribution License or equivalent. Every chapter published in this book has been scrutinized by our experts. Their significance has been extensively debated. The topics covered herein carry significant findings which will fuel the growth of the discipline. They may even be implemented as practical applications or may be referred to as a beginning point for another development.

The contributors of this book come from diverse backgrounds, making this book a truly international effort. This book will bring forth new frontiers with its revolutionizing research information and detailed analysis of the nascent developments around the world.

We would like to thank all the contributing authors for lending their expertise to make the book truly unique. They have played a crucial role in the development of this book. Without their invaluable contributions this book wouldn't have been possible. They have made vital efforts to compile up to date information on the varied aspects of this subject to make this book a valuable addition to the collection of many professionals and students.

This book was conceptualized with the vision of imparting up-to-date information and advanced data in this field. To ensure the same, a matchless editorial board was set up. Every individual on the board went through rigorous rounds of assessment to prove their worth. After which they invested a large part of their time researching and compiling the most relevant data for our readers.

The editorial board has been involved in producing this book since its inception. They have spent rigorous hours researching and exploring the diverse topics which have resulted in the successful publishing of this book. They have passed on their knowledge of decades through this book. To expedite this challenging task, the publisher supported the team at every step. A small team of assistant editors was also appointed to further simplify the editing procedure and attain best results for the readers.

Apart from the editorial board, the designing team has also invested a significant amount of their time in understanding the subject and creating the most relevant covers. They scrutinized every image to scout for the most suitable representation of the subject and create an appropriate cover for the book.

The publishing team has been an ardent support to the editorial, designing and production team. Their endless efforts to recruit the best for this project, has resulted in the accomplishment of this book. They are a veteran in the field of academics and their pool of knowledge is as vast as their experience in printing. Their expertise and guidance has proved useful at every step. Their uncompromising quality standards have made this book an exceptional effort. Their encouragement from time to time has been an inspiration for everyone.

The publisher and the editorial board hope that this book will prove to be a valuable piece of knowledge for researchers, students, practitioners and scholars across the globe.

List of Contributors

Panagiotis Zis, Sima Shende, Zuzana Walker and Andre Strydom
University College London, Division of Psychiatry, London, United Kingdom

Patrick McHugh
Division of Pharmacy and Pharmaceutical Sciences, School of Applied Sciences University of Huddersfield, Queensgate, Huddersfield, United Kingdom

Andrew McQuillin
University College London, Molecular Psychiatry Laboratory, London, United Kingdom

Domenico Praticò
Department of Pharmacology and Center for Translational Medicine, Temple University, Philadelphia, Pennsylvania, United States of America

Mark Dickinson
Enfield Integrated Learning Disability Team, Enfield, United Kingdom

Helma B. M. van Gameren-Oosterom, Minne Fekkes, Simone E. Buitendijk, Ashna D. Mohangoo, Jeanet Bruil and Jacobus P. Van Wouwe
Department Child Health, Netherlands Organization for Applied Scientific Research (TNO), Leiden, The Netherlands

Robin Roberson, Daniel Abebe, Laura Toso, Madeline Caballero and Catherine Y. Spong
Unit on Perinatal and Developmental Neurobiology, National Institute of Child and Human Development, National Institute of Health, Bethesda, Maryland, United States of America

Maddalena Incerti
Unit on Perinatal and Developmental Neurobiology, National Institute of Child and Human Development, National Institute of Health, Bethesda, Maryland, United States of America,
Department of Obstetrics and Gynaecology, University of Milano-Bicocca, Ospedale S. Gerardo, Fondazione MBBM, Monza, Italy

Kari Horowitz
Unit on Perinatal and Developmental Neurobiology, National Institute of Child and Human Development, National Institute of Health, Bethesda, Maryland, United States of America
Department of Obstetrics and Gynecology, University of Connecticut, Groton, Connecticut, United States of America

Vandana Rai, Upendra Yadav, Pradeep Kumar and Sushil Kumar Yadav
Human Molecular Genetics Laboratory, Department of Biotechnology, VBS Purvanchal University, Jaunpur, India,

Om Prakesh Mishra
Department of Pediatrics, Institute of Medical Sciences, Banaras Hindu University, Varanasi, India

Ewa Bieć, Joanna Zima and Dorota Wó jtowicz
Faculty of Physiotherapy, University School of Physical Education in Wroclaw, Wroclaw, Poland

Bożena Wojciechowska-Maszkowska and Krzysztof Kręcisz
Department of Biomechanics, The Opole University of Technology, Opole, Poland

Michał Kuczyński
Faculty of Physiotherapy, University School of Physical Education in Wroclaw, Wroclaw, Poland
Department of Biomechanics, The Opole University of Technology, Opole, Poland

Dorothy V. M. Bishop
Developmental Neuropsychology, University of Oxford, Oxford, United Kingdom

Alexander C. Phillips and Anthony J. Holland
Department of Psychiatry, University of Cambridge, Cambridge, United Kingdom

Stephen Morris and Saffron Karlsen
Department of Applied Health Research, University College London, London, United Kingdom

Nancy Chung
NHS Fetal Anomaly Screening Programme, University of Exeter, Exeter, United Kingdom

Melissa Hill and Lyn S. Chitty
Clinical and Molecular Genetics Unit, UCL Institute of Child Health and Great Ormond Street Hospital for Children NHS Foundation Trust, London, United Kingdom
Fetal Medicine Unit, University College London Hospitals NHS Foundation Trust, London, United Kingdom

Stephanie Kuhn and Walter Marcotti
Department of Biomedical Science, University of Sheffield, Sheffield, United Kingdom

Neil Ingham, Selina Pearson, Susan M. Gribble, Stephen Clayton and Karen P. Steel
Wellcome Trust Sanger Institute, Wellcome Trust Genome Campus, Hinxton, Cambridge, United Kingdom

Gloria Arque and Mara Dierssen
Genes and Disease Program, Center for Genomic Regulation (CRG), Pompeu Fabra University, Barcelona Biomedical Research Park (PRBB) and CIBER de Enfermedades Raras (CIBERER), Barcelona, Spain

Anna Casanovas
Department of Experimental Medicine and IRBLLEIDA, University of Lleida, School of Medicine, Lleida, Catalonia, Spain

Pongsathorn Chaiyasap
Interdepartment of Biomedical Sciences, Faculty of Graduate School, Chulalongkorn University, Bangkok, Thailand

Sissades Tongsima
Genome Institute, National Center for Genetic Engineering and Biotechnology, Khlong Nueng, Khlong Luang, Pathum Thani, Thailand

Supasak Kulawonganunchai
Interdepartment of Biomedical Sciences, Faculty of Graduate School, Chulalongkorn University, Bangkok, Thailand
Genome Institute, National Center for Genetic Engineering and Biotechnology, Khlong Nueng, Khlong Luang, Pathum Thani, Thailand

Chalurmpon Srichomthong, Kanya Suphapeetiporn and Vorasuk Shotelersuk
Center of Excellence for Medical Genetics, Department of Pediatrics, Faculty of Medicine, Chulalongkorn University, Bangkok, Thailand
Excellence Center for Medical Genetics, King Chulalongkorn Memorial Hospital, Thai Red Cross, Bangkok, Thailand

Claire Enea-Drapeau, Michè le Carlier and Pascal Huguet
Laboratoire de Psychologie Cognitive, Aix-Marseille University and Centre National de la Recherche Scientifique, Marseille, France

Taylor J. Jensen, Tricia Zwiefelhofer, Roger C. Tim, Zěljko Džakula, Sung K. Kim, Amin R. Mazloom, Zhanyang Zhu, John Tynan, Tim Lu, Paul Oeth and Cosmin Deciu
Research and Development, Sequenom Center for Molecular Medicine, San Diego, California, United States of America

Graham McLennan, Dirk van den Boom and Mathias Ehrich
Research and Development, Sequenom Inc., San Diego, California, United States of America

Glenn E. Palomaki and Jacob A. Canick
Women and Infants Hospital, Alpert Medical School of Brown University, Providence, Rhode Island, United States of America

Valerio Costa, Marianna Aprile, Roberta Esposito, Luigi Leone, Aldo Donizetti, Stefania Crispi and Alfredo Ciccodicola
Institute of Genetics and Biophysics "A. Buzzati-Traverso", CNR, Naples, Italy

Claudia Angelini
Istituto per le Applicazioni del Calcolo, Mauro Picone, CNR, Naples, Italy

Luciana D'Apice and Piergiuseppe De Berardinis
Institute of Protein Biochemistry, CNR, Naples, Italy

Margherita Mutarelli
Telethon Institute of Genetics and Medicine (TIGEM), Naples, Italy

Amelia Casamassimi and Monica Rienzo
Department of General Pathology and Excellence Research Centre on Cardiovascular Diseases, 1st School of Medicine, Second University of Naples, Naples, Italy

Linda Sommese
Section of Microbiology, Department of Experimental Medicine, 1st School of Medicine, Second University of Naples, Naples, Italy

Maria Assunta Gallo
Centro Diagnostico San Ciro, Portici, Italy

Berardo Sarubbi and Raffaele Calabrò
Cardiology Department of Second University of Naples, "Monaldi Hospital", Naples, Italy

Marco Picardi
Department of Biochemistry and Medical Biotechnology, University of Naples "Federico II", Naples, Italy

Paola Salvatore
Department of Cellular and Molecular Biology and Pathology "L. Califano", University of Naples "Federico II" and Ceinge Biotecnologie Avanzate s.c.a.r.l., Naples, Italy

Teresa Infante
Fondazione-SDN (Institute of Diagnostic and Nuclear Development), IRCCS, Naples, Italy

Claudio Napoli
Department of General Pathology and Excellence Research Centre on Cardiovascular Diseases, 1st School of Medicine, Second University of Naples, Naples, Italy
Fondazione-SDN (Institute of Diagnostic and Nuclear Development), IRCCS, Naples, Italy

Makiko Tsutsumi, Reiko Fujiwara, Hidehito Inagaki, Tamae Ohye, Takema Kato and Hiroki Kurahashi
Division of Molecular Genetics, Institute for Comprehensive Medical Science, Fujita Health University, Toyoake, Aichi, Japan

Haruki Nishizawa and Takuma Fujii
Department of Obstetrics and Gynecology, Fujita Health University, Toyoake, Aichi, Japan

Hiroshi Kogo
Department of Anatomy and Cell Biology, Gunma University Graduate School of Medicine, Maebashi, Gunma, Japan

Mayuko Ito
Division of Molecular Genetics, Institute for Comprehensive Medical Science, Fujita Health University, Toyoake, Aichi, Japan
Department of Obstetrics and Gynecology, Fujita Health University, Toyoake, Aichi, Japan

Lei Jin, Yun Bai and Minjun Yang
Shanghai-MOST Key Laboratory of Health and Disease Genomics, Chinese National Human Genome Center at Shanghai, Shanghai, China

Qimin Chen and Lijun Fu
Shanghai Children's Medical Center, Shanghai Jiao Tong University School of Medicine, Shanghai, China

Huasheng Xiao
National Engineering Center for Biochip at Shanghai, Shanghai, China

Chong Li, Guoping Zhao and Shengyue Wang
School of Life Science, Fudan University, Shanghai, China
Shanghai-MOST Key Laboratory of Health and Disease Genomics, Chinese National Human Genome Center at Shanghai, Shanghai, China

Michael A. Grassi, Vidhya Rao, Kathryn P. Winkler and Joseph D. Bogaard
Department of Ophthalmology & Visual Sciences, University of Illinois at Chicago, Chicago, Illinois, United States of America

Wei Zhang
Department of Pediatrics, University of Illinois at Chicago, Chicago, Illinois, United States of America

Siquan Chen
Cellular Screening Center, Institute for Genomics and Systems Biology, University of Chicago, Chicago, Illinois, United States of America

Jalees Rehman and Asrar B. Malik
Department of Pharmacology, University of Illinois at Chicago, Chicago, Illinois, United States of America

Nancy J. Cox
Section of Genetic Medicine, University of Chicago, Chicago, Illinois, United States of America

Bonnie LaCroix, Divya Lenkala and R. Stephanie Huang
Section of Hematology/Oncology, University of Chicago, Chicago, Illinois, United States of America

Jaclyn Vander Schilden, Anthony W. Bacon, John W. Bracey, Timothy Sowder, Robert A. Skinner, Frances L. Swain and William R. Hogue
Department of Orthopaedic Surgery, Center for Orthopaedic Research, University of Arkansas for Medical Sciences, Little Rock, Arkansas, United States of America

Kent D. McKelvey and Donna B. Leblanc
Department of Genetics, University of Arkansas for Medical Sciences, Little Rock, Arkansas, United States of America

Galen R. Wenger
Department of Pharmacology, University of Arkansas for Medical Sciences, Little Rock, Arkansas, United States of America

Tristan W. Fowler, Nisreen S. Akel, Dana Gaddy and Larry J. Suva
Department of Physiology & Biophysics, University of Arkansas for Medical Sciences, Little Rock, Arkansas, United States of America

Xiangdong Kong
Prenatal Diagnosis Center, the First Affiliated Hospital of Zhengzhou University, Henan, China

Lin Li
Department of Genetic Laboratory, Lin Yi People's Hospital, Shandong, China

Lei Sun, Kepeng Fu, Ju Long, Xunjin Weng, Xuehe Ye, Xinxiong Liu,
Shanhuo Yan, Haiming Ye and Zuqian Fan
Laboratory of Medical Genetics, Qinzhou Maternal and Child Health Care Hospital, Guangxi, China

Bo Wang
Genetics Laboratory, Hubei Maternal and Child Health Hospital, Hubei, China

Joanna Murray, Alex Bottle, Paul Aylin, Azeem Majeed and Sonia Saxena
Department of Primary Care and Public Health, Imperial College London, London, United Kingdom

Mike Sharland
Paediatric Infectious Diseases Unit, St. George's Hospital NHS Trust, London, United Kingdom

Neena Modi
Section of Neonatal Medicine, Department of Medicine, Imperial College London, London, United Kingdom

Christel Eckmann-Scholz and Walter Jonat
Department of Gynecology & Obstetrics, Christian-Albrechts-University Kiel & University Hospital Schleswig-Holstein, Kiel, Germany

Susanne Bens, Julia Kolarova, Sina Schneppenheim, Almuth Caliebe, Simone Heidemann, Reiner Siebert and Ole Ammerpohl
Institute of Human Genetics, Christian-Albrechts-University Kiel & University Hospital Schleswig-Holstein, Kiel, Germany

Monika Kautza
Praxis of Human Genetics, Kiel, Germany

Constantin von Kaisenberg
Institute of Human Genetics, Christian-Albrechts-University Kiel & University Hospital Schleswig-Holstein, Kiel, Germany
Department of Obstetrics, Gynecology and Reproductive Medicine, Hannover Medical School, Hannover, Germany

W. F. Tang
Department of Obstetrics and Gynaecology, Li Ka Shing Faculty of Medicine, The University of Hong Kong, Hong Kong Special Administrative Region, China

Sario S. Y. Chan and Simon C. K. Ding
Department of Obstetrics and Gynaecology, Queen Mary Hospital, Hong Kong Special Administrative Region, China

K. Y. Leung and Teresa Ma
Department of Obstetrics and Gynaecology, Queen Elizabeth Hospital, Hong Kong Special Administrative Region, China

Wing C. Leung
Department of Obstetrics and Gynaecology, Kwong Wah Hospital, Hong Kong Special Administrative Region, China

Anita S. Y. Kan, Elizabeth T. Lau, Kelvin Y. K. Chan, C. P. Lee, Pui Wah Hui and Mary H. Y. Tang
Department of Obstetrics and Gynaecology, Li Ka Shing Faculty of Medicine, The University of Hong Kong, Hong Kong Special Administrative Region, China
Department of Obstetrics and Gynaecology, Queen Mary Hospital, Hong Kong Special Administrative Region, China

Brian H. Y. Chung
Department of Obstetrics and Gynaecology, Queen Mary Hospital, Hong Kong Special Administrative Region, China
Department of Paediatrics and Adolescent Medicine, Queen Mary Hospital, Li Ka Shing Faculty of Medicine, The University of Hong Kong, Hong Kong Special Administrative Region, China

Homa Attar, Maryline Gagnebin, Yann Dupré, Christelle Borel, Samuel Deutsch, Emmanouil T. Dermitzakis and Stylianos E. Antonarakis
Department of Genetic Medicine and Development, University of Geneva Medical School, Geneva, Switzerland

Karen Bedard and Karl-Heinz Krause
Department of Pathology and Immunology, University of Geneva Medical School and University Hospitals, Geneva, Switzerland

Patrick Descombes
Genomics Platform, NCCR Frontiers in Genetics, University of Geneva Medical School, Geneva, Switzerland

Holger Prokisch, Thomas Meitinger and Divya Mehta
Institute of Epidemiology I, Helmholtz Zentrum München, German Research Center for Environmental Health, Neuherberg, Germany

Jean Maurice Delabar
Functional and Adaptive Biology, Universite´ Paris Diderot-Paris7 and CNRS, Paris, France

Erich Wichmann
Institute of Epidemiology I, Helmholtz Zentrum München, German Research Center for Environmental Health, Neuherberg, Germany
Institute of Medical Informatics, Biometry and Epidemiology, Chair of Epidemiology, Ludwig-Maximilians-Universität, Munich, Germany
Klinikum Grosshadern, Munich, Germany

Gary J. W. Liao, K. C. Allen Chan, Peiyong Jiang, Hao Sun, Rossa W. K. Chiu and Y. M. Dennis Lo
Centre for Research into Circulating Fetal Nucleic Acids, Li Ka Shing Institute of Health Sciences, The Chinese University of Hong Kong, Shatin, New Territories, Hong Kong, China
Department of Chemical Pathology, The Chinese University of Hong Kong, Shatin, New Territories, Hong Kong, China

Tak Y. Leung
Department of Obstetrics and Gynaecology, The Chinese University of Hong Kong, Shatin, New Territories, Hong Kong, China

Jonathan P. Bestwick, Wayne J. Huttly, Joan K. Morris and Nicholas J. Wald
Wolfson Institute of Preventive Medicine, Barts and the London School of Medicine and Dentistry, Queen Mary University of London, London, United Kingdom

Index